Psychiatric Intensive Care

Third Edition

Psychiatric Intensive Care

Third Edition

Edited by

Roland Dix
Gloucestershire Health and Care NHS Foundation Trust

Stephen Dye
Norfolk and Suffolk NHS Foundation Trust

Stephen M. Pereira
Keats House
NAPICU Chairman

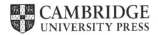

CAMBRIDGE
UNIVERSITY PRESS

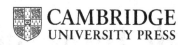

Shaftesbury Road, Cambridge CB2 8EA, United Kingdom

One Liberty Plaza, 20th Floor, New York, NY 10006, USA

477 Williamstown Road, Port Melbourne, VIC 3207, Australia

314–321, 3rd Floor, Plot 3, Splendor Forum, Jasola District Centre,
New Delhi – 110025, India

103 Penang Road, #05–06/07, Visioncrest Commercial, Singapore 238467

Cambridge University Press is part of Cambridge University Press & Assessment, a
department of the University of Cambridge.

We share the University's mission to contribute to society through the pursuit of
education, learning and research at the highest international levels of excellence.

www.cambridge.org
Information on this title: www.cambridge.org/9781108972376

DOI: 10.1017/9781108976770

First published 2001
Second edition 2008
Reprinted 2008
Third edition 2024

A catalogue record for this publication is available from the British Library

*A Cataloging-in-Publication data record for this book is available from the Library of
Congress*

ISBN 978-1-108-97237-6 Paperback

....

Every effort has been made in preparing this book to provide accurate and up-to-date
information that is in accord with accepted standards and practice at the time of
publication. Although case histories are drawn from actual cases, every effort has been
made to disguise the identities of the individuals involved. Nevertheless, the authors,
editors, and publishers can make no warranties that the information contained herein is
totally free from error, not least because clinical standards are constantly changing
through research and regulation. The authors, editors, and publishers therefore disclaim
all liability for direct or consequential damages resulting from the use of material
contained in this book. Readers are strongly advised to pay careful attention to
information provided by the manufacturer of any drugs or equipment that they
plan to use.

Contents

Contents

Contributors

James Baker
Psychiatric Clinical Decisions Unit
Caludon Centre
Clifford Bridge Road
Coventry, UK

Shanika Balachandra
Consultant Psychiatrist
Shannon ward PICU, St Charles Hospital, CNWL
CNWL PICU Trust Lead
NAPICU Deputy Director of Operations
London, UK

Elliott Carthy
Specialist Registrar in Forensic Psychiatry
Oxford Health NHS Foundation Trust
Oxford, UK

Khadija Chaudhry
Consultant Neuropsychologist
Kent and Medway NHS and Social Care Trust
Kent, UK

Rebecca Davies
Professional Head of Occupational Therapy for
Southwark Directorate
South London and Maudsley NHS Foundation
Trust
South London, UK
Executive Committee Member, National Association
of Psychiatric Intensive Care & Low Secure Units
(NAPICU)
Lead for the NAPICU Occupational Therapy
Network

Roland Dix
Editor
Approved Clinician
Consultant Nurse in Psychiatric Intensive Care
and Secure Recovery
Editor-in-Chief *Journal of Psychiatric Intensive Care*
NAPICU International Press
NAPICU Executive

Gloucestershire Health and Care NHS Foundation Trust
Montpellier Secure Recovery Service, Wotton Lawn
Hospital
Gloucestershire, UK

Stephen Dye
Editor
Consultant Psychiatrist, Suffolk Access
and Assessment Team, NSFT
Medical Member, First Tier Tribunal
(Mental Health)
Honorary Senior Lecturer, University
of East Anglia
Ipswich, UK

Harvey Gordon
Retired Consultant Forensic Psychiatrist
Broadmoor Hospital, Maudsley and Bethlem
Hospitals and
Littlemore Mental Health Centre
Oxford, UK

Jules Haste
Associate Divisional Director - Pharmacy Services
(West Sussex)
Sussex Partnership NHS Foundation Trust
Pharmacist Coordinator for IM section
of Medusa
West Sussex, UK

Bradley Hillier
Consultant Forensic Psychiatrist
West London Forensic Service
London, UK

Steve Ireland
Gloucestershire Health and Care NHS Foundation
Trust
Gloucestershire, UK

Sanjith Kamath
Executive Medical Director
St Andrew's Healthcare
Northampton, UK

Vishelle Kamath
Group Medical Director
CareTech
Potters Bar, UK

Thomas Kearney
Deputy Director
Medical Workforce
NHS England
London, UK

Marc Jonathon Kingsley
Consultant Clinical Psychologist
Strategic and Clinical Lead for Clinical Health
Psychology
NELFT NHS Foundation Trust
London, UK

Joana Ferreira Marques de Paiva
Psychiatry Core trainee
Oxford Health NHS Trust
Oxford, UK

Brian Malcolm McKenzie
Consultant Clinical and Forensic Psychologist
Bracton Centre
Oxleas NHS Foundation Trust
London, UK

Angus McLellan
Consultant Psychiatrist, Clinical Partners
Oxford, UK

Andrew Molodynski
Oxford Health NHS Foundation Trust
Department of Psychiatry, Oxford University
Oxford, UK

Chike I. Okocha
Consultant Psychiatrist
Nightingale Hospital London
London, UK

Mathew Page
Chief Operating Officer
Avon and Wiltshire Mental Health Partnership
NHS Trust
Bath NHS House
Newbridge Hill
Bath, UK

Reena Panchal
Consultant Forensic Psychiatrist
Warwickshire Team
Reaside Clinic, Birmingham and Solihull Mental
Health Foundation Trust
Birmingham, UK

Stephen M. Pereira
NAPICU Chairman
Consultant Psychiatrist and Cognitive Behaviour
Therapy Specialist
Keats House
London, UK

Emma Phillips
Consultant Liaison and Older Adult
Psychiatrist
Gloucestershire Health and Care NHS Foundation Trust
Gloucestershire, UK

Robert Rathouse
Clinical Specialist Psychiatric Intensive Care Unit
(PICU) Occupational Therapist
South London and Maudsley NHS Foundation Trust
London, UK

Ross Runciman
Gloucestershire Health and Care NHS
Foundation Trust
Gloucestershire, UK

Faisil Sethi
Chief Medical Officer and Consultant Psychiatrist
Dorset HealthCare University NHS
Foundation Trust
Dorset, UK

Wendy Sherwood
International Creative Ability
Network (ICAN)
Editorial Board, *Journal of Psychiatric
Intensive Care*
Honorary Fellow, St George's University
London, UK

Matthew Truscott
Head of Mental Health
South Western Ambulance Service NHS Foundation
Trust
Exeter, UK

Lucy M. Walker
RMN, Specialist Recovery Practitioner
Avon and Wiltshire Mental Health
NHS Trust
Bristol, UK

Brenda Wasunna-Smith
Gloucestershire Health and Care NHS
Foundation Trust
Gloucestershire, UK

Jim Welch
Registered Mental Health Nurse
Clinical and Operational Lead Nurse for
Gloucestershire Mental Health Liaison Services

Gloucestershire Health and Care NHS Foundation
Trust
Gloucestershire, UK

Karen Williams
Consultant Liaison Psychiatrist
Gloucestershire Health and
Care NHS Foundation Trust
Gloucestershire, UK

Foreword

In the realm of mental health care, the significance of psychiatric intensive care units (PICUs) cannot be overstated. These units stand as sanctuaries for people navigating the challenges and vulnerabilities of acute mental illness, providing a space where compassionate, safe and therapeutic care converges with expertise. This third edition delves into the intricacies of PICUs in the UK. Where appropriate, this volume draws upon evidence from the global PICU community thus unravelling the tapestry of challenges and triumphs woven within these specialised wards and facilities.

The first chapter sets the scene for interesting further reading. In exploring the development and definition of a PICU, this chapter delves into the evolution of mental health care and the crucial role that specialised units play in ensuring the safety and well-being of patients experiencing acute psychiatric crisis. By tracing the historical context and highlighting the contemporary challenges, the book aims to provide a comprehensive understanding of the complexities involved in shaping and defining these essential units within the broader landscape of mental health services.

As we embark on this PICU journey through the pages that follow, we find ourselves immersed in the inner workings of psychiatric care, navigating the delicate balance between understanding and intervention. The authors illuminate the unique role of PICUs, where every moment demands a nuanced approach, blending empathy with clinical precision.

In the United Kingdom, where the landscape of mental health care is ever-evolving, PICUs stand as resilient pillars, adapting to the diverse needs of those entrusted to their care. This book serves as a guide, navigating the distinctive elements that define the essence of PICUs.

The collaborative efforts of clinicians, researchers, and advocates in these units echo a commitment to reshaping the narrative surrounding mental health. Through shared insights and lessons learned, this book becomes a testament to the tireless dedication of those working within and alongside PICUs to foster healing, recovery, and ultimately, hope whilst improving the experience of patients.

The book also tackles some of the issues that has been in discussion for decades – the use of restrictive practices. Reducing the use of restrictive practices in psychiatric intensive care units is crucial for several reasons. Firstly, it promotes a more therapeutic environment, fostering trust between patients and healthcare staff. Additionally, minimising the use of restraints and seclusion aligns with a person-centred approach, and this book emphasises individualised care and respect for autonomy. Furthermore, decreased reliance on restrictive measures enhances the overall well-being of patients by reducing trauma and negative experiences associated with such interventions. It encourages the development of alternative strategies, such as de-escalation techniques and collaborative treatment plans, which contribute to improved long-term outcomes and recovery, and this is fully addressed in this third edition. Limiting the use of restrictive interventions in psychiatric care not only respects the rights and dignity of patients, but also enhances the therapeutic atmosphere, leading to better mental health outcomes.

May this book, with its intimate exploration into the intricacies of psychiatric intensive care units, not only deepen our understanding but also spark conversations that propel us toward a future where mental health care is both comprehensive and compassionate.

Chris Dzikiti
Director of Mental Health, Care Quality Commission

Preface to the Third Edition

Welcome to the third edition of *Psychiatric Intensive Care*, a comprehensive and authoritative resource that has been meticulously updated to reflect the latest developments in legislation, national surveys, clinical guidelines and emerging research.

This edition represents a significant milestone in our ongoing commitment to provide frontline clinicians with the most up-to-date and relevant information in the field.

In this edition, we are thrilled to introduce new chapters authored by leading experts in their respective fields. These additions broaden the scope of the book, encompassing the ever-evolving landscape of psychiatric intensive care. These chapters not only provide fresh insights but also address the contemporary challenges and opportunities that have emerged since the previous edition.

A hallmark of this edition is our dedication to incorporating the latest changes in legislation that impact the mental health arena, particularly psychiatric intensive care. As laws and regulations continue to evolve, we recognize the importance of presenting accurate and timely information, enabling our readers to navigate the complex legal landscape with confidence.

Additionally, the inclusion of new national surveys and clinical guidelines ensures that readers are equipped with the most current data and evidence-based recommendations. Our goal is to empower practitioners, researchers, students, and policymakers to make informed decisions and contribute effectively to their respective fields.

As we embark on this new edition, we extend our gratitude to our frontline clinical colleague contributors who have tirelessly worked to provide content that reflects the forefront of knowledge. We also express our appreciation to our readers for their continued support and engagement, which have driven us to deliver a third edition that meets and exceeds their expectations.

In conclusion, the third edition of *Psychiatric Intensive Care* stands as a testament to our commitment to excellence and relevance. We are confident that the updates, new chapters, and expert contributions will make this edition an indispensable resource for years to come. We hope that this book continues to serve as a trusted guide for those dedicated to advancing psychiatric intensive care practice and its related disciplines.

Stephen M. Pereira
NAPICU Chairman

Preface to the Second Edition

The first edition of this textbook was published in 2001 and its success surpassed our expectations. The editors have received many positive comments about the usefulness of the text and its relevance to everyday practice. The interest in the care of our most disturbed patients has been highlighted by both sales overseas and by the rapid translation of the text into Czech.

Since the publication of the first edition, the sub-specialities of psychiatric intensive care and low secure care have grown from strength to strength. The Department of Health adopted standards developed by members of National Association of Psychiatric Intensive Care and Low Secure Units (NAPICU) that outline the care that should be delivered in Psychiatric Intensive Care and Low Secure Units (PICUs and LSUs). The publishers of this book have supported NAPICU to develop the first ever journal dedicated to this field: the *Journal of Psychiatric Intensive Care* (http://journals.cambridge .org/jid JPI). The current chairman of NAPICU, Dr Stephen M. Pereira, played a central role in the development of the National Institute for Health and Care Excellence (NICE) guideline on the short-term management of violence; thus influencing the care of acutely disturbed patients beyond the speciality.

NAPICU continues to organise a successful annual national conference and quarterly regional miniconferences. The majority of UK mental health trusts are now members of NAPICU, and in order to support the infrastructure of a growing organisation, a permanent NAPICU office has been set up in Glasgow. NAPICU continues to produce a quarterly bulletin to keep members up to date with developments in the field. The development of a national clinical governance network, sponsored by the Department of Health, has also been supported and this has overseen clinical quality improvement projects in areas such as responding to emergencies, culture and diversity issues, and user and carer involvement. An award is given to the 'team of the year'. Each year, a travel bursary is awarded to fund a research, clinical audit or good practice project. A national audit of PICUs and LSUs conducted by Dr Pereira's team highlighted environmental issues that led to the Department of Health's investing capital monies to improve buildings.

This edition of the textbook has been expanded to include several new chapters. The interface between PICU/LSU and learning disabilities, child and adolescent psychiatry, general adult psychiatry and substance misuse are covered, as are multidisciplinary team working, the role of social work and user and carer involvement. All other chapters have been updated to include developments such as the publication of NICE guidelines. In the interests of space, the sample unit policies have been removed as most units have now developed their own, usually more comprehensive versions.

We hope that you find the additions to the textbook useful in your practice and look forward to further developments in the speciality of PICU/LSU care. Constructive comments on any aspect of the text are welcome and should be sent to the publisher.

Further details about NAPICU and its activities can be found on the official NAPICU website: www .napicu.org.uk.

The editors would like to thank Sarah Price (copy editor), and Jeanette Alfoldi and Chloe Wright from the Cambridge University Press Production team for all their help with the second edition.

M. Dominic Beer
Stephen Pereira
Carol Paton

Preface to the First Edition

'Why do we need a book about psychiatric intensive care?' 'What IS psychiatric intensive care?', 'Is there any difference between intensive care and general psychiatry?' 'Where is the distinction between forensic psychiatry and psychiatric intensive care?, 'What special skills do PICU staff require?' Our first attempt to address some of these questions came at the first national conference on psychiatric intensive care, held at Bexleyheath, England, in 1996. The enthusiasm of the delegates and their thirst for knowledge and networking has led to the publication of this book.

We, as editors, have attempted to cover as many elements of the psychiatric intensive care provision as is possible within one book. We are, however, aware of certain deficiencies. Where there is an evidence-base, we have attempted to use it. Where there is not, we have used personal experience and the experience of others to guide us. We believe that psychiatric intensive care is at the heart of psychiatry and its good practice requires a full multidisciplinary team, strong leadership and effective managerial support. We have, therefore, included a wide variety of chapters, all written by professionals who have extensive expertise in this area of care. We have included examples of sample policies, which can be used as a guide, but these obviously need to be adapted and scrutinised for use locally. The editors would welcome any comments and suggestions on this work.

The first section addresses treatment issues. Effective treatment requires input from a wide variety of professionals. We have included contributions on the role of medication, psychological treatments, therapeutic activities, and more controversially, the use of both restraint and seclusion. The development and definition of psychiatric intensive care and the management of the acutely disturbed patient and of the complex needs patient also warrant chapters in their own right.

The second section specifically addresses areas of risk and the interface with forensic services. Contributions from colleagues working in forensic services, we hope, will encourage the breaking down of unnecessary barriers between different services.

The third section addresses management issues such as how to set up and design a new psychiatric intensive care unit (PICU) and how to manage such a unit effectively once it has been established.

We believe that this book will be of use to all disciplines working in, or interacting with, PICUs, as well as managers who have the responsibility for commissioning, providing and monitoring this high risk area of care. Although the emphasis is on practice in the United Kingdom, the general principles should be relevant and applicable in any care setting where the disturbed psychiatric patient is managed.

We would like to thank all the contributors to the book; those who have assisted in the publishing, especially Geoff Nuttall, Nora Naughton, Kathleen Orr and Gavin Smith; our secretarial staff, Mrs Linda Wells, Mrs Lorraine Wright, Miss Michelle Gillham and Mrs Rosemary McCafferty for their considerable hard work; our patients and colleagues who have taught us much; and our families, especially Drs Naomi Beer and Preeti Pereira, for their support and patience through this project.

Dominic Beer
Stephen Pereira
Carol Paton
August, 2000

Acknowledgements

This book is dedicated to the memory of Dr Dominic Beer. Amongst his many achievements and contribution to improving services for people with acute mental health problems, Dominic was the inspiration as well as the lead editor of the 2 previous editions of this book.

Our gratitude goes to all the authors who made this book possible. Many of whom are practicing clinicians and leaders. We extend our sincere thanks for their determination, effort and patience in completing this project during a very difficult time for global health services. This book is also dedicated to patients with severe mental health problems and the frontline multidisciplinary PICU clinicians who constantly try and deliver the best to care to them.

Thanks also to Mr John Trevains for his encouragement and support for completing the project.

Roland Dix
Stephen Dye
Stephen Pereira

Psychiatric Intensive Care: Development and Definition

Stephen M. Pereira and Stephen Dye

Introduction

In this chapter, we outline the historical development of psychiatric intensive care as a specialty. Then, we present an overview of the current facilities and patients based on the most recent UK National Surveys and current admission criteria taken from national guidelines. Further, we discuss how psychiatric intensive care interfaces with general adult services, mental health secure estates, the criminal justice system and community mental health services. Finally, we present an outline of the future strategy for the development of the specialty.

Historical Development of PICU as a Specialty

The implication is that by reading this you have an interest in psychiatry, specifically psychiatric intensive care. There are chapters within this book that provide modern-day definitions and principles of practice which relate to illnesses, levels of disturbance, commissioning services and physical environments in which these services can be delivered. A question that you may wish to consider is 'how has this specialty evolved?' or even, 'has there always been a need for this type of care?'.

This chapter develops answers to these questions by reviewing the historical development of care provision for the seriously disturbed, mentally unwell individual. By reading it, you will have a better understanding of how and why such services have progressed into what we now understand as psychiatric intensive care. The chapter also looks to the future and reflects upon what it may bring to this specialty.

There are many books and articles that give a historical context to psychiatry. They may discuss specific diseases or symptoms, but few concentrate specifically on what we now understand to be psychiatric intensive care, a discipline that, although small, has given its expertise to the management of severely unwell people who pose risk to themselves and/or others.

Patterns of Care

Throughout history, there has been a cyclic pattern in the modes of care for people suffering from mental illness. Types of treatments have tended to be based on whether an individual's behaviour was considered normal or abnormal. This depended on the milieu within which the behaviour occurred and thus changed as a function of a particular time and culture. As such, uncommon behaviour or behaviour that deviated from sociocultural norms at that time has been used as a reason to control individuals. The more extreme the behaviour, the more significant the intervention. Turner (1996) wrote that historically, psychiatry has been judged by its management of the 'furiously mad'. Nearly 3,000 years ago the king of Babylon was put to pasture (literally) after he started to behave like a wild animal (Book of Daniel).

On the other hand, a less cultural relativist view of abnormal behaviour has focused on whether behaviour poses a threat to oneself or others or causes so much pain and suffering that it interferes with one's daily life and relationships, and treatment focused upon the level of threat.

Early History of Acute Mental Health Care

Cave art was found that originated from as early as 6500 BCE which depicted extreme sadness, and archaeologists have found skulls from around that time that display trephination (removal of sections within the skull). Some historians believe that this was a product of people who were experiencing hallucinations or who were chronically depressed (Farreras, 2021). In ancient Egypt (around 3500 BCE), a person suffering from psychological distress would be sent to a sanatorium, a sleep temple dedicated to healing. In the sanatorium, they would enter a dark cell and prepare for a 'therapeutic dream'. A hypnotic sleep state was induced by lamps and burning perfumed wood. Priests interpreted the dreams and consulted the 'Egyptian Dream Book' to find cures. This is not unlike segregation found in prisons or high-dependency units/seclusion suites found in modern-day psychiatric facilities receiving rapid tranquilisation to induce a calming state.

Throughout early history, mental illness was ascribed to supernatural powers, evil spirits or the wrath of gods. In Greek and Roman times, those marked with mental illness were often 'shunned, locked up, or on rare occasions put to death' (Corrigan, 2002). Sufferers were confined so that they would not cause injury to themselves or others, or damage to property. Two thousand years ago we read in the New Testament of a wild man wandering naked amidst the tombs, having broken the chains that bound him.

The ancient Greek philosopher Plato progressed matters. He suggested that the human soul had three parts, each one having its own home within the body. He remarked in the Timaeus that the body moulds and informs all three parts, and that even the rational part, albeit immortal, is affected by physical illnesses because it is confined to the head. Despite this, he also wrote 'If a man is mad, he shall not be at large in the city, but his family shall keep him in any way they can' (Meyer, 2015).

One of Plato's contemporaries, Xenophon, went further when he claimed to cite the teachings of Plato. He suggested that restraining a mentally ill person can be beneficial, but that a clear distinction must be made between people who are actually mad and people who are ignorant and foolish yet amenable to education and reasoning (Bonnette, 1994).

Western European accounts from the early part of the Middle Ages often blamed mental disorders on demons, an attribution that has precedents in the New Testament. Witch hunting and subsequent execution secondary to demonic possession became commonplace. As this practice diminished, it again became the individual's family that was held responsible for the actions of the mentally unwell. This led to people being hidden from the public by their families, often in states of neglect.

More recognised forms of segregation, motivated by the Christian duty of charity, developed towards the end of the Middle Ages. Somewhat akin to the ancient Egyptian sanitorium, religious houses took in 'lunatics'. In London, St Mary of Bethlehem (lastingly known as the Bethlem) was housing the mentally unwell by the late fourteenth century. By that time, the northern Belgian village of Gheel, with the shrine of St Dymphna, had achieved fame as a healing centre for insane and mentally defective individuals who were disturbed (Porter, 2002).

'Enlightened' Care

Before 1800, there was no country in which medical supervision was required for such asylums. The Bethlem became the national hospital for the disturbed mentally ill 750 years ago. The patient's parish of origin would pay for a stay of usually up to a year. Medical involvement did not automatically lead to good care, as the Bethlem institution showed. For example, the Monro of Fyrish family, who were associated with Bethlem Hospital, produced a dynasty of physicians in London who provided medical care in the eighteenth and nineteenth centuries and who, some suggest, regarded the treatment of madness as a family business as a means of generating wealth and status in society. The institution soon became known as 'Bedlam' as its conditions and practices were revealed. Violent patients were put on display like sideshow freaks for the public to view for the price of one penny; calmer patients were put out on the streets to beg for charity (Butcher, 2007).

Other countries began to follow suit and founded their own mental health facilities. San Hipolito was built in Mexico in 1566 and claims the title of the first asylum in the Americas. La Maison de Chareton was the first mental facility in France, founded in 1641 in a suburb of Paris. Constructed in 1784, the Lunatics' Tower in Vienna became a showplace. Many asylums were staffed by untrained individuals in conditions akin to prisons. A case study describes a typical scene at La Bicetre, a hospital in Paris, starting with patients shackled to the wall in dark, cramped cells. Iron cuffs and collars permitted just enough movement to allow patients to feed themselves but not enough to lie down at night, so they were forced to sleep upright. There were no visitors to the cell except to deliver food, and the rooms were never cleaned. Patients had to make do with a little amount of straw to cover the floor and were forced to be with their own excrement (Butcher, 2007).

'Treatment' followed practices typical of the time; purging and bloodletting being the most common. Other practices included drenching the patient in either hot or ice-cold water to shock them back into a normal state. The belief that patients needed to choose rationality over insanity led to techniques aiming to intimidate (Butcher, 2007): blistering, physical restraints, threats and straitjackets were employed to achieve this end. In the mid-1700s, Dr Boerhaave invented the 'gyrating chair', which became a popular tool in Europe and the United States. This 'was intended to shake up the blood and tissues of the body to restore equilibrium' but instead resulted in rendering the patient unconscious (Alexander and Selesnick, 1966).

Abuses, however, came to light; none better known than the case of William Norris in 1814, which prompted a parliamentary enquiry. This unfortunate American seaman had been admitted in 1800. In June 1804, he was permanently confined in an iron harness so that he could move no more than 12 inches. Ten years later he was still in the same spot. His isolation and constraints were described at the time as:

> a stout iron ring was rivetted round his neck, from which a short chain passed to a ring made to slide upwards or downwards on an upright massive iron bar, more than six feet high, inserted into the wall. Round his body a strong iron bar about two inches wide was rivetted; on each side of the bar was a circular projection, which being fashioned to and inclosing each of his arms, pinioned them close to his sides. This waist bar was secured by two similar bars which, passing over his shoulders, were rivetted to the waist bar both before and behind. The iron ring round his neck was connected to the bars on his shoulders, by a double link. From each of these bars another short chain passed to the ring on the upright iron bar. (Committee on Madhouses, 1815)

In the United Kingdom, under the 1828 Madhouse Act, the Metropolitan Commission in Lunacy was established. Several iterations of the Act ensued mainly dealing with the issue of management of pauper lunatics in Middlesex and surrounding areas, as no county asylum existed. Research by Argent (2023) suggests that in 1840 resident medical officers were required by law in houses with more than 100 patients.

Asylums were also established under religious auspices in eighteenth-century Liverpool, Manchester, Newcastle and York, and in 1845, the provision of county asylums was made mandatory. Up until then, affluence enabled segregation within 'private asylums' of all shapes and sizes as well as quality. The Lunacy Commission was a public body established by the Lunacy Act 1845 to oversee asylums and the welfare of mentally ill people in England and Wales. County lunatic asylums opened such as the ones found in Essex on 23 September 1853 with 450 beds. It had originally been planned to have 300 beds, but the Lunacy Commission felt this was inadequate. It was replaced by the still-utilised Goodmayes Hospital, London Borough of Redbridge, which opened in 1901 and still retains a psychiatric intensive care unit (PICU) called Pathways on Tagore for the most vulnerable mentally ill patients.

Evidence suggests that the abolition of mechanical restraints was 'a gradual process that occurred at the same time in a number of different institutions and that no single individual can be identified as the unequivocal initiator of this movement in the UK' (Haw and Yorston, 2004). Notable individuals include Robert Gardiner Hill, house surgeon, and Edward Charlesworth, physician and governor, at the Lincoln County Asylum in 1838, John Connolly at the Hanwell Asylum in 1839 and Thomas Prichard of the Northampton Asylum in 1857. However, Connolly, in his influential publication *Treatment of the Insane without Mechanical Restraints*, gave credit to Samuel Tuke of the Retreat at York and Phillipe Pinel at La Bicetre hospital in Paris as the 'men who led the way for the more complete system of non-restraint' (Connolly, 1856, p. 9). Despite his pleas for reform, Connolly remained in favour of seclusion: 'The great advantage of a padded room . . . . . . is that it renders both mechanical restraints and muscular force unnecessary for the control of even the most violent patients' (Connolly, 1856 p. 44).

The Mental Treatment Act 1930 introduced the concept of informal admission of patients and by 1938 such patients constituted 35% of all admitted patients (Jones, 1993). The Royal Commission on the Law Relating to Mental Illness and Mental Deficiency (1954–7) stressed that patients should be treated informally where possible. The Mental Health Act 1959 confirmed this and enacted strict guidelines for involuntary patients.

In the late 1950s, there was another important development in the care of the mentally ill. This was the introduction of chlorpromazine, the first pharmacological treatment for psychotic illness. The potent combination of effective antipsychotic drugs along with the introduction of patients' rights led to the unlocking of many hospital wards. The promise of community care was outlined by Enoch Powell in his 'Water Towers' speech when he stated: 'A hospital plan makes no sense unless the medical profession outside the hospital service will be able progressively to accept responsibility for more and more of that care of patients which today is given inside the hospitals.' Perhaps this paved the way for PICUs, as the occurrence of disturbed behaviour associated with mental illness in a small minority seemed to have been overlooked by politicians in their optimism when viewing care provision for the majority. Thus, the PICU function probably evolved as a pragmatic solution to the patient management problems encountered on the open wards.

Secure Provision in the 1970s in the United Kingdom

By the early 1970s, each health region was being encouraged to develop services in district general hospitals. These facilities could not adequately manage difficult patients. The latter joined the mentally abnormal offenders in asylums, prison or special hospitals.

The Department of Health and Social Security set up a working party in 1971 to review the existing guidance on security in National Health Service (NHS) psychiatric hospitals and make recommendations on the need for security. Consequently, the Glancy Report (Revised Report of the Working Party on Security in NHS Psychiatric Hospitals) was published (Department of Health and Social Services, 1974). The Report noted the almost total lack of secure facilities and recommended 1,000 places for England and Wales.

Perhaps the origin of what we now recognise as a PICU came from a man named Graham Young, who in 1971 at the age of 24 was working as a general handyman at a photographic instrument company in Hertfordshire, UK. In June, the head storeman, Bob Egle, was hospitalised with diarrhoea, nausea and numbness in his fingertips, and eight days later he died in hospital, apparently of broncho-pneumonia

and polyneuritis. Shortly afterwards, other employees at the company fell ill, apparently with food poisoning or what became known as the 'Bovingdon Bug'. After another man died, a meeting of management and staff at the company was addressed by a doctor who ruled out contamination by heavy metals (something the staff were worried about due to the chemicals at the company). But someone challenged him with a question: 'Do you not think that the symptoms are consistent with thallium poisoning?' The questioner was Graham Young. After speaking with him further, concerns grew regarding his apparent knowledge of toxicology and the police were subsequently called.

Following this, it was discovered that nine years previously, Graham Young had administered poison to his sister, father and a school friend, all of whom survived (he had also killed his stepmother by poisoning, which he later admitted, but for which he was never charged). Following this, at the age of 14, he was sent to Broadmoor (a high secure hospital) with a recommendation that he serve at least 15 years. Young spent eight years in Broadmoor before being discharged to community psychiatry services. He had applied for his job at the photographic instrument company stating that he had 'previously studied chemistry and toxicology'.

He was arrested, charged and subsequently convicted of two counts of murder, two counts of attempted murder and two counts of administering poison. Following this, the home secretary announced an immediate review of the control, treatment, assessment and release of mentally disordered offenders. The terms of reference of what became the Butler Committee were:

- To consider the criminal law in relation to mental disorder or abnormality and to recommend whether any changes in the powers and procedures were necessary.
- To recommend whether any changes were required in the provision of facilities and treatment for this group of patients.

The final report of the Butler Committee was presented to parliament in 1975 (Committee on Mentally Abnormal Offenders, 1975). It recommended the development of regional secure units (RSUs) (with central funding) in order to manage those mentally disordered offenders who do not need conditions of maximum security but cannot be managed by local psychiatric services. It suggested a figure of 2,000 secure beds. This was double the Glancy figure, which was based on the need for security among general psychiatric patients. It was envisioned that patients would remain within these units for 12–18 months prior to being discharged. It expected that these services would also be crucial in supporting the general psychiatric hospital as well as relieving overcrowding in special hospitals and providing a service to courts and prisons.

The RSUs were to be 50- to 150-bedded units closer to major centres of population than the special hospitals. Although this report addressed those patients who have offended, it did not refer to those mentally ill individuals who have not offended but present acute risk to others due to current mental state. A particular point that was made regarding difficult long-stay patients was that the RSUs should not be allowed to become blocked with such patients. If they did, then the problem which they were supposed to address would recur; however, no clear alternative model of care was proposed for these cases.

Subsequent to the Butler report, the Department of Health and Social Security very quickly made money available for 1,000 beds to be provided in RSUs and in interim secure units (ISUs) whilst the former were being built. These ISUs were usually converted psychiatric wards; most had a double door 'airlock' system to enter the unit and secure external exercise areas, as well as unbreakable glass and alarm systems. Bluglass (1976) proposed that the admission criteria should include any acutely ill patient whose illness was accompanied by difficult and dangerous behaviour but should exclude wandering demented patients, the severely learning disabled and the difficult acute patients.

Thus, historically, the RSU network has been centrally planned and funded, whereas locked beds for acutely ill, non-offender patients have not.

Development of PICUs Worldwide

The first publications which described locked PICUs came from the United States. Rachlin (1973) stated that 'an open-door policy cannot provide adequately for the treatment needs of all psychiatric patients'. He described the establishment of a 'locked intensive care unit' serving the Bronx area of New York 'to treat several types of patients who did not respond on open wards' (p. 829).

Half were referred because they were absconders. Crain and Jordan (1979) also reported on a PICU in

the Bronx which admitted mainly violent patients, 'who simply cannot be treated with an acceptable level of safety on a regular ward'. It also provided a more humane treatment setting, 'for such individuals whose behaviour ordinarily would provoke angry, punitive responses from the environment' (p. 197).

Other PICUs were described elsewhere in the world. Goldney et al. (1985) described a locked unit for acutely severely ill patients in Adelaide, Australia. Warneke (1986) described a PICU for acutely ill patients in a general medical hospital in Edmonton, Canada. The patients were mainly suicidal, and the unit was not locked, nor were the patients legally detained. Musisi et al. (1989) described a six-bedded unit in a provincial Toronto psychiatric hospital.

In England, the first designated PICU was opened in St James's Hospital, Portsmouth; Mounsey (1979) described the setting up of a twelve-bedded PICU in Salisbury. This was a lockable converted ward for disturbed patients referred from the rest of the psychiatric hospital.

In Scotland, Basson and Woodside (1981, p. 132) described the working of a mixed, 'secure/intensive care/forensic' ward and stated that, 'the pendulum has swung from "open door" hospitals back to a recognition for some security'.

Secure Provision in the United Kingdom in the 1980s and 1990s

The RSU model was first developed throughout England and Wales and then subsequently in Scotland. Several deficiencies of the RSU model have been noted. Snowden (1990) wrote that there is a group of patients who are not so dangerous that they require special hospital security but who are chronically ill or poor medication responders and who require a degree of security. Some of the more severely ill and disabled patients will not manage in the community and long-term care will not be available. The mentally ill who cannot manage in the community may become mentally ill offenders by default, and even if they do not, general psychiatric services could well put pressure on forensic services to take patients that would have been considered appropriate for RSU admission in the past.

In 1991, only 635 medium secure beds existed compared with 1,163 beds in 1986, according to the Reed Report; this review of health and social Services for mentally disordered offenders and others requiring similar services (Reed, 1992) proposed that 1,500 beds were needed. It also proposed that, 'access to local intensive care and locked wards should be available more widely' and that 'secure provision should include provision for those who require long-term treatment and/or care'. The Reed Report again referred to the lack of service provision.

Many offenders needing in-patient care can be accommodated in ordinary psychiatric provision. Although many offenders can be managed satisfactorily in 'open' wards, there must be also better access to local intensive care and locked wards (Annex J (local services 5.16 Hospital Services, p. 19)). The Report recognised, 'the need for each Health District to ensure the availability of secure provision … [which] should include provision for intensive care'. The Reed Report (Reed, 1992) referred to ICUs as low secure units (LSUs).

Smith et al. (1990) hypothesised that the role of the RSU was changing. They compared patients admitted to the Butler Clinic RSU in Southwest England in 1983 and 1989. In the 1983 population, there were significantly more patients who had been aggressive towards staff and had histories of absconding. The 1989 population was much more likely to have been referred from the criminal justice system. The authors speculated that the RSU was originally dealing with a 'backlog' of local hospital patients for whom there was no secure provision before the RSU opened.

A survey of RSU patient characteristics in 1994 confirmed that the RSU population had high levels of serious offending (McKenna, 1996) and warned that, 'The ability of the RSU to respond quickly, effectively or flexibly to acute difficulties in the services referring potential admissions must in turn be compromised.'

In order to respond quickly, NHS trusts have now used the low secure wards or PICUs to take up this demand for urgent forensic patients. Dix (1996) pointed out that this group does not necessarily present high levels of behavioural disturbance but requires a degree of security because of their charge or offence. James et al. (1996) also referred to a group of patients that had offended but did not require security. The suggestion is that local services should be able to provide low security in order to facilitate diversion of offenders from the criminal justice system and aid the rehabilitation of patients discharged from special hospitals.

As Dix (1996) writes, however, 'A significant number of PICUs do not consider themselves as "forensic units" and are reluctant to accept patients who, as a result of legal restrictions, cannot be discharged from the PICU when clinically indicated.' Cripps et al. (1995) describe a mixed PICU/forensic unit and discuss some of the advantages and disadvantages of this type of unit. Many would argue that the forensic role conflicts with the more dominant function of local LSUs, namely, the modus operandi outlined by Faulk (1995): 'The usual pattern is for the wards to accept the patient briefly, to get them over an acute disturbance, before returning them to the original ward.'

A third role which has been adopted by PICUs is the care of the chronically disturbed patient. Coid (1991a) noted that the private sector was being used increasingly for such patients because of the lack of NHS facilities and he also (Coid, 1991b) stated that 'the game of pass the parcel must stop' with reference to 'difficult to place patients'. The Mental Health Act Commission (1995) also reported on the lack of provision for patients who demonstrate longer-term behavioural problems.

The chief medical officer (CMO's Update, 1996) stated that the number of medium secure beds was planned to be 2,350 by the end of 1998 and that there was also a need for a greater diversity of secure beds, particularly those offering longer-term care at medium and low security levels. By 2001, there were some 2,000 beds (Sugarman, 2002).

PICUs in the United Kingdom in the 1990s

In the United Kingdom, PICUs have developed independently of the RSU network and have provided a range of services in line with local circumstances and needs. This development is wholly appropriate. Units may variably describe themselves as PICUs, extra care wards, intensive care, high dependency, special care, challenging behaviour, locked wards or LSUs. None of these terms have a universally agreed upon definition.

This was highlighted in a rather damming (but highly influential) paper by Zigmond (1995), who commented upon his personal experiences of such facilities in his role as a Mental Health Act commissioner and second opinion appointed doctor. He noted that the patients within such wards were different from those on open acute wards; they were amongst the sickest and displayed disturbed behaviour. Environments were usually poor, staff were isolated and unsupported with the development of a somewhat 'siege mentality' and patients were subject to a somewhat overpowering and regimented regime. He suggested several methods to improve such wards from philosophical, staffing, managerial and clinical perspectives. This could be seen as providing impetus for the development of standards for service provision.

Subsequent to Zigmond's criticisms, shoots started growing out of what eventually became the National Association of Psychiatric Intensive Care and Low Secure Units (NAPICU) (Dix et al., 1997). Whilst such services had developed independently, all attempted to provide a service to meet local needs. It seemed difficult to be prescriptive regarding the role of all these services. Perhaps it was better to focus on similarities, such as admission of patients too disturbed to be managed on acute wards due to aggression, self-harming behaviour or absconding. Despite this level of disturbance, patients were not under the purview of any criminal service and thus needed care within local psychiatric facilities. Secondary to their presentation, patients needed increased and intensive multiprofessional input as well as physical security. The initial definition of what we recognise as psychiatric intensive care was therefore conceived. Patients were generally too disturbed to be nursed on open wards (because of aggression, self-harming behaviour, unpredictability or absconding). There was, therefore, a need for increased nursing and multiprofessional input and perimeter security. Admissions and discharges were generally governed by symptoms and behaviour and not by the courts (Dix, 1996). In order to help patients served by and clinicians within this specialty, a group of like-minded psychiatric intensive care multidisciplinary clinicians formed NAPICU with the following aims:

- To advance psychiatric intensive care, low secure and other locked services
- To improve mechanisms for the delivery of emergency psychiatric intensive care
- To audit effectiveness and promote research
- To educate and develop best practice
- To raise awareness in the mental health and medical world about psychiatric intensive care.

PICU Developments Since the New Millennium

Within the United Kingdom, PICU National Minimum Standards were first published in 2002 and updated in 2014, recommending specific principles that should be adhered to when planning and managing psychiatric intensive care and low secure services (Pereira and Clinton, 2002; NAPICU, 2014). The objective of these standards is to provide users, clinicians, managers and commissioners with a dynamic framework for delivering high-quality services.

In 2012, NAPICU worked with the Department of Health to produce two draft good practice commissioning guides (Department of Health, 2012a, b) in the clinical areas of psychiatric intensive care and low secure care. This process highlighted a need to revise the clinical standards set in 2002 to reflect the current clinical processes in PICU and low secure care and to set the clinical framework for the coming decades in this challenging area.

The National Minimum Standards (NAPICU, 2014) looks at the clinical standards in PICU services. The project group was set up through the NAPICU executive, a group comprising multiple professional disciplines, patient and carer representatives and expertise in all types of PICU modality. The remit of the group was to revise the agreed-upon standards for psychiatric intensive care services and the general good practice guidance for each of these standards. The overall objective is to provide patients, carers, clinicians, managers and commissioners with a dynamic framework for delivering high-quality psychiatric intensive care services. These standards are derived from the clinical perspective, which in turn is driven by the achievement of a positive and empowering experience for patients in PICUS (these are further discussed elsewhere in this book).

Another important document regarding inpatient care, *Mental Health Policy Implementation Guide: Adult Acute Care Provision*, was published by the Department of Health in 2002. This guidance is addressed to all involved in acute mental health care and is useful to all who use, work in or commission these services. PICU practice is on the spectrum of inpatient care. It covers issues related to areas shown in Box 1.1.

The first textbook for psychiatric intensive care was published in 2001. It was authored and edited by multidisciplinary psychiatric care, low secure, forensic staff such as consultant psychiatrists, consultant nurses, nurse managers, charge nurses, staff nurses, therapy managers, nurse therapists, clinical psychologists and forensic psychologists, specialist registrars, occupational therapists, pharmacists and senior lecturers. It was the first evidence-based textbook to define the sub-specialty. The book was written by clinicians for clinicians. It was subsequently revised in 2009; you are currently reading the third revision.

In 2002, an innovative MSc programme in psychiatric intensive care was offered by London South Bank University; this is another milestone in the advancement of psychiatric intensive care. This programme was initiated and developed by Pathways Policy, Research and Development Group, Goodmayes Hospital, London Borough of Redbridge in collaboration with South Bank University, following a review of the training needs of PICU staff (Clinton et al., 2001). The programme aimed to examine a variety of frameworks for the delivery of safe and consistent approaches to psychiatric intensive care and provide practitioners with the necessary confidence to be fit for practice. The course covered in detail the assessment and management of clients in psychiatric intensive care settings together with the therapeutic interventions applied in such settings.

The MSc programme ran successfully for several years and is still being delivered as a short course in partnership with St George's University of London, covering key PICU-related topics such as risk management, mental health law, physical health, substance use, pharmacology, care involvement and restrictive practices (NAPICU, 2023).

In 2002, NAPICU produced a bulletin for its multidisciplinary membership in order to promote best practice and share information. This subsequently

formed the basis for the development of the *Journal of Psychiatric Intensive Care*, which continues to disseminate research devoted to the specialty.

In 2004, a study was commissioned by the UK Department of Health to evaluate the costs of addressing physical environment deficits in PICUs and LSUs in England (Pereira et al., 2006c). The results showed that approximately 37% of these units did not fulfil the National Minimum Standards for design. This critical study laid the evidence base for the UK government to release £160 million to address places of safety and for upgrading PICUs and LSUs to meet the National Minimum Standards in England (Pereira and Clinton, 2002).

To monitor the development of implementation of the National Minimum Standards, a National PICU Governance Network was created in 2004 as a joint venture of the National Institute of Mental Health in England (NIMHE), North East London Mental Health Trust (NELMHT) and NAPICU (Dye et al., 2005). The main aim of this network was to encourage the PICUs to work collaboratively to improve service provision, with an objective measurement of the benefits demonstrated. The collaborative nature of this project enabled the different PICUs to share experiences and difficulties and plan improvements, drawing upon expertise from both within and outside the network.

In 2005, NAPICU collaborated with the National Institute for Clinical Excellence in producing the clinical guideline, Violence: Short-term Management for Over 16s in Psychiatric and Emergency Departments. This guideline has been updated and replaced with NG10, Violence and aggression: short-term management in mental health, health and community settings, which was published in 2015 (NICE, 2015)

NAPICU continued to hold annual national conferences and quarterly meetings since formation, and during these years and it has been estimated that more than 10,000 multidisciplinary PICU and low secure clinicians have been involved in activities for sharing best practice and updating knowledge within the specialty.

In 2015, the National Minimum Standards for Psychiatric Intensive Care for Young People were published to ensure best practice in provision for young people (NAPICU, 2015).

Between 2009 and 2017, an accreditation programme was set up in collaboration between the

Royal College of Psychiatrists and NAPICU (NAPICU, 2009). Accreditation Inpatient Mental Health Services (AIMS) is an accreditation scheme, working with inpatient mental health services to assure and improve the safety and quality of services and their environments. AIMS-PICU is specifically designed for PICUs. It engages staff and service users in a comprehensive process of review, through which good practice and high-quality care are recognised.

Services are supported to identify areas for improvement and set achievable targets for change. Services that are performing well are accredited, assuring staff, service users and carers, commissioners and regulators of the quality of the service being provided. AIMS is an initiative of the College Centre for Quality Improvement. It is a collaboration between the Royal College of Psychiatrists, the British Psychological Society, the College of Occupational Therapists, the Royal College of Nursing and NAPICU, which means that it is led by the professional bodies of those staff most involved in inpatient care.

AIMS accreditation helps units to:

- demonstrate the quality of care they provide including:
  - dedicated, trained, and committed staff;
  - dedicated time with patients;
  - activity and therapy provision;
  - involvement of service users and carers; and
  - communication between services.
- demonstrate that they meet national standards, in line with national policy and guidance from the Department of Health, National Institute for Clinical Excellence (NICE) and the National Patient Safety Agency (NPSA)
- use the standards and assessment process as a framework to monitor contracts and develop service level agreements
- use information from the accreditation process in Trust Quality Accounts, as recommended by the National Quality Board

The accreditation process supports services to evaluate their performance and improve their practice through:

- Self-review of their service
- Peer-review identifying and discussing challenges with the visiting reviewers

- A detailed team report recognising areas of achievement and identifying areas for improvement
- Organised visits to other services supported by an experienced lead reviewer
- Report of national findings identifying trends and enabling benchmarking with other services
- Sharing good practice through newsletters, email discussion groups, annual conference and publication of resources
- Personal development through training in peer-reviewing and participation in the wider process
- Spread of learning beyond the participating unit to other services within the organisation

This is now being taken forward by the Royal College of Psychiatrists Centre for Quality Improvement.

In 2015, a position statement on seclusion was released entitled, 'NAPICU Seclusion position statement on the monitoring, regulation and recording of the extra care area, seclusion and long-term segregation use in the context of the Mental Health Act 1983: Code of Practice (2015)' (NAPICU, 2016).

Guidance was produced for commissioners in 2016 (NAPICU, 2016), closely followed by design guidance for the procurement of new builds to mitigate environmental risks associated with building design (NAPICU, 2017).

In 2018, a joint effort of the British Association of Psychopharmacology (BAP) and NAPICU produced Evidence-based Consensus Guidelines for the Clinical Management of Acute Disturbance: De-escalation and Rapid Tranquillisation (Patel et al., 2018), followed by COVID guidelines for safe management (NAPICU, 2020).

In summary, some of the major PICU developments of the modern era have included:

- Increased use of evidenced-based treatments. A greater emphasis has been placed on using treatments that are supported by research, and in the last 20 years has seen the publication of NICE guidelines for treatment and NICE technology appraisals suggesting the use of treatments as suggested by the National Minimum Standards (Pereira and Clinton, 2002; NAPICU, 2014) such as cognitive behaviour therapy, dialectical behaviour therapy and best practice in medication-assisted treatments

- A shift towards a more person-centered approach, with a focus on involving patients and carers in decision-making
- A shift towards single-sex units and away from mixed PICUs
- A focus on the design of the buildings to be safer and more therapeutic rather than containing, including the publication of national guidelines
- Improved staff training and safety measures. Staff training programmes have been developed to improve patient care and prevent burnout, including the AIMS PICU programme, and focusing on therapies such as the formation of a network of occupational therapists in PICUs (NAPICU, 2020)
- Focus on least restrictive practices
- Integration of technology. The use of technology such as remote consulting and electronic patient records has increased in PICUs, making it easier to monitor and treat patients and to coordinate care between different healthcare providers. Use of technology has also been utilised in PICUs, such as the introduction of sensory suites and some high-tech innovations in terms of digital walls in seclusion suites
- Expansion of community-based services, such as crisis/intensive/assertive outreach/home treatment and early intervention teams which have become more widely available, reducing the need for hospitalisation and allowing patients to receive care in a more community-based setting

Further developments in psychiatric intensive care include the Intensive Care in Special Hospitals (in press) and Prison Guidance endorsed by the Royal College of Psychiatrists (Dix and Woods, 2023).

Past and Present Surveys of Psychiatric Intensive Care

Although there was very little objective data concerning the service that these units provide, three surveys had been published prior to the development of NAPICU. Each of these surveys had a slightly different focus.

Ford and Whiffin (1991) surveyed the 169 health authorities in England and asked them 'about their units providing services to acutely ill clients who require close observation and frequent nursing observation' (p. 48). They identified 39 units in England which admitted in varying proportions those with acute or chronic problems such as aggression or self-harm (in the setting of mental illness) and those with a forensic history.

Mitchell (1992) surveyed psychiatric hospitals in Scotland to determine the numbers and characteristics of their patients. He identified 13 PICUs in Scotland with a total of 219 beds (3% of total inpatient psychiatric beds). Two-thirds of patients were compulsorily detained and half were younger than 30 years of age; schizophrenia was the most common diagnosis and comorbid substance abuse/personality disorder was present in 10% of patients younger than 30 years old.

Beer et al. (1997) identified 110 PICUs in the United Kingdom, 45 of which had been operational for less than three years. Eleven units were intensive care areas of four to five beds which formed part of acute admission wards; 18 units were mixed PICU/challenging behaviour or PICU/forensic. The remainder were dedicated PICUs. Bed occupancy rates were high at a level of 100%, particularly in the larger dedicated units.

There was a wide variation in the level of security provided, ranging from 11 units which were built to medium secure specifications to the 22 units which did not have permanently locked doors. Operational policies also differed widely, with many staff feeling that they might as well not have, for example, an admissions policy, because it was frequently overridden to accommodate difficult-to-manage patients who could not be placed elsewhere.

Units accepted patients from acute psychiatric wards, prisons, RSUs, special hospitals and the community in various combinations. Sixty-three units were willing to admit informal patients, and this was irrespective of whether the door was permanently locked. The terminology used to describe the patient group admitted was confusing. There was no accepted cut-off point between acute and chronic disturbance or between intensive care and challenging behaviour. The point at which a patient was described as 'forensic' is similarly blurred.

Medical staffing was also highly variable. Only 30 units had a dedicated consultant psychiatrist with no other inpatient beds. An equal number of units could be accessed by several consultants, none of whom had overall responsibility for the daily functioning of the unit. Junior doctor posts were not exclusively filled by experienced registrars; more than half the units accepted rotational senior house officers, often with no supervision from a more experienced staff grade doctor or senior registrar.

The multidisciplinary team working was less developed than in general adult psychiatry and written guidelines or policies covering high-risk areas such as rapid tranquilisation, control and restraint and seclusion were often absent, confirming the informal observations of Zigmond (1995). The implications of these findings have been further developed by Pereira et al. (1999).

National Surveys of Psychiatric Intensive Care and Low Secure Services

The first most comprehensive national survey on psychiatric intensive care and low secure services (Pereira et al., 2006a) identified 170 PICUs and 137 LSUs in the United Kingdom. This survey resulted in developing a national dataset for PICUs and low secure services together with a more comprehensive understanding of the service provision and patient characteristics (Pereira et al., 2006b) within these units.

In addition, it also highlighted some of the differences between PICUs and LSUs. The national survey builds upon an earlier London-wide survey conducted on PICUs and LSUs which described the service structure and functioning of PICUs and LSUs in London (Pereira et al., 2005a) along with the clinical characteristics of patients and the pathways for admission and discharge in the London units (Pereira et al., 2005b).

This national survey was revisited and replicated in 2015, with a view to examine how the service had changed over 10 years and to identify further research directions for the specialty (Pereira et al., 2021a, b).

Current UK Population of PICUs based on National Survey and Other Data

The aims were to update the benchmark from the 2006 national survey, comparing users of NHS PICU and LSU services, and to define 'locked rehabilitation unit' (LRU) patient characteristics. A cross-sectional census-day questionnaire (November 2016) with a six-month follow-up ending in May 2017 was utilised. Respondents included 104 NHS units: 73 PICUs, 644 patients; 17 LSUs, 190 patients; and 14 LRUs, 183 patients.

The typical PICU patient is younger, employed, stays for shorter periods and is more likely to suffer delayed discharge and mood disorder, have complex needs, had mental health admissions in the last 12 months, be on 1:1 or greater observations, and be prescribed fewer antipsychotic and physical health medications but more benzodiazepines. The typical LSU patient is an out-of-area transfer, least likely to have been admitted for self-harm or non-concordance and is of Black ethnic origin. The typical LRU patient is less likely to be married or have a long-term partner, has the lowest complex needs, and is most likely to have had physical examination and investigations.

There has been an increase in PICU and LSU patients from the Black and Minority Ethnic (BAME) population. Length of stay for PICU and LSU patients has doubled; there are lower rates of delayed transfers of care. These findings demonstrate that PICU and LSU services are providing care to the right patients as they were conceptualised in national guidance and provide a benchmark for LRU patients. Results are shown in Table 1.1.

Reasons for Admission to PICU

A referral from a mental health professional is typically required for admission to a PICU. Admission criteria vary, but generally patients are admitted if they meet the following criteria:

- Severe mental illness that requires close monitoring and management
- Risk of harm to self or others
- Acute symptoms that are not manageable in a less intensive setting
- Need for frequent assessment and reassessment of treatment options.
- Failure of previous treatment attempts
  Other factors that may be considered include:
- Medical stability
- History of violence or aggression
- Ability to follow safety protocols

Dix (1995) suggests that mental and behavioural characteristics requiring PICU admission will generally fall under one or more of the following headings:

- **Externally directed aggression.** A patient is assessed as posing a significant risk of harm to others or extreme aggression towards property.
- **Internally directed aggression.** A patient is assessed as posing a significant risk of suicide and the patient is unresponsive to preventative measures available.
- **Absconding.** These are patients who are detained under the Mental Health Act 1983, for whom the

Table 1.1 Respondents, demographic details, reason for admission and section status for NHS service users

	PICU n	2006 n	LSU n	2006 n	LRU n	x^2/f	p
By unit type	73	170	17	137	14		
SUs	644	1242	190	1583	183		
Demographics	% (n)	%	% (n)	%	% (n)		
Age (range in years)	↑ **37.0 (18–84)**	33	↓40.35 (18–78)	41	39.86 (19–78)	6.822	**.001**
Male	↑80 (506)	71.1	↑83 (158)	74.7	86 (143)	4.094	.129
Female	↓20 (129)	28.9	↓17 (32)	25.3	14 (23)		
Unemployed	↓88 (545)	89.5	↑ 94 (175)	90.5	94 (155)	9.770	**.008**
Employed	**12 (76)**		6 (11)		6 (10)		
Single	↑84 (528)	79.2	↑88 (163)	83.4	92 (152)	23.390	**.003**
Married/LT partner	↑9 (58)	8.9	↓ 3 (6)	4.1	**2 (3)**		
Divorced	3 (16)		6.5 (12)		4 (6)		
Separated	3 (14)		2 (4)		1 (2)		
Widowed	1 (7)		0.5 (1)		1 (2)		
Reason for admission							
Violence to others/property	↓58.5 (361)	60.4	↑68.8 (108)	46.5	52.9 (64)	42.410	**<.001**
Self-harm	↑6.3 (39)	0.5	↓**0.6 (1)**	8.6	5.0 (6)		
Absconding	↓3.2 (20)	9.2	↓1.3 (2)	5.7	6.6 (8)		
Non-compliance with medication	↑ 7.6 (47)		↑**1.9 (3)**		12.4 (15)		
Diagnostic Assessment	↑2.1 (13)		↑4.5 (7)		4.1 (5)		
Fire-setting	↑1.8 (11)		↑5.1 (8)		1.7 (2)		
Sexual behaviour	↓3.1 (19)	39.6	↓4.5 (7)	30.9	5.8 (7)		
Crisis/relapse	↑17.3 (107)	8.4	↑13.4 (21)	3.9	11.6 (14)		
Section status							
Informal	↓ 2.1 (13)	6.8	↓ 0.5 (1)	13.7	5.4 (8)	296.287	**<.001**
2	↑ 23.7 (145)	15.7	↓ 0.0 (0)	0.6	0.0 (0)		
3	↑65.4 (401)	61.4	↓38.5 (70)	51.4	51.7 (76)		
Forensic sections	↓ 6.2 (38)	12.4	↑**51.6 (94)**	33.5	32.0 (47)		
Prison transfer	↓ 2.6 (16)	3.3	↑9.3 (17)	2.0	10.9 (16)		

Arrows denote direction of change since (2006) (Pereira et al., 2021b)

Figures in bold denote statistically signficant results.

consequences of persistent absconding are serious enough to warrant treatment in the PICU. The PICU should not provide security for its own sake; there should always be a primary clinical reason for admission to prevent absconding.

- **Unpredictability**. These are patients whose behaviour is unpredictable, potentially posing a significant risk to self or others and requiring further assessment.

Definition of Psychiatric Intensive Care

Psychiatric intensive care is for patients who are in an acutely disturbed phase of a serious mental disorder. There is an associated loss of capacity for self-control with a corresponding increase in risk, which does not allow their safe, therapeutic management and treatment in a less acute or a less secure mental health ward. Care and treatment must be patient centred, multidisciplinary, intensive and have an immediacy of response to critical clinical and risk situations. Patients should be detained compulsorily under the appropriate mental health legislative framework, and the clinical and risk profile of the patient usually requires an associated level of security.

Psychiatric intensive care is delivered by qualified and suitably trained multidisciplinary clinicians according to an agreed philosophy of unit operation underpinned by the principles of therapeutic interventions and dynamic clinically focused risk engagement. Length of stay must be appropriate to clinical need and assessment of risk but would aim not to exceed eight weeks in duration (NAPICU, 2014).

Overall Service Model and Interface with Other Services

The service model of a PICU typically includes the following components:

- Multidisciplinary team: A PICU is staffed by a multidisciplinary team of mental health professionals, including psychiatrists, nurses, psychologists, occupational therapists and other support staff.
- Patient assessment: Upon admission, patients undergo a comprehensive assessment to determine their needs, risks and strengths. This assessment informs the development of an individualised treatment plan.
- Close monitoring and management: PICUs provide a high level of monitoring and management for patients who may be at risk of harm to themselves or others. This may include frequent observation and restriction of patients' movements as well as close monitoring of their mood and behaviour.
- Evidence-based treatments: PICUs offer a range of evidence-based treatments such as psychotherapy, medication management and occupational therapy, aimed at stabilising patients and reducing their risk of harm.
- Family involvement: PICUs typically involve family members in treatment planning and may offer family therapy and support.
- Discharge planning: The discharge of patients from a PICU is carefully planned, with the aim of ensuring that patients receive the appropriate level of care and support after leaving the unit.

- Collaboration and consultation: PICUs collaborate and consult with other mental health services, such as acute psychiatric units (APUs) and LSUs as well as with community-based services, such as crisis/intensive/assertive community treatment teams (ACTs) to coordinate care for patients and ensure that they receive the most appropriate level of care and support.

The overall goal of a PICU is to provide a safe and therapeutic environment for individuals with mental illness who require close monitoring and management and to support their recovery and well-being. The relationship between PICUs and other units and services is one of collaboration and coordination, aimed at ensuring that patients receive the most appropriate level of care and treatment for their specific needs and conditions. We examine the specific interfaces in the sections that follow.

General Adult Services

PICUs and APUs are both inpatient settings for treating individuals with serious mental illness, but they have some differences:

- Level of intensity: PICUs provide a higher level of intensity of care compared to APUs. Patients in PICUs require close monitoring and management, while those in APUs may have more stability.
- Type of patients: PICUs generally admit patients who are in crisis and at high risk of harm to self or others, while APUs may admit patients with less severe symptoms who still require inpatient treatment.
- Treatment focus: PICUs typically focus on stabilising a patient's symptoms and reducing their risk of harm, while APUs may offer more comprehensive treatment, including therapy and rehabilitation.
- Length of stay: PICUs tend to have shorter lengths of stay compared to APUs, as patients in PICUs are usually stabilised and transferred to a less intensive setting as soon as possible.
- Staffing and training: PICUs typically have more specialised staffing, with a higher proportion of mental health professionals, and staff are trained in crisis intervention and safety management. APUs may have a more generalist staffing model with a mix of mental health professionals and medical staff.

It's important to note that the differences between PICUs and APUs can vary depending on the facility, and some facilities may have a blended approach that incorporates elements of both. PICUs and APUs can interface in a number of ways:

- Patient transfer: Patients may be transferred from a PICU to an APU when they are stabilised and no longer require close monitoring and management. This can occur once their risk of harm to self or others has been reduced and they can be safely managed in a less intensive setting.
- Collaboration and consultation: Staff in PICUs and APUs may collaborate and consult with each other regarding patient care and treatment plans, especially when a patient is transferred between units.
- Joint treatment planning: PICUs and APUs may participate in joint treatment planning for patients, especially when a patient is transferred from one unit to the other, to ensure a seamless and effective continuation of care.
- Integration with community-based services: PICUs and APUs may interface with community-based services, such as ACT teams, to coordinate care for patients and ensure that they receive appropriate support and treatment after discharge.

PICU Interface with Other Mental Health Services

Low Secure Care

Low secure care is for patients who present with more prolonged disturbance or complex needs in the context of a serious mental disorder, requiring a 'low secure' level of physical, relational and procedural security. This may be due to an objective risk to others or because of associated criminal justice requirements. Low secure care is positioned between mainstream general adult psychiatric settings and forensic medium secure settings.

In general, there are three distinct patient types who may require low secure care:

- Those who require a step down in security from high or medium secure
- Those subject to requirements emanating from the criminal justice system

- Those who require rehabilitation due to prolonged challenging behaviour, treatment resistance and associated risk consistent with the need for low security

Care and treatment must be patient centred, multidisciplinary, primarily rehabilitation and recovery-focused and able to respond to critical clinical and risk situations. Patients should be detained compulsorily under the appropriate mental health legislative framework including parts II and III of the Mental Health Act (MHA, 1983).

Low secure care is delivered by qualified and suitably trained multidisciplinary clinicians according to an agreed philosophy of unit operation underpinned by the principles of clinically focused risk management. Length of stay must be appropriate to clinical need and assessment of risk and can generally range between six months and two years (NAPICU, 2014).

PICUs and LSUs are both types of inpatient facilities for individuals with serious mental illness, but they have some differences:

- Level of security: LSUs offer a lower level of security compared to PICUs, and patients are generally not at high risk of harm to self or others. PICUs are designed for patients who require close monitoring and management due to a high risk of harm.
- Treatment focus: PICUs focus on stabilising a patient's symptoms and reducing their risk of harm, while LSUs may offer more comprehensive treatment, including therapy and rehabilitation, aimed at long-term recovery.
- Length of stay: Patients in PICUs typically have shorter lengths of stay, while patients in LSUs may stay for several months or longer, depending on their progress and treatment goals (Pereira et al., 2021b).
- Staffing and training: Staff in PICUs are typically trained in crisis intervention and safety management, while staff in LSUs may have a more generalist training, including both mental health and medical training.
- Freedom of movement: Patients in LSUs generally have more freedom of movement and may be allowed to leave the unit for planned appointments or activities, while patients in PICUs may have more restrictions on their movement for safety reasons, although those in LSUs must often apply for Ministry of Justice agreement for leave which can be prolonged due to the nature of their offences.

It is important to note that the differences between PICUs and LSUs can vary depending on the facility and the specific needs of the patient. Some facilities may offer a blended approach that incorporates elements of both. PICUs and LSUs can interface in a number of ways:

- Patient transfer: Patients may be transferred from a PICU to an LSU when they are stabilised and no longer require close monitoring and management. This can occur once their risk of harm to self or others has been reduced and they can be safely managed in a less intensive setting.
- Collaboration and consultation: Staff in PICUs and LSUs may collaborate and consult with each other regarding patient care and treatment plans, especially when a patient is transferred between units.
- Joint treatment planning: PICUs and LSUs may participate in joint treatment planning for patients, especially when a patient is transferred from one unit to the other, to ensure a seamless and effective continuation of care.
- Integration with community-based services: PICUs and LSUs may interface with community-based services, such as ACT teams, to coordinate care for patients and ensure that they receive appropriate support and treatment after discharge.

Criminal Justice System

The interface between PICUs and the criminal justice system can occur in several ways:

- Court-ordered evaluations: PICUs may receive individuals who have been court ordered for psychiatric evaluations and treatment, particularly if they have been deemed not fit to stand trial or pose a danger to themselves or others.
- Inpatient treatment for offenders: PICUs may provide inpatient treatment for individuals who have committed crimes and have been diagnosed with a mental illness, with the goal of stabilising their symptoms and reducing their risk of harm.
- Forensic assessment and consultation: PICUs may provide forensic assessments and consultations to the criminal justice system to assist with decision-making regarding individuals with mental illness who have come into contact with the criminal justice system.

- Collaboration with forensic services: PICUs may collaborate with forensic mental health services, such as secure hospitals or prisons, to ensure the continuity of care for individuals with mental illness who have come into contact with the criminal justice system.

It is important to note that the interface between PICUs and the criminal justice system can vary depending on the jurisdiction and may be influenced by the availability of specialised forensic mental health services. The goal of the interface is to ensure that individuals with mental illness who have come into contact with the criminal justice system receive appropriate treatment and support, although evidence suggests that delays to hospital transfer remains a serious problem in England and Wales for all prison transfers (Woods et al., 2020).

Community Mental Health Services

The interface between PICUs and community mental health teams (CMHTs) can occur in several ways:

- Patient transfer: Patients may be transferred from a PICU to a CMHT for ongoing community-based treatment and support once they have stabilised and no longer require close monitoring and management.
- Collaboration and consultation: Staff in PICUs and CMHTs may collaborate and consult with each other regarding patient care and treatment plans, especially when a patient is transferred between the two.
- Joint treatment planning: PICUs and CMHTs may participate in joint treatment planning for patients, especially when a patient is transferred from one to the other, to ensure a seamless and effective continuation of care.
- Community-based services: PICUs may interface with community-based services, such as ACT teams, to coordinate care for patients and ensure that they receive appropriate support and treatment after discharge from the PICU.

Overall, the relationship between PICUs and CMHTs is one of collaboration and coordination, aimed at ensuring that patients receive the most appropriate level of care and treatment for their specific needs and conditions, both during their stay in the PICU and after discharge into the community.

Strategic Development for Future PICU Services

The future of PICUs will likely be shaped by several key strategic developments:

- Evidence-based practice: The focus on evidence-based practice will continue to drive the development of PICUs, with a focus on providing evidence-based treatments and interventions that are effective and have been shown to be effective in treating patients with mental illness.
- Integration with community-based services: PICUs will increasingly integrate with community-based services, such as ACT teams, to ensure that patients receive the most appropriate level of care and treatment both during their stay in the PICU and after discharge into the community.
- Quality and safety: Quality and safety will continue to be a priority for PICUs, with a focus on minimising the risk of harm to patients and staff and ensuring that patients receive high-quality care that supports their recovery and well-being.
- Collaboration with other mental health services: PICUs will continue to collaborate with other mental health services, such as APUs and secure units, to ensure that patients receive the most appropriate level of care and treatment for their specific needs and conditions.
- Use of technology: The use of technology, such as telepsychiatry and digital health, will continue to develop within PICUs in the future, with a focus on improving access to care and treatment, as well as monitoring and managing patients remotely.
- Workforce development: Workforce development will continue to be a key focus for PICUs, with a focus on ensuring that staff have the appropriate skills and knowledge to provide effective and high-quality care to patients.

Overall, the future of PICUs will be shaped by a focus on providing high-quality, evidence-based care that supports the recovery and well-being of patients with mental illness, and that integrates with other mental health services and community-based services to ensure a seamless and effective continuity of care.

Conclusion

Psychiatric intensive care is at the cutting edge of clinical psychiatry and is a continually developing specialty. Patients in these units are often very unwell and behaviourally disturbed.

The PICU clinical community has the responsibility to ensure that the collective cause of helping some of the most disadvantaged people in society achieve the best outcomes to their acute distress remains the highest of priorities. At the heart of this endeavour must be people coming together to share ideas and different points of view which can be processed into wisdom for the present and future (Dix, 2019). At times, debate and different perspectives can produce bumps on the road to advancement. PICU is one of the most challenging and rewarding areas of practice. The PICU is by design a place where people must come together, often in the most difficult of circumstances. This book seeks to address the principles and practice of meeting the needs of this group of patients.

References

Alexander,FG and Selesnick,S (1966) *The History of Psychiatry: An Evaluation of Psychiatric Thought and Practice from Prehistoric Times to the Present.* New York: Harper and Row.

Argent,V (2023) The 1832 Madhouse Act and the Metropolitan Commission in Lunacy from 1832. www.studymore.org.uk/3_06.btm#3.9.3.

Basson,JV and Woodside,M (1981) Assessment of a Secure/Intensive Care/Forensic Ward. *Acta Psychiatrica Scandinavica* 64: 132–41.

Beer,MD, Paton,C and Pereira,S (1997) Hot Beds of General Psychiatry: A National Survey of Psychiatric Intensive Care Units. *Psychiatric Bulletin* 21: 142–4.

Bluglass,R (1976) The Design of Security Units, the Type of Patient and Behaviour Patterns. *Hospital England* pp. 5–7.

Bonnette,A (1994) *Xenophon, Memorabilia*, trans. Amy L Bonnette. The Agora Editions. pp. 49–50. Ithaca: Cornell University Press.

Butcher,JN, Mineka,S and Hooley,JM (2007) *Abnormal Psychology*, 13th ed. Boston: Pearson Education.

Clinton,C, Pereira,S and Mullins,S (2001) Training Needs of Psychiatric Intensive Care Staff. *Nursing Standards* 15: 33–6.

CMO's update (1996) London Department of Health. In Snowden,P Regional Secure Units and Forensic Services. In Bluglass,R and Bowden,P (eds.), *Principles and Practice of Forensic Psychiatry*. London: Churchill Livingstone (1990) p. 1379.

Coid,JW (1991a) A Survey of Patients from Five Health Districts Receiving Special Care in the Private Sector. *Psychiatric Bulletin* 15: 257–62.

Coid,JW (1991b) Difficult to Place Patients. The Game of Pass the Parcel Must Stop. *British Medical Journal* **32**: 603–4.

Committee on Madhouses (1815) Report from the Committee on Madhouses in England, 1815 AD. www.bible .ca/psychiatry/report-from-the-committee-on-madhouses-in-england-1815ad.htm.

Committee on Mentally Abnormal Offenders (1975) *Report of the Committee on Mentally Abnormal Offenders*. London: HMSO.

Connolly,J (1856) *Treatment of the Insane without Mechanical Restraints*. London: Smith Elder & Co.

Corrigan,PW (2002) Empowerment and Serious Mental Illness: Treatment Partnerships and Community Opportunities. *Psychiatric Quarterly* **73** (3) 217–28.

Crain,PM and Jordan,EG (1979) The Psychiatric Intensive Care Unit – An In-hospital Treatment of Violent Adult Patients. *Bulletin of the American Academy of Psychiatry and the Law* **11** (2) 190–8.

Cripps,J, Duffield,G and James,D (1995) Bridging the Gap in Secure Provision: Evaluation of a New Local Combined Locked Forensic/Intensive Care Unit. *Journal of Forensic Psychiatry* **6**: 77–91.

Department of Health (2002) *Mental Health Policy Implementation Guide: Adult Acute Inpatient Care Provision*. London: HMSO.

Department of Health (2012a) *Psychiatric Intensive Care: Good Practice Commissioning Guide, consultation draft.* London: Department of Health

Department of Health (2012b) *Low Secure Services: Good Practice Commissioning Guide, Consultation Draft.* London: Department of Health

Department of Health (2015) *Mental Health Act 1983: Code of Practice.* London: Department of Health.

Department of Health and Social Services (1974) *Revised Report for the Working Party on Security in NHS Psychiatric Hospitals (Glancy Report).* London: DHSS.

Dix,R (1995) A Nurse-Led Psychiatric Intensive Care Unit. *Psychiatric Bulletin* **19**: 258–87.

Dix,R (1996) *An Investigation into Patients Presenting a Challenge to Gloucestershire's Mental Health Care Services.* Gloucester: Gloucestershire Health Authority.

Dix,R (2019) PICUs Problems and Progress: What Matters? *Journal of Psychiatric Intensive Care* **15** (2) 55–6.

Dix,R and Woods,L (2023) *The Referral and Admission of Prisoners to General Adult Psychiatric Intensive Care Units (PICU): Quality and Good Practice Guidance.* Glasgow: NAPICU Publishing.

Dye,S, Johnston,A and Pereira,S (2005) The National Psychiatric Intensive Care Governance Network 2004–2005. *Journal of Psychiatric Intensive Care* **1** (2) 97–104.

Farreras,IG (2021) History of Mental Illness. In Biswas-Diener,R and Diener,E (eds.), *Noba Textbook Series: Psychology.* Champaign, IL: DEF Publishers.

Faulk,M (1995) *Basic Forensic Psychiatry*, 2nd ed. Oxford: Blackwell.

Ford,I and Whiffin,M (1991) The Role of the Psychiatric ICU. *Nursing Times* **87** (51) 47–9.

Goldney,R, Bowes J, Spence,N, Czechowicz,A, and Hurley,R (1985) The Psychiatric Intensive Care Unit. *British Journal of Psychiatry* **146**: 50–4.

Haw,C and Yorston,G (2004) Thomas Prichard and the Non-restraint Movement at the Northampton Asylum. *Psychiatric Bulletin* **28** (4) 140–2.

James,AJ, Smith J, Hoogkamer,R, Laing,J and Donovan,M (1996) Minimum and Medium Security: The Interface: Use of Section 17 Trial Leave. *Psychiatric Bulletin* **20**: 201–4.

Jones,K (1993) *Asylums and After. A Revised History of the Mental Health Services: From the Early 18th Century to the 1900s.* London: Athlone Press.

McKenna,J (1996) In-Patient Characteristics in a Regional Secure Unit. *Psychiatric Bulletin* **20**: 264–68.

Mental Health Act (1983) HM Government. www.legisla tion.gov.uk/ukpga/1983/20/contents.

Mental Health Act Commission. 1995 Sixth Biennial Report. London: HMSO.

Meyer,SS (2015) *Clarendon Plato Series: Plato: Laws 1 and 2.* Oxford: Oxford University Press.

Mitchell,GD (1992) A Survey of Psychiatric Intensive Care Units in Scotland. *Health Bulletin* **50** (3) 228–32.

Mounsey,N (1979) Psychiatric Intensive Care. *Nursing Times* **75**: 1811–13.

Musisi,S, Wasylenski,DA and Rapp,MS (1989) A Psychiatric Intensive Care Unit in a Psychiatric Hospital. *Canadian Journal of Psychiatry* **34**: 200–4.

National Association of Psychiatric Intensive Care and Low Secure Care Units (NAPICU) (2009) AIMS PICU Accreditation programme. https://napicu.org.uk/publica tions/improve-your-unit/.

National Association of Psychiatric Intensive Care and Low Secure Care (2014) *National Minimum Standards for Psychiatric Intensive Care in General Adult Services.* Glasgow: NAPICU. https://napicu.org.uk/wp-content/uplo ads/2014/12/NMS-2014-final.pdf.

National Association of Psychiatric Intensive Care and Low Secure Units (NAPICU) (2015) *National Minimum Standards for Psychiatric Intensive Care for Young People.* Glasgow: NAPICU. https://napicu.org.uk/wp-content/uplo ads/2014/08/CAMHS_PICU_NMS_final_Aug_2015_cx. pdf.

National Association of Psychiatric Intensive Care and Low Secure Units (NAPICU) (2016) *Guidance for Commissioners* of Psychiatric Intensive Care Units (PICU). Glasgow: NAPICU. https://napicu.org.uk/wp-content/uploads/2016/04/Commissioning_Guidance_Apr16.pdf.

National Association of Psychiatric Intensive Care and Low Secure Units (NAPICU) (2016) Position Statement on the Monitoring, Regulation and Recording of the Extra Care Area, Seclusion and Long-term Segregation Use in the Context of the Mental Health Act Code of Practice (2015). Glasgow: NAPICU. https://napicu.org.uk/wp-content/uploads/2016/10/NAPICU-Seclusion-Position-Statement.pdf.

National Association of Psychiatric Intensive Care and Low Secure Units (NAPICU) (2017) Design Guidance for Psychiatric Intensive Care. Glasgow: NAPICU. https://napicu.org.uk/wp-content/uploads/2017/05/Design-Guidance-for-Psychiatric-Intensive-Care-Units-2017.pdf.

National Association of Psychiatric Intensive Care and Low Secure Units (NAPICU) (2020) Managing Acute Disturbance in the Context of COVID-19. Glasgow: NAPICU. https://napicu.org.uk/acute-disturbance-covid-19/, https://napicu.org.uk/wp-content/uploads/2020/12/NAPICU-Guidance_rev5_15_Dec.pdf.

National Association of Psychiatric Intensive Care and Low Secure Units (NAPICU) (2020) Occupational Therapists in PICU Network. https://napicu.org.uk/specialist-networks/ot-network/.

National Association of Psychiatric Intensive Care and Low Secure Units (NAPICU) (2023) Acute, Intensive and Emergency Psychiatry Course. https://napicu.org.uk/acute-intensive-and-emergency-psychiatric-care-short-course/.

National Institute for Health and Care Excellence (NICE) (2015) NG10 Violence and Aggression: Short-term Management in Mental Health, Health and Community Settings. www.nice.org.uk/guidance/ng10.

Patel,MX, Sethi,FN, Barnes,TR, Dix,R, Dratcu,L, Fox,B, et al. (2018) Joint BAP NAPICU Evidence-based Consensus Guidelines for the Clinical Management of Acute Disturbance: De-escalation and Rapid Tranquillisation. Journal of Psychopharmacology 32 (6) 601–40.

Pereira,S, Beer,MD, and Paton,C (1999) Good Practice Issues in Psychiatric Intensive Care Settings. Findings from a National Survey. Psychiatric Bulletin 23: 397–400.

Pereira,S and Clinton,C (2002) Mental Health Policy Implementation Guide: National Minimum Standards for General Adult Services in Psychiatric Intensive Care Units (PICU) and Low Secure Environments. London: Department of Health.

Pereira,S, Sarsam,M, Bhui,K and Paton,C (2005) The London Survey of Psychiatric Intensive Care Units: Psychiatric Intensive Care; Patient Characteristics and Pathways for Admission and Discharge. Journal of Psychiatric Intensive Care 1 (1) 17–24.

Pereira,S, Sarsam,M, Bhui,K and Paton,C (2005) The London Survey of Psychiatric Intensive Care Units: Service Provision and Operational Characteristics of National Health Service Units. Journal of Psychiatric Intensive Care 1 (1) 7–15.

Pereira,SM, Dawson,P and Sarsam,M (2006a) The National Survey of PICU and Low Secure Services: 2 Unit Characteristics. Journal of Psychiatric Intensive Care 2: 13–19.

Pereira,SM, Dawson,P and Sarsam,M (2006b) The National Survey of PICU and Low Secure Services: 1 Patient Characteristics. Journal of Psychiatric Intensive Care 2: 7–12.

Pereira,SM, Chaudhry,K, Pietromartire,S, Dale,C, Halliwell, J and Dix,R (2006c) Design in Psychiatric Intensive Care Units: Problems and Issues. Journal of Psychiatric Intensive Care 2: 70–6.

Pereira,SM, Walker,LM, Dye,S and Alhaj,H (2021) National Survey of Psychiatric Intensive Care, Low Secure and Locked Rehabilitation Services: NHS Patient Characteristics. Journal of Psychiatric Intensive Care 17 (2) 79–88.

Porter,R (2002) Madness: A Brief History. Oxford: Oxford University Press.

Rachlin,S (1973) On the Need for a Closed Ward in an Open Hospital: The Psychiatric Intensive-Care Unit. Hospital and Community Psychiatry 24: 829–33.

Reed,JL (1992) Review of Health and Social Services for Mentally Disordered Offenders and other Requiring Similar Services. Final Summary Report. London: Department of Health.

Smith,J, Parker,J and Donovan,M (1990) Is the Role of Regional Secure Units Changing? Psychiatric Bulletin 14: 713–14.

Snowden,P (1990) Regional Secure Units and Forensic Service in England and Wales. In Bluglass R, and Bowden,P (eds.), Principles and Practice of Forensic Psychiatry. pp. 1375–86. London: Churchill Livingstone.

Sugarman,P (2002) Home Office Statistical Bulletin 22/01: Statistics of MDOs 2000. Journal of Forensic Psychiatry & Psychology 13: 385–90.

Turner,T (1996) Commentary on 'Guidelines for the Management of Acutely Disturbed Patients'. Advances in Psychiatric Treatment 2: 200–1.

Warneke,L (1986) A Psychiatric Intensive Care Unit in a General Hospital Setting. Canadian Journal of Psychiatry 31: 834–7.

Woods,L, Craster,L and Forrester,A (2020) Mental Health Act Transfer from Prison to Psychiatric Hospital over a Six-Year Period in a Region of England. Journal of Criminal Psychology 10 (3) 219–31.

Zigmond,A (1995) Special Care Wards: Are They Special? Psychiatric Bulletin 19: 310–12.

Psychiatric Intensive Care in Mental Health Secure Units

Harvey Gordon

Introduction

Two chapters in the first and second editions of this book outlined the provision of intensive or special care units in forensic psychiatry (Anderson, 2001, 2008; Gordon, 2001, 2008). In the 13 years since the second edition, neither general nor forensic psychiatry, nor their interface, has stood still. The main issues in forensic psychiatry since 2008 include the growth of medium secure units (MSUs) to become the hub of the sub-speciality, and the reduction in high-security beds (Gunn and Taylor, 2014). The high secure hospitals provide for those patients when at high risk and are the protective shield around the entire psychiatric system (Gordon, 2008). The ongoing development of the low secure sector provides a vital resource for many patients in short-term crisis and for many with chronic mental illness (Beer, 2008; Longdon et al., 2018; Pereira et al., 2021). Forensic psychiatric services have also continued to develop in the community (Humber et al., 2011; Khosla et al., 2014). There is also an ongoing contribution to forensic services by the charitable and independent sector (Nimmagadda et al., 2008; Dickens et al., 2010).

Major changes have also occurred with the UK National Health Service (NHS) having taken full responsibility for mental health services in prisons, where many of those imprisoned suffer from some form of mental disorder(s) (Fazel and Seewald, 2012; Harty et al., 2012). Prisons are not covered by the Mental Health Act but offer an opportunity for the assessment and treatment of prisoners. A joint prison and hospital endeavour called the Dangerous and Severe Personality Disorder (DSPD) programme that was set up in 2008 has now ended (Duggan, 2011); however, it has been replaced by new services for those with personality disorder, which is no longer

viewed as a diagnosis of exclusion (Saradjian et al., 2013; Skett et al., 2017). The treatment of patients with personality disorder is appropriate (Tyrer, 2020), but health professionals know how hard it often is (Chandler et al., 2017) and have to brace themselves for lack of success in many cases with higher levels of recidivism (Conlin and Braham, 2018). Embedded into psychiatric care in these years has also been diversion of mentally disordered offenders to hospital from the community (Kane et al., 2020) and from prison (Sharpe et al., 2016).

A change of some note in general and forensic psychiatry has also been the reversion to single-sex wards, though there are exceptions (Nadkarni et al., 2012). The integration of wards began in the 1960s (Taylor and Swan, 1999), but the safety especially of female patients was a concern (Lawn and McDonald, 2009). The more recent pressing social issue of how best to respond to gender identity adds further complexity when in prison (Marlow et al., 2015; Nulty et al., 2019) or secure hospital (Hill et al., 2020). If gender transition has been completed, patients in secure hospitals have generally been placed on wards for patients of the gender to which the patient has transitioned (Gordon, 2012). But where a self-declaration has yet to be accompanied by biological alteration, placement has generally been in wards for patients of the patient's gender at birth.

Aggression and violence may occur on any psychiatric ward but are known to be extensive in secure units. A study of violent incidents in an NHS MSU from 1980 to 1996 found 2,180 violent incidents (Rutter et al., 2004). Another study in a private hospital of medium and low secure units over a 15-month period in 2008–9 noted 3,133 incidents of violence to others or self (Dickens et al., 2013). A study at Rampton high secure hospital found

5,658 violent incidents over a 16-month period in 2007–8 (Uppal and McMurran, 2009). If such violence occurred in the community, it might well, at least initially, be a matter for the police. Should psychiatric inpatients be referred to the police when they are assaultive? Should psychiatric patients have a free pass when their behaviour in any other circumstances may constitute a criminal offence? Or is such behaviour the intrinsic business of psychiatry, the violence a product of the mental disorder? If all such incidents required police intervention, why not incorporate a police station in the hospital? A reminder to patients that they are also citizens and have rights but also responsibilities. In practice, psychiatry is generally expected to pursue its task without recourse to the police, but there are exceptions. In the nineteenth century, homicides in local lunatic asylums were recorded (Gordon, 2012; Ion et al., 2014). They are now much rarer but occur from time to time (Blom-Cooper et al., 1995). Indeed, the police must also be called for any serious violent or sexual assault. Whether the police and the Crown Prosecution Service then prosecute depends on whether there is enough evidence for a realistic prospect of conviction and whether it is in the public interest (Janicki, 2009; Young et al., 2009; Clark et al., 2012; Wilson et al., 2012; Gupta et al., 2018). When offences are committed by the mentally disordered their criminal responsibility may be absent if severely psychotic or severely learning disabled, but in most cases it is diminished or reduced. And there is a victim and the victim's family and the effects on the community to consider. Prosecution of a mentally disordered offender already detained in a psychiatric hospital may result in a new order for detention, perhaps now with a restriction order imposed. Alternatively, prosecution may result in conviction and a prison sentence, especially when the patient suffers from a severe personality disorder. But personality disorder is a mental disorder, is it not?

History and Development of PICUs within Secure Mental Health Facilities

There was a time in human history when there were no psychiatric intensive or special care units; indeed, there weren't any psychiatric hospitals at all. But there were the mentally ill and sometimes they were disturbed in their behaviour and at times violent. The New

Testament may not be a scientific publication, but it tells the story of the man living in the tombs, possessed by an evil spirit so violent he needed restraint in chains from which he broke free. Secluded from his community, Jesus approached the man and commanded the evil spirit to depart. This it did, entering a herd of pigs, which then all rushed over a cliff to their deaths (Gold et al., 1995). The inclusion of this narrative is a tribute to the memory of Dominic Beer, an editor of the previous editions of this book and a devoted Christian (Beer and Pocock, 2006). Two centuries later in the second century AD the Roman emperor, Marcus Aurelius, advised that an insane man who had killed his mother should not be punished but kept under observation and in chains if necessary (Crichton, 2015). Chains continued to be used for the mad if frenzied or dangerous for many centuries and this remains the case in much of the world, though only marginally in Britain. The community resorted to restraint to keep itself safe from the mad and the mad from themselves (MacDonald, 1981).

Such mechanical restraint was used, at least initially, in the Bethlem Hospital, which opened the first criminal lunatic wing of a hospital in the world in 1816. By the time of its closure in 1864 and the opening of Broadmoor, mechanical restraint had largely fallen into disuse following the movement to abolish it in Britain and its replacement by seclusion (Scull et al., 1996; Gordon, 2012). From the outset, Broadmoor had a ward for its most refractory patients and continues to have one today, as do all the high secure hospitals, including Rampton, Ashworth and the State Hospital, Carstairs, Scotland (Larkin et al., 1988; Coldwell and Naismith, 1989; Mason and Chandley, 1995; Brook and Coorey, 1996; Thomson et al., 1997; Gordon et al., 1998).

From the mid-1970s, MSUs also noted the need to provide areas within the unit for patients posing a high risk to others or themselves. This especially applied to those patients on civil orders transferred from local psychiatric hospitals as too difficult to manage, though offender patients also required the facility (Crichton, 1995; Dolan and Lawson, 2001; Green and Robinson, 2001; Adams and Clark, 2008; Kasmi, 2010). Scotland managed without MSUs until opening its first one in November 2000 (Nelson, 2003; Gow et al., 2010), whilst Northern Ireland followed in 2005 (McLean, 2010). Scotland also took its own course, opting for a Risk Management Authority instead of a DSPD programme (Darjee and Crichton, 2002; Tuddenham and Baird, 2007) and legislation allowing appeals against levels of security (Bennett et al., 2013; Roy and Thomson, 2017). Psychopaths haven't officially been admitted to secure psychiatric hospitals in Scotland, but in practice there are such patients in the State Hospital (Thomson, 2010) and as elsewhere issues of treatability have arisen (Crichton et al., 2001). Northern Ireland also does not have psychopathic disorder in its mental health legislation (Thomson, 2010). It also is the only nation in the United Kingdom to have introduced fusion legislation regarding mental incapacity into the criminal justice system (Campbell and Rix, 2018). Many forensic psychiatrists, the current author included, are doubtful that mental capacity should determine detention and treatment of mentally disordered offenders.

The open-door policy of the 1960s, beneficial for many patients, had left psychiatric hospitals less able to manage patients manifesting challenging behaviour or absconding (Rollin, 1966). In the early 1990s, the joint Department of Health and Home Office Committee on mentally disordered offenders chaired by John Reed advised the reopening of locked wards, thereby stimulating the development of psychiatric intensive care units (PICUs) and low secure units (Cripps et al., 1995; Beer et al., 2009, Aimola et al., 2016; Johnson et al., 2019; Pereira et al., 2021).

As the 1990s progressed, it emerged that gaps and complexities of provision were present in the medium secure sector and later to an extent in low secure units as well. The Butler Committee's intention was for MSUs to have a length of stay of no more than two years (Home Office and Department of Health and Social Security (1975). However, long-stay patients could be found in local psychiatric hospitals (Mann and Cree, 1976) and had always been an aspect of high secure hospitals (Gordon, 2012). After 20 years of the operation of MSUs, they also became aware that some patients needed longer than two years (Taylor et al., 1996; Reed, 1997; Shah et al., 2011; Vollm et al., 2017; Kasmi et al., 2020).

The medium and low secure units also came to recognise that provision was required for four further types of patients: children and adolescents, learning disabled, female patients and patients with personality disorder. A fifth might be added, patients with autistic spectrum disorders, and even a sixth, elderly mentally disordered offenders.

Child and adolescent mentally disordered offenders lie on the interface between child and adolescent psychiatry and forensic psychiatry. The high-security hospitals had taken small numbers of patients younger than sixteen years and, separately, occasionally babies had been born in Broadmoor to female patients pregnant on admission (Gordon, 2012). Child and adolescent secure forensic units have progressed since the 1990s (Bailey et al., 1994; Dimond and Chiweda, 2011; Hindley et al., 2017; White et al., 2017; Hill et al., 2019; Livanou et al., 2020).

Patients with learning disability also make up a proportion of those passing through the criminal justice system (Isherwood et al., 2007; Jones and Talbot, 2010; Hassiotis et al., 2011). Rampton continues to provide high security where appropriate for patients with learning disability (Taylor and Morrissey, 2012) but is now accompanied by medium secure (Halstead et al., 2001; Yacoub et al., 2008) and low secure provision (Reed, 2004).

Wards in high secure hospitals had always been segregated by gender for patients, but the MSUs arose at a time when integration had taken place in the NHS. Integrated wards afforded more normal living conditions, but there are risks attached to mixed units, including issues of privacy, safety, sexual contact both voluntary and by coercion, sexually transmitted infections and pregnancy (Taylor and Swan, 1999). Towards the end of the 1990s, policy began to revert to single-sex wards in the NHS, such that MSUs located male and female patients separately (Women in Special Hospitals, 2000; Bartlett and Hassell, 2001; Allan and Beech, 2010; Long et al., 2015; Tully et al., 2019). Characteristics of women in secure services, as described by Sarkar and di Lustro (2011), are that they are more likely than male patients to have been on civil detention orders, to have been transferred from the NHS, to suffer from personality disorder, to have been convicted of fewer violent offences and only rarely convicted of sex offences, to have fewer previous convictions, to victimise family rather than strangers, and to manifest aggression to staff and deliberate self-harm. In addition, they are less likely than men to reoffend on discharge.

The reluctance of the MSUs to take patients with personality disorder was brought to an end by the Department of Health's insistence that personality disorder could not be a reason for exclusion (Department of Health, 2003). Units in MSUs were subsequently established (McCarthy and Duggan,

2010; Long et al., 2015; Horgan et al., 2019; Tully et al., 2019). Note should also be taken that patients with personality disorder often have comorbidity with mental illness (Blackburn et al., 2003; Milton et al., 2007). The DSPD, though disbanded, gave rise to the new initiative of an offender personality pathway (O'Laughlin, 2014; Minoudis and Kane, 2017; Skett et al., 2017; Cohen et al., 2019).

Patients with autistic spectrum disorders can be found in small numbers in secure hospitals (Scragg and Shah, 1994; Dein and Woodbury-Smith, 2010; Murphy, 2010, 2020). Recently it has been suggested that both learning disability and autistic spectrum disorders be removed from the Mental Health Act (Hollins et al., 2019). People with autism can also be found in prisons (McCarthy et al., 2019). If such patients could not be detained in secure hospitals they would have to be located somewhere else if convicted, probably prison. This does not seem preferable (Courtenay, 2020). Autistic spectrum disorders can occur without any other mental disorder, but they also show comorbidity (Ghaziuddin et al., 1998; Murphy, 2007; North et al., 2008; Pina-Camacho et al., 2016; McCarthy et al., 2019). A few specialised units for autistic spectrum disorders can be found in the private sector (Dein and Woodbury-Smith, 2010).

Elderly people with mental disorders can be found in prisons (Taylor and Parrott, 1988; Fazel et al., 2001; Purewal, 2020) and in secure hospitals (Coid et al., 2002; O'Sullivan and Chesterman, 2007; Yorston and Taylor, 2009; Lightbody et al., 2010; Girardi et al., 2018; di Lorito et al., 2019; Walker et al., 2021). In some cases, elderly forensic patients may need placement in an intensive care unit (McLeod et al., 2008).

Female patients may be more challenging than male patients in secure hospitals, but the level of risk posed by female patients is generally less than that of male patients. In 2007, Broadmoor closed its female wing, transferring those female patients who still needed high security to Rampton and the remainder to either MSUs or to a new provision known as enhanced MSUs for women (Women in Special Hospitals, 1999; Sarkar and di Lustro, 2011; Harty et al., 2012; Bartlett and Somers, 2017; Edge et al., 2017; Walker et al., 2019).

Admission and Discharge Criteria

Within secure provision, intensive or special care units provide a mechanism for patients to receive treatment in a higher-staffed environment, with less emotional arousal from fewer interactions with fellow patients and away from the pressures of mainstream wards where patients have to exercise more personal responsibility (Kasmi, 2010). The more acutely disturbed or psychiatrically distracted by inner perceptions and emotions, the less self-control and the more the need for more external control by the institution to prevent harmful behaviour. Patients admitted to these forensic units differ from those in local psychiatric hospital PICUs in that most will have criminal convictions usually for violent offences, or are civilly detained patients who have been transferred from a local psychiatric hospital because their level of violence could not be safely managed there (Kasmi, 2010). Though most incidents in forensic intensive or special care units are in the less severe category, more serious incidents may also occur especially in high security. In MSUs the average length of stay in an intensive care unit is between two and three months (Dolan and Lawson, 2001; Kasmi, 2010), whilst in high security it is four to six months, but some stays are much longer (Larkin et al., 1988; Gordon et al., 1998). The objective is to reduce the patient's level of violence and this is generally achieved, though readmissions may occur.

The interface between general and forensic psychiatry is characterised by both tension and mutual cooperation (Gunn, 1977, 2008; Snowden et al., 1999; Buchanan, 2002; Coid et al., 2007; O'Grady, 2008; Turner and Salter, 2008; Holloway, 2011; Humber et al., 2011; Gordon et al., 2014; Khosla et al., 2014). The same applies to the forensic interfaces linking high, medium and low secure units and community forensic psychiatry. In fact they apply to any interface within psychiatry, including child and adolescent to general adult (Singh et al., 2010; Paul et al., 2013; Collins and Munoz-Solomanda, 2018), general adult to old age (Hilton, 2015; Khrypunov et al., 2018) and learning disability and general adult psychiatry (Hawramy, 2020), or even between psychiatry and medicine, including old age psychiatry and geriatric medicine (Fisher and Teodorczuk, 2017; Thacker et al., 2017), and psychiatry and neurology / neuroscience (Crossley et al., 2015; David and Nicholson, 2015; Fitzgerald, 2015; Ron, 2018).

While some forensic patients may be relatively harmless, some civilly detained patients may pose a considerable risk to themselves and others, and in their past may have accrued criminal convictions. Patients admitted to forensic intensive or special care units include a proportionately higher number on civil sections (Coid et al., 2001; Gordon, 2008; Kasmi, 2010; Galappathie et al., 2017). In the nineteenth century, one aspect of preventive psychiatry was the need to prevent 'lunatics' becoming 'criminal lunatics' (Nicolson, 1878). In modern practice, most forensic psychiatric patients have previously been managed in general psychiatric services and most will be transferred back there (Gordon, 2008).

Within the forensic sector, admission into the intensive or special care unit is best undertaken by staff consensus rather than by formal assessment carrying the potential for acceptance or rejection. The corollary of this is that transfer from intensive or special care is also a matter for dialogue. The main criteria are the level and severity of the patient's harm to others and/or to their self. In some cases, transfer out may need to be to a different mainstream ward to avoid retraumatisation of any patient or staff who may have been injured by the patient's behaviour.

It should be noted that violence to others and self requires close supervision. The direction of hostility may vary from external to internal or even both may be present concurrently (Gordon, 2002; Pluck and Brooker, 2014; Gunn, 2019).

Interventions Used in Forensic Intensive or Special Care Wards

Forensic units, including their intensive or special care wards, have the objective of achieving therapeutic improvement of patients whilst rendering patients, staff and visitors safe. Methods to achieve this include ongoing treatment in the context of the relational security of the milieu provided by the multidisciplinary team (Chester et al., 2017), procedural security provided by the policies of the unit (Gunn and Taylor, 2014) and physical security to contain patients in the therapeutic space (Kennedy, 2002; Crichton, 2009). All need to be undertaken in a framework consistent with the human rights of patients (Curtice and Exworthy, 2010) but also of those who may be affected by their behaviour (Gordon, 2012).

Most patients in secure units at all levels of security suffer from schizophrenia, personality disorder or substance abuse with frequent comorbidity (Taylor et al., 1998; Blackburn et al., 2003; Milton et al., 2007; Kasmi, 2010). Some patients may also have affective disorders (Busch, 2009; Oakley et al., 2009) or paraphilias (Saleem et al., 2001; Darjee and Russell,

2012; Winder, 2014; Khan et al., 2017; Lewis et al., 2017; Rix, 2017; Yakeley and Wood, 2017).

The main biological method of treatment is by medication, though electroconvulsive therapy (ECT) is also used where indicated (Kristensen et al., 2012; Lally et al., 2016). For treatment-resistant cases of psychosis, clozapine has a clear edge over other options (Swinton and McNamee, 2003; Beer et al., 2007) and has also been used for some cases of personality disorder (Swinton, 2001; White et al., 2017). Instances of and debate about the administration of clozapine without the patient's consent by nasogastric tube are also recorded (Barnes, 1999; Pereira et al., 1999; Silva et al., 2017). This author also knows of a patient in a high-security hospital where ECT was used without the patient's consent followed by his taking clozapine with his consent, which he had earlier refused, all authorised by a second-opinion doctor from the Mental Health Act Commission. Possibly, the recent availability of intramuscular clozapine may alleviate these types of situations (Henry et al., 2020).

All forms of psychotherapy are available in secure hospitals, but their use in intensive or special care units may depend on the level of the patient's behavioural disturbance. These include psychodynamic psychotherapy (Yakeley, 2018; Gibson et al., 2019), cognitive behavioural therapy (Howells, 2010) and cognitive analytic therapy (Withers, 2008). Allied therapies include arts therapy (Klugman, 1999), drama therapy (Cox, 1992) and music therapy (Mezey et al., 2015). Music especially has been known for many centuries to soothe the troubled mind (Downie, 2012; Wilkinson, 2019).

Delivering all treatment whether biological or psychological involves various members of the multidisciplinary team, including nursing (Mason et al., 2008, Allen and Beech, 2010; Jordan, 2011), clinical psychology (Gudjonsson and Young, 2007; Crichton and Towl, 2015), occupational therapy (Cordingley and Ryan, 2009; Connell, 2016), education (Taylor and Healy, 2001) and social work (Buckle, 2005). Liaison with family and friends is undertaken and may include family therapy where appropriate, though this may be difficult as frequently the victim of the index offence is a family member (Geelan and Nickford, 1999; Davies et al., 2014). Full recognition needs to be afforded to the religious and spiritual affiliations of patients as an important part of their identity (Poole, 2020).

Forensic psychiatry is a sub-speciality of psychiatry, which in turn is a branch of medicine. General and forensic psychiatric patients have higher rates of morbidity and mortality as a result of physical ill-health factors including cardiovascular disease, obesity and type 2 diabetes (Cormac et al., 2005; Haw and Rowell, 2011; Haw and Stubbs, 2011; Long et al., 2016; Puzzo et al., 2017). The decision to ban smoking in psychiatric hospitals including secure hospitals has removed one risk factor for physical ill health (Cormac et al., 2010; Shetty et al., 2010). The architectural environment of secure units can facilitate more healthy lifestyles and well-being by availability of secure outside areas for fresh air and exercise and gym facilities within the unit.

An essential but sometimes insufficiently emphasised aspect of patients' health also includes attention to enabling of adequate and restful sleep. Psychological function is altered but does not stop during sleep (Wilson and Argyropoulis, 2012; Selsick and O'Regan, 2018; Van Veen et al., 2020). Night staff need to observe for any insomnia or any sleep disorder that may be present. Sleep disorders involving violent or sexually assaultive behaviour are known (Leschziner, 2019) but are not so far recorded in secure hospitals, presumably as a result of the patient sleeping alone and subject to night observations.

In secure units, threatened or actual violence is preferably prevented by conflict resolution (Bowers, 2014) or de-escalated if possible (Goodman et al., 2020). Where they are not possible or have not succeeded, methods of restraint include geographical, biological or physical means. Methods of restraint vary across the world. It is far from clear that the ethics of any one method is any better than that of another. Much is determined by tradition.

- Geographical restraint

  - segregation is isolation from fellow patients, supervised by staff. It had been used in high security but was first recorded as being used in medium security in 1993 in the form of an Extra Care Area (ECA) (Kinsella et al., 1993) and is generally not used for highly disturbed patients (Long et al., 2010). Segregation can be long term and is defined in the Code of Practice (Department of Health, 2015) as a situation where in order to reduce a sustained risk of harm posed by the patient to others, which is a constant feature of their presentation, a multidisciplinary review and a representative

from the responsible commissioning authority determines that a patient should not be allowed to mix freely with other patients on the ward or unit on a long-term basis.

  - seclusion is the placement of a patient in a space from which they cannot wilfully exit. It is defined in the Code of Practice (Department of Health, 2015) as supervised confinement and isolation of a patient away from other patients in an area from which the patient is prevented from leaving, where it is of immediate necessity for the purpose of containment of severe behavioural disturbance which is likely to cause harm to others. The door of a seclusion room is usually locked, but in the nineteenth century a male nurse of large stature may simply have blocked egress. Seclusion may often result in the calming of a patient by reducing arousal from interpersonal interaction and afford time for the patient to reflect on their behaviour if rational enough to do so. There are some risks associated with seclusion, including its perception by some patients that it is punitive (Keski-Valkama et al., 2010), that it may breach human rights (McSherry, 2017), and that death may occur (Prins et al., 1993). There is also the view that seclusion could be abolished without increasing levels of behavioural disturbance (Department of Health, 1992), with some calling for not only the abolition of seclusion but also the closure of Ashworth Hospital.

Seclusion, however, is not so easy to dispense with (Gaskin et al., 2007; Cohen et al., 2008; Ching et al., 2010; Maguire et al., 2011; Newton-Howes, 2013). Some studies have shown that seclusion can be reduced without any concomitant increase in aggressive incidents, but to do so requires attention to unit architecture, access to secure outside areas, reduced overcrowding where needed, more staff resources and training and managerial emphasis on such a policy (Quraschi et al., 2010; Newton-Howes, 2013; van der Scharf et al., 2013; Long et al., 2015). As stated by one of the editors of this book, seclusion and restraint are probably the longest running debate in psychiatry (Dix, 2014).

- Two further aspects of seclusion

  - Seclusion programmes – these have been used only in high secure hospitals. They have been applied to a small number of patients in intensive or special care units where the level of behavioural disturbance is repetitive, severe and otherwise irremediable. Such patients do not require a fresh initiation for each seclusion but can be allowed to mix with others when safe to do so and returned to seclusion when needed. It was argued that such seclusion programmes were contrary to the Code of Practice of the Mental Health Act Commission. However, the case of Munjaz was heard in 2005 in the House of Lords, which found that the Code of Practice was guidance not law and account had to be taken of the actual circumstances on the ground (Seligman and Feery; Curtice, 2009).

- Routine night-time seclusion – this only applies in high secure hospitals and had been the usual practice until the early 1990s. It was reintroduced in 2003 for DSPD and in 2011 for high security as a whole (Silva and Shepherd, 2019). It was challenged on grounds that seclusion should only be used where clinically appropriate (Szmukler, 2019) but defended on the basis that it produced no adverse effects and that it was a sensible use of nursing resources (Chu et al., 2015; Thomson, 2019). Perhaps nurses could read patients bedtime stories!

- Transfer to a more secure hospital – this is also a geographical method of managing the containment of an uncontrollable patient (Anderson, 2008). It becomes impossible or almost so at the buffer point of the intensive or special care unit of a high-security hospital. The only exception is a homicide or near homicide by a patient with personality disorder. Even then it is debatable whether it is appropriate to reverse divert a hitherto psychiatric patient to a prison, but nonetheless it has been undertaken in the past (Gordon et al., 1997). A rare example would be an incident in 1977 in the special care unit at Broadmoor when two patients killed a third patient in a context of homosexual interaction. Both perpetrator patients were charged with murder, remanded in prison custody, subsequently convicted of murder and sentenced to life imprisonment. One of them later killed again in prison (Gordon et al., 1997). In cases of psychopaths detained in hospital who remain dangerous but untreatable, Scotland amended its law in 1999 to prevent discharge of such patients on

grounds of public safety (Darjee and Crichton, 2003). Reverse diversion is also in effect when a sentenced prisoner is transferred back to prison from a secure hospital when stable, though there is a higher risk of future reoffending on release from prison (Doyle et al., 2014; Igoumenou, 2019).

- Biological restraint – most patients in secure psychiatric hospitals will be on some form of medication, as comorbidity is frequent in this population (Vollm et al., 2012). During a behavioural crisis, intramuscular Haldol or a benzodiazepine is commonly used (Gunn and Taylor, 2014). However, rapid tranquillisation (Joint BAP NAPICU, 2018) is used less in secure hospitals because patients tend to become calmer in seclusion, especially when persuaded to take oral medication. All medications have side effects, including, albeit uncommonly, sudden death, especially when arousal levels are high (Farnham and Kennedy, 1997; Abdelmawla and Mitchell, 2006).

- Physical restraint

  - manual restraint – the therapeutic relationship between patients and nursing staff can be affected by manual restraint (Knowles et al., 2015). Manual restraint is not without risks (Hollins and Stubbs, 2011).
  Some patients may perceive manual restraint as punitive and in others it may evoke flashbacks of past trauma. Some patients have even reported that they provoked restraint in order to feel more contained (Sequeira and Halstead, 2002). Deaths in physical restraint have been reported in police and prison custody and psychiatric hospitals (Parkes, 2002). In 2004, a patient died in an MSU in manual restraint, possibly due to positional asphyxia (Blofeld et al., 2004). Staff may also be injured whilst restraining (Stubbs, 2008).

Britain's abolition of mechanical restraint in the nineteenth century (Conolly, 1856) was not followed by Europe or the United States. It also removed a means of protecting a patient from repeated self-harm, such as trichotillomania in the learning disabled or head banging. In practice, head guards may need to be used and so may be forms of protective clothing to prevent shredding of clothing to be used for self-harm.

In the 1990s, sporadic instances of the use of mechanical restraint were noted in high-security hospitals (Mason and Chandley, 1995; Gordon et al., 1999). Such equipment can either fix the patient to a bed or be ambulatory, enabling some movement. It prevents violence to others or self, with the exceptions of biting, spitting or head banging. The occasional use of mechanical restraint in high secure hospitals has continued, including in the State Hospital, Carstairs, Scotland (Walker and Tulloch, 2020).

- other mechanical restraint – the use of handcuffs for patients in high secure hospitals transferred to general medical hospitals has also attracted attention (Curtice and Sandford, 2010).

There is also one report of a patient in a low secure unit being immobilised by a taser by police (Little and Burt, 2013).

It is unclear whether GPS tracking can be regarded as a form of coercion. It enables psychological restraint at a distance and has been used in some MSUs (Murphy et al., 2017) and affords clinicians more confidence to agree to a patient's leave (Tully et al., 2014, 2016). It has also been used in old age psychiatry to keep track of patients with dementia who may wander off (Miskelli, 2004).

Evidence and Data

Levels of incidents of aggressive behaviour towards others and self are high in all grades of security, including low (Muthukumaraswamy et al., 2008), medium (Kasmi, 2010) and high (Uppal and McMurran, 2009) secure units, forensic adolescent units (Hill et al., 2019) and forensic units housing learning disabled patients (Dickens et al., 2013). Though most incidents are by male patients, female patients are involved in proportionately higher numbers (Muthukumaraswamy et al., 2008). Patients on civil sections account for proportionately higher numbers of incidents than those on forensic sections (Coid et al., 2001). Incidents of deliberate self-harm occur more frequently in female patients than in male patients (Newton-Howes, 2013). A small number of patients account for a high number of incidents (Dolan and Lawson, 2001). Levels of violence are high on secure intensive or special care units (Green and Robinson, 2001; McCulloch et al., 2020). Lengths of stay in intensive or special care units are about two and a half months in medium security (Dolan and Lawson, 2001; Kasmi, 2010) and four to six months in

high security (Gordon, 1998), though there are shorter and longer outliers; a few are much longer and some require readmission. One patient known to the author whose placement in the special care unit in high security lasted about seven years before transfer to a mainstream ward stated he could only think of killing himself or those around him at the peak of his psychotic state. He ascribed his still being alive to the restrictions imposed on him.

Standards and Policy Framework

Mental health provision, especially when undertaken on an involuntary basis, is subject to human rights principles emanating variously from the United Nations, European Convention on Human Rights or the 1998 Human Rights Act. The main aspects affecting forensic psychiatry include the right to life, prohibition of torture and inhumane or degrading treatment, right to liberty and security, right to a fair trial, right to respect for private and family life, right to freedom of thought, conscience and religion, right to marry and right of freedom from discrimination (Puri et al., 2005; Curtice and Exworthy, 2010; Kelly, 2016). In each case, these principles require professional and sometimes legal judgement.

A range of relevant guidelines affecting secure hospitals including psychiatric intensive or special care units have been issued (Royal College of Psychiatrists, 2013, 2018; Department of Health, 2014, 2015; NAPICU, 2014, 2016; NICE, 2015; Patel et al., 2018). The Care Quality Commission emphasises the need to avoid unnecessary or disproportionate restraint and inappropriate restriction of liberty. Services are judged on parameters of safety, efficacy, caring, responsiveness to needs and capability of professional and managerial leadership (Radar Healthcare, 2021).

COVID-19 and Its Effect on Forensic Psychiatry

Infectious diseases have long been known to have profound effects on society, the criminal justice system and forensic psychiatric care. The plague in 1348 contributed to the Peasants' Revolt of 1381 (Ashton, 2020). In 1750, typhus in Newgate Prison led to the deaths of lawyers, judges and even the Lord Mayor of London (Beattie, 1986). In 1890, an outbreak of flu emanating from Russia affected patients and staff in Broadmoor (Gordon, 2012). The so-called Spanish flu of 1919, which didn't actually come from Spain, is said to have resulted in the deaths of many people in prisons (Finney et al., 2014). In the early phase of the COVID-19 pandemic, an outbreak occurred in a prison in the Chinese province of Hubei (Liebrenz et al., 2020). As there is potential for rapid spread of COVID-19 in prisons, early vaccination when available is appropriate (Edge et al., 2021), but that would advantage prisoners over people of similar age in the community.

Psychiatry and infectious disease are both conditions affecting public health for which legislation enables detention if appropriate (Dawson and Verweij, 2007; Bhugra et al., 2018; Duggan, 2019). COVID-19 and lockdown led to delays of criminal trials, suspension of jury trials, longer stays on remand, suspension of prison visits, restriction of occupational prison activities and other effects of staff shortages (Hewson et al., 2020). Cases of COVID-19 have also been reported in some forensic psychiatric units (Simpson et al., 2020; Carthy and Sen Gupta, 2021; Thomson, 2021), and a format for assessing forensic psychiatric patients at risk of becoming COVID-19 positive has been identified on the basis of underlying health conditions such as hypertension, obesity and diabetes (Basrak et al., 2021). The use of telepsychiatry, already available in forensic psychiatry (Khalifa et al., 2008), expanded during the COVID-19 pandemic to interview prisoners and patients, with all its advantages and disadvantages (Sales et al., 2018; Gunn et al., 2020; Smith et al., 2020). Guidelines for the management of COVID-19 in secure institutions have been issued (Royal College of Psychiatrists, 2021), but it is acknowledged that some patients may find it hard to follow advice. The long-term effects of COVID-19 are also yet to be clarified (Ashton, 2020; British Medical Journal, 2020; Hotopf et al., 2020). Neurological symptoms have been noted in the short term (Mao et al., 2020; McLoughlin et al., 2020). The 1919 pandemic gave rise to encephalitis and parkinsonism in some patients (Ashton, 2020) and a few cases were linked to patients admitted to Broadmoor (Gordon, 2012).

Some concern has been expressed during the COVID-19 pandemic of a possible increase in domestic violence (Anurudran et al., 2020; Chandon et al., 2020). Some have anticipated an increase in suicide and self-harm (Lennon, 2020; Sher, 2020). However, such early predictions are not necessarily accurate (Ashton, 2021; Hewson et al., 2021) and in prisons reduced social contact may limit interpersonal stress and suicidal ideation and acts (Hewson et al., 2020). If COVID-19 results in exacerbation of poverty and social disadvantage, these will also contribute to worsening mental health and criminality (Knifton and Inglis, 2020). Much has been learned regarding the management of COVID-19 in prisoners and forensic psychiatric patients, but each new pandemic has its own characteristics and course.

Conclusion

Intensive or special care is an ongoing aspect of general and forensic psychiatry, as it is in general medicine. When mental disorder reduces or negates sound judgement and limits self-control, patients may need close observation and treatment in a more secure location. Subject to appropriate safeguards, secure units enable patients to return to the less constrained conditions in the mainstream hospital and later to the community. This author still remembers the patient who said that the tight security he was under for some years probably saved his own life and that of others.

References

Abdelmawla,N and Mitchell,AJ (2006) Sudden Cardiac Death and Antipsychotics. Part 1. Risk Factors and Mechanisms, and Part 2. Monitoring and Prevention. *Advances in Psychiatric Treatment* **12**: 35–44 and 12: 100–9.

Adams,J and Clark,T (2008) Hot Beds of Forensic Psychiatry: Psychiatric Intensive Care Units within Medium Security. *Journal of Psychiatric Intensive Care* **4** (1–2) 59–63.

Aimola,L, Jasim,S, Tripathi,N, Holder,S, Quirk,M and Crawford,MJ (2016) Quality of low Secure Services in the UK: Development and Use of the Quality of Environment in Low Secure Services (QELS) Checklist. *Journal of Forensic Psychiatry and Psychology* **27** (4) 504–16.

Allen,S and Beech,A (2010) Exploring Factors that Influence Nurses: Judgements of Violence Risk in a Female Forensic Population. *British Journal of Forensic Practice* **12** (1) 4–14.

Anderson,J (2001) The Interface with Forensic Services. In Beer,MD, Pereira,SM and Paton,C (eds.), *Psychiatric Intensive Care.* pp. 239–52. London: Greenwich Medical Media Ltd.

Anderson,J (2008) The Interface with Forensic Services. In Beer,MD, Pereira,S and Paton,C (eds.), *Psychiatric Intensive Care,* 2nd ed. pp. 191–200. Cambridge: Cambridge University Press.

Anurudran,A, Yared,L, Comrie,C, Harrison,K and Burke,T (2020) Domestic Violence and COVID-19. *Gynaecology and Obstetrics* **150** (2) 255–6.

Ashton,J (2020) COVID-19 and the Summer of Blood of 1381. *Journal of Royal Society of Medicine* **113** (10) 410–11.

Ashton,J (2020) Long COVID – What Doesn't Kill You May Not Make You Stronger. *Journal of Royal Society of Medicine* **113** (11) 466–7.

Ashton,J (2021) Mental Health, the Hidden Crisis of the COVID-19 Pandemic. *Journal of Royal Society of Medicine* **114** (2) 96–7.

Bailey,SM, Thornton,L and Weaver,AB (1994) The First 100 Admissions to an Adolescent Secure Unit. *Journal of Adolescence* **17**: 207–20.

Barnes,TRE (1999) Commentary . . . The Risks of Enforcing Clozapine Therapy. *The Psychiatrist* **23**: 656–7.

Bartlett,A and Hassell,Y (2001) Do Women Need Special Secure Services? *Advances in Psychiatric Treatment* **7**: 302–9.

Bartlett,A and Somers,A (2017) Are Women Really Difficult? Challenges and Solutions in the Care of Women in Secure Services. *Journal of Forensic Psychiatry and Psychology* **28** (2) 226–41.

Basrak,N, Mulcrone,N, Sharifuddin,S, Ghumman,Z, Bechan,N, Mohammed,E, et al. (2021) COVID-19 in Forensic Psychiatry Settings: The Unique Vulnerability of Patients in Secure Services. Poster online at Forensic Faculty of Royal College of Psychiatrists Annual Conference 3–5 March 2021.

Beattie,JM (1986) *Crime and the Courts in England 1660–1800*. Princeton, New Jersey: Princeton University Press.

Beer,MD (2008) Psychiatric Intensive Care and Low Secure Units: Where Are We Now? *Psychiatric Bulletin* **32** (12) 441–3.

Beer,MD, Khan,AA and Ratnajothy,K (2007) The Effect of Clozapine on Adverse Incidents in a Low Secure Challenging Behaviour Unit. *Journal of Psychiatric Intensive Care* **2**: 65–70.

Beer,MD, Muthukumaraswamy,A, Khan,AA and Musabbir,MA (2009) Clinical Predictors and Patterns of Absconding in a Low Secure Challenging Behaviour Mental Health Unit. *Journal of Psychiatric Intensive Care* **5** (2) 81–7.

Beer,MD and Pocock,ND (2006) *Mad, Bad or Sad? A Christian Approach to Antisocial Behaviour and Mental Disorder*. London: Christian Medical Fellowship.

Bennett,DM, Skilling,G, Brown,K and Thomson,LDG (2013) Appeals against Detention in Conditions of Excessive Security in Scotland. *Journal of Forensic Psychiatry and Psychology* **24** (3) 386–402.

Bhugra,D, Bhui,K, Yeung,S, Wong,S and Gilman,SE (2018) *The Oxford Textbook of Public Mental Health*. Oxford: Oxford University Press.

Blackburn,R, Logan,C and Donnelly,J (2003) Personality Disorders, Psychopathy and Other Mental Disorders. Comorbidity among Patients at English and Scottish High Secure Hospitals. *Journal of Forensic Psychiatry and Psychology* **14**: 111–37.

Blofeld,J, Sallah,D, Sashidaran,S, Stone,R and Struthers,J (2004) *Independent Inquiry into the death of David Bennett*. Cambridge: Norfolk, Suffolk and Cambridgeshire Strategic Health Authority.

Blom-Cooper,L, Hally,H and Murphy,E (1995) *The Falling Shadow: One Patient's Mental Health Care 1978 – 1993*. London: Gerald Duckworth and Co Ltd.

Bowers,L (2014) Safeguards: A New Model of Conflict and Containment on Psychiatric Wards. *Journal of Psychiatry and Mental Health Nursing* **21**: 499–508.

Brook,R and Coorey,PR (1996) An Acute ICU in a Maximum Secure Hospital. *Psychiatric Bulletin* **20**: 306–11.

Buchanan,A (ed.) (2002) *Care of the Mentally Disordered Offender in the Community*. Oxford: Oxford Medical Publications.

Buckle,D (2005) Social Work in a Secure Environment: Towards Social Inclusion. *Journal of Psychiatric Intensive Care* **1** (1) 37–43.

Busch,FN (2009) Anger and Depression. *Advances in Psychiatric Treatment* **15** (4) 271–8.

Campbell,P and Rix,K (2018) Fusion Legislation and Forensic Psychiatry: The Criminal Justice Provisions of the Mental Capacity Act (Northern Ireland) 2016. *BJ Psych Advances* **24** (3) 195–203.

Chandler,RJ, Newman,A and Butler,C (2017) Burnout in Clinicians Working with Offenders with Personality Disorder. *British Journal of Forensic Practice* **19** (2) 139–50.

Chester,V, Alexander,RT and Morgan,W (2017) Measuring Relational Security in Forensic Mental Health Services. *BJ Psych Bulletin* **41** (6) 358–63.

Ching,H, Daffern,M, Martin,T and Thomas,S (2010) Reducing the Use of Seclusion in a Forensic Psychiatric Hospital: Assessing the Impact on Aggression, Therapeutic Climate and Staff Confidence. *Journal of Forensic Psychiatry and Psychology* **21** (5) 737–60.

Chu,S, McNeill,K, Wright,KM, Hague,A and Wilkins,T (2015) The Impact of a Night Confinement Policy on Patients in a UK High Secure Inpatient Mental Health Service. *British Journal of Forensic Practice* **17** (1) 21–30.

Clark,CR, McInerny,BA and Brown,I (2012) The Prosecution of Psychiatric Inpatients: Overcoming the Barriers. *Journal of Forensic Psychiatry and Psychology* **23** (3) 371–81.

Cohen,DP, Akhtar,MS, Siddiqui,A, Shelley,C, Larkin,C, Kinsella,A, et al. (2008) Aggressive Incidents on a Psychiatric Intensive Care Unit. *Psychiatric Bulletin* **32** (12) 455–8.

Cohen,R, Trebilcock,J, Weaver,T and Moran,P (2019) The Offender Personality Disorder Pathway for Women in England and Wales: A Hopeful New Development? *Criminal Behaviour and Mental Health* **29** (5–6) 257–60.

Coid,J, Fazel,S and Kahtan,N (2002) Elderly Patients Admitted to Secure Forensic Psychiatry Services. *Journal of Forensic Psychiatry* **13**: 416–27.

Coid,J, Kahtan,N, Gault,S, Cook,A and Jarman,B (2001) Medium Secure Forensic Psychiatry Services: Comparison of Seven English Health Regions. *British Journal of Psychiatry* **178**: 55–61.

Coid,JW, Hickey,N and Yang,M (2007) Comparison of Outcomes Following After-care from Forensic and General Adult Psychiatric Services. *British Journal of Psychiatry* **190**: 509–14.

Coldwell,JB and Naismith,IJ (1989) Violent Incidents on Special Care Wards in a Special Hospital Medicine. *Science and Law* **29** (2) 116–23.

Collins,A and Munoz-Solomando,A (2018) The Transition from Child and Adolescent to Adult Mental Health Services with a Focus on Diagnosis Progression. *BJ Psych Bulletin* **42** (5) 188–92.

Conlin,A and Braham,L (2018) Comparison of Outcomes of Patients with Personality Disorder to Patients with Mental Illness Following Discharge from Medium Secure Hospital: Systematic Review. *Journal of Forensic Psychiatry and Psychology* **29** (1) 124–45.

Conolly,J (1856) *The Treatment of the Insane without Mechanical Restraint*. London: Smith and Elder.

Cormac,I, Creasey,S, McNeill,A, Ferriter,M, Huckstep,B and D'Silva,K (2010) Impact of a Total Smoking Ban in a High Secure Hospital. *The Psychiatrist* **34** (10) 413–17.

Cormac,I, Ferriter,M, Benning,R and Saul,C (2005) Physical Health and Health Risk Factors in a Population of Long-Stay Psychiatric Patients. *Psychiatric Bulletin* **29**: 18–20.

Courtenay,K (2021) The Case for Removing Intellectual Disability and Autism from the Mental Health Act. *British Journal of Psychiatry* **218**: 64–5.

Cox,M (ed.) (1992) *Shakespeare Comes to Broadmoor: The Actors Are Come Hither*. London: Jessica Kingsley Publishers.

Crichton,J (1995) *Psychiatric Patient Violence: Risk and Response*. London: Gerald Duckworth and Co Ltd.

Crichton,JHM (2009) Defining High, Medium and Low Security in Forensic Mental Healthcare: The Development of the Matrix of Security in Scotland. *Journal of Forensic Psychiatry and Psychology* **20** (3) 333–53.

Crichton,JHM (2015) Could Marcus Aurelius be the Missing Link in the Insanity Defence? *British Journal of Psychiatry* **207** (4) 362.

Crichton,JHM, Darjee,R, McCall-Smith,A and Chiswick,D (2001) Mental Health (Public Safety and Appeals) (Scotland) Act 1999: Detention of Untreatable patients with Psychopathic Disorder. *Journal of Forensic Psychiatry* **12**: 647–61.

Crighton,DA and Towl,GJ (2015) *Forensic Psychology BPS Textbooks in Psychology*, 2nd edition. Chichester: Wiley.

Cripps,J, Duffield,G and James,D (1995) Bridging the Gap in a Secure Provision: Evaluation of a New Local Combined Locked Forensic/Intensive Care Unit. *Journal of Forensic Psychiatry* **6** (1) 77–91.

Crossley,NA, Scott,J, Ellison-Wright,I and Mechelli,A (2015) Neuroimaging Distinction between Neurological and Psychiatric Disorders. *British Journal of Psychiatry* **207** (5) 429–34.

Curtice,M (2009) Article 8 of the Human Rights Act 1998: Implications for Clinical Practice. *Advances in Psychiatric Treatment* **15** (1) 23–31.

Curtice,M and Sandford,J (2010) Article 3 of the Human Rights Act 1998 and the Treatment of Prisoners. *Advances in Psychiatric Treatment* **16** (2) 105–14.

Curtice,MJ and Exworthy,T (2010) FREDA: A Human Rights-Based Approach to Healthcare. *The Psychiatrist* **34** (4) 150–6.

Darjee,R and Crichton,J (2003) Personality Disorder and the Law in Scotland: A Historical Perspective. *Journal of Forensic Psychiatry and Psychology* **14**: 394–425.

Darjee,R and Crichton,JHM (2002) The MacLean Committee: Scotland's Answer to the Dangerous People with Severe Personality Disorders Proposals. *Psychiatric Bulletin* **26**: 6–8.

Darjee,R and Russell,K (2012) What Clinicians Need to Know before Assessing Risk in Sexual Offenders. *Advances in Psychiatric Treatment* **18** (6) 467–78.

David,AS and Nicholson,T (2015) Are Neurological and Psychiatric Disorders Different? *British Journal of Psychiatry* **207** (5) 373–4.

Davies,A, Mallows,L, Easton,R, Morrey,A and Wood,F (2014) A Survey of the Provision of Family Therapy in Medium Secure Units in Wales and England. *Journal of Forensic Psychiatry and Psychology* **25** (5) 520–34.

Dawson,A and Verweij,M (eds.) (2007) *Ethics, Prevention and Public Health*. Oxford: Clarendon Press

Dein,K and Woodbury-Smith,M (2010) Asperger's Syndrome and Criminal Behaviour. *Advances in Psychiatric Treatment* **16** (1) 37–43.

Department of Health (1992) *Report of the Committee of Inquiry into Complaints about Ashworth Hospital*. London: HMSO.

Department of Health (2003) *Personality Disorder: No Longer a Diagnosis of Exclusion – Policy Implantation Guidance for the Development of Services for People with Personality Disorder*. London: Department of Health.

Department of Health (2014) *Positive and Proactive Care: Reducing the Need for Restrictive Interventions*. London: Department of Health.

Department of Health (2015) *The Mental Health Act 1983: Code of Practice 2015*. London: Department of Health.

Department of Health and Home Office (1992) *Report into Mentally Disordered Offenders and Others who Require Similar Services (Reed Report)*. London: HMSO.

Dickens,G, Picchioni,M and Long,C (2013) Aggression in Specialist Secure and Forensic Inpatient Mental Health Care: Incidence across Care Pathways. *Journal of Forensic Practice* 15 (3) 206–17.

Dickens,G, Sugarman,P, Picchioni,M and Long,C (2010) HoNOS-Secure: Tracking Risk and Recovery for Men in Secure Care. *British Journal of Forensic Practice* 12 (4) 36–46.

Dickinson,SC, Odell-Miller,H and Adlam,J (2013) *Forensic Music Therapy: A Treatment for Men and Women in Secure Hospital Settings*. London: Jessica Kingsley Publishers.

DiLorito,C, Dening,T and Vollm,B (2018) Ageing in Forensic Psychiatric Secure Settings: The Voice of Older Patients. *Journal of Forensic Psychiatry and Psychology* 29 (6) 934–60.

Dimond,C and Chiweda,D (2011) Developing a Therapeutic Model in a Secure Forensic Adolescent Unit. *Journal of Forensic Psychology and Psychology* 22 (2) 283–305.

Dix,R (2014) Mechanical Restraint and Seclusion: Earning a Place at the Debating Table. *Journal of Psychiatric Intensive Care* 10 (2) 261–3.

Dolan,M and Lawson,A (2001) A Psychiatric Intensive Care Unit in a Medium Security Unit. *Journal of Forensic Psychiatry* 12 (3) 684–93.

Downie,R (2012) Paying Attention: Hippocratic and Askeplian Approaches. *Advances in Psychiatric Treatment* 18 (5) 363–8.

Doyle,M, Coid,J, Archer-Power,L, Dewa,L, Hunter-Didrichsen,R, Stevenson,R, et al. (2014) Discharges to Prison from Medium Secure Psychiatric Units in England and Wales. *British Journal of Psychiatry* 205 (3) 177–82.

Duggan,C (2011) Dangerous and Severe Personality Disorder. *British Journal of Psychiatry* 198 (6) 431–3.

Duggan,C (2019) Looking from the Outside: No Substitute for Rigorous Evaluation. *Criminal Behaviour and Mental Health* 29 (4) 189–95.

Edge,C, Lewer,D, Hayward,A, Braithwaite,I and Hard,J (2021) Early Vaccination in Jails Will Reduce Mortality and Protect Prisoners' Rights. *British Medical Journal* 3–10

Edge,D, Walker,T, Meacock,R, Wilson,H, McNair,L, Shaw,J, et al. (2017) Secure Pathways for Women in the UK: Lessons from the Women's Enhanced Medium Secure Services (WEMMS) Pilots. *Journal of Forensic Psychiatry and Psychology* 28 (2) 206–25.

Farnham,FR and Kennedy,HG (1997) Acute Excited States and Sudden Death. *British Medical Journal* 315: 1107–8.

Fazel,S, Hope,T and O'Donnell,I (2001) Hidden Psychiatric Morbidity in Older Prisoners. *British Journal of Psychiatry* 179: 535–9.

Fazel,S and Seewald,K (2012) Severe Mental Illness in 33,588 Prisoners Worldwide: Systematic Review and Meta-Regression Analysis. *British Journal of Psychiatry* 200 (5) 364–73.

Finney,T, Copley,V, Hall,I and Keach,S (2014) An Analysis of Influenza Outbreaks in Institutions and Closed Societies. *Epidemiology and Infection* 142 (1) 107–13.

Fisher,J and Teodorczuk,A (2017) Old Age Psychiatry and Geriatric Medicine: Shared Challenges, Shared Solutions? *British Journal of Psychiatry* 210 (2) 91–3.

Fitzgerald,M (2015) Do Psychiatry and Neurology Need a Close Partnership or a Merger? *BJ Psych Bulletin* 39 (3) 105–7.

Galappathie,N, Khan,ST and Hussain,A (2017) Civil and Forensic Patients in Secure Psychiatric Aettings: A Comparison. *BJ Psych Bulletin* 41 (3) 156–9.

Gaskin,CJ, Elsom,SJ and Happell,B (2007) Interventions for Reducing the use of Seclusion in Psychiatric Facilities: Review of the Literature. *British Journal of Psychiatry* 191 (4) 298–303.

Geelan,S and Nickford,C (1999) A Survey of the Use of Family Therapy in Medium Secure Units in England and Wales. *Journal of Forensic Psychiatry* 10: 317–24.

Ghaziuddin,M, Werdmer-Michail,E and Ghaziuddin,N (1998) Comorbidity of Asperger's Syndrome: A Preliminary Report. *Journal of Intellectual Disability Research* 4: 279–83.

Gibson,R, Till,A and Adshead,G (2019) Psychotherapeutic Leadership and Containment in Psychiatry. *BJ Psych Advances* 25 (2) 133–41.

Girardi,A, Snyman,P, Natarajan,M and Griffiths,C (2018) Older Adults in Secure Mental Health Care: Health Social Well-Being and Security Needs Measured with HONOS-Secure across Different Age Groups. *Journal of Forensic Psychiatry and Psychology* 29 (5) 824–43.

Gold,VR, Hoyt Jr,TL, Ringe,SH, Thistlewaite,SB, Throckmorton Jr,BH and Withers,BA (1995) *The New Testament and Psalms: An Inclusive Version*. Oxford: Oxford University Press.

Goodman,H, Brooks,CP, Price,O and Barley,EA (2020) Barriers and Facilitators to the Effective De-escalation of Conflict Behaviours in Forensic High-Secure Settings: A Qualitative Study. *International Journal of Mental Health Systems* 14: 59.

Gordon,H (2001) The Provision of Intensive Care in Forensic Psychiatry. In Beer,MD, Pereira,SM and Paton,C (eds.), *Psychiatric Intensive Care*. pp. 253–62 London: Greenwich Medical Media Ltd.

Gordon,H (2002) Suicide in Secure Psychiatric Facilities. *Advances in Psychiatric Treatment* 8: 408–17.

Gordon,H (2008) The Provision of Intensive Care in Forensic Psychiatry. In Beer,MD, Pereira,S and Paton,C (eds.), *Psychiatric Intensive Care.* pp. 183–90. Cambridge: Cambridge University Press.

Gordon,H (2012) *Broadmoor.* London: Psychology News Press.

Gordon,H, Hammond,S and Veeramani,R (1998) Special Care Units in Special Hospitals. *Journal of Forensic Psychiatry* 9 (3) 571–87.

Gordon,H, Hindley,N, Marsden,A and Shivayogi,M (1999) The Use of Mechanical Restraint in the Management of Psychiatric Patients. Is It Ever Appropriate? *Journal of Forensic Psychiatry* 10 (1) 173–86.

Gordon,H and Khosla,V (2014) The Interface between General and Forensic Psychiatry: A Historical Perspective. *Advances in Psychiatric Treatment* 20 (5) 350–8.

Gordon,H, Oyebode,O and Minne,C (1997) Death by Homicide in Special Hospitals. *Journal of Forensic Psychiatry* 8 (3) 602–19.

Gow,RL, Choo,M, Darjee,R, Gould,S and Steele,J (2010) A Demographic Study of the Orchard Clinic: Scotland's First Medium Secure Unit. *Journal of Forensic Psychiatry and Psychology* 21 (1) 139–55.

Green,B and Robinson,L (2001) A Further 12-Month Study of Violent Incidents Within a Medium Secure Psychiatric Unit (and a Comparison with the Previous 12 Months). *British Journal of Forensic Practice* 3 (3) 13–22.

Gudjonsson,GH and Young,S (2007) The Role and Scope of Forensic Clinical Psychology in Secure Unit Provision: A Proposed Model for Psychological Therapies. *Journal of Forensic Psychiatry and Psychology* 18 (4) 534–56.

Gunn,J (1977) Management of the Mentally Disordered Offender: Integrated or Parallel. *Proceedings of Royal Society of Medicine* 70: 877–80.

Gunn,J (2008) Forensic Psychiatry and General Psychiatry: Re-examining the Relationship. *Psychiatric Bulletin* 32 (5) 197.

Gunn,J (2019) Extended Suicide, or Homicide Followed by Suicide. *Criminal Behaviour and Mental Health* 29 (4) 239–46.

Gunn,J and Taylor,PJ (2014) *Forensic Psychiatry: Clinical, Legal and Ethical Issues,* 2nd ed. London: CRC Press. Taylor and Francis Group.

Gunn,J, Taylor,PJ, Forrester,A, Parrott,J and Grounds,A (2020) Telemedicine in Prisons: A Crime in Mind Perspective. *Criminal Behaviour and Mental Health* 30 (2–3) 65–7.

Gupta,S, Akyuz,EU, Flint,J and Baldwin,T (2018) Violence and Aggression in Psychiatric Settings: Reporting to the Police. *BJ Psych Advances* 24 (3) 146–51.

Halstead,S, Cahill,A, Fernando,L and Isweran,M (2001) Discharges from a Learning-Disability Medium Secure Unit: What Happens to Them? *British Journal of Forensic Practice* 3 (1) 11–21.

Harty,M, Jarrett,M, Thornicroft,G and Shaw,J (2012) Unmet Needs of Male Prisoners under the Care of Prison Mental Health Inreach Services. *Journal of Forensic Psychiatry and Psychology* 22 (3) 285–96.

Harty,M, Somers,N and Bartlett,A (2012) Women's Secure Hospital Services: National Bed Numbers and Distribution. *Journal of Forensic Psychiatry and Psychology* 23 (5–6) 590–600.

Hassiotis,A, Gazizova,D, Akinionu,L, Bebbington,P, Meltzer,H and Strydom,A (2011) Psychiatric Morbidity in Prisoners with Intellectual Disabilities: Analysis of Prison Survey Data for England and Wales. *British Journal of Psychiatry* 199 (2) 156–7.

Haw,C, Muthu-Veloe,A, Suett,M, Ibodor,O and Picchioni,M (2016) Monitoring Antipsychotic Side-Effects: A Completed Audit Cycle Conducted in a Secure Hospital. *British Journal of Forensic Practice* 18 (3) 182–8.

Haw,C and Rowell,A (2011) Obesity and its Complications: A Survey of Inpatients at a Secure Psychiatric Hospital. *British Journal of Forensic Practice* 13 (4) 270–7.

Haw,C and Stubbs,J (2011) What Are We Doing about Weight Management in Forensic Psychiatry? A Survey of Forensic Psychiatrists. *British Journal of Forensic Practice* 13 (3) 183–90.

Hawramy,M (2020) Interface between Community Intellectual Disability and General Adult Psychiatry Services. *BJ Psych Advances* 26 (5) 299–305.

Henry,R, Massey,R, Morgan,K, Deeks,J, MacFarlane,H, Holmes,N and Silva,E (2020) Evaluation of the Effectiveness and Acceptability of Intramuscular Clozapine Injection: Illustrative Case Series. *BJ Psych Bulletin* 44: 239–43.

Hewson,T, Green,R, Shepherd,A, Hard,J and Shaw,J (2021) The Effects of COVID-19 on Self-Harm in UK Prisons. *BJ Psych Bulletin* 45 (3)131–3.

Hewson,T, Shepherd,A, Hard,J and Shaw,J (2020) Effects of the COVID-19 Pandemic on the Mental Health of Prisoners. *Lancet Psychiatry* 7 (7) 568–69.

Hill,SA, Ferreira,J, Chamorro,V and Hosking,A (2019) Characteristics and Personality Profiles of First 100 Patients Admitted to a Secure Forensic Adolescent Hospital. *Journal of Forensic Psychiatry and Psychology* 30 (2) 352–66.

Hill,SA, Thorpe,A, Petrauskarte,R and Wilson,S (2020) Characteristics of Patients with Gender Dysphoria Admitted to a Secure Forensic Adolescent Hospital. *Journal of Forensic Psychiatry and Psychology* 31 (6) 854–67.

Hilton,C (2015) Age Inclusive Services or Separate Old Age and Working Age Services? A Historical Analysis from the Formative Years of Old Age Psychiatry c1940 - 1989. *BJ Psych Bulletin* 39: 90–5.

Hindley,N, Lengua,C and White,O (2017) Forensic Mental Health Services for Children and Adolescents: Rationale and Development. *BJ Psych Advances* 23 (1) 36–43.

Hollins,S, Lodge,K-M and Lomax,P (2019) The Case for Removing Intellectual Disability and Autism from the Mental Health Act. *British Journal of Psychiatry* 215 (5) 633–5.

Hollins,L and Stubbs,B (2011) Managing the Risks Associated with Physical Intervention: A Discussion Paper. *British Journal of Forensic Practice* 13 (4) 257–63.

Holloway,F (2011) Gentlemen, We Have No Money, Therefore We Must Think – Mental Health Services in Hard Times. *The Psychiatrist* 35 (3) 81–3.

Home Office and Department of Health and Social Security (1975) *Report of the Committee on Mentally Abnormal Offenders (Butler Report)*. London. Home Office and Department of Health and Social Security.

Horgan,H, Charteris,C and Ambrose,D (2019) The Violence Reduction Programme: An Exploration of Post Treatment Risk Reduction in a Specialist Medium Secure Unit. *Criminal Behaviour and Mental Health* 29 (5–6) 289–95.

Howells,K (2010) The 'Third Wave' of Cognitive Behavioural Therapy and Forensic Practice. *Criminal Behaviour and Mental Health* 20 (4) 251–6.

Humber,N, Hayes,A, Wright,S, Fahy,T and Shaw,J (2011) A Comparative Study of Forensic and General Community Psychiatric Patients with Integrated and Parallel Models of Care in the UK. *Journal of Forensic Psychiatry and Psychology* 22 (2) 183–202.

Igoumenou,A, Kallis,C, Huband,N, Hague,O, Coid,JW and Duggan,C (2019) Prison v Hospital for Offenders with Psychosis: Effects on Reoffending. *Journal of Forensic Psychiatry and Psychology* 30 (6) 939–58.

Ion,R, Pegg,S and Moir,J (2014) Nineteenth Century Newspaper Accounts of a Murder Committed by an Inmate of a Scottish Asylum. *Journal of Forensic Psychiatry and Psychology* 25 (2) 152–63.

Isherwood,T, Burns,M, Naylor,M and Read,S (2007) 'Getting into Trouble': A Qualitative Analysis of the Onset of Offending in the Accounts of Men with Learning Disabilities. *Journal of Forensic Psychiatry and Psychology* 18 (2) 221–34.

Janicki,N (2009) Prosecuting Inpatient Violence: Perceptions of Staff, Patients and Others in a Woman's Enhanced Medium Secure Service. *British Journal of Forensic Practice* 11 (4) 27–38.

Johnson,O, Andrew,A and Connolly,T (2019) Outcomes in a Low Secure Unit: Pre-admission and Post-discharge Comparisons. *Journal of Forensic Psychiatry and Psychology* 30 (2) 203–19.

Jones,G and Talbot,J (2010) No One Knows: The Bewildering Passage of Offenders with Learning Disability and Learning Difficulty through the Criminal Justice System. *Criminal Behaviour and Mental Health* 20 (1) 1–7.

Jordan,M (2011) Therapeutic Relationships with Offenders: An Introduction to the Psychodynamics of Forensic Mental Health Nursing. *British Journal of Forensic Practice* 13 (3) 213–4.

Kane,E, Evans,E, Mitsch,J and Jilani,T (2020) Are Liaison and Diversion Interventions in Policing Delivering the Planned Impact: A Longitudinal Evaluation in Two Constabularies. *Criminal Behaviour and Mental Health* 30 (5) 256–67.

Kasmi,Y (2010) Profiling Medium Secure Psychiatric Intensive Care Unit Patients. *Journal of Psychiatric Intensive Care* 6 (2) 65–71.

Kasmi,Y, Duggan,C and Vollm,B (2020) A Comparison of Long-Term Medium Secure Patients within NHS and Private and Charitable Sector Units in England. *Criminal Behaviour and Mental Health* 30 (1) 38–49.

Kelly,BD (2016) *Mental Illness, Human Rights and the Law.* London. Royal College of Psychiatrists.

Kennedy,HG (2002) Therapeutic Uses of Security: Mapping Forensic Mental Health Services by Stratifying Risk. *Advances in Psychiatric* Treatment 8: 433–43.

Keski-Valkama,A, Koivisto,A-M, Eronon,M and Riitakertuj,K-H (2010) Forensic and General Psychiatric Patients View of Seclusion: A Comparison Study. *Journal of Forensic Psychiatry and Psychology* 21 (3) 446–61.

Khalifa,N, Saleem,Y and Stankard,P (2008) The Use of Telepsychiatry within Forensic Practice: A Literature Review on the Use of Video Link. *Journal of Forensic Psychiatry and Psychology* 19 (1) 2–13.

Khan,O, Ferriter,M, Huband,N, Powney,MJ, Dennis,JA and Duggan,C (2017) Pharmacological Interventions for Those Who Have Sexually Offended or Are at Risk of Offending. *BJ Psych Advances* 23 (6) 360.

Khosla,V, Davison,P, Gordon,H and Verghese,J (2014) The Interface between General and Forensic Psychiatry: The Present Day. *Advances in Psychiatric Treatment* 20 (5) 359–65.

Khrypunov,O, Aziz,R, Al-Kaissy,B, Jethwa,K and Joseph,V (2018) Interface between General Adult and Old Age Psychiatry. *BJ Psych Advances* 24 (3) 188–94.

Kinsella,C, Challoner,C and Brosnan,C (1993) An Alternative to Seclusion. *Nursing Times* 89 (18) 62–4.

Klugman,S (1999) Art Therapy and Art Education within a Secure Setting. *Journal of British Association of Art Therapists* 4: 29–34.

Knifton,L and Inglis,G (2020) Poverty and Mental Health: Policy, Practice and Research Implications. *BJ Psych Bulletin* 44: 193–6.

Knowles,SF, Hearne,J and Smith,I (2015) Physical Restraint and the Therapeutic Relationship. *Journal of Forensic Psychiatry and Psychology* 26 (4) 461–75.

Kristensen,O, Brandt-Christensen,M, Ockelmann,HH and Jorgensen,MB (2012) The Use of Electroconvulsive Therapy in a Cohort of Forensic Psychiatric Patients with Schizophrenia. *Criminal Behaviour and Mental Health* **22**: 148–56.

Lally,J, Tully,J, Robertson,D, Stubbs,B, Gaughran,F and McCabe,JH (2016) Clozapine with Electroconvulsive Therapy in Treatment Resistant Schizophrenia: A Systematic Review and Meta-analysis. *Schizophrenia Research* **171**: 215–24.

Larkin,E, Murtagh,S and Jones,S (1988) A Preliminary Study of Violent Incidents in a Special Hospital (Rampton). *British Journal of Psychiatry* **153**: 226–31.

Lawn,T and McDonald,E (2009) Developing a Policy to Deal with Sexual Assault on Psychiatric In-Patient Wards. *Psychiatric Bulletin* **33** (3) 108–11.

Lennon,JC (2020) What Lies Ahead: Elevated Concerns for the Ongoing Suicide Pandemic. *Psychological Trauma* **12** (s1) s118–19.

Leschziner,G (2019) *The Nocturnal Brain, Nightmares, Neuroscience and the Secret World of Sleep.* London. Simon and Schuster.

Lewis,A, Grubin,D, Ross,CC and Das,M (2017) Gonadotrophin – Releasing Hormone Agonist Treatment for Sexual Offenders: A Systematic Review. *Journal of Psychopharmacology* **31** (10) 1281–93.

Liebrenz,M, Bhugra,D, Buadze,A and Schleifer,R (2020) Caring for Persons in Detention Suffering with Mental Illness during the COVID-19 Outbreak. *Forensic Science International: Mind and Law* **1**: 100013.

Lightbody,E, McCall Smith,A, Crichton,J and Chiswick,D (2010) A Survey of Older Adult Patients in Special Secure Psychiatric Care in Scotland from 1998 to 2007. *Journal of Forensic Psychiatry and Psychology* **21** (6) 966–74.

Little,JD and Burt,M (2013) Tasers and Psychiatry: The Use of a Taser on a Low Secure Unit. *Journal of Psychiatric Intensive Care* **9** (1) 56–8.

Livanou,MI, Lane,R, D'Souza,S and Singh,SP (2020) A Retrospective Case Note Review of Young People in Transition from Adolescent Medium Secure Units to Adult Services. *British Journal of Forensic Practice* **22** (3) 161–72.

Long,C, Rowell,A, Rigg,S, Livesey,F and McAllister,P (2016) What is Effective in Promoting a Healthy Lifestyle in Secure Psychiatric Settings? A Review of the Evidence for an Integrated Programme that Targets Modifiable Health Risk Behaviours. *British Journal of Forensic Practice* **18** (3) 204–15.

Long,CG, Dolly,O and Hollin,CR (2015) Treatment Progress in Medium Security Hospital Settings for Women: Changes in Symptoms, Personality and Service Need from Admission to Discharge. *Criminal Behaviour and Mental Health* **25** (2) 99–111.

Long,CG, Silaule,P and Collier,N (2010) Use of an Extra Care Area in a Medium Secure Setting for Women: Findings and Implications for Practice. *Journal of Psychiatric Intensive Care* **6** (1) 39–45.

Long,CG, West,R, Afford,M, Collins,L and Dolley,O (2015) Reducing the Use of Seclusion in a Secure Service for Women. *Journal of Psychiatric Intensive Care* **11** (2) 84–94.

Longdon,L, Edworthy,R, Resnick,J, Byrne,A, Clarke,M, Cheung,N, et al. (2018) Patient Characteristics and Outcome Measurement in a Low Secure Forensic Hospital. *Criminal Behaviour and Mental Health* **28** (3) 255–69.

MacDonald,M (1981) *Mystical Bedlam: Madness, Anxiety and Healing in Seventeenth-Century England.* Cambridge. Cambridge University Press.

Maguire,T, Young,R and Martin,T (2011) Seclusion Reduction in a Forensic Mental Health Setting. *Psychiatric and Mental Health* Nursing **19** (2) 97–106.

Mann,S and Cree,W (1976) 'New' Long-Stay Psychiatric Patients: A National Sample Survey of Fifteen Mental Hospitals in England and Wales 1972/73. *Psychological Medicine* **6**: 603–16.

Mao,L, Jin,H, Wang,M, Hu,Y, Chen,S and He,Q (2020) Neurological Manifestations of Hospitalized Patients with Coronavirus Disease 2019 in Wuhan, China. *Journal of American Medical Association. Neurology* **77**: 683–90.

Marlow,K, Winder,B and Elliott,HJ (2015) Working with Transgendered Sex Offenders: Prison Staff Experiences. *British Journal of Forensic Practice* **17** (3) 241–54.

Mason,T and Chandley,M (1995) The Chronically Assaultive Patient: Benchmarking Best Practices. *Psychiatric Care* **2** (5) 180–3.

Mason,T, Lovell,A and Coyle,D (2008) Forensic Psychiatric Nursing: Skills and Competencies: I. Role Dimensions. *Journal of Psychiatric Mental Health Nursing* **15** (2) 118–30.

McCarthy,J, Chaplin,E, Forrester,A, Underwood,L, Hayward,H, Sabet,J, et al. (2019) Prisoners with Neurodevelopmental Difficulties: Vulnerabilities for Mental Illness and Self-Harm. *Criminal Behaviour and Mental Health* **29** (5–6) 308–20.

McCarthy,L and Duggan,C (2010) Engagement in a Medium Secure Personality Disorder Service: A Comparative Study of Psychological Functioning and Offending Outcomes. *Criminal Behaviour and Mental Health* **20** (2) 112–28.

McCulloch,S, Stanley,C, Smith,H, Scott,M, Kana,M, Ndubuisi,B, et al. (2020) Outcome Measures of Risk and Recovery in Broadmoor High Secure Forensic Hospital: Stratification of Care Pathways and Moves to Medium Secure Hospitals. *BJ Psych Open* **6**: 4e74.

McLaughlin,BC, Miles,A, Webb,TC, Knopp,P, Eyres,C, Falobri,A, et al. (2020) Functional and Cognitive Outcomes after COVID-19 Delirium. *European Geriatric Medicine* **11**: 857–62.

McLean,RJ (2010) Assessing the Security Needs of Patients in Medium Secure Psychiatric Care in Northern Ireland. *The Psychiatrist* **34** (10) 432–6.

McLeod,C, Yorston,G and Gibb,R (2008) Referrals of Older Adults to Forensic and Psychiatric Intensive Care Services: A Retrospective Case-Note Study in Scotland. *British Journal of Forensic Practice* **10** (1) 36–43.

McSherry,B (2017) Regulating Seclusion and Restraint in Healthcare Settings: The Promise of the Convention on the Rights of Persons with Disabilities. *International Journal of Law and Psychiatry* **53**: 39–44.

Mezey,G, Durkin,C and Krljes,S (2015) Finding a Voice – The Feasibility and Impact of Setting Up a Community Choir in a Forensic Secure Setting. *Journal of Forensic Psychiatry and Psychology* **26** (6) 781–97.

Milton,J, Duggan,C, McCarthy,L, Costley-White,A and Mason,L (2007) Characteristics of Offenders Referred to a Medium Security NHS Personality Disorder Service: The First Five Years. *Criminal Behaviour and Mental Health* **17** (1) 57–67.

Minoudis,P and Kane,E (2017) It's a Journey, not a Destination – From Dangerous and Severe Personality Disorder (DSPD) to the Offender Personality Disorder (OPD) Pathway. *Criminal Behaviour and Mental Health* **27** (3) 207–13.

Miskelly,F (2004) A Novel System of Electronic Tagging in Patients with Dementia and Wandering. *Age and Ageing* **33**: 304–6.

Murphy,D (2007) Hare Psychopathy Checklist Revised Profiles of Male Patients with Asperger's Syndrome Detained in High Security Psychiatric Care. *Journal of Forensic Psychiatry and Psychology* **18** (1) 120–6.

Murphy,D (2010) Extreme Violence in a Man with an Autistic Spectrum Disorder: Assessment and Treatment within High-Security Psychiatric Care. *Journal of Forensic Psychiatry and Psychology* **21** (3) 462–77.

Murphy,D (2020) Autism: Implications for High Secure Psychiatric Care and Move Towards Best Practice. *Research in Developmental Disability* **100**: 103615.

Murphy,P, Potter,L, Tully,J, Hearn,D, Fahy,T and McCrone,P (2017) A Cost Comparison Study of Using Global Positioning System Technology (Electronic Monitoring) in a Medium Secure Forensic Psychiatric Service. *Journal of Forensic Psychiatry and Psychology* **28** (1) 57–69.

Muthukumaraswamy,A, Beer,MD and Ratnajothy,K (2008) Aggression Patterns and Clinical Predictors of Inpatient Aggression in a Mental Health Low Secure Unit. *Journal of Psychiatric Intensive Care* **4** (1–2) 9–16.

Nadkarni,J, Blakelock,DJ, Jha,A, Tiffin,P and Sullivan,F (2012) The Clinical Profile of Young People Accessing a Low Secure Adolescent Unit. *British Journal of Forensic Practice* **14** (3) 217–26.

National Association of Psychiatric Intensive Care and Low Secure Units (NAPICU) (2014) *National Minimum Standards for Psychiatric Intensive Care in General Adult Services.* Glasgow: NAPICU.

National Association of Psychiatric Intensive Care and Low Secure Units (NAPICU) (2016) *NAPICU Position on the Monitoring, Regulation and Recording of the Extra Care Area, Seclusion and Long-Term Segregation Use in the Context of the Mental Health Act 1983: Code of Practice (2015).* Glasgow: NAPICU.

Nelson,D (2003) Service Innovations: The Orchard Clinic: Scotland's First Medium Secure Unit. *Psychiatric Bulletin* **27**: 105–7.

Newton-Howes,G (2013) Use of Seclusion for Managing Disturbance in Patients. *Advances in Psychiatric Treatment* **19** (6) 422–8.

National Institute for Health and Care Excellence (NICE) (2015) *Violence and Aggression: Short-Term Management in Mental Health, Health and Community Settings [NG10].* London: NICE.

Nicholson,D (1878) The Measure of Individual and Social Responsibility in Criminal Cases: The Responsibility of Society: The Prevention of Criminal Lunacy. *Journal of Mental Science* **24**: 1–25 and 249–73.

Nimmagadda,SR, Sugarman,P, Duggan,LM and McAlister, HM (2008) Growth in Independent Hospitals: An Opportunity for Training beyond the NHS. *Psychiatric Bulletin* **32** (2) 41–3.

North,AS, Russell,AJ and Gudjonsson,GH (2008) High Functioning Autism Spectrum Disorders: An Investigation of Psychological Vulnerabilities during Interrogative Interview. *Journal of Forensic Psychiatry and Psychology* **19** (3) 323–34.

Nulty,JE, Winder,B and Lopresti,S (2019) 'I'm not different, I'm still a human being (..) but I am different': An Exploration of the Experiences of Transgender Prisoners using Interpretative Phenomenological Analysis. *British Journal of Forensic Practice* **21** (2) 97–111.

Oakley,C, Hynes,F and Clark,T (2009) Mood Disorders and Violence: A New Focus. *Advances in Psychiatric Treatment* **15** (4) 263–270

O'Grady,J (2008) Time to talk. Commentary on . . . Forensic Psychiatry and General Psychiatry. *Psychiatric Bulletin* **32** (1) 6–7.

O'Laughlin,A (2014) The Offender Personality Disorder Pathway: Expansion in the Face of Failure? *Howard Journal of Criminal Justice* **53** (2) 173–92.

O'Sullivan,PCJ and Chesterman,LP (2007) Older Adult Patients Subject to Restriction Orders in England and Wales: A Cross-Sectional Survey. *Journal of Forensic Psychiatry and Psychology* **18** (2) 204–20.

Parkes,J (2002) A Review of the Literature on Positional Asphyxia as a Possible Cause of Sudden Death during Restraint. *British Journal of Forensic Practice* **4** (1) 24–30.

Patel,M, Sethi,FN, Barnes,TR, Dix,R, Dratcu,L, Fox,B, et al. Joint BAP NAPICU Evidence-Based Consensus Guidelines for the Clinical Management of Acute Disturbance: De-escalation and Rapid Tranquilisation. *Journal of Psychopharmacology* 32 (6) 601–40.

Paul,M, Ford,T, Kramer,T, Islam,Z, Harley,K and Singh,SS (2013) Transfers and Transitions between Child and Adult Mental Health Services. *British Journal of Psychiatry* **202** (s54) s36–40.

Pereira,S, Beer,D and Paton,C (1999) Enforcing Treatment with Clozapine. Survey of Views and Practice. *The Psychiatrist* 23: 342–5.

Pereira,SM, Walker,L and Dye,S (2021) A National Survey of Intensive Care, Low Secure and Locked Rehabilitation Units. *Mental Health Practice*. **24** (4) 24–34.

Pina-Camacho,L, Parallada,M and Kyriakopoulos,M (2016) Autism Spectrum Disorder and Schizophrenia: Boundaries and Uncertainties. *BJ Psych Advances* 22 (5) 315–24.

Pluck,G and Brooker,C (2014) Epidemiological Survey of Suicide Ideation and Acts and Other Deliberate Self-Harm among Offenders in the Community under Supervision of the Probation Service in England and Wales. *Criminal Behaviour and Mental Health* 24 (5) 358–64.

Poole,R (2020) The Sacred versus the Secular in UK Psychiatry. *BJ Psych Advances* 26 (5) 285–86.

Prins,H, Backer-Holst,T, Francis,E and Keitch,I (1993) *Report of the Committee of Inquiry into the Death in Broadmoor Hospital of Orville Blackwood and a Review of the Deaths of Two Other Afro-caribbean Patients: Big, Black and Dangerous?* London. Special Hospitals Service Authority.

Purewal,R (2020) Dementia in UK Prisons: Failings and Solutions? *Criminal Behaviour and Mental Health* **30** (2–3) 53–8.

Puri,BK, Brown,RA, McKee,HJ and Treasaden,IH (2005) *Mental Health Law: A Practical Guide*. London. Heather Arnold.

Puzzo,I, Gable,D and Cohen,A (2017) Using the National Diabetes Audit to Improve the Care of Diabetes in Secure Hospital In-Patient Settings in the UK. *Journal of Forensic Psychiatry and Psychology* 28 (3) 400–11.

Quraschi,I, Johnson,D, Shaw,J and Johnson,B (2010) Reduction in the Use of Seclusion in a High Secure Hospital: A Retrospective Analysis. *Journal of Intensive Care* 6 (2) 109–15.

Radar Healthcare (2020) What are the 5 CQC Standards. Website. https://radarhealthcare.com/news-blogs/what-are-the-5-cqc-standards/.

Reed,J (1997) The Need for Longer Term Psychiatric Care in Medium or Low Security. *Criminal Behaviour and Mental Health* 7: 201–12.

Reed,S (2004) People with Learning Difficulties in a Low Secure In-Patient Unit: Comparison of Offenders and Non-Offenders. *British Journal of Psychiatry* **185**: 499–504.

Rix,K (2017) Pharmacological Interventions for Sex Offenders: A Poor Evidence Base to Guide Practice: Commentary on . . . Cochrane Corner. *BJ Psych Advances* **23** (6) 361–5.

Rollin,HR (1966) Mental Hospitals without Bars: A Contemporary Paradox. *Proceedings of Royal Society of Medicine* 59: 701–4.

Ron,MA (2018) The Neuropsychiatry of Multiple Sclerosis. *BJ Psych Advances* 24 (3) 178–87.

Roy,C and Thomson,L (2017) Appeals against Detention in Conditions of Excessive Security: Outcomes and Decision-Making. *Journal of Forensic Psychiatry and Psychology* **28** (5) 674–93.

Royal College of Psychiatrists (2013) Prevention and Management of Violence. Guidance for Mental Health Care Professionals. College Report CR177. London.

Royal College of Psychiatrists (2018) Restrictive Interventions in In-Patient Intellectual Disability Services: How to Record, Monitor and Regulate. CR220. London.

Royal College of Psychiatrists (2021) COVID-19: Secure Hospital and Criminal Justice Settings. London. Rcpsych.ac.uk/about-us/responding to Covid-19-guidelines for clinicians/community-and-inpatientservices/secure-hospital-and-criminal-justice-settings.

Rutter,S, Gudjonsson,G and Rabe-Hesketh,S (2004) Violent Incidents in a Medium Secure Unit: The Characteristics of Persistent Perpetrators of Violence. *Journal of Forensic Psychiatry and Psychology* 15 (2) 293–302.

Saleem,R, Kaitiff,D, Treasaden,I and Vermeulen,J (2011) Clinical Experience of the Use of Triptorelin as an Antilibidinal Medication in a High Security Hospital. *Journal of Forensic Psychiatry and Psychology* **22** (2) 243–51.

Saradjian,J, Murphy,N and McVey,D (2013) Delivering Effective Therapeutic Interventions for Men with Severe Personality Disorder within a High Secure Prison. *Psychology, Crime and Law* 19 (5-6) 433–47.

Sarkar,J and di Lustro,M (2011) Evolution of Secure Services for Women in England. *Advances in Psychiatric Treatment* 17 (5) 323–31.

Scragg,P and Shah,A (1994) Prevalence of Asperger's Syndrome in a Secure Hospital. *British Journal of Psychiatry* **165**: 679–82.

Scull,A, Mackenzie,C and Hervey,N (1996) *Masters of Bedlam: The Transformation of the Mad Doctoring Trade*. Chichester: Princeton University Press.

Seligman,M and Feery,D (2006) Seclusion: Lord Steyn's Lament. *Journal of Psychiatric Intensive Care* 2 (2) 111–7.

Selsick,H and O'Regan,D (2018) Sleep Disorders in Psychiatry. *BJ Psych Advances* 24 (4) 273–83.

Sequiera,H and Halstead,S (2002) Control and Restraint in the UK: Service User Perspectives. *British Journal of Forensic Practice* 4 (1) 9–18.

Shah,A, Waldron,G, Boast,N, Coid,JW and Ullrich,S (2011) Factors Associated with Length of Admission at a Medium Secure Forensic Psychiatric Unit. *Journal of Forensic Psychiatry and Psychology* 22 (4) 496–512.

Sharpe,R, Vollm,B, Akhtar,A, Puri,R and Bickle,A (2016) Transfers from Prison to Hospital under Section 47 and 48 of the Mental Health Act between 2011 and 2014. *Journal of Forensic Psychiatry and Psychology* 27 (4) 459–75.

Sher,L (2020) The Impact of the COVID-19 Pandemic on Suicide Rates. *International Journal of Medicine* 113 (10) 707–12.

Shetty,A, Alex,R and Bloye,D (2010) The Experience of a Smoke-Free Policy in a Medium Secure Hospital. *The Psychiatrist* 34 (7) 287–9.

Silva,E and Shepherd,A (2019) Tick, Tock, Lock: Night Time Confinement in High Security – History, Practice, Ethics and Practicalities. *BJ Psych Bulletin* 43 (1) 1–3.

Silva,E, Till,A and Adshead,G (2017) Ethical Dilemmas in Psychiatry: When Teams Disagree. *BJ Psych Advances* 23 (3) 231–9.

Simpson,AIF, Chatterjee,S, Darby,P, Jones,RM, Maheandiran,M, Penney,SR, et al. (2020) Management of COVID-19 Response in a Secure Forensic Mental Health Setting. *Canadian Journal of Psychiatry* 65 (10) 695–700.

Singh,SS, Paul,M, Ford,T, Kramer,T, Weaver,T, McClaren,S, et al. (2010) Process, Outcome and Experience of Transition from Child to Adult Mental Healthcare: Multiperspective Study. *British Journal of Psychiatry* 197 (4) 305–12.

Sivan,M and Taylor,S (2020) NICE Guideline on Long COVID. *British Medical Journal* 371: m4938.

Skett,S, Goode,I and Barton,S (2017) A Joint NHS and NOMS Offender Personality Disorder Pathway Strategy: A Perspective from 5 Years of Operation. *Criminal Behaviour and Mental Health* 27 (3) 214–21.

Smith,K, Ostinelli,E, MacDonald,O and Cipriani,A (2020) COVID-19 and Telepsychiatry: Development of Evidence-Based Guidance for Clinicians. *JMIR Mental Health* 7 (8) e21108.

Snowden,P, McKenna,J and Jasper,A (1999) Management of Conditionally Discharged Patients and Others Who Represent Similar Risks in the Community. *Journal of Forensic Psychiatry* 10: 583–96.

Stubbs,B (2008) Injuries to Staff from Implementation of Physical Interventions: Could Poor Manual Handling Be at Fault? *British Journal of Forensic Practice* 10 (4) 12–14.

Swinton,M (2001) Clozapine in Severe Borderline Personality Disorder. *Journal of Forensic Psychiatry* 12: 580–91.

Swinton,M and McNamee,H (2003) Clozapine in Forensic Settings: Persuading Patients. *British Journal of Forensic Practice* 5 (2) 33–8.

Szmukler,G (2019) Night-Time Confinement is an Unacceptable Hospital Practice *BJ Psych Bulletin* 43 (1) 35–7.

Taylor,J and Healy,P (2001) Education in Secure Psychiatric Units. *British Journal of Forensic Practice* 3 (4) 3–7.

Taylor,J and Morrisey,C (2012) Integrating Treatment for Offenders with an Intellectual Disability and Personality Disorder. *British Journal of Forensic Practice* 14 (4) 302–15.

Taylor,PJ, Leese,M, Williams,D, Butwell,M, Daly,R and Larkin,E (1998) Mental Disorder and Violence: A Special (High Security) Hospital Study. *British Journal of Psychiatry* 173: 218–26.

Taylor,PJ, Maden,A and Jones,D (1996) Long-Term Medium Security Hospital Units: A Service Gap of the 1990s. *Criminal Behaviour and Mental Health* 6: 213–19.

Taylor,PJ and Parrott,JM (1988) Elderly Offenders: A study of Age-Related Factors among Custodially Remanded Prisoners. *British Journal of Psychiatry* 152: 340–6.

Taylor,PJ and Swan,T (1999) *Couples in Care and Custody.* Oxford: Butterworth Heinemann.

Thacker,S, Skelton,M and Harwood,R (2017) Psychiatry and the Geriatric Syndromes – Creating Constructive Interfaces. *BJ Psych Bulletin* 41 (2) 71–5.

Thomson,L (2019) Night-Time Confinement and the Practice of Realistic Medicine. *BJ Psych Bulletin* 43 (1) 32–4.

Thomson,L (2021) NHS Scotland Forensic Network: Response to COVID-19. Talk given online at Forensic Faculty of Royal College of Psychiatrists. Annual Conference 4 March 2021.

Thomson,L, Bogue,J, Humphreys,M, Owens,D and Johstone,E (1997) The State Hospital Survey: A Description of Psychiatric Patients in Conditions of Special Security in Scotland. *Journal of Forensic Psychiatry* 8: 263–84.

Thomson,LDG (2010) Personality Disorder and Mental Health Legislation in the UK: Commentary on . . . Personality Disorder and the Mental Health Act 1983 (Amended). *Advances in Psychiatric Treatment* 16 (5) 336–8.

Tracy,DK (2020) Keeping the Brain in Mind: Why Neuroscience Matters to 21st Century Psychiatrists. *BJ Psych Advances* 26 (6) 331–2.

Tuddenham,L and Baird,J (2007) The Risk Management Authority in Scotland and the Forensic Psychiatrist as Risk Assessor. *Psychiatric Bulletin* 31 (5) 164–6.

Tully,J, Cappai,A, Lally,J and Fotiadou,M (2019) Follow-up Study of 6.5 Years of Admissions to a UK Female Medium Secure Forensic Psychiatric Unit. *BJ Psych Bulletin* 43 (2) 54–7.

Tully,J, Cullen,AE, Hearn,D and Fahy,T (2016) Service Evaluation of Electronic Monitoring (GPS 'Tracking') in a Medium Secure Unit. *Journal of Forensic Psychiatry and Psychology* 27 (2) 169–76.

Tully,J, Hearn,D and Fahy,T (2014) Can Electronic Monitoring (GPS 'Tracking') Enhance Risk Management in Psychiatry? *British Journal of Psychiatry* 205 (2) 83–5.

Turner,T and Salter,M (2008) Forensic Psychiatry and General Psychiatry: Re-examining the Relationship. *Psychiatric Bulletin* 32 (1) 2–6.

Uppal,G and McMurran,M (2009) Recorded Incidents in a High-Secure Hospital: A Descriptive Analysis. *Criminal Behaviour and Mental Health* 19 (4) 265–76.

Van der Schaaf,PS, Dusseldorp,E, Keuning,FM, Janssen, WA and Noorthoorn,EO (2013) Impact of the Physical Environment of Psychiatric Wards on the Use of Seclusion. *British Journal of Psychiatry* 202 (2) 142–9.

Van Veen,MM, Karsten,J, Verkes,RJ and Lancel,M (2020) Sleep Quality is Associated with Aggression in Forensic Psychiatric Patients, Independent of General Psychopathology. *Journal of Forensic Psychiatry and Psychology* 31 (5) 699–713.

Vollm,BA, Chadwick,K, Abdelrazak,T and Smith,J (2012) Prescribing of Psychotropic Medication for Personality Disordered Patients in Secure Forensic Settings. *Journal of Forensic Psychiatry and Psychology* 23 (2) 200–16.

Vollm,B, Edworth,R, Holley,J, Talbot,E, Majid,S and Duggan,C (2017) A Mixed-Methods Study Exploring the Characteristics and Needs of Long-Stay Patients in High and Medium Secure Units in England: Implications for Service Organisation. *Health Services Delivery Research.* pp. 5–11.

Walker,H and Tulloch,L (2020) A 'Necessary Evil': Staff Perspectives of Soft Restraint Kit Use in a High-Security Hospital. *Frontiers in Psychiatry* 11: 357.

Walker,K, Griffiths,C, Yates,J and Vollm,B (2021) Service Provision for Older Forensic Mental Health Patients: A Scoping Review of the Literature. *Journal of Forensic Psychiatry and Psychology* 32 (1) 29–50.

Walker,T, Shaw,J, Edge,D, Senior,J, Sutton,M, Meacock,R, et al. (2019) A Qualitative Study of Contemporary Secure Mental Health Services: Women Service Users' Views in England. *Journal of Forensic Psychiatry and Psychology* 30 (5) 836–53.

White,O, Hill,SA, Coleman,R and Delmage,E (2017) Effect of Clozapine on Rates of Risk Incidents and Functioning in Female Adolescents with a Diagnosis of Severe Emerging Emotionally Unstable Personality Disorder. *Journal of Forensic Psychiatry and Psychology* 28 (6) 737–52.

Wilkinson,G (2019) Bartholomew the Englishman: On the Properties of Things – Wikipedia of the Middle Ages. *British Journal of Psychiatry* 215 (5) 635.

Wilson,S and Argyropoulis,S (2012) Sleep in Schizophrenia: Time for Closer Attention. *British Journal of Psychiatry* 200 (4) 273–4.

Wilson,S, Murray,K, Harris,M and Brown,M (2012) Psychiatric In-Patients, Violence and the Criminal Justice System. *The Psychiatrist* 36 (2) 41–4.

Winder,B, Lievesley,R, Kaul,A, Elliott,HJ, Thorne,K and Hocken,K (2014) Preliminary Evaluation of the Use of Pharmacological Treatment with Convicted Sexual Offenders Experiencing High Levels of Sexual Preoccupation, Hypersexuality and/or Sexual Compulsivity. *Journal of Forensic Psychiatry and Psychology* 25 (2) 176–94.

Withers,J (2008) Cognitive Analytic Therapy (CAT): A Therapy in a Medium Secure Hospital for a Mentally Disordered Offender with a Personality Disorder. *British Journal of Forensic Practice* 10 (3) 24–32.

Women in Special Hospitals (2000) *Consultation with Women Patients in Secure Mental Health Settings. Report on Independent Evaluation.* London. WISH.

Yacoub,E, Hall,I and Bernal,J (2008) Secure In-Patient Services for People with Learning Disability: Is the Market Serving the User Well? *Psychiatric Bulletin* 32 (6) 205–7.

Yakeley,J (2018) Psychodynamic Approaches to Violence. *BJ Psych Advances* 24 (2) 83–92.

Yakeley,J and Wood,H (2014) Paraphilias and Paraphilic Disorders: Diagnosis, Assessment and Management. *Advances in Psychiatric Treatment* 20 (3) 193–201.

Yorston,G and Taylor,PJ (2009) Older Patients in an English High Security Hospital: A Qualitative Study of the Experiences and Attitudes of Patients Aged 60 years and Over and Their Care Staff in Broadmoor Hospital. *Journal of Forensic Psychiatry and Psychology* 20 (2) 255–67.

Young,C, Brady,J, Iqbal,N and Browne,F (2009) Prosecution of Physical Assaults by Psychiatric In-Patients in Northern Ireland. *Psychiatric Bulletin* 33 (11) 416–19.

Chapter 3

National Standards and Good Practice

Stephen Dye

Introduction

Although much has changed since the previous edition of this book, the underlying principles of providing the correct care to the right patient at the best time remain. In order to perform this, robust standards must underpin the framework within which clinicians work. Such benchmarks should be accurate, meaningful and accessible to clinicians, patients and carers alike.

Over time there have been many standards, policies and guidelines that impact psychiatric intensive and low secure care. A multitude of organisations, both statutory and non-statutory, have developed these. The documents have various aims; some are specifically orientated towards practices prevalent within PICUs, a good example of which includes guidance for the management of disturbed behaviour (NICE, 2015), whilst others have a broader focus within psychiatry but can apply within most subspecialities, like the Mental Health Act 1983 (MHA) Code of Practice (Department of Health and Social Care, 2015). Some led to policy development, others to practice guidance, and a few may seem aspirational and challenging to meet within day-to-day practice. Policies are designed to be followed at all times but could well be inappropriate in specific clinical situations. For example, Figure 3.1 shows improper use of a clinical policy developed within initial COVID-19 pandemic stages (a man with no air entry/exit via mouth/nose who, due to policy, was wearing a face mask).

Good clinical practice must be the base from which to develop policies and guidance. This chapter outlines clinical standards designed by clinicians within the National Association of Psychiatric Intensive Care and Low Secure Units (NAPICU) (NAPICU, 2014) and points to some other relevant advice and guidance.

Development of PICU Standards

Publication of the first UK National Minimum Standards (NMS) (Department of Health, 2002) gave clinicians, managers and commissioners a framework to deliver high-quality services and care to some of the most severely and acutely unwell patients treated by the mental health system. Developed by a PICU and low secure practice development network (consisting of a multidisciplinary group of professionals and user representatives from around the United Kingdom), they gave general good practice guidance for psychiatric intensive care and low secure services.

Subsequently, commissioning arrangements further separated PICUs from low secure services, the latter lying within forensic psychiatry instead of general adult psychiatric services. To reflect this, in 2012, NAPICU worked with the Department of Health to produce a draft good practice commissioning guide in the clinical area of psychiatric intensive care. This highlighted a need to revise the clinical standards to reflect up-to-date clinical processes and set the clinical framework for the upcoming decades. Therefore in 2014, NAPICU (a multidisciplinary organisation with user and carer representation) produced revised standards which reflected changes and developments within psychiatric intensive care (NAPICU, 2014).

Format of National Minimum Standards

The NMS supply an all-encompassing framework on which to base services; they provide transparency regarding expectations as to what should be delivered and give guidance on how to provide care in a challenging area of psychiatric practice.

The document offers clear operational definitions of both psychiatric intensive and low secure care.

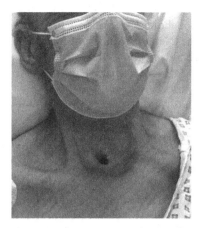

Figure 3.1 Inappropriate application of a policy: 'You must wear a mask . . .'

A mutually agreed definition leads to service operation consistency and is the most crucial factor for the efficiency of such services. It is essential to define roles within the framework of psychiatric care provision in a locally sensitive fashion. Failure to do so is an invitation to potential poor practice. The interface between acute psychiatry, intensive care, long-term and low secure services, intensive rehabilitation and forensic psychiatry must be straightforward. The definitions provided by the NMS go some way to address this.

Service definitions constitute the first of 21 sections (see Box 3.1). Following these, the references and a list of contributors, there are also two appendices: one provides a specific list of topics necessary for staff training and education, and the other provides standards for practice within places of safety (aka, Section 136 suites) when a PICU operationally oversees them.

The structure of each section is akin to the previous NMS version; each divided into:

- the rationale for developing standards of that nature
- standards pertaining to that topic
- good practice guidance surrounding the topic

Within each of these subheadings, there are numerical references that ensure easy auditing and communication. This arrangement gives every reader a simple reference point with which to convey information to others. For example, standard 12.2.1 states that 'Staff supervision should occur at a minimum of once every four weeks or more frequently as per professional guidance'.

Box 3.1 Sections of the PICU National Minimum Standards

1. Definitions
2. Admission criteria
3. Core interventions
4. Multidisciplinary team service structure and personnel
5. Operations and clinical leadership
6. PICU core pathways
7. Physical environment
8. Patient involvement
9. Carer involvement
10. Documentation
11. Ethnicity, culture and gender
12. Supervision
13. Liaison with other agencies
14. Policies and procedures
15. Clinical audit and monitoring
16. Staff training
17. Continuing professional development
18. Security and risk assessment
19. PICU support infra structure
20. Other types of psychiatric intensive care
21. Staffing levels

Individual standards within the NMS also lead to clarification of practice issues in many different areas, and these are addressed further within the document. Many of the topics are covered elsewhere in this book (e.g. physical environment, multidisciplinary working, liaison with other agencies). Perhaps one of the most challenging standards to produce was one that many clinicians and some service managers had thought was an oversight from the previous version of the NMS: actual nursing staff numbers required. This is a challenging and somewhat 'thorny' issue, but the guidance gives an explicit recommendation based upon clinical and operational experience in standard 12.2.11 (see Box 3.2).

Other Guidance

As stated in this chapter's introduction, there has been the publication of many different guidance documents that provide standards. After the revised NMS, NAPICU itself published other standards and guidance.

Box 3.2 PICU National Minimum Standards: Nursing Staffing Levels

- The nursing staff establishment on PICUs should be at least one third higher than on general acute psychiatric wards (weighted per bed).
- On each shift, a third of the nursing staff should be qualified, and no less than two per shift.
- As an example, minimum shift staff numbers for 10 patients in a male PICU should not fall below six for the early and late shift, and four for the night shift. These numbers should not include management and other specific therapy staff.

These included collaborating with other recognised expert agencies to produce:

- The joint British Association of Pharmacology (BAP) and NAPICU 'Evidence-based consensus guidelines for the clinical management of acute disturbance: De-escalation and rapid tranquillisation' (Patel et al., 2018).
- The NAPICU and Design in Mental Health Network (DIMHN) 'Design Guidance for Psychiatric Intensive Care Units' (NAPICU and DIMHN, 2017).

Also, following the revision of the Mental Health Act Code of Practice (Department of Health, 2015), there appeared to be confusion regarding the definition and regulation of seclusion. Clinical staff working on PICUs raised several questions concerning:

- Definition of seclusion not involving a patient locked alone in a room
- In the absence of a seclusion room with a locked door, the point at which seclusion monitoring would begin
- Understanding of long-term segregation and its interface with seclusion monitoring

The NAPICU executive team consulted with the Department of Health and CQC and subsequently produced a position statement which clarified matters (NAPICU, 2016b). It defines 'Traditional Seclusion' and an 'Extra Care Area' and how this and the care provided within it fits within seclusion and long-term segregation and associated monitoring within both processes.

As mentioned within the NMS (chapter 20), the model of care in general adult PICUs has evolved into other specialties such as medium security and child and adolescent PICUs. Further minimum standards

have been/are planned to be developed for these (always produced collaboratively, with a wide range of stakeholders). The 'National Minimum Standards for Psychiatric Intensive Care Units for Young People' (NAPICU, 2015) is formatted in a similar way to the standards for adults and provides standards of care for patients younger than 18 years who are admitted to a PICU setting. Clinical challenges presented by young people cared for in PICUs and the variability of service provision underlined the need for agreed and standardised care for the young people in such restrictive environments. As stated within the forward: 'Through addressing standards for referral, assessment and admission, with clear care and treatment planning, ensuring full young person and carer participation through to safe discharge, these standards also encompass management of risk and the importance of the built and relational environment together with the best evidence base for medicine optimisation and psychological therapies.' The standards help ensure the highest quality of care for young people in child and adolescent PICUs and enable provider organisations to define and organise services.

It is not only clinicians or patients who need access to standards and guidance. Often those who commission such services do so in the absence of clinical experience and expertise. Thus, in collaboration with the Mental Health Commissioners Network, NAPICU developed further appropriate 'Guidance for Commissioners of Psychiatric Intensive Care', which provides relevant detail to help (NAPICU, 2016a). These are intended to support and enable, and not to be an additional burden to those in commissioning or providing services. It does this by, amongst other things, providing examples and giving guidance to support commissioning decisions on potential service reconfiguration for PICUs, set out a model of care, establish service principles governing the overall approach to the provision of a safe environment and by advocating key performance indicators for operation and quality of care delivery.

Of course, other organisations in the United Kingdom have produced relevant guidance for use within a PICU setting. Perhaps the most appropriate guidance for services caring for individuals forcibly detained in hospital (in the United Kingdom, under provisions of the Mental Health Act) is the Mental Health Act Code of Practice (Department of Health, 2015). Given the restrictions imposed by a PICU setting, all patients admitted should be appropriately legally detained. Thus, the Code of Practice provides a set of standards that should be adhered to. It ensures that anyone experiencing mental disorder and being treated under the Act gets the right care, treatment and support. It states that all patients, including those who may present with behavioural disturbance, should receive treatment in a safe and therapeutic environment. It also provides guidance for providers, professionals and practitioners on the particular issues related to managing disturbed behaviour which may present a risk to the patient or to others. The guidance affirms that any restrictive interventions (e.g. restraint, seclusion and segregation) must be undertaken only in a manner that is compliant with human rights. As described previously, some clinicians found the specifics describing exact methods to be used in such situations to be unclear and thus NAPICU produced a position statement clarifying details (NAPICU, 2016a).

Although the Code of Practice itself is not statutory guidance in treating those detained under the Mental Health Act, it describes legislative functions and duties. The Code also assists those responsible for inspecting or monitoring the quality of services, including statutory inspectors (such as the Care Quality Commission in the United Kingdom), commissioners and local authorities. Departures from the Code could give rise to legal challenges, thus any divergence should be clearly recorded. It states that courts will scrutinise such reasons to ensure that there is sufficiently convincing justification in the circumstances. This was demonstrated in the case of a patient at Ashworth high secure hospital who challenged legality of the seclusion policy. The House of Lords judgement stated that the Code of Practice guidance 'should be given great weight': 'It is not instruction, but it is much more than mere advice which an addressee is free to follow or not as it chooses. It is guidance which any hospital should consider with great care, and from which it should depart only if it has cogent reasons for doing so' (Munjaz v United Kingdom, no. 2913/06, 44 § 2, ECHR, 2012) Another guidance document especially relevant to PICU is the National Institute for Health and Care Excellence's (NICE) guide NG10: 'Violence and aggression: short term management in mental health, health and community settings' (NICE, 2015). This replaced a previous version (CG25) (NICE, 2005) and will be updated according to

protocol. It covers principles for managing violence and aggression, including anticipating, preventing and managing it both within mental health and other settings. Within the United Kingdom, organisations commissioning and providing services are expected to take recommendations within NICE clinical guidelines into account when planning and delivering services. NICE has produced many clinical guidelines and meeting them demonstrates to regulators that good care is being practised. Thus, the demonstration of auditing services with NICE guidelines as a benchmark is crucial. Sometimes this is hard to effectively validate in a straightforward fashion as, by the very nature of the guidelines, some things are left to clinical judgement. For example, using 'the least intrusive level of observation necessary' may appear quite vague. It highlights the need for consistency across services and within the training of staff and the NMS may help achieve this.

There are organisations and societies interested in clinical practices that occur within mental health inpatient settings and particularly in PICUs. Some have produced guidance that clinicians and managers should take heed of. One project that was developed by a charity led by an inspirational user of services was called 'Star Wards' (www.starwards.org.uk/download-star-wards/). This gave each ward practical ideas for improving the daily experiences and treatment outcomes for mental health inpatients and developed a standard that introducing these ideas could be measured against. A different guideline developed by practitioners that focuses upon processes is entitled 'Safe Wards' (www.safewards.net/). The process encourages staff and patients on wards to work together to reduce conflict and containment as much as possible. It portrays a model with six domains identifying the critical influences over conflict and containment rates: the patient community, patient characteristics, the regulatory framework, the staff team, the physical environment and outside hospital. It then describes specific interventions that if implemented can help modify the domains. Interventions include having 'clear mutual expectations' and using 'positive words'. These standards can easily be incorporated within a PICU setting to improve the care provided and care outcomes for patients within them.

Another example of a charity that develops standards is the Restraint Reduction Network (https://restraintreductionnetwork.org/). This has a vision to help services reduce reliance on restrictive practices and hopes to achieve this by sharing learning as well as developing quality standards and practical tools that support reduction. It has developed training standards for use that ensure training promotes human rights and supports cultural change necessary to reduce reliance on restrictive practices (rather than focus on technical skills purely).

This section has demonstrated that standards for use within a PICU service can originate from many sources. Some encompass the totality of PICU, whilst others encompass only a proportion, and a few are statutory, but most have implications upon practice. A number are appropriate to monitor the service, and a few provide guidance for improving quality. The next section addresses quality within PICUs.

Quality Improvement

Quality improvement is central to health care, and the PICU is no different. The term refers to a systematic attempt to strive for continuous improvement in patients' quality of care and outcomes.

Quality in healthcare, defined by the *NHS Next Stage Review* (Department of Health, 2008), has the following criteria:

- safety: doing no harm to patients
- experience of care: this should be characterised by compassion, dignity and respect
- effectiveness of care: preventing people from dying prematurely, enhancing the quality of life, and helping people recover following ill health episodes

Quality improvement has been described in several ways. For instance, the Royal College of General Practitioners (Royal College of General Practitioners, 2015) has a lengthy definition: 'a commitment to continually improving the quality of healthcare focusing on the preferences and needs of the people who use services. It encompasses a set of values (including self-reflection, shared learning, partnership, leadership, the use of theory, and understanding of context) and a set of methods (including measurement, understanding variation, cyclical change, benchmarking and a set of tools and techniques)'. However, a more succinct definition is: 'the systematic use of methods and tools to continuously improve patients' outcomes and the patient experience'.

Although there are many different approaches to quality improvement, there is no evidence that any one is better than the others. Instead, it is having a systematic process and consistent application of that process which is essential (Ross and Naylor, 2017). There are some fundamental principles common to approaches which include:

- Staff training in systems
- Collection and use of appropriate data
- Involvement of all staff in contribution and action of improvement ideas
- Using smaller scale tests of improvement strategies as learning opportunities
- Maintaining a focus on the needs and experiences of individuals served by the system (Ham et al., 2016)

Quality improvement goes above and beyond traditional management, target setting and policymaking. It uses the subject matter expertise of people closest to the issue (especially staff and service users/carers) to identify potential solutions and test them. Figure 3.2 depicts a useful illustration of the quality improvement cycle.

'Context and culture' refers to having a group that is keen to experiment and supportive of trying something new. This is essential to enable change to occur and to be sustained.

The figure depicts various steps:

- Diagnose – assess the area of your practice needing improvement and generate baseline data
- Plan and test – decide the aims, methods and monitoring of the change

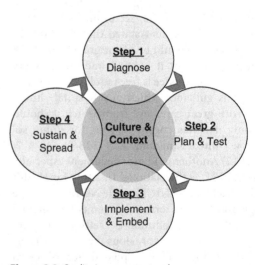

Figure 3.2 Quality improvement cycle

- Implement and embed – make any successes part of your systems or processes
- Sustain and spread – consider how aims or intervention can continue to be implemented on a larger scale, if appropriate, and how the conclusions can be made more widely available

Quality improvement can be (inter)national, specialty or individually service based.

National

A national survey discovered variances in the physical monitoring of patients who had received rapid tranquillisation (Loynes et al., 2013) (*Diagnose*). Subsequently, around the time of the joint BAP/NAPICU consensus guidelines pertaining to rapid tranquillisation, the Prescribing Observatory for Mental Health (POMH) within the Royal College of Psychiatrists' Centre for Quality Improvement (CCQI) decided to perform a national clinical audit upon rapid tranquillisation and the subsequent physical monitoring of patients who had been subjected to it. This was with a view to quality improvement (*Plan and Test*). The subsequent publication of the POMH/NAPICU guidelines also coincided with distributing further information from the CCQI to organisations upon the need for physical monitoring (*Implement and Embed*). The audit was published (Paton et al., 2019) and copies sent to participating organisations (*Sustain and Spread*). This found that physical health monitoring still did not reach the minimum recommended level in most episodes and postulated reasons why and speculated on potential barriers to implementation (*Diagnose*).

Specialty

COVID-19 presented challenges for the care and engagement of mental health patients presenting with acute disturbance and who are also a possible infection risk. Of particular concern are those who are experiencing acute disturbance and represent COVID-19 infection risk to others or are in a high-risk group for infection or are in a ward that is 'locked down' or 'self-isolating' (*Diagnose*). NAPICU produced guidance for staff and organisations in a timely fashion (March 2020) (NAPICU, 2020) (*Plan and Test*). This was publicised and distributed to member PICUs (*Implement and Embed*) and a specific forum established. In conjunction with the virus, the guidance continued to evolve and was revised on many occasions (*Sustain and Spread*).

Unit

Quality improvement and clinical audit go hand in hand, and the NMS provides standards that can easily be audited. Indeed, it has a specific chapter on clinical auditing and monitoring. Individual units demonstrate quality improvement at NAPICU events, and there are many published papers within the *Journal of Psychiatric Intensive Care* that attest to such progress. Perhaps a good example is the development of a Psychiatric Intensive Care/Low Secure Governance Network which focused on four specific key areas: multidisciplinary working, diversity, service user/carer involvement and responding to emergencies. Using the NMS as a benchmark, and through project working, positive changes in services for patients, with demonstrable benefits via a system of audit and review, were demonstrated (Dye et al., 2005). Such a project's collaborative nature allowed PICUs/low secure units (LSUs) to share experiences and difficulties and plan improvements drawing on expertise from both within and outside the network. Through individual units demonstrating successful and sustainable improvements to patient care and sharing these with other units in a similar position, the Governance Network helped in not only monitoring standards but also disseminating positive change occurring as a result of their development.

Conclusion

A clear and defined system of operating within any environment fosters good practice and confidence. The NMS provide a template that aids in developing such a system: they demystify the PICU role, which leads to transparency of practice and encourages self-critical and innovative methods of working rather than reinforcing traditional views of what constitutes PICU practice. The NMS are crucial for each unit to improve and monitor their own ways of working. The NMS are guidelines to 'inform' practice and not to 'instruct' it, but they were developed with the best interests of both patients and staff in mind and should be commended for this. There is something for any stakeholder or staff member associated with PICUs to take from the NMS (this is a testament to the wide-ranging consultation and involvement of different groups of individuals in their formation). For instance, junior staff members may wish to concentrate on admission criteria and documentation, commissioners of services would find the physical environment of units and personnel service structure useful, and clinical governance departments can be guided by the section on clinical audit and monitoring. The NMS thus promote psychiatric intensive care and provide a foundation from which to base good practice and quality improvement within any such unit.

It is heartening to note that the most recent PICU and low secure services study (Pereira et al., 2021) revealed improvements in essential areas of practice and care standards. For example, one survey demonstrated that only 4% of PICUs were willing to admit patients not detained by law (compared to 58% in a previous survey) (Pereira et al., 2006). Also, units that receive input from psychology staff increased by 60%. Despite many other improvements, there remain characteristics that display diversity between PICUs. For instance, only 54% had a dedicated area for children/family visits, and only 84% had a dedicated consultant providing responsible clinician duties.

As psychiatric services continue to mature and expand, they must appreciate the fluid nature of standards informed by quality improvement. With good practice and quality remaining at the top of the agenda, 'our target now is to ensure that as this specialism [psychiatric intensive care] grows, it is not an ivory tower but bridges with other services and countries' (Pereira and Dalton, 2006). Further development of robust crisis, home treatment and outreach services will lead to robust intensive community services. The focus of psychiatric intensive care perhaps should shift away from the physical environment in which care is given to the specific type of care provided to the most unwell individuals treated within psychiatric services.

Not only must services recognise changeable standards, but they also need to account for 'marketplace' development of sometimes ill-defined services. Development of facilities that do not clearly describe the type of individual they undertake to serve can only be detrimental to patients and practitioners alike (Dye et al., 2016). Sometimes, although practitioners well understand the clinical characteristics of patients serviced by PICUs, these characteristics are not accurately captured by the data collected. This could be because the methods used to capture clinical severity and patient need are ineffective and possibly invalid (Dye, 2017). This will lead to misunderstanding from a managerial perspective and perhaps to funding disparities when developing or improving services in the future. Despite advances in treatment for psychiatrically unwell individuals, there will always remain those whose illness severity and acuity will indicate the need for psychiatric intensive care. This needs to be clearly defined to enable them to receive the most appropriate care of the best quality in the most suitable environment.

In conjunction with other available guidance, it is evident that the NMS have been significant in establishing and highlighting the standards to which all PICUs should practice. It is essential that this valuable document is used appropriately in conjunction with other relevant guidance and that, in the spirit of quality improvement, standards of care continue to improve.

References

Department of Health (2002) National Minimum Standards for General Adult Services in Psychiatric Intensive Care Units (PICU) and Low Secure Environments. In Pereira,S and Clinton,C (eds.), *Mental Health Policy Implementation Guide*. London: Department of Health.

Department of Health (2008) *High Quality Care for All: NHS Next Stage Review Final Report*. London: Department of Health.

Department of Health (2015) *Mental Health Act 1983: Code of Practice*. London: Department of Health.

Dye,S, Johnston,A, and Pereira,S (2005) The National Psychiatric Intensive Care Governance Network 2004–2005. *Journal of Psychiatric Intensive Care* 1 (2) 97–104.

Dye,S, Smyth,L and Pereira,S (2016) 'Locked Rehabilitation': A Need for Clarification. *BJPsych Bulletin* 40 (1) 1–4.

Dye,S (2017) Can Mental Health Clusters Be Replaced By Patient Typing? *British Journal of Health Care Management* 23 (5) 229–37.

Ham,CM, Alderwick,H, Dunn,P and McKenna,H (2017) *Delivering Sustainability and Transformation Plans*. London: Kings Fund.

Loynes,B, Innes,J, and Dye,S (2013) Assessment of Physical Monitoring Following Rapid Tranquillisation: A National Survey. *Journal of Psychiatric Intensive Care* 9 (2) 85–90.

Munjaz v United Kingdom, no. 2913/06, 44 § 2, ECHR 2012 [Online]. www.globalhealthrights.org/wp-content/uploads/2013/02/ECtHR-2012-Munjaz-v-United-Kingdom.pdf.

National Association of Psychiatric Intensive Care and Low Secure Units (NAPICU) (2014) *National Minimum Standards for Psychiatric Intensive Care in General Adult Services*. Glasgow: NAPICU. https://napicu.org.uk/wp-content/uploads/2014/12/NMS-2014-final.pdf.

National Association of Psychiatric Intensive Care and Low Secure Units (NAPICU) (2015) *National Minimum Standards for Psychiatric Intensive Care Units for Young People.* Glasgow: NAPICU. https://napicu.org.uk/wp-con tent/uploads/2014/08/CAMHS_PICU_NMS_final_Au g_2015_cx.pdf.

National Association of Psychiatric Intensive Care and Low Secure Units (NAPICU) (2016a) *Guidance for Commissioners of Psychiatric Intensive Care Units (PICU).* Glasgow: NAPICU. https://napicu.org.uk/wp-content/uplo ads/2016/04/Commissioning_Guidance_Apr16.pdf.

National Association of Psychiatric Intensive Care and Low Secure Units (NAPICU) (2016b) *NAPICU Position on the Monitoring, Regulation and Recording of the Extra Care Area, Seclusion and Long-Term Segregation Use in the Context of the Mental Health Act 1983: Code of Practice (2015).* Glasgow: NAPICU. https://napicu.org.uk/wp-con tent/uploads/2016/10/NAPICU-Seclusion-Position-Statem ent.pdf.

National Association of Psychiatric Intensive Care and Low Secure Units (NAPICU) (2020) *Managing Acute Disturbance in the Context of COVID-19.* Glasgow: NAPICU. https://napicu.org.uk/wp-content/uploads/2020/ 12/NAPICU-Guidance_rev5_15_Dec.pdf.

National Association of Psychiatric Intensive Care and Low Secure Units (NAPICU) and Design in Mental Health Network (DIHMN) (2017) *Design Guidance for Psychiatric Intensive Care Units.* Glasgow: NAPICU. https://napicu.org .uk/wp-content/uploads/2017/05/Design-Guidance-for-Psy chiatric-Intensive-Care-Units-2017.pdf.

National Institute for of Health and Care Excellence (NICE) (2005) *Violence: Short-Term Management for Over 16s in Psychiatric and Emergency Departments.* London: NICE.

National Institute of Health and Care Excellence (NICE) (2015) *Violence and Aggression: Short-Term Management in Mental Health, Health and Community Settings [NG10].* London: NICE. www.nice.org.uk/guidance/ng10.

Patel,MX, Sethi,FN, Barnes,TR, Dix,R, Dratcu,L, Fox,B, et al. (2018) Joint BAP NAPICU Evidence-Based Consensus Guidelines for the Clinical Management of Acute Disturbance: De-escalation and Rapid Tranquillisation. *Journal of Psychopharmacology* **32** (6) 601–40.

Paton,C, Adams,C, Dye,S, et al. (2019) Physical Health Monitoring after Rapid Tranquillisation: Clinical Practice in UK Mental Health Services. *Therapeutic Advances in Psychopharmacology* 9: 1–12.

Pereira,S and Dalton,D (2006) Integration and Specialism: Complementary Not Contradictory. *Journal of Psychiatric Intensive Care* 2 (1) 1–5.

Pereira,S, Dawson,P and Sarsam,M (2006) The National Survey of PICU and Low Secure Services: 2. Unit Characteristics. *Journal of Psychiatric Intensive Care* **2** (1) 13–19.

Pereira,SM, Walker,L and Dye,S (2021) A National Survey of Psychiatric Intensive Care, Low Secure and Locked Rehabilitation Units. *Mental Health Practice.*

Ross,S and Naylor,C (2017) *Quality Improvement in Mental Health.* London: Kings Fund.

Royal College of General Practitioners (2015) *Quality Improvement for General Practice: A Guide for GPs and the Whole Practice Team.* London: Royal College of General Practitioners. https://elearning.rcgp.org.uk/pluginfile.php/ 174184/mod_book/chapter/519/RGCP-QI-Guide-260216% 20%285%29.pdf.

Chapter 4

Commissioning and Developing a PICU

Thomas Kearney and Mathew Page

Introduction

This chapter provides an overview of the commissioning and development of a psychiatric intensive care unit (PICU).

In this context commissioning can be defined as:

the process of assessing needs, planning and prioritising, purchasing and monitoring health services, to get the best health outcomes. (NHS, 2022)

Once the need for a PICU has been established, the work of designing and building begins, but the physical environment is only one aspect of the task. Creation of policies and procedures, recruitment of the right personnel and establishment of processes to ensure the quality of the service are as equally important as the building.

This volume provides a wealth of guidance on what constitutes a good PICU and this chapter describes the beginning of the journey.

Commissioning

It is a common misconception that commissioning is merely involved in the initial understanding of demand, funding and setting up of services. This is only partly true because to be truly effective commissioning needs to continue to run in parallel with a service provision.

Good commissioning of a PICU should be seen as a delivery and performance monitoring function which understands the changing nature and evolution of needs over time. The commissioning function should modify funding, infrastructure and performance measurement and shape the future service in line with changing needs so that the service fully meets the demand profile. Therefore, it is imperative that commissioning is a facilitative and organic process.

Generally speaking, any PICU provision will have a commissioning organisation. This may be government or an independent body with a mandate to independently contract PICU services. Commissioning will create an understanding of the need, first and foremost on a demographic demand profile. Next, there will need to be consideration of national clinical standards required, such as the National Association of Psychiatric Intensive Care and Low Secure Units (NAPICU) National Minimum Standards (NMS) (NAPICU, 2014), and estates needs based on standards such as the Design Guidance for Psychiatric Intensive Care Units (NAPICU Design in Mental Health Network, 2017).

The cost of provision is then established based on the following four clear factors:

- Demand profile and need
- Clinical standards required
- Human resources required
- Estates

Once the cost has been established, this service may then be tendered in line with requirements for fair and open business competition laws within the country, such as European and UK procurement regulations (Official Journal of the European Union, 2022)

Once an open and transparent tendering process has been completed and service delivery has commenced, commissioning the PICU service is an ongoing process. In terms of commissioning, the PICU may be perceived as straightforward with relatively low financial envelope compared to some other services (such as community mental health services). For these reasons, there is a danger that a single PICU may not receive the commissioning focus required for it to be properly considered or understood. From a commissioning perspective, it is strongly advised that the PICU demand profile is constantly evaluated so that the population's needs can be met.

Assessing the Population for a PICU

The following steps should be taken to establish demand profile:

1. If a PICU does not exist within a given acute mental health pathway, then the first port of call should be public health reviews. These should help to establish the mental illness prevalence within the population that the PICU will be expected to service. Within the given demographic area, the mental health needs should then be projected forward for at least the next decade. This can be based on several factors, including population growth, age, employment and so on. For example, in the United Kingdom, this is covered within Joint Strategic Needs Assessments (Department of Health and Social Care, 2022).

2. The second source of information which is equally important is the number of patients within the defined service area who have used a PICU within the last three years at any given time. It is very likely that these patients were sent out of area by the current provider(s) of mental health services without a PICU.

3. Third and more subjectively, but also equally important, is to involve the existing mental health service providers in a review of patients who needed support/interventions of the type that a PICU provides. Examples of PICU-type interventions include 1:1 level observation, seclusion (or other restrictive intervention), rapid tranquilisation, absconding prevention and so on. An assessment of the level of requirement for these interventions should be undertaken establishing needs during the course of the last two years. Finally, completing a process for establishing how many of these patients the general adult service consider would have benefited from a PICU if one were available in the area.

Using a Project Approach to Establish a PICU

The development of any new ward represents an infrequent opportunity to provide a significant improvement in the care of patients. A new physical environment is usually associated with a new clinical team and therefore new ways of providing better care and treatment. Delivering such a substantial task requires significant investment in every sense. In financial terms, this means investment in the salaries of the clinicians and administrators, the cost of enabling services and, most significantly, capital investment, that even in the case of a modest refurbishment, will often run into several million pounds.

Because of the opportunity this represents to do things better and the financial risks arising from it going wrong, considerable thought must be given to how the task will be orchestrated and by whom.

In most industries, it is now generally accepted that a tested project management methodology should be employed when investing significantly. There are several tools available, each of which have merits; whichever is chosen will generally be dependent on the strategy of the organisation and what methodology staff have been trained in.

Selecting a Commissioning Approach

Each jurisdiction will have approaches to macro level policy developments with recommended project management tools. It is advisable to spend time researching the current evidence and experience with using an approach most likely to suit the proposed development. Within the United Kingdom, National Health Service (NHS) England and NHS Improvement have published a comprehensive suite of documents to enable organisations to approach projects. It describes a six-stage approach:

1. Start out
2. Define and scope
3. Measure and understand
4. Design and plan
5. Implement
6. Handover and sustain (NHS England and NHS Improvement, 2021)

A project such as commissioning a new PICU is of a much greater scale and complexity than many other tasks a healthcare provider might approach. As such, the level of detail of documentation and rigour of assurance must be at a high level.

It is not possible to provide a full synopsis of project management within this chapter, however, there are a few key elements which are worth spotlighting.

Making the Business Case

All organisations will require a business case which may be used with external partners in order to justify the outlay and ensure the project is necessary and well-thought through.

There are several areas which require comprehensive analysis within a business case. The UK government standard template recommends consideration of five:

1. Strategic
2. Economic
3. Commercial
4. Financial
5. Management (Department for Digital, Culture, Media and Sport, 2017)

Taking a PICU Development Forward: Project Initiation Document

The content of the business case which should be comprehensive and relatively exhaustive will be useful in then developing a project initiation document (PID), which provides all the detail of the 'who/what/when/where/how' of getting the job done. NHS England and NHS Improvement provide a template of what should be included:

1. Project rationale
2. Project objectives
3. Costs and benefits
4. Project approach and work streams
5. Project plan – indicative timescales
6. Project management team structure and roles
7. Risks management (NHS England and NHS Improvement, 2021)

The PID will then form the basis of the project and should always be available for people to read and gather an overall summary of what is happening. Almost all projects are subject to some change (e.g. in relation to timelines or costs) and any alterations to the initial case and project summary need to be subject to the organisation's governance structure to ensure they are properly agreed upon.

Making Decisions

Different organisations will have various ways of delegating decision-making. In establishing a project to develop a new PICU, one of the most important initial duties is to assign roles and responsibilities.

A common structure would be for a single person to take overall charge, often referred to as a senior responsible officer (SRO), who will lead a project board which will have several work streams reporting to it. These would each be individually led and would include issues such as workforce, clinical model, building design and so on. Depending on the complexity of the task, any of the work streams could involve other subsets of activity.

A vital element of any project is defining where actual decisions are to be made. This is to distinguish between the governance functions (discussed further later in the chapter) of running a project and the actual executive decisions such as unit type, location and budget, which will be held elsewhere.

To this end, an SRO and project team will need to be clear on specific decision-making points and who has responsibility for them. Examples of decisions which would need to be made (based on recommendations from the experts within the project) would be workforce composition, clinical model and building design.

Quality Impact Assessment

Organisations will have structures and process for evaluating the viability and benefits of plans. One exercise that is usually undertaken is a quality impact assessment (QIA). This will include consideration of such factors as:

- Patient experience
- Patient safety
- Clinical quality (NHS Providers, 2015)

Other impact assessments that can be undertaken include equality and data protection. The role of these impact assessments, how they are considered and how they are endorsed should be clearly understood at the beginning of the project.

An important point here is to ensure that the project team is not left to unilaterally do the work and make the decisions. Whatever project method an organisation uses and whether it is subject to the NHS QIA approach or not, there must be a process whereby external scrutiny is applied and the decision is owned through the organisation up to its executive and non-executive board.

Making Progress

The adage that 'time is money' is as true in health care as in any other sector. It is vital that clear timelines are planned, the risks affecting them understood and appropriate mitigations considered. Any change in the pace of progress can lead to wasted labour costs and increased capital costs. In addition to these types of risks within the project itself, other indirect costs, reputational damage and most significantly patient confidence and experience can all be affected.

A rigorous and comprehensive project structure should ensure that all the objectives are met on time. If they are not, this must be escalated within the project and organisational structure.

For some frontline PICU clinicians who may be unfamiliar with project methodology, the process can at times seem laborious. This can even extend to feeling that the process is unnecessarily bureaucratic, however, the metaphor that a majority of resources should go into a building foundation before building the house should be remembered. Every piece of scrutiny, measuring and checking at the planning phase for a new PICU is likely to significantly reduce the risk of clinical or regulatory issues further down the line. Alongside this of course, the project team must ensure that processes add value and are efficient in achieving the outcome.

Designing and Developing the Physical Environment

The topic of PICU design is comprehensively covered elsewhere in this volume (Chapter 5), so will not be repeated here. The National Minimum Standards (NMS) (NAPICU, 2014) and Design Guidance for Psychiatric Intensive Care Units (NAPICU and Design in Mental Health Network, 2017) should be the basis of all design discussions and considerations.

Existing Estate and New Builds

Probably the most significant immediate issue is whether the opportunity is available for a new purpose-built building or whether the project team is expected to make use of an existing estate and oversee a refurbishment to create a PICU.

Where money is not a limiting factor, the preference would probably be for a new build, for pure ease of development. A refurbishment of perhaps a vacated acute or older peoples ward is not impossible but is likely to either be costly or result in compromises in the design. These calculations must be considered carefully. Depending on local variables, it can be more costly to develop an existing building than to create a new one.

Conversion versus New Builds

In the United Kingdom, a considerable amount of mental health inpatient provision is now around 30 years old, having replaced the old asylums, which were closed in the 1980s and 1990s. While three decades is not long in building terms, it is a considerable period in terms of mental health ward design. The theory of how we use space, available technology and changes in single-sex and infection control requirements mean that many buildings are no longer desirable as good quality clinical spaces.

Where a vacant estate is being considered, a comprehensive analysis against the NMS (NAPICU, 2014) must be undertaken to consider viability and any necessary compromises.

Where the costs of a new unit can run into millions of pounds, the availability of capital investment must be considered at the outset. The lifespan of the building will also need to be considered and, where possible, incorporating as much flexibility as possible is recommended to ensure the best potential for future innovations to be utilised.

Background to Opening a New Service

A programme of recruitment for the PICU should be enacted well in advance of the expected operational date. It is preferable that staff specifically apply for or show interest in working within the PICU rather than simply being redeployed or being 'required' to work in the PICU.

Any project structure should ensure that there are processes in place extending beyond the completion of the physical building work. While the tradespeople have been busy on the 'bricks and mortar' side of the project, other subsets of the project team are required to ensure the clinical model, policy and standard operating procedure (SOP) have been agreed upon.

In many respects, receiving the new building is just the start of the process of establishing a new PICU. As with any new service, the first weeks and months will be punctuated by issues, problems and learning. It is preferable that the new PICU team is directly involved in policy and procedure development well in advance of the service becoming operational.

Despite any pressure to the contrary, PICU leaders must ensure that the PICU development towards becoming operational is well paced and should ensure it is not expected to be fully operational immediately.

New buildings will often have minor 'snagging' issues of carpentry, plumbing and wiring, which can be problematic to fix/repair if the ward is full of patients, but perhaps more significantly, there will be learning from the way people begin to use the building and making sure that the procedures reflect this.

Simple issues like where meals are served from may seem minor but can often have an impact on patient safety and experience. A prudent approach of admitting patients gradually enables these issues to be tested and resolved.

The project plan should take account of this type of learning and incorporate review points for such issues as SOPs and workforce numbers and skill mix.

Testing a New PICU Build

There are examples of clinical staff and service leaders spending a few days living in a new build before it becomes fully operational. This process can be very effective in identifying areas that require addressing before the PICU becomes operational.

Developing the Operational Policy

A clear and defined care pathway describing exactly how a person enters and leaves a PICU is required. An operational policy should include a clear description of the stages of care including an outline of journeys which involve psychiatric intensive care. Further, it should also include a description of how the PICU supports the overall system, including its limitations.

The operational policy should be a clear document which controls how the PICU should work in relation to the rest of the system, that is, a reflection of its core purpose and the service specification which has been articulated by commissioning based on national clinical standards and the required capacity.

Moreover, the operational policy of the PICU should encompass the SOPs for admission, treatment and discharge from the PICU but also clear escalation to commissioning when there is an identified need which the PICU may not be able to meet.

Because of the intrinsic complexity associated with PICUs, the longer-term needs of patients together with any legal restrictions to their care and discharge must be understood within the operational policy framework. This should include the route to escalate clinical concerns when the placement is no longer appropriate.

Team Identification and Defining Induction Programme

All PICUs should have input from professionals in the following disciplines within the context of core team skills (NAPICU, 2014):

- Responsible clinician (often a consultant psychiatrist and a trainee psychiatric doctor)
- Nursing (a team of specialist inpatient nurses, both qualified nurses, healthcare support workers and assistant practitioners)
- Management (a manager and deputy with relevant clinical expertise)
- Occupational therapy (a specialist in psychiatric inpatient care)
- Psychology (a specialist clinical psychologist)
- Pharmacy (a specialist pharmacist with experience in acute psychiatric inpatient settings)
- Social work (access to a social worker to address holistic care needs)
- Activity, physical health and engagement (e.g. physiotherapist, sports therapist, dietician).

Team cohesion is an essential factor in the development of the team. Team skills should be developed in line with the needs of patients. Investment will be required in organisational development and 'team building' from an early stage of the project. Team skill set and the interventions required within a PICU should be outlined within the quality schedule of the contract for the PICU and then reflected throughout, including into individual professional development reviews and training budgets.

Induction Programme for a New Team

A staff induction programme, often of several weeks' duration, is required before the new PICU service becomes operational. This is an opportunity to test and become familiar with the building, further develop/promote ownership for the operation policy and for the team to become familiar with each other. A comprehensive induction programme can be very cost effective when compared to the costs of rectifying problems that have occurred because of a poorly prepared team.

The induction within the PICU should use the SOPs in highlighting admission, treatment and discharge and how the PICU works including service expectations, security and safety. Professionals working on the unit should be able to influence this induction process and its subsequent improvements, feeding into an evolutionary service provision.

The team should have an operational clinical culture which promotes the development of the service and offers the best possible care to patients. These services should promote good governance by engaging the overall team in such a way that every voice is heard, especially in relation to quality, safety and delivery issues.

The selection of the right staff, induction and team development are key to running a successful PICU.

Establishing Benchmarking, Performance and Outcome Measures

The aims of a PICU at the macro level are very straightforward: to support and care for patients in a safe and effective way in order that they can be transferred to an acute ward environment as soon as possible. However, a range of approaches can be used to ensure the highest standards are upheld.

'Benchmarking' (assessing against the activity of comparable services) is a common exercise undertaken by commissioners and providers to establish the effectiveness of a health care service. While there will be some local variation, data should include basic activity information, including admissions, discharges, average length of stay and numbers of serious incidents. This information can then be discussed more widely as care pathway issues, such as the interface with forensic services, are explored and developed.

Some specific issues may warrant attention at a given point in time. For instance, use of restrictive practices (such as restraint and seclusion) is a particular area where accurate data is essential. Properly understanding this information will inform a range of clinical and delivery discussions. High-functioning teams manage acuity and disturbance effectively and if managed well have lower incident rates. They also have lower turnover as the staff feel supported and happier in their work in the service.

Key Performance Indicators

While benchmarking compares services, any PICU should also have its own suite of key performance indicators (KPIs) which can be monitored at team, organisation and system levels, monitoring progress and improvement over time. There is a relatively limitless number of things that can be monitored as a KPI, however, these may fall into several broad areas.

Quality and Safety

- Clinical outcomes
- Patient feedback and satisfaction
- Incident rates
- Audits and quality control
- Use of restrictive practices

Workforce

- Staff support – Compliance with staff safety including rate of debriefs completed after all incidents
- Staff feedback – Support and active management intervention when there are issues in culture
- Turnover
- Recruitment and retention

Finance

- May best be considered as a cost per patient admission (total cost of running a PICU per year divided by number of admissions)

In the arena of mental health care, measures which apply to individual patients is an area of continual development. These measures will fall into one of three categories:

- Clinician-rated outcome measures
- Patient-rated outcome measures
- Patient-rated experience measures

These are scientifically validated tools which should be used to inform both the care of individuals and wider service delivery. In England, several core patient-rated experience measures are being agreed upon for use in community settings. While the PICU is not specifically included, a review of such tools as Recovering Quality of Life: ReQoL-10 (University of Sheffield, 2022) show that they may have benefit during all stages of the care pathway, including inpatient services.

Conclusion

This chapter introduced the commissioning and development of a PICU. While contexts may vary between nations and over time, the principles of establishing the need, using robust processes to develop a unit and long-term rigour to ensure quality apply everywhere.

This book provides clinicians, commissioners and managers with comprehensive considerations for providing the best possible service. In commissioning and developing a PICU it is anticipated that the full wealth of expertise and evidence base is used in order to ensure the best possible outcomes for those who use the service.

References

Department for Digital, Culture, Media and Sport (2017) Business Case Template. Gov.UK. www.gov.uk/govern ment/publications/libraries-alternative-delivery-models-to olkit/stage-6-business-case.

Department of Health and Social Care (2022) *Statutory Guidance on Joint Strategic Needs Assessments and Joint Health and Wellbeing Strategies*. https://assets.publishing.s ervice.gov.uk/government/uploads/system/uploads/attach ment_data/file/1099832/Statutory-Guidance-on-Joint-Strat egic-Needs-Assessments-and-Joint-Health-and-Wellbeing-Strategies-March-2013.pdf.

National Association of Psychiatric Intensive Care and Low Secure Units (NAPICU) (2014) *National Minimum Standards for Psychiatric Intensive Care in General Adult Services*. Glasgow: NAPICU. https://napicu.org.uk/wp-con tent/uploads/2014/12/NMS-2014-final.pdf.

National Association of Psychiatric Intensive Care and Low Secure Units (NAPICU) and Design in Mental Health Network (DIMHN) (2017) *Design Guidance for Psychiatric Intensive Care Units*. Glasgow: NAPICU. https://napicu.org .uk/wp-content/uploads/2017/05/Design-Guidance-for-Psyc hiatric-Intensive-Care-Units-2017.pdf.

National Health Service England (2022) What is Commissioning? www.england.nhs.uk/commissioning/wh at-is-commissioning/.

National Health Service England and National Health Service Improvement (2021) *Project Initiation Document*. www.england.nhs.uk/wp-content/uploads/2021/03/qsir-pr oject-initiation-document.pdf.

National Health Service England and National Health Service Improvement (2022) *Project Management Overview*. www.england.nhs.uk/wp-content/uploads/2022/02/qsir-pr oject-management-an-overview.pdf.

National Health Service Providers (2015) *Good Practice Quality Impact Assessment*. https://nhsproviders.org/media/ 1160/prepprog-good-practice-qias-2.pdf.

Official Journal of the European Union (2022) European & UK Procurement Regulations. ojeu.eu. www.ojeu.eu/Direc tives.aspx.

University of Sheffield (2022) Recovering Quality of Life (ReQoL) for Users of Mental Health Services. www .reqol.org.uk/p/overview.html.

PICU Design, Environment and Security

Roland Dix and Mathew Page

Introduction

Knowledge underpinning effective design and security of psychiatric intensive care units (PICUs) has developed significantly since the first and second editions of this book. In the second edition (Dix, 2001; Dix and Page, 2008), PICU design was considered in the context of the National Minimum Standards (NMS) for General Adult Services in Psychiatric Intensive Care Units and Low Secure environments (DOH, 2002). The NMS were later reviewed (NAPICU, 2014), this version then informing the comprehensive Design Guidance for Psychiatric Intensive Care Units (NAPICU and DIMHN, 2017).

Any book chapter such as this must recognise that the evidence, technology and other driving factors for PICU development will change over time. It is not therefore advisable to set out a list of standards to be met, as those could quickly become obsolete. In this chapter, we provide advice and set out core considerations for designers of PICUs and the staff who operate them. We explore some supporting evidence for how PICUs should be physically configured. Further, we explore the core equipment needed for PICU service delivery and some of the procedures/specifications for maintaining PICU levels of security.

Who Is Involved with PICU Design?

Smith (1999) cites four sets of stakeholders whose needs must be considered in the design of a building:

- The patients
- Those caring for the patients
- The commissioning organisation
- Those managing the building

Those leading the development of a new service are well advised to begin by developing a shared set of values where the safety and wellbeing of patients should be paramount. In achieving a consensus around such principles, the needs of all concerned are likely to be met

because the reality is that a safe and well-accommodated group of patients will lead to a happy and motivated group of clinicians and managers.

In addition to PICU specific guidance, documents such as the Design Guide: Medium Secure Psychiatric Units (NHS Estates, 1993), the Royal College of Psychiatrists Standards for Medium Secure Units (2019) and Environmental Design Guide: Adult Medium Secure Services (2011) may also be of value when considering PICU common issues. Overall, this chapter provides the clinical context within which PICU design should be considered.

PICU Design Underpinning Principles

The location, size, operational policy and patient population will vary amongst units. Issues such as geography and a desire to keep patients as close as possible to their home communities will often be in tension with viable PICU size and will require careful consideration and negotiation.

PICUs can be specialised for particular needs or patient groups, including general adult, gender specific, older people, young people and 'forensic' patients. An effective PICU physical environment needs to be based on broad principles that reflect the type of service one is proposing.

Opportunities for New Builds

In any new development, there is opportunity to embrace new technology and design concepts. Of particular interest is the potential for developing mental health units which contribute to organisations delivering net zero for carbon consumption. Skilful design which optimises natural light, minimises solar thermal gain and insulates against heat loss will add to the pleasant ambience of the PICU. In addition, systems which ensure energy efficiency and potentially energy generation are also becoming common features.

PICU Core Design Outcomes

Commissioning of a new service is an opportunity to ensure that the project is informed by a collaboration between patients who are experts by experience and front-line staff. Expert by experiences should be involved in all aspects of the design from the outset. Insights achieved having spent time as a patient in a PICU must be considered on par with, or even outweigh, many other driving factors and opinions.

For the purposes of this chapter, the following statements constitute core outcomes for PICU design. The PICU will:

- allow a range of therapeutic activities to take place
- provide adequate space and facilities for a homely environment in which a patient can spend the majority of their day
- be effective in providing increased safety, particularly mitigation against aggressive, impulsive and unpredictable behaviour
- offer impediments to absconding and the methods necessary for absconding will be predictable

These broad statements should be relevant to any PICU serving a variety of patient groups.

PICU Position and Layout

The PICU should be preferably on the ground floor. This will:

- assist in the admission of acutely disturbed patients by not having to navigate stairs or a lift
- facilitate access to gardens and fresh air
- reduce risk of injury from absconding attempts from upper floors

One possible benefit often argued for locating the PICU on the first floor is that it may discourage absconding through windows, although the risk of injury to someone exiting via a first-floor window is high. The benefits of locating the unit at ground level are significant, and window specifications should prevent absconding.

General Layout

For PICUs that are part of or on the site of larger hospitals, an entrance to the PICU that does not necessitate travelling through the rest of the hospital should be provided.

Multiple corridors should be avoided to promote unobtrusive observation. Creating shallow curved alcoves in corridors does not inhibit observation but does create a less harsh institutional-looking environment. There should be a central general circulation point within the unit from which most other areas can be easily seen.

Space and Unit Feel

The amount of space to which patients have access is considered an important design factor. Palmstierna et al. (1991) investigated the relationship between overcrowding and aggressive behaviour in a PICU. They concluded that aggressive behaviour was more likely to occur in areas where people tend to gather.

Further evidence that PICUs need ample space is provided by Pereira et al. (2021) who recognise that the issue may be compounded when the length of stay in the PICU is not as brief as may be expected. Jenkins et al. (2014) studied the effects of moving from an inferior PICU to a new building and observed that the physical environment has a significant impact on levels of arousal and aggression.

Ulrich et al. (2018) comprehensively analysed the effect of physical environment based on recognition that patient stress is a primary factor in much aggression. In designing mental health wards to reduce stress, the study recommended the following considerations:

- Reduction of crowding stress
  - Single-patient rooms with private bathrooms
  - Communal areas with movable seating and ample space to regulate relationships
  - Design for low social density (at least one room per patient)
- Reduction of environmental stress
  - Noise-reducing design
  - Design for personal (patient) control (e.g. audio device volume)
- Stress-reducing positive distractions
  - Garden accessible to patients
  - Nature window views
  - Nature art
  - Daylight exposure
- Design for observation
  - Communal spaces and bedroom doors observable from central area

The NHS Estates (1993) design guidance for medium secure units (MSUs) suggested a medium secure PICU should offer 30 square metres of free access space per

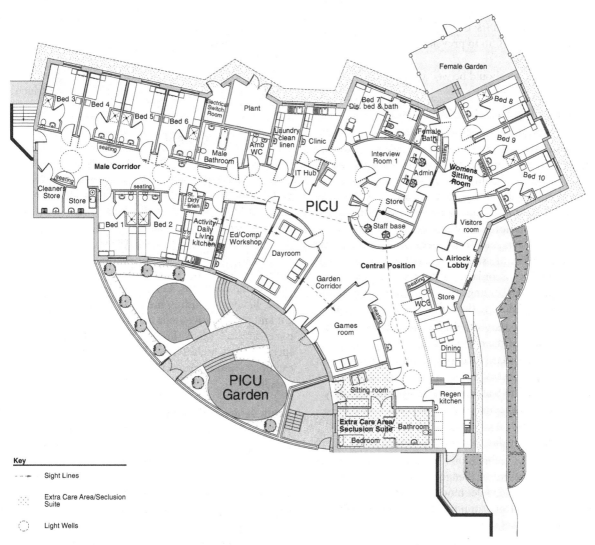

Figure 5.1 PICU suggested diagram courtesy of Quattro Design Architects

patient. MSU design guidance (2011) suggested that the design should enable a full range of social, clinical and therapeutic spaces to be provided (in addition to a range of core areas that staff will need to support the operation of the service). When assessing the available space for patients in a PICU, the mistake of including staff areas in square metres should be avoided.

Bed Numbers

The Design Guidance for PICUs suggests a maximum of 14 beds with 10 considered to be the most manageable number (NAPICU and DIMHN, 2017). There should also be access to an enclosed garden (Dix and Williams, 1996)

Effective designs share a number of general characteristics (e.g. utilities and heating are securely hidden). Other important characteristics are listed here and illustrated in Figure 5.1.

1. There is a central focal point within the unit from which most other areas can be seen.
2. Wherever possible, there should be clear lines of sight. This should also be possible around corners by means of aligned interior windows or convex (parabolic) mirrors.
3. Corridors should be wide enough to allow four abreast comfortably.
4. Ceiling height can be extended in some areas, giving the feeling of space.

5. The design should allow increased daylight into the main corridors; these should be fitted with suitable glass/film to prevent excessive solar thermal gain.
6. The building should be well ventilated.

Single- and Mixed-Gender PICUs

The CQC report *Sexual Safety on Mental Health Wards* (2018) identified the scale of this issue by describing more than 1,100 sexual incidents within English mental health wards over a three-month period during 2017. Of particular concern to hospital designers was the finding that ward environments did not always promote sexual safety of patients.

At the design stage, it is essential to consider how the principles of single-sex accommodation will be upheld in accordance with national and local requirements (NHS England and NHS Improvement, 2019). At a minimum, this will mean ensuring that:

- no one will share sleeping accommodation with a member of the opposite sex
- no one will share toilet or bathroom facilities with the opposite sex
- no one has to walk through an area occupied by patients of the opposite sex to reach toilets or bathrooms
- women-only day rooms are provided

Given the admission criteria, mixed-gender PICUs can present challenges in maintaining sexual safety. If a mixed-gender model is used, then there will need to be clear supporting policies specifically addressing sexual safety.

PICU Security Levels

Forensic PICUs

Level of interior and perimeter security is influenced by whether the unit is serving the general adult population or the forensic population. PICUs within or serving an MSU will have security characteristics consistent with the NHS Estates design guides (1993, 2011) for MSUs. The same applies for units located within a high secure hospital.

General Adult and Other Specialist PICUs

For units serving the general adult population, all recommendations laid out by the Design Guidance for PICU should be considered (NAPICU and DIMHN, 2017). It is easy to either over or

underestimate levels of security for the general adult PICU. Care should be taken to ensure there is a difference between medium security and the general adult PICU.

PICU core security considerations are described throughout this chapter in the specific areas to which they apply.

Security Assessment

When considering the likely methods that may be used by a patient to abscond, it is a useful exercise to spend time either in the existing building or reviewing plans for new builds to specifically consider potential means of absconding.

The views of experts by experience who have spent time within PICU, as well as inspection of incident reports, will provide useful information on which to base design decisions. Following this exercise, many of the likely absconding methods will become apparent and preventative steps may be employed. Security issues are described throughout this chapter in the specific areas addressed. All security measures, for example, window restrictors, should be as discreet as possible.

Secure Garden and Perimeter Security

The level to which the garden is secure will largely be a matter for the PICU planning group. Standard operating procedure (SOP) will generally require a staff presence when the garden is in use. A sensible balance should be drawn between the construction/height of the fence and the oppressive image created by fencing.

Garden furniture should be secured in a location where it cannot be used to assist absconding or climbing.

Consideration should be given to the proposed patient group and the intended garden use. Having the garden of sufficient size to accommodate an activity area, as well as seating and more horticultural areas, is advisable.

Perimeter Security

For the determined and skilled individual, it will often be possible to climb or defeat most perimeter walls and fences. The objective of effective design is to make this difficult, allowing more time for staff to intervene in the case of absconding attempts.

Where fencing/walling is used, the minimum height should be 3 metres. Single-weld mesh can be an effective perimeter (NAPICU and DIMHN, 2017).

Flat-faced, solid timber, close-boarded fencing can be effective with good anti-climb performance as well as providing a less oppressive image. Additional anti-climb measures are available which can be added to various locations within, on top of and around the overall fence/wall structure.

Entrance and Exit

Main Entrance

An air lock design is recommended for the main entrance. This means that the entrance comprises two pairs of doors set opposite each other. Once a person has entered through the first set, the second will not open until the first has closed. This may be achieved by means of magnetic lock systems or by synchronised mechanical locks.

Main Entrance Location

The main entrance should be located away from the main clinical area. This will help prevent absconding when the entrance is in use. It also helps to remove attention from the main entrance, which is often a focus in absconding attempts.

Main Entrance Locking Systems

An airlock system utilising magnetic locks which may be operated via electronic proximity keys at each door and via switches in the unit office is preferable. As digital options continue to develop, alternatives to key fobs/cards, such as biometrics, will become more readily available.

Care should be taken to avoid reliance on traditional mechanical keys, which, by their nature, cannot be deactivated, thus creating a significant problem in the event of a key being mislaid. In many units, magnetic plate locks have proved effective and quiet in operation.

Doors that open inwards will help withstand very determined attempts to force them open.

Main entrance doors should be of a robust and solid construction. If they are locked along the top width only, then they will need to be sufficiently solid/rigid to reduce excessive flexion or warping at the bottom.

Main Entrance 'Air Lock' Operation

The airlock control system should allow for the following methods of operation:

- Touch/proximity card key

- Push-button operation for both doors located within a staff-only station
- An emergency override allowing both doors to be opened at the same time, providing for large numbers of staff to move quickly through the entrance in cases of emergency

Units which include the provision of administration areas should aim, where possible, to have these areas independently accessed from outside of the PICU. This is to ensure that clinical staff are not expected to see visitors solely attending meetings in and out of the airlock entrance.

Fire Exits

Fire safety and security are frequently in tension. The local fire officer must be involved at an early stage of planning (NHS Estates, 1993) and the relevant issues worked through until consensus is achieved.

It is possible for fire exits to be secured on magnetic locks that become inactive when the fire alarm is activated (Dix and Williams, 1996), however, there can be several problems with this arrangement. Firstly, the system will need to be disconnected from the fire alarm test procedure. Secondly, patients may soon become familiar with this system and activate the fire alarm in order to abscond. Collaboration is required with the fire safety officer to consider time-delayed opening of the access control system and mechanical locking. In any scenario, there must be a clear procedure for evacuation in the event of fire.

PICU Evacuation Standard Operating Procedure

Fire policies will vary from unit to unit. However, a phased horizontal evacuation approach is likely to be the most pragmatic. For instance, in the event of fire, moving all patients and personnel behind one fire door is likely to provide adequate protection in most emergencies.

In the event of a prolonged emergency, withdrawal to the unit's secure garden may be the next step before evacuating altogether. A contingency which makes the nearest (preferably lockable) ward available for evacuation is advisable. In the event of fire exits being used, it may be beneficial if they open into a secure area or garden, as the level of confusion caused by an emergency creates an ideal opportunity to abscond.

A clear fire evacuation procedure known to all is required for all locked door environments. This should also be discussed and agreed upon with the local fire officer.

Doors

All doors should be of solid core construction and at least 45-mm-thick. Such doors will be durable against abuse and offer good sound proofing. Lillywhite et al. (1995) highlighted the benefits of interview room doors opening outwards, including preventing patients from barricading themselves in and promoting an easy exit.

For the interior of the unit, it can be beneficial for some doors to open both ways.

Aggression and Access through Doors

Areas in which people gather are often the locations of aggressive incidents (Palmstierna et al., 1991). Double doors should provide access to areas from which a patient may require relocation using physical intervention-type techniques. This will provide enough width to allow access for three staff and a patient to pass through.

Several authors have identified the dining area and specifically mealtimes as a focus point for aggressive incidents (Fottrell, 1980; Kennedy et al., 1995; Hunter and Love, 1996). Kennedy et al. (1995) found that of 80 incidents of aggression that took place away from the main residential unit, 74 took place in the dining room. As a general principle, double doors should be installed in rooms such as the day room, dining room, activities room and other areas in which more than two patients gather. For bedrooms, a half-leaf arrangement is useful for allowing improved access.

PICU Locks and Keys

Modern mental health units now routinely use some type of electronic access control system. This system has advantages of remote operation, easy changing of access rights and deactivation in the event of a change or loss of a security pass. This results in reduced risks and costs compared to replacing traditional mechanical keys and locks.

Assessment, planning and adequate levels of investment are required to ensure access control systems are appropriate for the task. Consideration is also required for issues such as fire procedure (see above) and business continuity contingencies in the event of power or IT failure.

Use of numerical keypads is now generally discouraged due to the major disadvantage of unmortised people soon becoming familiar with the combination (Dix and Williams, 1996).

Electronic Lock Performance

Specification for an electronic access control system must take account of time delays in locks opening and re-engaging. Any system where the door can appear closed and yet not have locked carries an inherent risk of a staff member assuming a door to be secure and neglecting to prevent someone else 'tailgating' their exit from the unit.

An access control system which produces doubts about its efficacy or reliability will add to anxiety of those working in the unit and potentially create a regular opportunity for patients subverting access control arrangements.

Keys and Access Control

Electronic proximity keys (PKs) are recommended. Mechanical keys cannot be deactivated if lost. PKs also have the advantage of being programable with different authorities for access and egress. Patients can be allocated an electronic key to their own room and potentially other areas of the unit depending upon risk assessment.

Mechanical locks can still be useful in providing a backup in the event of electronic system failure.

Staff Key Handling and Tracker Systems

PICUs and other similar services require specific procedures and dedicated equipment for handling keys and other security equipment (e.g. personal alarms). Equipment is available that will provide for storage and electronically tracked allocation and return of keys/other items required on a shift basis. These systems improve security, save time and reduce equipment loss. They also mitigate the common problem of equipment being taken home by staff.

Biometrics

As biometric technology develops, access control applications such as face recognition and fingerprint have become readily available and reliable (Le et al., 2022). This provides opportunities for more responsive security systems and possibly greater freedom for patients to move around unescorted, which should be encouraged and explored.

Biometrics for access control also has the advantage of diminishing the extent to which keys need to be carried or controlled and reducing the potential of losing them.

Where Should Locks be Fitted?

It is desirable for as many rooms as possible to be access controllable. Rooms such as the day and dining area can remain open for free access most of the time. There may be times however when it will be necessary for these rooms to be temporarily restricted.

Windows

Dolan and Snowden (1994) concluded that the majority of escapes from an MSU occurred through windows. While windows offer an obvious target for absconding, they also help the unit to feel less claustrophobic. In some sitting areas, some windows can be placed 700 to 800 mm above the floor to allow seated outside views.

Any unit design should aim for as much natural daylight as possible into the main clinical areas. The design suggested in Figure 5.1 includes ample outside windows in all rooms and, where appropriate, interior windows across rooms. Because of the need for clear lines of sight, outside windows directly into the main corridor are difficult to achieve (see Figure 5.1). To overcome this, ceiling sky lights or light wells may be used, providing the unit is without a second floor. While windows are an obvious focal point in unit security, Bowers et al. (2000) found that observability and levels of security within wards are not clear correlates for absconding; it was hypothesised that the quality of nursing interventions is more significant.

Window Design

Robust anti-ligature specialised window designs are required. Manufacturers are constantly improving window products with combined glass, metal and plastic construction. The resulting window can be extremely robust. It is also important for the frame to withstand very determined attempts at dismantling.

All fixtures and fittings should be considered in the context of a systematic ligature risk assessment of the unit (Reena, 2022). Areas with inherent difficulties with windows, such as seclusion rooms, may be located out of reach or consideration may be given to light wells, which allow natural light to be transferred through roof spaces.

Where reduced ligature curtain arrangements are problematic, such as in the extra care area (ECA) (see below), integral window blinds may be used instead.

Windows and Ventilation

Ventilation is also very important (Mueller, 1983). Windows without other built-in security features should have a restricted opening of no more than 125 mm.

Windows are now available with a built-in, non-obtrusive, durable, perforated metal grill which allows for ventilation whilst preventing object exit and ingress.

Kitchen, Bathrooms and Toilets

Kitchens

The kitchen area presents particular problems and should always be considered a potentially dangerous area. A clear operational policy should describe the use of the kitchen, including the circumstances in which access may be restricted.

Bathrooms and Toilets

Obviously, the bathrooms and toilet will need to be lockable from the inside. Staff must be able to override these locks from the outside, with keys held by staff only.

Bedrooms

Bedrooms may also be locked from the inside with the same precautions as for kitchens and bathrooms. It may be useful in promoting least restriction and reducing conflict to provide patients with access control to their own rooms. This should only be done with the provision of an override system operated by staff. In any room that can be locked from the inside, care should be taken to ensure that the override system will work, even if the interior side of the lock is held.

Observation and Design

Types of Observations

The National Institute for Health and Care Excellence (2015) describes the following types of observation:

- Low-level intermittent observation: the baseline level of observation in a specified psychiatric setting. The frequency of observation is once every 30 to 60 minutes.
- High-level intermittent observation: usually used if a service user is at risk of becoming violent or aggressive but does not represent an immediate

risk. The frequency of observation is once every 15 to 30 minutes.

- Continuous observation: usually used when a service user presents an immediate threat and needs to be kept within eyesight or at arm's length of a designated nurse, with immediate access to other members of staff if needed.
- Multiprofessional continuous observation: usually used when a service user is at the highest risk of harming themselves or others and needs to be kept within eyesight of two or three staff members and at arm's length of at least one staff member.

The need for higher levels of observation is a frequently quoted reason for admission to the PICU. Continuous observation sometimes referred to as 'specialing' or '1:1' is a familiar and often unpopular practice amongst many patients and staff. Green and Grindle (1996) found one-to-one close observation to be common practice in 80 psychiatric hospitals in the United States. In their analysis, the authors identified several disadvantages, including secondary gain and behavioural escalation by the patient. Other authors have also identified higher-level observation as a problematic procedure lacking clear empirical evaluation of its effectiveness (Macpherson et al., 1996; Ashaye et al., 1997; Page, 2006a). The Mental Health Act Code of Practice considers higher levels of observation as a restrictive intervention which should only be used when clearly required (MHA Cop, 2015).

Collins et al. (2022) found that there could be value in continuous observation. However, this was dependent upon the patient–staff relationship, staff's interpersonal skills and qualities, collaboration, practical modifications and inclusion of activities. In their retrospective study, Shugar and Rehaluk (1990) concluded that one-to-one observation in excess of 72 hours was particularly problematic and should be avoided. Bowers et al. (2000) found that while close observation was common practice in UK hospitals, policies were often unhelpful and inconsistent.

Design Features Reducing Need for Obtrusive Observation

Empirical evidence, nursing experience and, most importantly, experiences described by patients who have been subject to observation all point to the need for designing units in such a way that intrusive non-therapeutic observation can be kept to an absolute minimum.

Figure 5.1 offers a suggestion for a unit design that allows for high levels of unobtrusive observation. Design characteristics likely to diminish the need for obtrusive observation include:

- A central main area within the unit from which most other communal areas can be easily seen.
- As many clear lines of sight as possible should be available, avoiding numerous corners and corridors (see Figure 5.1). Interior windows should be aligned where possible (as shown in Figure 5.1) to allow observation across a number of rooms.
- Most doors (except for the bathrooms and toilets) should be fitted with a robust glazed panel. This will enhance safety when moving around the unit by ensuring that the staff and patients can see the other side of doors.
- Bedrooms and bathrooms should be fitted with a louver-type window controlled from the outside by a key mechanism available to staff only.
- Bedroom lights should be controlled by switches with a dimmer, located inside and outside of the room. This will allow for night-time observation.
- Where corridors meet, and in other areas without clear lines of sight, convex mirrors can be fitted at ceiling level to allow views around corners.

Observation and Technology

The use of technology in maintaining patient safety and meeting some of the functions of nursing observation has rapidly developed over the last two decades. One of the first innovations was in using infrared closed-circuit television (CCTV) for less intrusive night-time observation (Dix, 2002; Dix and Meiklejohn, 2003; Page et al., 2004). Subsequent research found that when patients were able to exercise choice over how they were observed, the technology had some therapeutic benefit (Warr et al., 2005; Page, 2007).

CCTV

CCTV can have value in several areas. Its advantages in the ECA are discussed later in the chapter. CCTV can be used to monitor activity in the unit garden and entrances to the unit, and a high-level camera will enable unobtrusive observation of patients on unescorted leave in the grounds. Having a system which provides a photographic record of all visitors as well as any suspicious activity, such as dropping illicit substances into the unit garden.

Appenzeller et al. (2019) questioned the value of CCTV in communal areas for improving safety or security. PICU NMS (NAPICU, 2014) summarise the use of CCTV in PICU as:

- Additional options for observation in difficult to supervise areas (e.g. gardens, smoking areas)
- A means of evidence, recording untoward incidents, potential offences or investigating allegations
- An additional means by which staff can review and learn from the management of difficult situations

Up-to-date pictures of patients who may have absconded and are considered at risk

Body-Worn Cameras

The use of body-worn cameras (BWCs) by clinical staff has been trialled in some mental health settings. Most staff reported being generally supportive or neutral about their use (Hakimzada et al., 2020). Similar to use of this technology amongst emergency services, the intention is to reduce incidents by acting as a deterrent and providing a clear record of what has occurred for reflection, training and audit purposes.

Despite enthusiasm for this logic from some quarters, the evidence base is currently very limited and assessments of the effectiveness of this technology in mental health settings are equivocal (Wilson et al., 2022). As technology further improves and research is considered across the full range of domains including patient safety, experience and clinical practice, the arguments for more routine use may increase.

Life Sign Observations Monitoring

As technology continues to develop and become more affordable, further opportunities for its use in ensuring patient safety are becoming available. Barrera et al. (2020) described a system which uses optical sensors and artificial intelligence to conduct intermittent and hourly night-time observations, including life sign detection.

Such systems appear to have some merit in reducing disruption for patients when necessary checks are being undertaken. This has also been proposed to be of value, particularly for those subject to seclusion.

Facilities for Managing the Most Acutely Disturbed Patient

Seclusion Rooms

For many years, the use of seclusion has been questioned for its clinical, ethical and practical value (Hamil, 1987; Angold, 1989; Tooke and Brown, 1992; Kinsella and Brosnan, 1993).

Patients who demonstrate extremely unpredictable and assaultive behaviour present particular management problems. Throughout the history of mental health care, traditional seclusion (locked alone in a room) was often the solution for this type of behaviour (Renvoize, 1991). Seclusion is considered in detail elsewhere in this volume. The focus here is on physical environment considerations.

Some units may opt for a non-traditional seclusion policy and rely upon the ECA for managing disturbance rather than locking the patient alone in a single room (Dix, 2019). The NHS Estates building note no. 35 (1996), advises the project group for a new PICU to decide on the need for a traditional seclusion room.

The use of seclusion has been advanced as an alternative to prolonged restraint following deaths due to postural asphyxiation (Patterson and Leadbetter, 2004; Howe and Sethi, 2018). Careful consideration of design features is required for seclusion facilities given the circumstances in which they are required.

Extra Care Area (ECA)

The use of an ECA has been proposed as an alternative to traditional seclusion (Dix, 2017, 2019; Long et al., 2009). The ECA is defined as a closely supervised living space, away from the main clinical area, in which a single patient may be nursed apart from the other patients (Dix, 1995). It differs from traditional seclusion in that the patient remains with staff and is not locked alone in a room (Dix, 2017).

Extra Care Area Location

The ECA should be part of, or in very close proximity to, the main unit and not physically separated in a way that would render it completely isolated. In terms of the number of staff needed, there is a danger of creating a ward within a ward.

Figure 5.1 shows an ECA separated by double doors, which could be fixed open to allow the ECA to become part of the unit. In the ECA, a higher level of safety is needed than anywhere else in the unit. All features of the ECA should be, so far as possible, robust and tamperproof. Care is necessary to ensure that items which could be used as a weapon are avoided.

Extra Care Area Composition

The ECA should be able to provide for the daily living needs of a single patient. This will require the following to be in close proximity to each other:

- A seclusion or de-escalation room (see below)
- A toilet and shower facility
- A sitting room with simple furnishings
- An entrance to the ECA directly from outside the unit for the admission of acutely disturbed patients
- Access to the garden
- Built-in entertainment equipment (e.g. TV, radio, music, games console, etc.)
- A very well-ventilated area with air conditioning to mitigate overheating during physical intervention
- An intercom system to the main office.

Seclusion Room Location

Rather than stand alone, it is increasingly accepted that any seclusion room should be located within a dedicated 'seclusion suite' including a variety of related facilities (Kaar et al., 2017). A seclusion suite is effectively the same as an ECA, other than it includes a room into which the patient can be locked alone. In contrast, the ECA instead includes a de-escalation room in which the staff remain with the patient. Curran et al. (2005) provide detailed guidance on the composition and design of a seclusion suite/ECA.

Seclusion Room Core Features

The National Institute for Health and Care Excellence (NICE) Guidelines (2015) recognise that use of seclusion is a restrictive practice and therefore it should be minimised. Noting that it is not used in all settings/ organisations, the guidance suggests that if present it should:

- allow staff to clearly observe and communicate with the service user
- be well insulated and ventilated, with temperature controls outside the room
- have access to toilet and washing facilities
- have furniture, windows and doors that can withstand damage

It is also required that any fixtures or fittings within the room are either tamperproof to a very high level or out of reach, including by standing on the bed.

Figure 5.1 shows an ECA, which could also include a seclusion room or, if preferred, a de-escalation room in which staff remain with the patient rather than the patient being locked in alone.

Design of Seclusion/De-escalation Room

- This room should be located in the ECA of the unit.
- It should have a single very robust moulded vinyl safety bed.
- The size should be around 15 m^2 with a ceiling clearance that cannot be reached by jumping or standing on the safety bed.
- The room must be able to withstand very determined attack and damage.
- The walls and floors should be lined with a welded-seam vinyl surface or other high-performance covering.
- The door should be of solid core design and thick enough to withstand a very determined attack.
- The door should be fitted with a robust observation panel.
- It should be possible to see into the whole room from the observation panel, without any hidden corners.
- Ventilation/heating should be anti-tamperproof and underfloor or out of reach. Noise levels generated by this equipment must also be minimised.
  - The placement of infrared CCTV cameras in this area enables staff in the ward office to monitor the room. A recording system may also be useful for reflection/debrief and as protection for both staff and patients as evidence of what occurred.

Interior Equipment Communication and Monitoring

- Built-in electronic life sign monitoring systems are available and should be considered for installation within seclusion rooms.

- A vandal-resistant patient controllable media outlet should be considered for the room.
- An intercom or equivalent means of communication between those outside the room and the patient within must be available.
- The room should have an integral ensuite which can be remotely access controlled if necessary.
- A means of telling the time and date should be provided within the room or in an easily viewable location.

Facilities for Engagement, Activity and Physical Health

The value of planned therapeutic activity amongst patients in institutional settings has long been accepted (Aumack, 1968). There is strong evidence that psychiatric institutions are poor performers in ensuring that therapeutic activity is high on the agenda (Drinkwater and Gudjonsson, 1989; Standing Nursing and Midwifery Advisory Committee, 1999).

Correlation between aggression and inactivity has also long been established (Lloyd, 1995). With the inevitable preoccupation surrounding safety and containment, a PICU may be amongst the most vulnerable of mental health settings in failing to provide an adequate environment or resources for therapeutic activity (Zigmond, 1995). Pereira et al. (2021) noted a 'pleasing increase' in the number of psychologists, occupational therapists and social workers on PICUs over the last decade.

Several authors have highlighted the value of activity for bringing about positive changes to disturbed behaviour in the PICU setting (Best, 1996; Antonysamy, 2017).

An effective PICU design will give provision of therapeutic activity an equal status to safety and security, as the former is a key component of the latter.

Specific Rooms for Recreation/Activity

Figure 5.1 includes:
- A games/exercise room containing equipment such as a pool table, table tennis, exercise bike, treadmill and so on
- A skills/activities room containing electronic and other games, art supplies, musical instruments and other equipment
- A skills kitchen

- A dayroom and sitting room equipped with television and video
- Access to an enclosed garden area.

Recreation Activity Supporting Procedures

Within the PICU, activities will often be undertaken with direct support of staff. Individual assessments will indicate the amount of staff intervention required (Best, 1996). When not in use, or as clinically indicated, these areas may be locked. Use of activity equipment and facilities should be supported by SOPs (see below). Activity programmes must include collaboration between Nursing staff, Occupational and Sports Therapists.

Individual Multimedia Outlets

Robust and patient-controllable media outlets in bedrooms should be installed, although there should be the provision for them to be centrally controlled/disconnected by staff if required. These media outlets have the advantage of reducing need for patients to bring their own TVs, music equipment and so on.

Furniture and Fittings

The unit environment should be made as homely as possible. Wall-mounted pictures, potted plants and non-moulded furniture promote a relaxed environment without presenting a major risk to safety. Poster-type pictures may be fixed to the wall on a back-board covered with polycarbonate.

Television and other media devices should be safely installed to reduce the likelihood of damage without the need to use oppressive-looking protection which can impede viewing enjoyment and cause frustration.

Decor and Art

The unit should be decorated in pleasant, homely colours. Paint must be tolerant of scrubbing in case of dirty marks, stains or graffiti. Shaw et al. (2018) demonstrated the value of creative artwork and decor in a PICU. Service planners are advised to review the literature around the use of artwork in PICUs.

Acoustics

Carpets should also be used where possible to reduce an 'institutional look' and mitigate amplified acoustics from hard surfaces (NAPICU & DIMHN, 2017). Carpets must be of a high quality and should be both burn and stain resistant. Carpet performance in helping to manage acoustics and providing a softer look can outweigh infection control and need for cleaning in a PICU.

Ceilings can also be specified with high acoustic-absorbing performance.

Alarm Systems, Staff and Patient Safety

Personal alarm systems carried by staff that, when activated, alert others to an emergency are essential within a PICU.

The basic principle of these systems is that a signal is sent from a hand unit to a wall- or ceiling-mounted sensor which can process audio-visual output. These units operate by either ultrasonic, infrared or radio signals (or often a combination of these technologies). Simple 'attack alarms' which emit a very loud sound can also be reliable and effective for alerting others to the need for emergency assistance.

Alarm Systems' Performance Characteristics

The technology in this area is rapidly developing, and new products are constantly entering the market. When considering which product will be most effective, a demonstration by the manufacturer is a necessary step. The following common problems should be avoided:

- Systems that are too directionally sensitive, resulting in the need to point the hand set directly at the receiver
- Systems where the handset is overpowered, resulting in the activation of several receivers confusing the exact location of the emergency
- Systems that are under-sensitive, resulting in the need to press the hand unit several times before the alarm is sounded.

Fixed/Wall-Mounted Emergency Alert Systems

Wall-mounted emergency buttons which are integrated into the overall alarm system are also necessary. These should be installed in addition to the handheld systems, as they also offer protection for the patients.

A button should be placed in all rooms and at regular intervals in corridors. There should be the provision for the system to be managed centrally in the event of persistent inappropriate use.

Alarm/Security Management Systems and Audit

Most systems are now managed by sophisticated software which can be used to achieve a variety of tasks, including various configurations, audit and monitoring.

A fully integrated alarm/security system should allow for many functions including:

- Control/isolation of water and electricity to bedrooms
- Alarm configuration and audit
- Integrated CCTV
- Access control
- Making a pre-recorded telephone call on the hospital's emergency system announcing a psychiatric emergency.

Searching

Consideration is required for how the unit's search policy will be implemented. This may need to extend to the provision of a dedicated search room close to the unit's main entrance. Consideration of privacy and monitoring of such areas is required.

A variety of detection equipment is available and requires planning for storage or, in the case of fixed scanners, mounting.

Laidlaw et al. (2017) conducted a randomised controlled trial of the use of metal detection in mental health. It concluded that commonly used handheld equipment failed to detect 95% of items searched for. Newer technology such as ferromagnetic scanners demonstrated a 100% success rate for finding items when investigated under scientific conditions.

Communication Systems

Methods of two-way communication for several applications are essential within a PICU.

Two-way radios are recommended, as these are useful for communication around the hospital and while engaged in escorted leave. They are also of value in other situations, for example, searching for a patient who has absconded. Radios can be configured on a hospital network, allowing instant communication with staff around the hospital.

A variety of products are available, with new equipment entering the market. For extended range, it is necessary to install a booster transmitter on top of the building.

Standard industrial hand units are relatively inexpensive and offer good reliable performance at shorter ranges. With booster units, these radios can work over a distance of several kilometres. Regular servicing is imperative, as batteries need replacing every 12–18 months. For longer-distance escorted leave, a mobile phone is recommended. It should be preprogrammed with the numbers of the ward, the hospital reception and the police.

Patient Available Communications and Wi-Fi

Most patients will have their own telephone and thus a local policy for their usage is needed. Many units will also need to agree on a policy position for recording and use of smartphone cameras.

For those unable to access a personal phone, a unit patient telephone should be provided. A location for the unit patient telephone that allows people to talk with appropriate privacy must be considered.

Unit-wide guest Wi-Fi which can be tracked in terms of activity is recommended.

Transport

Access to a dedicated unit vehicle is recommended. It should be of a suitable size without having an institutional look. So-called multi-purpose vehicles (MPVs) or people carriers are ideal and more comfortable than minibuses.

The vehicle should be suitable for a variety of purposes, such as taking patients on escorted leave and searching for and returning an absconded patient.

Robustness is a consideration, as inevitably the vehicle will have a harder working life than when in domestic use.

Safety must be considered, and a vehicle with a high European safety rating is preferred.

Infection Prevention and Control

The COVID-19 pandemic created many significant challenges for mental health services. Fundamental amongst these was difficulty maintaining a high standard of infection prevention and control (IPC) practice amongst a cohort of patients unable or unwilling to comply with restrictions or unable to understand the consequences of non-compliance.

McLean and Forrester (2020) set out the core considerations for PICUs and other acute mental health in patient units. These include:

- Staff donning and doffing areas
- Staff showers
- Personal protective equipment (PPE) storage space

- Spacious and well-ventilated ensuite bedrooms with adequate facilities to live in for several days in the event of the need to isolate
- Adequate hand washing facilities
- Bedroom areas where clusters of rooms can be separated by a locked door so that infected individuals can be cohorted
- Visiting areas which can be cleaned and separated via a screen or window if necessary
- Ventilation management which does not increase the risk of spreading airborne viruses

The issue of physical intervention infection control is a concern for clinicians. Dix et al. (2021) found that various levels of available PPE had similar efficacy in limiting contact contamination, but that provision of an additional layer of clothing (such as overalls) which can be removed and washed was particularly helpful.

Standard Operating Procedures

The value of equipment and managing the physical environment may be optimised by developing SOPs, which are widely used by organisations faced with complex management situations. They describe a standard response to situations that commonly occur and for which contingency plans are needed. They are designed to promote confidence in the staff for using equipment, dealing with difficult situations and maximising the therapeutic options that may be considered. The following is an example of an SOP in the event of safety concerns emerging during escorted leave.

1. During every episode of escorted leave, the escort will carry a radio and/or mobile telephone. The mobile phone must also be carried if the patient's destination is more than 2 kilometres miles away.

2. Before leaving the unit, the escort will ensure a second radio is held by a member of staff and that both radios are switched on and working. The escort will state the intended destination and approximate duration of leave.

3. If there is a deviation from the stated plan or expected duration of leave, the escort will inform the unit.

4. If safety concerns emerge, including attempts to leave the escort or if the patient refuses to return:

   - attempt verbal negotiation to resolve the situation
   - follow the patient at a safe distance and contact other staff by radio with situation reports at 5-minute intervals

SOPs are used to support staff in using equipment and maintaining a safe environment. They should be kept as simple as possible and taught to all the unit staff. In terms of the physical environment, the development of SOPs should be considered for:

1. Preparing the ward environment for admission of a patient who is displaying features of acute disturbance
2. Managing the main entrance
3. Interviewing or negotiating with a potentially aggressive patient
4. Using the extra care area

Future Innovations

Technological advancement progresses at pace. Any new development presents a myriad of opportunities for installing systems not used previously.

There have been significant developments in the use of monitoring technology in mental health care, including the use of artificial intelligence. It is likely that technology which is applicable to mental health will continue to develop rapidly. It is imperative that service planners remain aware of new developments and the effectiveness/ethical considerations of how these might help patients.

Conclusion

It is not possible to describe every detail of the ideal PICU physical environment or security features. The design guidance offered here is not overly prescriptive but is intended to provide the principles on which PICU design can be based (NAPICU & DIMHN, 2017).

The physical environment, design and security measures within mental health inpatient facilities have long been recognised as centrally important to improving outcomes. During her study of nurses' perceptions of a new PICU, Gentle (1996) identified dissatisfaction with the physical environment as a major issue. Taj and Sheehan (1994) also found high levels of dissatisfaction in the architectural design of a new acute unit. They recommended major design changes after only six months.

It is essential that the planning of a new PICU or improving an existing service involves a detailed and careful analysis of the physical environment and equipment required and clear supporting procedures for their use.

For those planning a new PICU development, it is highly recommended that several visits are made to established units to consider the environment's strengths and weaknesses. Collaboration between clinicians, experts by experience and architects is also essential. A design will only be a success if all parties work collaboratively. Once a new unit is operational, it should be considered as an inherent part of planning that the physical environment will be modified and developed.

References

Angold,A (1989) Seclusion. *British Journal of Psychiatry* **154**:437–44.

Antonysamy,A (2017) How Can We Reduce Violence and Aggression in Psychiatric Inpatient Units? *BMJ Quality Improvement Reports* **2**: u201366.w834.

Appenzeller,Y, Appelbaum,P and Trachsel,M (2019) Ethical and Practical Issues in Video Surveillance of Psychiatric Units. *Journal of Psychiatric Services.* https://doi.org/10.1176/appi.ps.201900397

Ashaye,O, Ikkos,G and Rigby,E (1997) Study of Effects of Constant Observation of Psychiatric In-Patients. *Psychiatric Bulletin* **21** (3) 145–7.

Aumack,L (1968) The Patient Activity Checklist: An Instrument and an Approach for Measuring Behaviour. *Journal of Clinical Psychology* **25**: 134–7.

Barrera,A, Gee,C, Wood,A, Gibson,O, Bayley,D and Geddes,J (2020) Introducing Artificial Intelligence in Acute Psychiatric Inpatient Care: Qualitative Study of Its Use to Conduct Nursing Observations. *Evidence-Based Mental Health* **23**: 34–8.

Best,D (1996) The Developing Role of Occupational Therapy in Psychiatric Intensive Care. *British Journal of Occupational Therapy* **59**: 161–4.

Bowers,L, Gournay,K and Duffy,D (2000) Suicide and Self-Harm on Inpatient Psychiatric Units: A National Survey of Observation Policies. *Journal of Advanced Nursing* **32**: 437–44.

Bowers,L, Jarret,M, Clark,N, Kiyimba,F and McFarlane,L (2000) Determinants of Absconding by Patients on Acute Psychiatric Wards. *Journal of Advanced Nursing* **32** (3) 644–9.

Care Quality Commission (2018) *Sexual Safety on Mental Health Wards.* London: CQC

Collins,E, Lawson,M and Sheeran,A (2022) Enhanced Observation: How Therapeutic Are They Within a Medium Secure Forensic Mental Health Setting? *The Journal of Forensic Psychiatry & Psychology* **33** (1) 68–88.

Curran,C, Adnett,C and Zigmond,T (2005) Seclusion: Factors to Consider When Designing and Using a Seclusion

Suite in a Mental Health Hospital. *Hospital Development* **36** (1) 19–26.

Department of Health (2002) *Mental Health Policy Implementation Guide: National Minimum standards for General Adult Services in Psychiatric Intensive Care Units and Low Secure Environments.* London: DOH.

Dix,R (1995) A Nurse Led Psychiatric Intensive Care Unit. *Psychiatric Bulletin* May: 285–7.

Dix,R. (2001) The Physical Environment. In Beer,D., Pereira,S and Paton,C (eds.), *Psychiatric Intensive Care.* Cambridge: Cambridge University Press.

Dix,R (2002) Observation and Technology: Logical Progression or Ethical Nightmare. *National Association of Psychiatric Intensive Care Units Bulletin* **2** (4) 22–9.

Dix,R (2017) Seclusion: What's In a Name? *Journal of Psychiatric Intensive Care* **13** (2) 57–9. https://doi.org/10.2 0299/jpi.2017.012.

Dix,R (2019) Restrictive Interventions and Seclusion: Time for Another Look. *Journal of Psychiatric Intensive Care* **15** (1) 1–3 doi:10.20299/jpi.2019.006.

Dix,R and Meiklejohn,C (2003) Observation and Technology: Questions and Answers. *National Association of Psychiatric Intensive Care Units Bulletin* **3**:39–49.

Dix,R and Page,M (2008) Physical Environment. In Beer,D., Pereira,S and Paton,C (eds.), *Psychiatric Intensive Care.* Cambridge: Cambridge University Press.

Dix,R, Straiton,D, Metherall,P, Laidlaw,J, McLean,L, Hayward,A, et al. (2021) COVID-19: A Systematic Evaluation of Personal Protective Equipment (PPE) Performance during Restraint. *Medicine, Science, and the Law* **61** (4) 275–85.

Dolan,M and Snowden,P (1994) Escapes from a Medium Secure Unit. *Journal of Forensic Psychiatry* **5** (2) 275–86.

Dix,R and Williams,K (1996) Psychiatric Intensive Care Units, a Design for Living. *Psychiatric Bulletin* **20**:527–9.

Drinkwater,J and Gudjonsson,G (1989) The Nature of Violence in Psychiatric Hospitals. In Howells,K and Hollin, C (eds.), *Clinical Approaches to Violence.* Chichester: Wiley.

Environmental Design Guide Adult Medium Secure Services (2011) *Secure Services Policy Team.* London: Department of Health.

Fottrell,E (1980) A Study of Violent Behaviour Amongst Patients in Psychiatric Hospitals. *British Journal of Psychiatry* **136**:216–21.

Gentle,J (1996) Mental Health Intensive Care Units: The Nurses' Experience and Perceptions of a New Unit. *Journal of Advanced Nursing* **24** (1) 1194–1200.

Goldney,R, Bowes,J, Spence,N, Czechowicz,A and Hurley,R (1985) The Psychiatric Intensive Care Unit. *British Journal of Psychiatry* **146**:50–4.

Green,J and Grindel,C (1996) Supervision of Suicidal Patients in Adult Inpatient Psychiatric Units in General Hospitals. *Psychiatric Services* **47** (8) 859–63.

Hakimzada,M, O'Brien,A and Wigglesworth,H (2020) Exploring the Attitudes of the Nursing Staff Towards the Use of Body Worn Cameras in Psychiatric Inpatient Wards. *Journal of Psychiatric Intensive Care* **16** (2) 75–84.

Hamil,K (1987) Seclusion: Inside Looking Out. *Nursing Times* **83** (5) 174–9.

Howe,A and Sethi,F (2018) Seclusion: The Untold Legacy of the Non-Restraint Movement in the UK. *Journal of Psychiatric Intensive Care* **14** (1) 5–13.

Hunter,M and Love,C (1996) Total Quality Management and the Reduction of Inpatient Violence and Costs in a Forensic Psychiatric Hospital. *Psychiatric Services* **47** (7) 751–4.

Jenkins,O, Dye,S and Foy,C (2014) A Study of Agitation, Conflict and Containment in Association with Change in Ward Physical Environment. *Journal of Psychiatric Intensive Care* **10** (1) 1–9.

Kaar,S, Walker,H, Sethi,F and McIvor,R (2017) The Function and Design of Seclusion Rooms in Clinical Settings. *Journal of Psychiatric Intensive Care* **13** (2) 83–91.

Kennedy,J, Harrison,J, Hillis,T and Bluglass,R (1995) Analysis of Violent Incidents in a Regional Secure Unit. *Medicine Science and the Law* **35** (3) 255–60.

Kinsella,C and Brosan,C (1993) An Alternative to Seclusion. *Nursing Times* **89** (18) 62–4.

Laidlaw,J, Dix,R, Slack,P, Foy,C, Hayward,A, Metherall,A, et al. (2017) Searching for Prohibited Items in Mental Health Settings: A Randomised Controlled Trial of Two Metal Detecting Technologies. *Medicine, Science and the Law* **57** (4) 167–74. https://doi.org/10.1177/ 0025802417725642.

Le,QD, Vu,TTC and Vo,TQ (2022) Application of 3D Face Recognition in the Access Control System. *Robotica* **40** (7) 2449–67.

Lillywhite,A, Morgan,N and Walter,E (1995) Reducing the Risk of Violence to Junior Psychiatrists. *Psychiatric Bulletin* **19**: 24–7.

Lloyd,C (1995) *Forensic Psychiatry for Health Professionals.* Therapy in Practice. London: Chapman & Hall. pp. 46–6.

Long,C, Silaule,P and Collier,N (2010) Use of an Extra Care Area in a Medium Secure Setting for Women: Findings and Implications for Practice. *Journal of Psychiatric Intensive Care* **6** (1) 39–45.

Macpherson,R, Anstee,B and Dix,R (1996) Guidelines for the Management of Acutely Disturbed Patients. *Advances in Psychiatric Treatment* **2**: 194–201.

McLean,L and Forrester,L (2020) COVID-19, Infection Prevention and Control within Acute Inpatient Mental Health Facilities: A New Challenge Requiring a New

Approach. *Journal of Psychiatric Intensive Care* **16** (2) 69–74. doi: https://doi.org/10.20299/jpi.2020.015.

Mueller,CW (1983) Environmental Stressors and Aggressive Behavior. *Aggression: Theoretical and Empirical Reviews* **2**: 51–76.

Musisi,S, Wasylenki,D and Rapp,M (1989) A Psychiatric Intensive Care Unit in a Psychiatric Hospital. *Canadian Journal of Psychiatry* **34** (3) 200–4.

National Association of Psychiatric Intensive Care and Low Secure Units (NAPICU) (2014) *National Minimum Standards for Psychiatric Intensive Care in General Adult Services.* Glasgow: NAPICU.

National Association of Psychiatric Intensive Care and Low Secure Units (NAPICU) and Design in Mental Health Network (DIMHN) (2017) *Design Guidance for Psychiatric Intensive Care Units.* Glasgow: NAPICU.

National Institute for Health and Care Excellence (NICE) (2015) *Violence and Aggression: Short-Term Management in Mental Health, Health and Community Settings.* London: NICE.

NHS England and NHS Improvement (2019) *Delivering Same-Sex Accommodation.* London.

NHS Estates (1993) *Design Guide: Medium Secure Psychiatric Units.* Leeds.

NHS Estates (1996) *Accommodation for People with Mental Illness, Health Building Note 35: Part 1 – The Acute Unit.* Leeds: HMSO.

Page,M (2006) Low Secure Care: A Description of a New Service. *Journal of Psychiatric Intensive Care* **1** (2) 89–96.

Page,M (2007) Engaging the Disengaged: Collecting the Views of Patients in a Low Secure Unit on Methods of Observation. *Journal of Psychiatric Intensive Care* **3** (1) 13–20.

Page,MJ (2006) Methods of Observation in Mental Health Inpatient Units. *Nursing Times* **102** (22) 34–5.

Page,M, Meiklejohn,C and Warr,J (2004) CCTV and Night-Time Observations. *Mental Health Practice* **7** (10) 28–31.

Palmstierna,T, Huitfeldt,B and Wistedt,B (1991) The Relationship between Crowding and Aggressive Behaviour in the Psychiatric Intensive Care Unit. *Hospital and Community Psychiatry* **42** (12) 1237–40.

Patterson,B and Leadbetter,D (2004) Learning the Right Lessons. *Mental Health Practice* **7** (7) 12–15.

Pereira, SM, Walker,L and Dye,S (2021) A National Survey of Psychiatric Intensive Care, Low Secure and Locked Rehabilitation Units. *Mental Health Practice* **24** (4) 24–34.

Reena,P, Baker,J, Scally,R and Attard,J (2022) The Ligature Assessment Tool: The Development of a Structured Tool to Improve Quality of Reporting of Ligature Incidents. *Journal of Psychiatric Intensive Care* **18** (1) 45–51.

Renvoize,E (1991) The Association of Medical Officers of Asylums and Hospitals for the Insane, the Medico-Psychological Association, and Their Presidents. In Berrios, G and Freeman,H (eds.), *150 Years of British Psychiatry 1841–1991.* London: Gaskell. pp. 29–75.

Royal Collage of Psychiatrists (2019) Standards for Forensic Mental Health Services: Low and Medium Secure Care – Third Edition Quality Network for Forensic Mental Health Services Publication Number: CCQI304.

Shaw,T, White,N, Butler,S, Shannon,G, Smale,E, Corrigan, M, et al. (2018) Art Inspires and Transforms the PICU. Conference: NAPICU Annual Conference 2018. www.researchgate.net/publication/348917511_Art_Inspires_and_Transforms_the_PICU.

Shugar,G and Rehaluk,R (1990) Continuous Observation for Psychiatric Inpatients. *Comprehensive Psychiatry* **30** (1) 48–55.

Smith,M (1999) Designed for Living. *Mental Health Care* **2** (11) 367–9.

Standing Nursing and Midwifery Advisory Committee (1999) *Mental Health Nursing: "Addressing Acute Concerns."* London: SNMAC.

Taj,R and Sheehan,J (1994) Architectural Design and Acute Psychiatric Care. *Psychiatric Bulletin* **18**: 279–81.

Tooke,K and Brown,J (1992) Perceptions of Seclusion: Comparing Patient and Staff Reactions. *Journal of Psychosocial Nursing* **30** (8) 23–6.

Ulrich,R, Bogren,L, Gardiner,S and Lundin,S (2018) Psychiatric Ward Design Can Reduce Aggressive Behaviour. *Journal of Environmental Psychology* **57**: 53–66.

Warr,J, Page,M and Crossen-White,H (2005) *The Appropriate Use of Closed Circuit Television (CCTV) Observation in a Secure Unit.* Bournemouth: Bournemouth University.

Wilson,K, Eaton,J, Foye,U, Ellis,M, Thomas,E and Simpson, A (2022) What Evidence Supports the Use of Body Worn Cameras in Mental Health Inpatient Wards? A Systematic Review and Narrative Synthesis of the Effects of Body Worn Cameras in Public Sector Services. *International Journal of Mental Health Nursing* **31** (2) 260–77.

Zigmond,A (1995) Special Care Wards: Are They Special? *Psychiatric Bulletin* **19**: 310–12.

Team Resilience

Thomas Kearney and Stephen Dye

Introduction

The concept of team resilience within acute mental health, especially when dealing with challenging behaviour, is something not given enough attention. This is illustrated by a paucity of studies in the healthcare context.

Defining resilience is moot unless we identify the context in which the resilience pertains. For the purposes of this chapter, and working with challenging behaviour, team resilience is defined as:

> The ability of a team to expeditiously adapt to change and proactively address challenging behaviour in clinical situations, whilst minimising stress on the patient and team members.

This definition aims to address the common demands placed upon teams working in an environment of challenging behaviour in health care.

When we talk about 'the team' in relation to challenging behaviour, who and what do we mean? The team must involve the entire spectrum of multidisciplinary staff who engage with patients exhibiting challenging behaviour and clinically contribute to the delivery of care. The holistic approach and joint delivery of care is justifiable in relation to resilience for several reasons. Firstly, multidisciplinary team (MDT) approaches within secure environments remain, idealistically at least, a cornerstone of quality care provision. Department of Health and healthcare governance publications have continuously re-emphasised the benefits of collaborative working augmenting care delivery (Department of Health, 1999, 2000, 2001, 2007, 2010, 2011, 2012; NAPICU, 2014). Secondly, implementing and positively operating MDT interventions and approaches remain a continuing goal within all clinical environments. Within a secure environment, the collective MDT jointly provides the basis for interventions and interactions with patients. The nature of an MDT will bring a variety of clinical approaches and styles which are intended to enhance care delivery and experience. This is in the interest of changing patient behaviour to enhance their experience of interpersonal interactions and societal normalisation.

If the clinical team works well together and has a unified purpose, a clear ethos, set standards and good leadership, it will normally function well (Borrill, 2000a; Lewis, 2011). This chapter outlines core ingredients essential to the quality of team approaches whilst considering the potential additional emotional and interprofessional demands placed upon the team and its members when working with individuals who display challenging behaviour. Mechanisms which successfully support and maintain these team approaches are core to continuous success and team resilience. The maintenance and development of such core MDT strength are the premises of this chapter in the face of the demanding clinical environment of challenging behaviour.

Development of an MDT Approach

The notion of the MDT in health care has its roots in lessons learned from the airline industry, particularly how a cockpit team of a large airliner functions (Powell and Hohenhaus, 2006). Several air crash disasters during the 1970s brought to light the extremely complex interrelationship between professional autonomy/authority of the captain with that of other crew members. Cockpit resource management (CRM) represented an idea for a highly developed team function based on effective communication and full utilisation of all team members' skills towards a single goal (Baker et al., 2006).

Parallels were drawn with health care in which the consultant doctor was seen to have similarities with the aircraft captain. To minimise errors and maximise team reliability, much of the philosophy of CRM was imported directly into the healthcare setting, representing the philosophical as well as operational underpinning for the modern MDT.

Definitions of an MDT in wider literature often do not accurately describe the nature of MDT working in the context of mental health or, even more specifically, in relation to challenging behaviour. Ovretveit (1995) described MDT working as 'a group of practitioners with different professional training working together to treat one or more clients within a given clinical area'. He added that although diverse, teams need a tightly defined purpose or ethos, design and consistent management to be effective.

In mental health, the MDT working ethos has largely emanated from community settings to permeate inpatient settings. We have moved away from large asylum-based treatment to smaller bed bases and greater specialism across the range of psychiatric care in both community and inpatient settings. This move was intended to provide more focused care and transitional support for recovery. It has required more of individual clinical specialities within psychiatry with the purpose of enhancing treatment outcomes. There have been implications for the development of MDTs across all these specialities. One of these implications has been a drive towards greater efficiency (implied faster recovery); others include care transitions and patient throughput. Collective MDT approaches have had to mesh quickly in order to provide holistic care planning and enhanced outcomes for patients. This has meant the development into specific aspects of service delivery, delivery which has grown beyond medical-based approaches within inpatient environments (in line with longer established community approaches) into a multidimensional care provision mechanism. This has required support, integration, truly joint approaches and a high degree of effective leadership in order to harness the potential of MDT approaches to meet demand.

The makeup, dynamics and cohesion of the clinical team are affected by several factors that ultimately impact the team's effectiveness in intervention. These factors include communication, clinical approaches and modalities, joint care planning, roles within the unit, team integration and geographical base (i.e. based on the unit or off).

Team Development and Key Attributes of Successful Teams

It is important to recognise that there is little evidence to support the contention that MDT approaches are more effective than alternatives at meeting demand in health care (Johnston and Dye, 2008). It seems that strategic and legislative drivers have been largely responsible for the emphasis on MDT approaches. This is opposed to a progressive development based on foundations of evidence for its effectiveness. The logic for desirability of the MDT may be underpinned by ideology that collective intelligence and specialisms offer a larger range and expert perspective on what patients need than in any alternative model. This seems to concur with common sense and is difficult to argue with. Furthermore, the idea of harnessing the collective power of teams is extremely well established in organisational effectiveness and operational delivery, so why shouldn't this be the same in health care (Collins, 2001)?

The argument is therefore that the key aspects of high-performing teams should be as equally applicable and adapted to face the demands of healthcare environments to make this 'efficient and enhanced delivery' a reality (Gallup, 2007).

The core behaviours and presuppositions of high-performing teams that are resilient in therapeutic engagement with patients who display challenging behaviour are based on the following:

- A clear unity of purpose
- The group being self-conscious about its operations
- The group having set clear and demanding performance goals
- An informal, relaxed and comfortable atmosphere
- Consistent discussion about issues in which all staff members feel free to participate (this is particularly important when considering specific challenging behaviours)
- People being free to air feelings as well as ideas
- Disagreement (which is encouraged) that is comfortable and quickly resolved with clear resolution, direction and purpose
- Collective decision-making around general agreement with a consensus viewpoint more often carried forward
- Collectively held expectations that are always maintained by all members of the team
- Frequent and frank criticism that is well received in the interests of making things better and comfortable
- Shifting of group leadership as necessary

(Oynett et al., 1997; Borrill et al., 2000b; Katzenbach and Smith, 2005; Barr and Dowding, 2012).

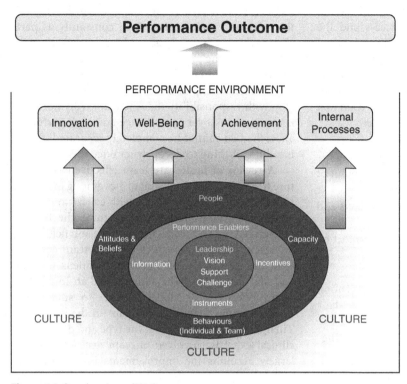

Figure 6.1 Based on Jones (2010)

The preceding model advocates that agreeing on a clear way of working, clear end points and sharing responsibility allows teams to perform better and be better protected from whatever they face; this is essential for team resilience in the face of any challenge. Jones (2010) reinforces this through extensive research on what supports high-performing teams and their continued success. This is visually represented in Figure 6.1.

Emphasis is placed on ensuring that conditions and drivers are in place for teams, as these components are essential building blocks of team resilience. A team's consistency and reliability are founded on its resilience and commonality, built upon a positive and supportive culture in which common goals drive behaviours rather than conflicting messages and different perspectives influencing interpretation and therefore understanding. The research on team resilience is sparse, but studies do show a link between team resilience and social 'capital', that is, the team's ability to trust in the collective team members' joint understanding and trust in each other (Lewis, 2011). This contributes to the collective confidence that a team can succeed in the face of adversity and that members will support each other. This ability for support and trust would seem an

augmented need within the context of challenging behaviour environments.

Difficulties Faced within Challenging Behaviour Settings

Resilience is a well-explored dimension within the wealth of literature on individual development. However, the mediums through which teams operate have not been separated from the studies. Neither have studies concentrated specifically on highly emotionally stressful environments whilst trying to care for individuals who may be verbally or physically abusive.

A core part of patient management within this environment is consistent reinforcement and education around the appropriateness of behaviour. This necessitates the consistent maintenance of boundaries by all staff members in order to be effective. Otherwise, splitting occurs, and the 'weak spots' within the staff group are exposed.

The need to consistently, calmly, sensitively and safely challenge patients within this environment is a key factor to the success of the unit and the team that works within it. Furthermore, the consistent ability of a team to repeatedly perform this task holistically and unanimously is central to clinical success and the perceived quality of care. The repeatability of central functions to performance whilst maintaining the well-being of the team is the very definition of resilience.

The additional factors which need enhanced attention in relation to disturbed behaviour and a team that works within units that provide care include:

- Team leadership which is perceived to be intimately connected to the 'real' issues facing the team and is also observable at the specific point of engagement with challenging behaviour
- Clarity of purpose interwoven into care plans and interactions with all patients
- Daily review of interactions within the context of these actions
- Team unity in delivery for consistency
- Staff support for each other in active intervention and post intervention through handover and daily emotional recognition and debriefs
- Review of the effect of 'challenge with tact' using involvement from patients and carers
- Consideration of all staff opinion and intervention to crystallise a collective approach for all patients
- Active challenge of those staff who do not actively maintain these principles and actions

This all sounds, and probably is, relatively simplistic. However, the nature of challenging behaviour environments means that the leadership and boundaries of clinicians and team members will be constantly tested. Consistency within approach and outcome is the powerful mechanism by which most behaviour is formed and changed. Therefore, setting the conditions for successful meshing of the MDT and developing the team to cope with pressures becomes of paramount importance. Creating the right conditions can enhance the delivery of care and allow the team to strengthen in order to work with the additional demands of challenging behaviour.

An overriding mechanism in the development and maintenance of resilience is the 'embeddedness' and reinforcement of a core ethos of proven techniques to an end goal which gives demonstrable results. This bolsters team approach, mentality and confidence in interventions that benefit both patients and staff. Put simply, the team will be more resilient if they believe in what they are doing and are empowered to do so, even in the face of adversity. The key to this is demonstrating the power of the techniques and reinforcing them when developing the team and maintaining them constantly as part of a positive culture. This can be achieved through simple operating procedures, process maps, supervision, debriefs and staff and patient engagement. This requires leadership dedication and devolved ownership with responsibility that the team truly holds. It is also the crossover of resilience and high performance; the two cannot be completely separated. Belief is a difficult thing to deconstruct once it is created.

A review of healthcare team effectiveness literature from 1985 to 2004 distinguishes among intervention studies that compare team with usual (non-team) care; intervention studies that examine the impact of team redesign on team effectiveness; and field studies that explore relationships between team context, structure, processes, and outcomes (Lemieux-Charles and McGuire, 2006). The authors used an Integrated Team Effectiveness Model (ITEM) to summarise research findings and identify gaps in the literature. Their analysis suggested that the type and diversity of clinical expertise involved in team decision-making largely accounts for improvements in patient care and organisational effectiveness. The study did not specify how these multi-perspectives were incorporated, channelled or controlled. It was suggested that perhaps the reason for lack of cohesive evidence for the efficiency of care could be partly attributable to the lack of wholehearted embracing of joint decision-making and why psychiatrists are still looked to, by default of authority and qualification, to override/make the final decision over patient care. Although this could be considered by some to be a natural process, 'the "responsible clinician" carries the responsibility' is an oft-quoted phrase from both medical and non-medical personnel. However, this detracts from the ability of a team to become more resilient, as it relies on individuals rather than the sum of the component parts. A team must become more than individuals and embody the belief and ethos it holds dear to become truly resilient.

Collaboration, conflict resolution, participation and cohesion are most likely to influence staff satisfaction and perceived team effectiveness. The studies examined here underscore the importance of considering the contexts in which teams are embedded.

An example of this approach can be seen when examining the management of the case example in Box 6.1.

Box 6.1 Case Study

A 33-year-old female (Patient J) was admitted to a low secure forensic environment. She had committed an index offence of actual bodily harm (ABH) and there was a history of chronic assaultive behaviour. Initially, Patient J had been given multiple diagnoses ranging from acute psychosis to bipolar affective disorder. Over time, these diagnoses were less supported after extensive assessment and treatment within inpatient wards. Her medication had been benzodiazepines, atypical antipsychotics and a number of mood stabilisers.

This admission occurred following an assault on a member of the public, Patient J's third offence in a year. She was initially re-admitted into a general adult ward under provisions of section 3 of the England and Wales Mental Health Act 1983 (MHA) (UK Government, 1983). After a period of weeks, following several assaults upon patients and staff, Patient J was referred and accepted by a low secure unit (LSU) for a period of continuing treatment and rehabilitation. At the time of admission to that service, she was receiving quetiapine 400 mg per day (as a mood stabiliser) and benzodiazepines as required.

When admitted to the low secure service, Patient J was very angry at still being detained. She refused to comply with requests from staff, and there were multiple outbursts and altercations, including spitting at (and on one occasion punching) other patients. This behaviour and altercations with other patients led to staff having to intervene seven times in Patient J's first 48 hours on the ward. She also had to be restrained four times. She subsequently began to spit at staff members and refused to engage in conversation or de-escalation. Due to the length of one of her restraint periods and her level of aggression, Patient J was placed in seclusion. Here, she ran at the door from the far side of the room, hitting the door with her head; she then had to be removed and restrained again to avoid self-harm.

De-escalation was a main management strategy. For large parts of the day Patient J refused to communicate with many staff and often stated she would only speak to the ward manager whom she said was the only person who understood her. There became an emerging pattern of behaviour of Patient J telling various staff members different things about what the previous shift had stated.

Team Approach Issues Arising from Case Example

The preceding clinical example has several facets which could reasonably be considered to represent significant challenges to team cohesion, functioning and resilience. There would also likely be the concern of attrition arising from the collective effect of the behaviours upon individuals and the team.

Some of the most difficult facets of this presentation may include:

- Dealing with aggression (effects on individuals)
- Spitting (a particularly offensive challenging behaviour)
- Potential for splitting of team members
- The possibility that involvement of the criminal justice system may improve team cohesion
- The way the ward manager handles being the only one that Patient J would talk to. There is a fine balance between taking the required legitimate role as the official leader against disempowering other team members and their function

Team Approach

A meeting held with all members of the MDT for Patient J outlined specific aspects of her presentation. The agreed-upon diagnosis based on assessment was one of emotionally unstable personality disorder, borderline type with antisocial traits.

It was important that the main influential staff within the team (these may not be the most senior by grade) with the strongest views were identified and made central to any process of deciding on the appropriate care plan.

Aim

The agreed-upon overall treatment aim was to manage behaviour and suggest alternatives which did not result in aggressive outbursts and work within a psychoeducation and mentalisation framework.

Management Strategy

Through discussion, the team determined that the main trigger for Patient J's aggressive outbursts was her perception that her requests to staff were not being met. Also identified were issues with Patient

J giving various versions of interactions that had occurred. There was a suggestion that Patient J was manipulating or completely misinterpreting staff communication. It was important that this issue be understood and accepted by the team.

A wellness recovery action plan (WRAP) (Copeland, 2002) was initiated to identify initial triggers and coping strategies. A collective decision was made to document Patient J's daily requests, which she countersigned each shift. Patient J was actively involved in this decision. One-to-one sessions would specifically focus on the interpretation of Patient J's interactions and possible misinterpretations and other ways of handling specific situations. Baselines of incidents were taken from Patient J's stay in the challenging behaviour unit and from the open acute ward. These were examined for triggers and the application of any coping strategy. These, too, were monitored and reviewed in one-to-ones with Patient J once a week. She was also encouraged to talk about any other coping mechanisms she wished to learn more about and provided with appropriate literature. Medication was reduced using an agreed-upon plan which was reviewed weekly alongside the success of the application of learnt coping strategies.

Clinical Outcomes

Within one month, there was a 50% reduction in weekly incident rates, and Patient J had been taught and applied 12 variants of immediate coping strategies for situations she found difficult. This was a significant improvement from previous interactions, and this continued to improve over her stay within the unit.

The staff discussed the emotional impact from certain patients, including Patient J, in daily handover, and interactional goals for shifts with all patients were introduced at the request of staff. Staff agreed to support each other immediately after difficult interactions with all patients as standard before any debrief that was necessary. Also, staff discussed how they could have handled things better for the patient.

A graded exposure aspect to care planning was introduced, including increased responsibility for Patient J within the unit as well as her financial planning, psychotherapy one-to-one sessions and extended leave.

Aggressive incidents continued to reduce and so did medication titration until Patient J was medication free after a six-month period.

Team Outcomes

Evident throughout the treatment plan were the elements required for the promotion of team resilience and cohesion while engaging with severe challenging behaviour. Whilst discrete resilience-building activities such as formal specific individual supervision, specific debrief meetings and group supervision are well practiced and useful interventions, they do not substitute for team resilience considerations built innately into the clinical care plan.

In Patient J's case, the following can be identified as clear components in the overall approach and specific treatment plan:

- Giving every member of the team an opportunity to contribute to the care plan
- Hearing and understanding the views of all ward staff by the unit and service leadership
- Allowing team members to contribute to defining care plans and limits
- Setting a context within which the criminal justice service could be involved
- Possible staff supervision groups
- Leadership from the front with direct clinical input by the ward manager

Conclusion

Team resilience is not just an idea or a trait but a set of behaviours demonstrated and driven by underpinning mechanisms. Resilience is driven by faith in idealistic and non-maleficent premises and benevolence within a clinical context.

It requires setting conditions of empowerment, belief and leadership throughout a team, not to be held by singular clinicians. It is maintained by reinforcement and demonstration of the benefits to patients and staff of behaviours. It is continued by ways of working which bolster management of difficult engagement and challenges within a challenging behaviour setting to allow change for the clinical benefit of patients and harmony of the clinical medium.

The emotional effects of these difficult challenges do not diminish but are offset and regulated by the ethos of the collective group and strong support mechanisms which underpin it, including supervision, debriefing, the processes and system and, most importantly, collective ownership from both staff and patients of the aforementioned expectant behaviours.

A team which uses these mechanisms, built around these core beliefs, will be far more resilient in coping with both internal and external challenges by having this wealth of culture and systems driving quality of clinical care and the confidence to deal with difficulties that arise.

References

Baker,DP, Day,R and Salas,E (2006) Teamwork as an Essential Component of High-Reliability Organizations. *Health Services Research* **41** (4) 1576–98.

Barr,J and Dowding,L (2012) *Leadership in Health Care*, 2nd ed. London: Sage Publications Limited.

Borrill,C, Carletta,J, Carter,AJ, Dawson,JF, Garrod,S, Rees, A, et al. (2000a) *The Effectiveness of Health Care Teams in the National Health Service Report*. Scotland: Glasgow University Press.

Borrill,C, West,M, Shapiro,D and Rees,A (2000b) Team Working and Effectiveness in Healthcare. *British Journal of Healthcare Management* **6** (8) 364–71.

Collins,J (2001) *Good to Great*. London: Random House Business Books.

Copeland,ME (2002) Wellness Recovery Action Plan. *Occupational Therapy in Mental Health* **17** (3–4) 127–50.

Department of Health (1999) *National Service Framework for Mental Health: Modern Standards and Service Models*. London: HMSO.

Department of Health (2000) *The NHS Plan: A Plan for Investment, a Plan for Reform*. London: HMSO.

Department of Health (2001) *Health and Social Care Act 2001*. London: TSO.

Department of Health (2002) National Minimum Standards for General Adult Services in Psychiatric Intensive Care Units (PICU) and Low Secure Environments. In Pereira,S and Clinton,C (eds.), *Mental Health Policy Implementation Guide*. London: Department of Health Publications.

Department of Health (2010) *Essence of Care*. London: HMSO.

Department of Health (2011) *The Operating Framework for the NHS in England 2012/13*. London: TSO.

Department of Health (2012) *The Health and Social Care Act 2012*. London: TSO.

Johnston,A and Dye,S (2008) *Multidisciplinary Teams within PICUs/LSUs*. in Beer,DM, Pereira,S and Paton,C (eds.), *Psychiatric Intensive Care*, 2nd ed. pp. 322–39. Cambridge: Cambridge University Press.

Jones,G (2010) A Context for Success: Creating the High-Performance Environment. *Business Finance* **16** (3) 26.

Katzenbach,JR and Smith,DK (2005) *The Wisdom of Teams: Creating the High-Performance Organization*. Boston: Harvard Business School Press.

Lemieux-Charles,L and McGuire,WL (2006) What Do We Know about Health Care Team Effectiveness: A Review of the Literature. *Medical Care Research and Review* **63** (3) 263–300.

Lewis,R, Donaldson-Feilder,E and Pangallo,A (2011) *Developing Resilience: An Evidence-Based Guide for Practitioners*. London: Chartered Institute of Personnel and Development.

Mallak,LA (1998) Measuring Resilience in Health Care Provider Organizations. *Health Manpower Management* **24** (4–5) 148–52.

UK Government (1983) Mental Health Act 1983. legislation.gov.UK. www.legislation.gov.uk/ukpga/1983/20/contents.

Onyett,S, Pillinger,T and Muijen,M (1997) Job Satisfaction and Burnout among Members of Community Mental Health Teams. *Journal of Mental Health* **6** (1) 55–66.

Powell,S and Hohenhaus,S (2006) Multidisciplinary Team Training and the Art of Communication. *Journal of Clinical Paediatric Emergency Medicine* **7** (4) 238–40.

Scott,K and Mensik,JS (2010) Creating the Conditions for Breakthrough Clinical Performance. *Nurse Leader* **8** (4) 48–52.

Tuckman,B (1965) Developmental Sequence in Small Groups. *Psychological Bulletin* **63** (6) 384–99.

White,A (2009) *From Comfort Zone to Performance Management*. Belgium: White & MacLean Publishing.

Chapter

7

Principles and Practice for Management of Acutely Disturbed Patients

Stephen M. Pereira and Lucy M. Walker

Introduction

In this chapter, we describe the nature of the acutely disturbed patient and their associated symptoms and behaviours, followed by an overview of general challenges for managing such disturbance. We present a philosophy for dealing with disturbed patients, followed by a section on appropriate assessment and care planning. We also present a brief outline of the range of appropriate interventions, including verbal de-escalation and reducing institutional escalation, medication, physical intervention, seclusion and segregation. Further, we discuss how to develop activity and engagement programmes for acute disturbance, followed by an outline of the staff levels of training and experience required for effective management. We conclude the chapter with a brief outline of the roles of multidisciplinary team (MDT) members in the management of acute disturbance.

Violence and Aggression

Violence and aggression are relatively common and serious occurrences in health and social care settings. Between 2013 and 2014, there were 68,683 assaults reported against National Health Service (NHS) staff in England: 69% in mental health or learning disability settings, 27% against ambulance staff, 25% involving primary care staff and 26% involving acute hospital staff. Violence and aggression in mental health settings occur most frequently in inpatient psychiatric units and most acute hospital assaults take place in emergency departments (NICE, 2015).

Violence is a serious concern in the psychiatric inpatient and emergency setting (Zeng et al., 2013; Cheung et al., 2017; Olashore et al., 2018). Systematic reviews of workplace violence suggest prevalence rates of violence range from 11.4% to a staggering 97.6% (Joo Jang et al., 2022), with a one-year prevalence of verbal and/or physical workplace violence around

84.2% (Lu et al., 2019). This high prevalence is believed to be caused by differences in healthcare settings, healthcare service delivery, the common aspect of caring for patients and specific characteristics of the psychiatric ward and psychiatric patients (Ferri et al., 2016; Ruben et al., 2019).

Psychiatric intensive care unit (PICU) staff are frequently called upon to manage patients who are violent or potentially violent; more than half of all admissions (58.5%) are for violence to others/damage to property (Pereira et al., 2021). It is vital that staff work together in an informed and supported environment to minimise the potential risks to themselves and others.

The Acutely Disturbed Patient: Symptoms and Behaviours

Acute behavioural disturbance requires urgent intervention. It usually manifests with mood, thought or behavioural signs and symptoms and can be transient, episodic or long lasting. It can have either a medical or psychological etiology and may reflect a person's limited capacity to cope with social, domestic or environmental stressors. The use of illicit substances or alcohol can accompany an episode of acute disturbance or can be causative Dyer (1996). (See Chapter 9, Section 3 for further information.)

Disturbed behaviour is often transient and associated with the severity of the underlying psychiatric disorder. As the illness responds to treatment, so does the behaviour. Acute disturbance can also become chronic disturbance. Such patients are often described as exhibiting 'challenging behaviour' and may require longer admission and a wide range of pharmacological and psychological treatments. Some patients in this group have associated cognitive deficits (e.g. head injury) or severe problems with impulse control (e.g. borderline personality disorder).

Acutely disturbed patients can exhibit a wide range of symptoms and behaviours that can vary depending on the underlying cause of their disturbance. The following are some common symptoms and behaviours that may be observed in an acutely disturbed patient:

- **Agitation**: Patients may become restless, irritable or fidgety and may exhibit signs of increased activity, such as pacing or restlessness.
- **Aggression**: Patients may become verbally or physically abusive and/or aggressive, which can pose a risk to themselves or others. This abuse may involve threatened or actual violence towards others, destruction of property, emotional upset or psychological distress. More than one patient may be involved and everyday objects such as chairs, table knives or broken cups may be used to threaten or cause damage to others or to property.
- **Delusions**: Patients may exhibit delusional thinking, such as paranoia, grandiosity or bizarre beliefs.
- **Hallucinations**: Patients may experience auditory or visual hallucinations, which can be frightening and disorienting.
- **Confusion**: Patients may become confused and disoriented and may have difficulty with memory, attention and decision-making.
- **Disorganised behaviour**: Patients may exhibit disorganised behaviour, such as odd or inappropriate speech, dressing inappropriately for the weather or exhibiting poor hygiene. They may be disinhibited, exposing themselves or masturbating in public areas and exhibit extreme overactivity.
- **Self-harm**: Patients may engage in active self-harming behaviours, such as cutting or burning themselves, or they may express suicidal thoughts or intent or threats to self-harm.
- **Substance abuse**: Patients may exhibit symptoms of substance abuse or withdrawal, which can exacerbate their other symptoms.

It is important to note that these symptoms and behaviours can be caused by a variety of underlying conditions, including psychiatric disorders, medical conditions or drug use, among others. It's crucial that acutely disturbed patients receive a thorough evaluation and appropriate treatment to address the underlying cause of their symptoms and behaviours.

General Challenges for Managing Acute Disturbance

Managing acute disturbance in patients can present several challenges for healthcare professionals, including the following:

- **Safety concerns**: Acutely disturbed patients can pose a risk to themselves or others, which can be challenging to manage. Healthcare professionals need to ensure the safety of both the patient and those around them while providing appropriate care.
- **Communication difficulties**: Acutely disturbed patients may have difficulty communicating their needs and may have impaired decision-making ability. Healthcare professionals need to be skilled in communicating with patients who are experiencing acute disturbance and finding alternative methods of communication when necessary.
- **Diagnostic uncertainty**: It can be difficult to determine the underlying cause of a patient's acute disturbance, particularly if they have no prior psychiatric history or present with atypical symptoms. This can make it challenging to provide appropriate treatment and care.
- **Time pressure**: Acutely disturbed patients often require immediate intervention to ensure their safety and prevent harm to others. Healthcare professionals need to work quickly to assess the patient, determine the appropriate course of action and initiate treatment promptly.
- **Resource limitations**: Managing acutely disturbed patients can be resource-intensive, requiring specialised training, equipment and personnel. Limited resources can make it challenging to provide the necessary level of care, particularly in settings with high patient volumes or limited access to mental health resources.

The following summarises the relevant issues in PICUs:

- PICU staff should be familiar with the procedures to be followed to facilitate the safe admission of an acutely disturbed patient.
- PICU staff should be trained in risk assessment and in the prediction, prevention and management of aggression.
- The PICU should have a written policy for the management of aggression. This should include advice on psychological and pharmacological interventions and when to involve the police.

- Ward policies on aggression should be communicated to patients as soon as is appropriate after admission.
- Incident forms should be completed after all aggressive incidents. These incident forms should be regularly reviewed and feedback should be provided to staff.
- Time and resources should be provided for formal debriefing after incidents. Specialist counselling may be required for victims of serious incidents.
- Sufficient appropriately staffed units to manage disturbed behaviour should be available across all levels of security.

Addressing these challenges requires a collaborative approach that involves a multidisciplinary team, including physicians, nurses, social workers and other healthcare professionals. Training in crisis intervention, de-escalation techniques and communication strategies can help healthcare professionals manage acutely disturbed patients effectively while maintaining a safe and therapeutic environment. These issues are also considered in detail elsewhere in this volume.

Preparing the Ward for the Arrival of an Acutely Behaviourally Disturbed Patient

While many patients admitted to PICUs are already well known to the service, a significant proportion will be being admitted for the first time. A standard admissions procedure will help staff to feel more in control and reduce the variability in approaches that may occur when less experienced staff or staff unfamiliar with the ward are on duty. Such a procedure could be written as a bulleted list and displayed in a prominent position in the nursing office, as is shown here.

- Ideally, the patient should have been assessed prior to admission by PICU staff and a management plan should be in place.
- All PICU nursing staff should be alerted.
- If the patient is waiting in a police vehicle, they should remain there until the PICU is ready to receive them.
- If there is no dedicated 'reception suite', ensure that the unit is safe (e.g. lock the servery, TV room, etc.).
- Remove all other patients from the reception area.

- Ensure staff are prepared (e.g. that staff trained in de-escalation and physical intervention is available if required). Decide which member of staff will be talking to the patient.
- Inform medical staff/prescriber and discuss any immediate requirement in advance, if possible (e.g. a medical examination if the patient is already sedated or a rapid assessment if the patient is still very disturbed and requires sedation).

Nursing Observations

Ideally, prior to admission, PICU staff should have assessed the patient and a clear nursing plan should be in place. For new admissions unknown to staff, the level of nursing observations should be negotiated between the clinicians on duty involved with the admission.

Observation/engagement levels and national guidance/local policy will dictate the exact terminology used. The levels of observations are outlined in the following sections.

Level 1: Nominal Supervision
- Awareness of expected whereabouts of patient at all times

Level 2: Close Attention
- Specified randomised checks commonly ranging from every 5, 15 and 30 minutes to hourly

Level 3: Constant Care
- Continual line-of-sight observation, but privacy granted for specific reasons (e.g. bathing)

Level 4: Intensive Observations
- Continual presence of nursing staff and constant, direct visual observation sometimes within a specified distance (e.g. within arm's reach)

On admission, it is wise to be cautious. It is easier to reduce observation levels if the patient is more settled than anticipated than to deal with the consequences of inadequate observation. Close observation can also be distressing for the patient and at times can be the specific cause of escalation. These issues should be assessed, and the best balance drawn between safety and imposing restriction.

The level of observation should be determined by the multidisciplinary team (MDT) and reviewed at least once each nursing shift. Staff should be appropriately trained for carrying out close observation. It should be recognised that special observation can exacerbate behavioural disturbance and unobtrusive monitoring can sometimes be used effectively. Episodes of continuous observation lasting less than 72 hours have been shown to help two-thirds of patients (Shugar and Rehaluk, 1990).

Mental Health Act Status

Ideally the PICU should have a policy in place which clearly defines the legal status of patients who may be admitted. This should be subject to local agreement. According to the most recent UK national survey of PICUs, 65.4% of admissions were detained under the Mental Health Act 1983 (UK Government, 1983) Section 3, 23.7% under Section 2, 6.2% from forensic sections, 2.6% from prison transfer and 2.1% were informal admissions (Pereira et al., 2021).

Informal patients are sometimes admitted, although this should be the exception rather than the rule (Department of Health, 2002).

In the United Kingdom, if patients are resisting, aggressive and refusing treatment or wishing to leave the ward without agreement and their status is still informal, then an assessment for eligibility for detention under the Mental Health Act (MHA) should be arranged. If it is immediately necessary, for example to prevent significant injury, intramuscular medication can be given under common law (under the doctrine of necessity). This requires careful consideration and clear documentation because professionals may be open to prosecution for assault by an informal patient.

Within the United Kingdom, any hospital doctor or 'approved clinician' may use Mental Health Act (1983) Section 5(2) to detain a patient for up to 72 hours, or any registered mental health nurse can use Section 5(4) to detain a patient for up to 6 hours. However, medication cannot be given against the patient's will under Section 5, but it can be given under Sections 2, 3 or 4 (as in Section 2, but involving only one doctor and valid for up to 72 hours). It is considered good practice to audit the use of these sections in a PICU; they should never be relied upon for routine care. (See Chapters 19 and 20 for the use of physical intervention and seclusion.)

Ensuring a Safe Environment

Ensuring a safe environment requires:

- good visibility in all areas of the unit
- alarms always within easy reach and, ideally, worn about the person

- consistent staff response to alarms
- minimal movable objects; those that exist should be of safe size and construction
- provision of structured activities (e.g. gym, garden, games)

(See Chapter 4 and NAPICU, 2014.)

Philosophy for Management

There are various philosophies that guide the management of acute disturbance in healthcare settings. Some of these philosophies include:

- **Person-centred care**: This philosophy emphasises the importance of viewing the acutely disturbed patient as a whole person rather than simply a collection of symptoms. It involves actively involving the patient in their care and treatment and working collaboratively to develop a care plan that addresses their individual needs and preferences (Corrigan, 2015).
- **Trauma-informed care**: This philosophy recognises that many acutely disturbed patients have experienced significant trauma in their lives, which can impact their behaviour and ability to cope. It involves creating a safe, supportive environment that avoids re-traumatising the patient and prioritises their emotional and psychological well-being (McKenna et al., 2019).
- **Recovery-oriented care**: This philosophy emphasises the possibility of recovery and encourages a patient-centred, strengths-based approach to treatment. It involves supporting the patient in their journey toward recovery, helping them identify and build on their strengths and focusing on their goals for the future (Laranjeira and Querido, 2022).
- **Harm reduction**: This philosophy recognises that some acutely disturbed patients may engage in risky or harmful behaviours, such as substance abuse or self-harm. It involves prioritising harm reduction strategies that help minimise the risks associated with these behaviours, such as providing clean needles for injection drug use or implementing suicide prevention protocols (Lev-Ran, S. et al., 2014).
- **Evidence-based practice**: This philosophy emphasises the importance of using the best available evidence to guide decision-making and treatment planning. It involves regularly reviewing the latest research and incorporating it

into clinical practice to ensure that patients receive the most effective and appropriate care (Norcross et al., 2006).

Overall, the philosophy for managing acute disturbance should prioritise the safety and well-being of the patient while providing compassionate, individualised care that considers the patient's unique needs and circumstances. It should also emphasise the importance of working collaboratively with the patient and their family, as well as other healthcare professionals, to ensure that the patient receives the best possible care and support.

Management after an Aggressive Incident/Debriefing

After all aggressive incidents, formal debriefing should be offered (NICE, 2015, 2017), focusing on practical and emotional issues at the time; although there is some controversy about the effectiveness of debriefing (Rick et al., 1998), victims need sympathy, support and reassurance.

For professionals who are assaulted, it is advisable for them to return to work as soon as possible to prevent 'the incubation of fear'. Usually, the team working at the time of the incident is sufficient to deal with the debriefing known as a 'hot debrief' (Gilmartin et al., 2020). However, in the case of very serious incidents, it may be useful to have an external person to ensure that sufficient counselling is provided, particularly to anyone who has sustained significant physical or emotional injury; debriefing tools can be used to structure the session (Sugarman et al., 2021).

At the time of a serious aggressive incident, immediate safety issues must take precedence over any investigation. The latter should attempt, as sensitively as possible, to compile detailed reports of the incident to understand its causes, context and consequences.

Dealing with the Aftermath of an Incident If You Are the Victim

- Acknowledge that you may experience some symptoms of stress and be aware that these may be delayed for several hours.
- Do not become helpless; be explicit about what you want or do not want in the way of support.
- Do not blame yourself; try and learn from the experience.

- Try to return to work soon.
- Accept the necessary management investigations.
- Follow procedures carefully.
- Ensure that you get support, both formal and informal.

What Colleagues and Friends Can Do

- At the time, give the victim unconditional reassurance.
- Show that you are willing to talk at any time.
- Reassure the victim's family and ensure that the victim is not left alone after work; for example, offer a lift home.
- Help the victim to assimilate the experience and keep a sense of proportion, bearing in mind the nearly universal problem of unrealistic guilt.
- Do not treat victims as if they have an infectious disease (they do report being ignored).

What Teams and Ward Managers Can Do

- Consider the need both for support and debriefing.
- Allow time to talk as a group.
- Consider what worked well/went wrong and how to prevent/deal with similar incidents in the future.
- Consider the feelings involved and make sure you have a chance to express them.
- Act on any suggestions which come out of the post-incident debriefing, given the tendency of organisations to experience denial after traumatic events.

Whether to Charge a Patient after an Incident

This is often a very difficult decision, and it may require considerable time and effort on the part of the clinical team to even persuade the local police service to interview the patient. It is essential for the MDT to decide whether to press charges, as there will be issues for the victim if they are part of the clinical team.

The victim of the attack will need the support of colleagues because there may be emotions such as guilt, which need to be worked through. Factors that may influence the team's decision to press charges may include:

- The patient's mental state
- The capacity of the patient to form intent
- The degree of harm inflicted
- The likely effect on the patient
- Perceived need for more secure placement

Based on a literature review by Leeuwen and Harte (2011), it is advised to report and investigate a case when the incident results in severe injury, the incident is a sexual offence or when a patient repetitively causes violent incidents. Moreover, it appears that, although many studies have been published on violence in psychiatry, the prosecution of violent psychiatric patients has received little attention in the international literature.

Advantages of Criminal Justice Engagement

Advantages of involving the criminal justice system include:

- The possible therapeutic effect for the patient who may understand the concept and value of boundaries.
- The responsibility for managing difficult behaviour is shared with court/criminal justice system professionals.
- The patient may get a criminal record/hospital order/restriction order, which will alert others to possible danger in the future.
- Resources may be more forthcoming for the treatment of such a patient.
- Formal documentation of an incident is made.
- The patient has the opportunity to defend theirself if they feel wrongly accused.
- It may increase the chance of compensation for the victim.

'Organisation-Wide' Issues Regarding Management of Disturbed Behaviour

- The PICU should have policies on the management of aggression.
- Staff should be trained in the management of aggression.
- Incident forms should be completed for all aggressive incidents.
- These incident forms should be regularly analysed, and feedback provided to staff.
- Time and resources should be available for formal debriefing after incidents.

- Time and resources should be provided for specialist counselling of those victims of a serious incident.
- The MDT should be expected to engage and counsel patients who exhibit repeated episodes of disturbed behaviour.
- Ward policies on aggression designed for patients should be communicated to them as soon as appropriate after admission.
- Anger management groups should be provided for patients.
- Ensure that staff understand and have experience in risk assessment.
- Ensure that there is good cooperation between health and social services.
- Ensure that there is good record-keeping and communication between community and inpatient facilities.
- Ensure that there are sufficient units to manage disturbed behaviour (e.g. intensive care units which are well staffed and arrange training of staff in the assessment and management of the acutely disturbed patient).

Leadership is essential. Basic skills in risk assessment and confidence in the management of disturbed behaviour are core skills that should be shared by all staff working in PICUs.

Evidenced-Based Guidelines

There are several evidence-based guidelines for managing acute behavioural disturbance in healthcare settings, including:

- *The National Institute for Health and Care Excellence (NICE) Guidelines for Violence and Aggression (NG10)*: These guidelines provide recommendations for the assessment and management of violence and aggression in healthcare settings, including the use of physical interventions, pharmacological interventions and psychological interventions (NICE, 2015).
- *The National institute for Health and Care Excellence (NICE) Guidelines for Self-Harm: Assessment, Management and Preventing Recurrence (NG225)*: This guideline covers assessment, management and preventing recurrence for children, young people and adults who have self-harmed. It includes those with a mental health problem, neurodevelopmental disorder or learning disability and applies to all

sectors that work with people who have self-harmed (NICE, 2022).

- *The Royal Australian and New Zealand College of Psychiatrists' Guidelines on the Management of Deliberate Self-Harm*: These guidelines provide recommendations for the assessment and management of patients who have engaged in deliberate self-harm, including the use of psychological and pharmacological interventions and the implementation of suicide prevention strategies (Carter et al., 2016).
- *The Crisis Prevention Institute's Nonviolent Crisis Intervention Training Program*: This program provides evidence-based training in crisis prevention and de-escalation techniques, including strategies for managing acute behavioural disturbance in healthcare and other settings (Godin et al., 2003).
- *The Joint NAPICU and British Association of Psychopharmacology Consensus Guidelines for the Clinical Management of Acute Disturbance: De-escalation and Rapid Tranquillisation*: This guideline includes recommendations for clinical practice and an algorithm to guide treatment by healthcare professionals with various options outlined according to their route of administration and category of evidence. Fundamental overarching principles are included and highlight the importance of treating the underlying disorder (Patel et al., 2018).

Overall, these guidelines emphasise the importance of using evidence-based interventions to manage acute behavioural disturbance, as well as the need for a collaborative and multidisciplinary approach that involves healthcare professionals, patients and their families in the care and treatment process.

It is important to note the following points regarding guidelines:

- They may vary by geographic location and healthcare setting, and healthcare professionals should consult local guidelines and policies for the most up-to-date recommendations.
- They are subject to updates and may vary by country. They may have different recommendations for specific interventions and may have various levels of evidence for each of their recommendations. The most recent version of the guidelines in your specific region should be consulted for the most accurate information.

- They are meant to be prescriptive and should be used as a resource to inform clinical decision-making rather than dictate it. It is always recommended to consider the patient's individual needs and circumstances in making treatment decisions.

It is important to ensure that you consult the guideline in conjunction with other sources of information and seek the guidance of senior colleagues or supervisory bodies when dealing with complex or difficult cases.

Assessment

Staff Safety

Staff working in PICUs should be aware of the basic rules to follow to reduce the risk to themselves. They should also ensure that other staff who may visit the ward on a sessional basis are aware of these rules.

- When interviewing a patient who has potential for aggressive behaviour always inform colleagues of your intentions and location.
- Try to conduct joint medical and nursing assessments to protect interviewers and to reduce stimulation to the patient.
- Ensure that there are always alarms close by.
- Consider providing staff with personal alarms that have the facility to alert others to an emergency and its location.
- Sit at an angle to the patient at a safe distance away and near the exit.
- Avoid interviewing with the patient between you and the door.
- Call the police if necessary.

Research performed in PICUs (Walker and Seifert, 1994) has shown that a disproportionately high number of violent incidents are perpetrated by a few patients (two patients were responsible for 15 of the 37 violent incidents considered in the study). Mortimer (1995) also showed that a few patients caused many incidents. As more staff were trained in control and restraint, the number of incidents decreased. It is often very difficult to predict accurately who these patients will be, but patients who score heavily on the factors in the lists below should be deemed those most at risk of disturbed behaviour.

Assessment of acute behavioural disturbance involves a comprehensive evaluation of the patient's presenting symptoms, medical history, mental health status and risk factors for harm to self or others. Here are some key components of the assessment process:

- **Physical assessment**: should be performed to rule out any underlying medical conditions that may be contributing to the patient's symptoms. This may include vital signs, neurological examination and drug or alcohol screening.
- **Mental health assessment**: should be conducted to evaluate the patient's current mental state, including their mood, affect, thought content and level of distress. This may involve standardised assessment tools such as the Brief Psychiatric Rating Scale (BPRS) or the Global Assessment of Functioning (GAF) scale.
- **Comprehensive substance misuse assessment**: this should be used to evaluate the patient's use of any drugs and/or alcohol This should also include motivational assessment and urinalysis if necessary and indicated (see Chapter 9 on Substance Misuse).
- **Risk assessment**: should be conducted to evaluate the patient's risk of harm to self or others. This may involve assessing the patient's history of violence, access to means of harm and level of impulsivity.
- **Environmental assessment**: should be conducted to identify any factors that may be contributing to the patient's symptoms, such as proximity of bedroom to nursing office for monitoring/noise levels, overcrowding, overstimulation by noise or other stressors.
- **Collateral information**: should be obtained from family members, friends or other healthcare providers who have knowledge of the patient's history and current status.
- **Cultural considerations**: should be include language barriers, cultural beliefs and other factors that may impact the assessment process and treatment plan.

Occupational and Social Assessment

An occupational and social assessment can help to identify the patient's strengths, challenges and needs related to their occupational performance and social functioning. This type of assessment can be particularly important for patients experiencing acute behavioural disturbance, as occupational and social factors can contribute to the development and maintenance of the patient's symptoms.

Here are some components that may be included in an occupational and social assessment:

- **Occupational history**: An occupational therapist can gather information about the patient's past and present work, leisure and self-care activities. This can help to identify areas of strength and challenge related to the patient's occupational performance.
- **Functional assessment**: An occupational therapist can assess the patient's functional abilities related to self-care, work and leisure activities. This can help to identify areas where the patient may need support or intervention to improve their occupational performance.
- **Environmental assessment**: An occupational therapist can assess the patient's physical and social environment to identify factors that may be contributing to the patient's symptoms or impairing their occupational performance. This can include factors such as noise/lighting, their home environment or social environmental support.
- **Social history**: A social worker or other social services provider can gather information about the patient's social history and functioning, including their relationships with family and friends, social support networks and community involvement.
- **Social and emotional functioning**: A social worker or other mental health professional can assess the patient's social and emotional functioning, including their coping skills, emotional regulation and social skills.
- **Personal strengths and resources**: The assessment can also identify the patient's personal strengths and resources, such as skills, interests and hobbies, which can be used to support their occupational performance and social functioning.

An occupational and social assessment can help to identify areas where the patient may need support or intervention to improve their occupational performance and social functioning. This information can be used to develop a comprehensive care plan that addresses the patient's physical, emotional and environmental needs.

Overall, the assessment process should be thorough and tailored to the individual needs and circumstances of the patient. It should involve collaboration between healthcare professionals, the patient and their family members, and should be conducted in a supportive and non-threatening environment. The assessment findings should guide the development of an individualised care plan that addresses the patient's acute behavioural disturbance as well as any underlying medical or mental health conditions and occupational or social care needs.

Risk Factors for Violent Behaviour

A systematic meta-analysis study showed that almost one in five patients admitted to acute psychiatric units may commit acts of violence. Being male, diagnosed with schizophrenia, substance use and a history of aggression were factors linked to violence (Lozzino et al., 2015). Important factors from the patient's history, which may indicate an increased risk of violence (Royal College of Psychiatrists, 1995; College Research Unit, 1998), include:

- Previous violence towards others or self (Anderson and Bukor, 2012; Witt et al., 2013; Gintalaite-Bieliauskiene et al., 2020)
- Being young and male (Witt et al., 2013)
- Previous forensic history; history of imprisonment, recent arrest for any offence or history of conviction for a violent offence (O'Driscoll, 2012; Burca et al., 2013; Witt et al., 2013)
- Substance misuse (Dyer, 1996)
- Antisocial, explosive or impulsive personality traits (Howard et al., 2013; Witt et al., 2013)
- Poor compliance with treatment or services, particularly psychological therapies and medication (Witt et al., 2013)
- Association with a subculture prone to violence
- Evidence of social restlessness or rootlessness
- Recent homelessness/unstable accommodation, history of homelessness (Witt et al., 2013; Trevedi et al., 2022)
- Presence of precipitants (e.g. loss events)
- Access to any named potential victims identified in mental state

The characteristics in Box 7.1. have been identified as predicting the 'potential for immediate violence/aggression' (College Research Unit, 1998) and have been evidenced/updated with further research since that time, such as systematic reviews and meta-regression analyses of 110 studies of risk factors for violence in psychosis (Witt et al., 2013).

Box 7.1 Violence Risk Characteristics

Primary Characteristics

- Previous history of assaults/aggression or violence, overtly aggressive acts or forensic history (Witt et al., 2013)
- Hostile, threatening verbalisation, boasting of prior abuse
- Suspicious, paranoid ideation
- Delusions of control or hallucinations with violent content
- Poor impulse control/lack of self-control (Woessner and Sneider, 2013)
- Non-verbal expression of hostile intent such as increased motor activity, pacing, invading an other's personal space, angry facial expression
- Refusal to communicate
- Poor concentration or unclear thought processes
- Possession of a weapon

Secondary Characteristics

- Fear, anger, anxiety and pain
- Inappropriate and unrealistic demands
- Exacerbation of psychotic illness, particularly changes in life events, low self-esteem or vulnerability to interpersonal stress
- Inability to verbalise feelings
- Boredom (Kustermans, 2016)
- Previous substance abuse (see Chapter 9, Section 3)
- Low self-esteem (Woessner and Sneider, 2013)
- History of parenting problems (Woessner and Sneider, 2013)
- History of violent victimisation in childhood (Witt et al., 2013)
- Experienced physical or sexual abuse in childhood (Witt et al., 2013)
- Parental history of criminal involvement (Witt et al., 2013)
- Parental history of alcohol misuse (Witt et al., 2013)

Related Factors and Considerations

- Hypomanic excitement
- Confusional states
- Psychiatric or psychological motivation for problematic behaviour
- Goal structure for aggressive/problematic behaviour
- Lower socio-economic status (Witt et al., 2013)
- Lacking insight (Witt et al., 2013)

Precipitants of Violent Incidents on Wards

- Enforcement of ward rules
- Denial of patient's requests
- Confrontational or irritable manner of staff

Staff Factors Related to Incidents

- Staff stability
- Staff training (young untrained more likely to be victims)
- Poor leadership
- Inadequate staff resources

There are also some behavioural clues which have been identified as being predictors of imminent violence (Wykes and Mezey, 1994). These are mainly intuitive and include dishevelled appearance, smell of alcohol, signs of increased physiological arousal, pacing, gesticulating and violent gestures, increased muscle tension such as clenched fists and teeth, flared nostrils, escalating volume of speech, swearing, direct threats, labile affect and appearing frightened, confused and disorientated (see Box 7.2).

Older, more experienced staff (Hodgkinson et al., 1985; James et al., 1990; Carmel and Hunter, 1991) and those that have been trained in the prevention and management of violence (Carmel and Hunter, 1990) are less likely to be physically assaulted. Research has found that employees at high risk of assault are younger, less experienced, less formally trained, predominately females, trainees and more experienced nurses during restraint and seclusion procedures (Flannery et al., 2006)

Systematic reviews examining 20 years of research with 2,891 inpatient staff victims (Flannery et al., 2011) including 67% (1,565) mental health workers, 26% (606) nurses, 5% (103) clinicians and 14% (46) other support staff or students (14%) found that 87% (2,034) were subject to physical assaults, 1% (26) to sexual assaults, 2% (25) to acts of nonverbal intimidation and 5% (119) to verbal treats. Restraints were employed in 41% (951) incidents.

Injuries to staff included:

- 45% (1,049) bruises
- 15% (339) head and/or back injuries
- 6% (139) bone/tendon/ligament injuries
- 13% (292) open wounds or scratches

- 1% (26) abdominal wounds
- 18% (410) incidents of psychological fright

In terms of severity, 300 (34%) of these assaults mild, 400 (34%) were moderate and 164 (14%) were more severe. A gender analysis of the inpatient victims suggested that male staff were more likely to be physically assaulted (92%) than female staff, whereas female staff were more likely to be victims of verbal threat (7%) and to experience greater psychological distress (21%). These differences were statistically significant for type of assault [$x^2(5) = 37.04$; P < .0001] and type of injury [$x^2(7) = 32.89$; P < .0001].

Agency staff (James et al., 1990) are more likely to be assaulted, particularly when they are unfamiliar with ward routines (Katz and Kirkland, 1990). Several studies support an association between aggression and overcrowding on wards (Palmstierna et al., 1991; Tietelbaum et al., 2016). (See Chapter 4 for more information.)

- Access to weapons
- No fresh air
- Lack of privacy
- Environment that is too hot or too cold
- Uncared-for environment
- Lots of hidden corners in the building
- Overcrowding
- Unclear staff functions
- Unpredictable routines and structure
- Overstimulation
- Authoritarian conditions

(Katz and Kirkland, 1990; Palmstierna et al., 1991; College Research Unit, 1998, Tietelbaum et al., 2016.)

Medical Causes

Some medical or neurological conditions may present with disturbed behaviour and treatment of the underlying problem is vital. Such problems need to be excluded when accepting an unknown patient into the PICU. The exact screening tests required in any individual patient would depend, of course, on the clinical presentation.

Examples of medical conditions that can present in this way are shown below:

- Head injury with vascular lesions, especially subdural haematoma

- Delirium tremens
- Intoxication with illicit drugs or alcohol
- Overdose with prescribed drug (e.g. anticholinergics)
- Meningitis
- Encephalitis
- Hypoglycaemia
- Diminished cerebral oxygenation of any aetiology (e.g. vascular, metabolic or endocrine)
- Hypertensive encephalopathy
- Wernicke's encephalopathy
- Temporal lobe epilepsy
- Neoplastic conditions
- Dementia

On admission, or ideally prior to admission, a comprehensive history should be obtained from as many sources as possible. This may include the patient, family, police, general practitioner, social worker, community psychiatric nurse and previous notes.

Mental State Examination

Mental state examination should cover the mental state factors known to be associated with violence. These are:

- Evidence of any 'threat/control override' symptoms especially persecutory delusions and delusions of passivity
- Emotions related to violence especially irritability, anger, hostility and suspiciousness
- Erotomania or morbid jealousy symptoms
- Misidentification phenomena
- Command hallucinations

The severity and nature of the patient's symptoms in the acute situation often limit history taking and detailed examination of the mental state. However, this should be carried out at the first available opportunity.

In the mental state examination, special attention should be paid to the level of consciousness, attention and concentration, memory, language abnormalities and mood and affect. Brief and quantifiable tests such as the Mini Mental State Examination can be useful for monitoring the progress of such patients (Cockrell and Folstein, 2002). Signs of acute organic brain syndrome (delirium) should be suspected until proven otherwise if the following are present:

- Disorientation (especially if worse at night)
- Clouding of consciousness

- Abnormal vital signs
- No previous psychiatric history (especially if older than 40 years)
- Visual hallucinations

Other signs and symptoms include an acute onset (hours to days), a reversed sleep–wake cycle, labile mood, shifting delusions, disjointed thoughts, poor attention and impaired memory.

Suicide Risk

Some patients are admitted to PICUs because they pose a risk to themselves. The PICU does not offer significant advantages over general acute wards in the management of many suicidal patients. However, in those patients where absconding from the ward in order to self-harm is potentially problematic, then the additional security of the PICU confers additional protection.

Predictors of suicide specific to different diagnostic groups of patients (Beer, Pereira and Paton, 2008) include:

Depression

- Male
- Older
- Single
- Separated
- Socially isolated
- Previous deliberate self-harm/suicide attempt
- Insomnia/hypersomnia
- Self-neglect
- Memory impairment
- Agitation
- Guilt
- Bleakness about the future
- Severe depression

Schizophrenia

- Male
- Younger
- Socially isolated
- Unemployed
- Previous deliberate self-harm/suicide attempt
- Depressive episode
- Severe and relapsing illness
- Insight and fear of deterioration in mental state

Alcohol Problems

- Male
- Aged 40–60 years
- Depression
- Previous deliberate self-harm/suicide attempt
- Bereavement
- Poor physical health

A NICE consultation report (2011) found that the following factors predicted non-fatal repetition of self-harm in adults:

- Prior self-harm
- Depression symptoms
- Schizophrenia and related symptoms
- Alcohol misuse
- Other psychiatric history
- Unemployment and 'registered sick'
- Female gender (mixed and poor-quality evidence)
- Unmarried status (narrative evidence only; not predictive in pooled analysis)
- Younger age

The following symptoms predicted suicide among adults with prior self-harm:

- Suicide intent/intent to die
- Male gender
- Psychiatric history
- Older age
- Violent methods of self-harm
- Physical health problems (mixed evidence)
- Alcohol abuse (mixed evidence)

Risk factors for repeated self-harm among young people were like those identified for adults.

Care Planning

A care plan for acute behavioural disturbance should be tailored to the individual needs and circumstances of the patient and should address both the immediate symptoms of agitation and any underlying medical or mental health conditions that may be contributing to the disturbance.

Here are some key components of a care plan for acute behavioural disturbance:

- **De-escalation techniques**: The first step in managing acute behavioural disturbance is often to use de-escalation techniques to help calm the patient and reduce their level of agitation. These techniques may include verbal reassurance, active listening, offering choices and avoiding confrontational language or behaviour.
- **Medication**: Medication may be used to help manage acute agitation, particularly in cases where non-pharmacological interventions have been unsuccessful or are contraindicated. The choice of medication should be based on the patient's clinical presentation and medical history and should be prescribed in accordance with evidence-based guidelines.
- **Psychological interventions**: Psychological interventions, such as cognitive-behavioural therapy or trauma-focused therapy, individual and group therapy may be used to help address underlying emotional and psychological issues that may be contributing to the disturbance.
- **Environmental modifications**: These include care-planning time in quiet spaces, quiet lounges, sensory rooms, tactile considerations, weighted blankets/clothing, special sensory-minimising visual stimuli, providing calm-down activities and ensuring a supportive/understanding environment. Research has found that sensory modulation reduced the percentage of patients needing seclusion as well as patient distress levels along with positive feedback from patients and staff (Alhaj and Trist, 2023).
- **Collaborative care**: A collaborative care approach, involving healthcare professionals, the patient and their family members or caregivers, can help to ensure that the patient receives appropriate and coordinated care that addresses their immediate needs as well as any ongoing medical or mental health issues.
- **Follow-up care**: Follow-up care, including regular monitoring and assessment, can help to ensure that the patient's symptoms are effectively managed over time and that any ongoing needs are addressed.

Consider developing a safety plan in partnership with people who have self-harmed. Safety plans should be used to:

- Establish the means of self-harm.
- Recognise the triggers and warning signs of increased distress, further self-harm or a suicidal crisis.
- Identify individualised coping strategies, including problem-solving any factors that may act as a barrier.

- Identify social contacts and social settings as a means of distraction from suicidal thoughts or escalating crisis.
- Identify family members or friends to provide support and/or help resolve the crisis.
- Include contact details for the mental health service, including out-of-hours services and emergency contact details.
- Keep the environment safe by working collaboratively to remove or restrict lethal means of suicide (NICE, 2022).

Overall, a care plan for acute behavioural disturbance should be individualised and evidence-based and should prioritise the safety and well-being of the patient while addressing any underlying medical or mental health conditions.

Range of Interventions

The management of acute disturbance should prioritise the use of the least restrictive interventions possible. This means that interventions should be used only to the extent necessary to ensure the safety and well-being of the individual and those around them.

It is important to note that the least restrictive interventions may vary depending on the individual's situation, condition and the severity of the disturbance, so a tailored approach is necessary. Also, the safety of the individual and others should always be considered, and the least restrictive approach should not compromise it.

Here are a few examples of least restrictive ways to manage acute disturbance:

- **Activity and engagement programs**: Occupational therapists can develop individualised activity programs to promote relaxation and positive coping strategies, such as guided imagery, deep breathing and art therapy. (See Chapter 7, Section 2 for further information.)
- **Verbal de-escalation techniques**: Trained staff can use verbal techniques to help calm a patient and reduce agitation. This may involve active listening, validating the patient's feelings and using a calm and non-judgmental tone of voice. (See Chapter 8, Section 2 for further information.)
- **Time off the ward**: If Section 17 leave allows, time off the ward often helps reduce the patient's level of agitation and, on return, they are often less agitated and more at ease. Positive risk taking

(Stickley and Felton, 2006) and relational security approaches to risk management, such as the use of the relational security explorer (RCP, 2023) particularly with staff and the patients outside connections are key considerations here for safety.

- **Providing 1:1 time**: Patients can be offered time away from the main shared parts of the ward, time in the garden and so on. Some PICUs have staff allocated directly to garden observation duties to ensure that patients can access the garden at any time during daytime hours and outside of any set times, if necessary, as averting a possible violent/self-harm incident is always preferable to maintaining the ward routine of set garden access times. Engagement can be as simple as playing cards, board games or chess, watching TV with the patient, playing pool (if accessible), cooking, or console gaming to overcome the links of violent behaviour with boredom (Kustermans, 2016).
- **Social interventions**: Social workers can work with the patient to address social and environmental factors that may be contributing to their symptoms. This may include providing resources for housing, financial assistance or connecting the patient with community support services.
- **Environmental modifications**: Making changes to the environment can help to reduce agitation and promote relaxation. This may include reducing noise and sensory stimuli, adjusting lighting or providing a private space for the patient to rest.
- **Medication management**: Psychiatric providers can prescribe medication to help manage symptoms of acute behavioural disturbance, but it is important to start with the lowest effective dose and monitor the patient for side effects.

It is important to prioritise the least restrictive interventions whenever possible to avoid the negative consequences of more restrictive interventions such as seclusion and restraint. The least restrictive approach is also more likely to promote recovery and improve long-term outcomes for the patient.

Occupational Interventions

Occupational interventions can be an important part of a comprehensive care plan for acute behavioural disturbance. Occupational therapy can help to identify and address underlying factors that may be contributing to the patient's symptoms, such as occupational performance issues, environmental factors or social and emotional difficulties.

Here are some occupational interventions that may be included in a care plan for acute behavioural disturbance:

- **Activity analysis**: An occupational therapist can perform an activity analysis to identify activities that the patient finds meaningful or enjoyable and that can be used to promote relaxation, reduce stress or improve mood. Activities may include hobbies, crafts or exercise (Reitz and Scaffa, 2020).
- **Environmental modifications**: An occupational therapist can assess the patient's physical environment and make modifications that can help to reduce stress and improve the patient's sense of safety. Modifications may include adjusting lighting, reducing noise or organising the physical space to promote calm and comfort (Reitz and Scaffa, 2020).
- **Sensory interventions**: Sensory interventions, such as deep pressure therapy, music therapy or aromatherapy, can be used to promote relaxation and reduce stress. Occupational therapists can work with patients to identify sensory preferences and develop sensory-based interventions that are tailored to the individual's needs and preferences (Crasswell et al., 2021).
- **Self-regulation techniques**: An occupational therapist can teach the patient self-regulation techniques, such as deep breathing, mindfulness or progressive muscle relaxation, to help reduce anxiety, improve mood and promote relaxation (Fix and Fix, 2013).
- **Education and training**: Occupational therapists can provide education and training to patients and their caregivers on stress management, coping strategies and other skills that can help to reduce the risk of future acute behavioural disturbances.

Overall, occupational interventions can play a key role in helping patients manage their symptoms of acute behavioural disturbance and improve their overall quality of life. Occupational therapists can work closely with other healthcare professionals to develop a comprehensive care plan that addresses the patient's physical, emotional and environmental needs.

Social Interventions

Social interventions can also be an important part of a comprehensive care plan for acute behavioural disturbance. Social interventions can help to address the patient's social and emotional needs and provide support and resources to help them manage their symptoms.

Here are some social interventions that may be included in a care plan for acute behavioural disturbance:

- **Peer support**: Programs can provide the patient with a supportive network of individuals who have had similar experiences and can offer guidance and encouragement (Bouchard et al., 2010).
- **Family education and support**: Education and support for the patient's family can help to improve family functioning and communication, reduce caregiver stress and improve overall patient outcomes (Carr, 2009).
- **Social skills training**: This can help the patient develop effective communication and social interaction skills and reduce social anxiety (Kolko et al., 1990).
- **Employment support**: Employment programs can help the patient find and maintain employment, which can improve their self-esteem, social connections and financial stability (Hendricks, 2010).
- **Housing support**: Housing programs can help the patient find and maintain stable housing, which can improve their overall sense of security and well-being.

Overall, social interventions can help to address the patient's social and emotional needs, reduce social isolation and improve their overall quality of life. Social interventions can be provided in conjunction with other interventions, such as medication and therapy, to help the patient manage their symptoms of acute behavioural disturbance and prevent future episodes.

Verbal De-escalation and Reducing Institutional Escalation

Verbal de-escalation is an important tool for managing acute behavioural disturbance and can help prevent the need for more restrictive interventions, such as physical or pharmacological interventions. The goal of verbal de-escalation is to calm the patient down and reduce their level of agitation by engaging them in a non-threatening manner.

Acutely disturbed behaviour can sometimes be anticipated; informing patients of their detention under the MHA, denial of requests to leave hospital or enforcing medication against a patient's will are all potentially provocative actions. Disturbance can also be unpredictable. A member of staff or another patient may say or do something that is misinterpreted by a paranoid patient who then lashes out. The underlying thought processes may not be obvious to others.

NICE (2015) identifies the following framework for anticipating and identifying ways to reducing violence and aggression and the use of restrictive interventions on inpatient wards:

- Ensure that the staff work as a therapeutic team by using a positive and encouraging approach, maintaining staff emotional regulation and self-management and encouraging good leadership.
- Ensure that service users are offered appropriate psychological therapies, physical activities, leisure pursuits such as film clubs and reading or writing groups, and support for communication difficulties.
- Recognise possible teasing, bullying, unwanted physical or sexual contact or miscommunication between service users.
- Recognise how each service user's mental health problem might affect their behaviour (e.g. their diagnosis, severity of illness, current symptoms and past history of violence or aggression).
- Anticipate the impact of the regulatory process on each service user (e.g. being formally detained, having leave refused, having a failed detention appeal or being in a very restricted environment such as a low, medium or high secure hospital).
- Improve or optimise the physical environment (e.g. use unlocked doors whenever possible, enhance the décor, simplify the ward layout and ensure easy access to outside spaces and privacy).
- Anticipate that restricting a service user's liberty and freedom of movement (e.g. not allowing service users to leave the building) can be a trigger for violence and aggression.
- Anticipate and manage any personal factors occurring outside the hospital (e.g. family disputes or financial difficulties) that may affect a service user's behaviour.

The Safewards model of care and containment suggests that violence and aggression can be managed via having clear mutual expectations understood, using soft-words, talk-down strategies and positive words, being sensitive when delivering bad news (bad-news mitigation), knowing each other's initiatives on the ward so staff and service users can start to build therapeutic relationships, initiating mutual help meeting between service users to build trust and mutual respect, having readily accessible calm-down methods (such as a calm-down box containing sensory items) and using reassurance and a discharge tree where patients can write discharge messages of hope for those still detained on the unit (see Figure 7.1).

The model consists of six domains which identify the key influences over conflict and containment rates:

1. Patient community
2. Patient characteristics
3. Regulatory framework
4. Staff team
5. Physical environment
6. Outside hospital

These domains give risk to flashpoints that have the capacity to trigger conflict and/or containment.

Staff interventions can modify these processes by reducing the conflict originating factors.

- Preventing flashpoints from arising
- Cutting the link between flashpoint and conflict
- Choosing not to use containment
- Ensuring that containment use does not lead to further conflict

A description of the model and how it can be used to devise strategies for promoting the safety of patients and staff can be found at www.safewards.net.

Some general principles for verbal de-escalation include:

- **Remain calm**: The staff member should remain calm and composed, speaking in a clear and measured tone.
- **Listen actively**: The staff member should listen actively to the patient's concerns and feelings, acknowledging and validating their emotions.
- **Use non-threatening language**: The staff member should avoid using threatening or aggressive language and use non-judgmental language that is supportive and empathic.
- **Establish rapport**: The staff member should establish a rapport with the patient, creating a positive environment where the patient feels respected and heard.

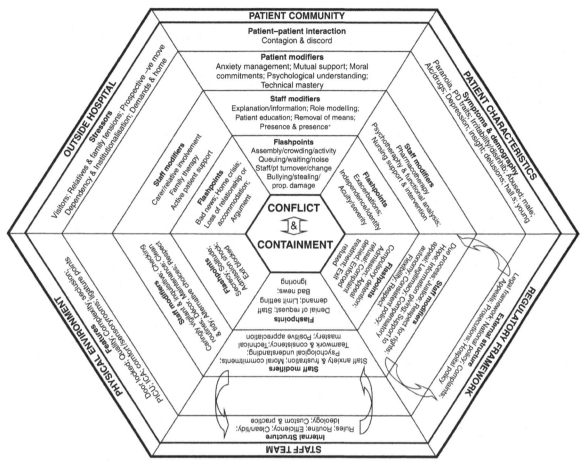

Figure 7.1 Safewards model

- **Use collaborative problem-solving**: The staff member should work collaboratively with the patient to identify and address the underlying causes of their distress.

The Joint NAPICU BAP consensus guidelines (Patel et al., 2018) provide guidance for effective evidence-based de-escalation components, including:

- Continual risk assessment
- Self-control techniques
- Avoidance of provocation
- Respect of individual space
- Management of the environment – moving others away, offering activities, self-soothing
- Passive intervention and watchful waiting
- Empathy
- Reassurance
- Respect and avoidance of shame
- Appropriate use of humour

- Identification of any unmet needs
- Distraction
- Negotiation
- Reframing events for patients
- Non-confrontational limit setting

Reducing institutional escalation involves creating a therapeutic environment that is designed to prevent the escalation of behaviours and minimise the use of restrictive interventions. This can include strategies such as creating a calm and supportive environment, promoting patient autonomy and choice and providing ongoing education and training for staff members.

Here are some general principles for reducing institutional escalation:

- **Promote a culture of respect**: The healthcare environment should be built on a foundation of mutual respect and empathy, where patients are treated with dignity and staff members are valued for their contributions.

- **Provide ongoing education and training**: Staff members should receive ongoing education and training in the management of acute behavioural disturbance, including strategies for verbal de-escalation and non-restrictive interventions.
- **Involve patients in their care**: Patients should be involved in the planning and delivery of their care, with an emphasis on patient autonomy and choice.
- **Create a therapeutic environment**: The healthcare environment should be designed to promote calm and relaxation, with a focus on reducing stressors that may contribute to the escalation of behaviours.
- **Implement risk reduction strategies**: Strategies should be in place to identify and manage high-risk patients and prevent the escalation of behaviours that may require more restrictive interventions.

By implementing these strategies, healthcare providers can create a therapeutic environment that promotes patient safety and well-being, while minimising the need for restrictive interventions.

Use of Medication

Medication may be necessary to manage acute behavioural disturbance when less restrictive measures, such as verbal de-escalation or environmental interventions, have failed. However, medication should always be used in conjunction with other interventions and as a last resort, and the patient's rights and dignity must be respected throughout the process.

Here are some general principles for the use of medication in managing acute behavioural disturbance:

- **Medication review**: Reviewing current medications to identify if any are contributing to the acute disturbance and adjusting or discontinuing them if necessary.
- **Use the least restrictive medication first**: Before using more potent medications, less restrictive medications should be tried, such as benzodiazepines or antipsychotics.
- **Use the minimum effective dose**: When medication is necessary, the minimum effective dose required to safely manage the situation should be used. Research reviewing eight cases of sudden death in detained patients concluded that

'the risk of sudden cardiotoxic collapse in response to neuroleptic medication given during a period of high physiological arousal should be widely publicized' (Banerjee et al., 1995).

- **Monitor for side effects**: Patients should be monitored for any potential side effects of medication and the medication should be adjusted as necessary. Pulse oximetry should always be used following an episode of rapid tranquillisation and increased nursing observations may be necessary if sedating PRN medications are utilised (NMS, 2014, 2015).
- **Involve appropriate staff members**: Medication should be prescribed and administered by staff members who are appropriately trained and qualified to do so.
- **Respect the patient's rights and dignity**: Throughout the medication process, the patient's rights and dignity should be respected. The medication should be prescribed and administered in a manner that is least restrictive and least intrusive to the patient's autonomy (NMS, 2014, 2015).
- **Document the medication intervention**: Medication interventions should be documented, including the medication prescribed, the dose and any side effects or adverse reactions.

It is important to note that medication should only be used when necessary and in compliance with legal and ethical standards. Healthcare providers should always consider the risks and benefits of using medication and use it as a last resort after other interventions have failed.

The reader here is referred to the National Institute for Health and Care Excellence (NICE, 2015) guideline (NG10): Violence and Aggression and the Joint British Association of Psychopharmacology and NAPICU Consensus Guideline for Management of Acute Disturbance (Patel et al., 2018), both of which cover pharmacological management of agitation and aggression.

The *Maudsley Prescribing Guidelines in Psychiatry* (Taylor et al., 2021) is a widely used resource for the prescribing of psychotropic medications in the United Kingdom. It provides guidance on the use of medications in the management of acute disturbance and various mental health conditions.

The guidelines recommend the use of atypical antipsychotics, such as olanzapine, quetiapine and risperidone, as first-line treatment for the management of acute disturbance, including agitation, aggression and psychosis. The guidelines also recommend the use of benzodiazepines, such as lorazepam or diazepam, as a second-line treatment option. (See Chapters 17 and 18 for more specific guidance on psychopharmacology and rapid tranquillisation.)

Physical Intervention

Physical intervention may be necessary to manage acute behavioural disturbance when less restrictive measures have failed and the patient poses a significant risk to themselves or others. However, physical intervention should always be used as a last resort, and the patient's rights and dignity must be respected throughout the process.

Here are some general principles for physical intervention:

- **Use the least restrictive measures first**: Before physical intervention is used, less restrictive measures should be tried, such as verbal de-escalation, diversion or medication.
- **Use the least amount of force necessary**: When physical intervention is necessary, the minimum amount of force required to safely manage the situation should be used. The intervention should be proportionate to the level of risk posed by the patient.
- **Use safe and appropriate techniques**: Physical intervention should be carried out using safe and appropriate techniques that do not cause unnecessary harm or injury to the patient or staff. Staff members should be trained in these techniques and use them in a consistent manner.
- **Involve appropriate staff members**: Physical intervention should be carried out by staff members who are appropriately trained and qualified to carry out such interventions. There should be adequate staffing levels to ensure that physical intervention can be carried out safely and effectively.
- **Respect the patient's rights and dignity**: Throughout the physical intervention process, the patient's rights and dignity should be respected. The intervention should be carried out in a manner that is least restrictive and least intrusive to the patient's autonomy.
- **Monitor and document the intervention**: Physical intervention should be monitored and documented to ensure that it is carried out in

a safe and appropriate manner. Any injuries or incidents should be documented, and a debriefing should be carried out following the intervention.

It is important to note that physical intervention should only be used when absolutely necessary and in compliance with legal and ethical standards. Healthcare providers should always consider the risks and benefits of using physical intervention and use it as a last resort after other interventions have failed. (See Chapter 12, Section 2 for more detailed information.)

Seclusion and Segregation

Seclusion and segregation are restrictive interventions used to manage acute behavioural disturbance when less restrictive measures have failed and the patient is at risk of harming themselves or others. These interventions involve isolating the patient in a room or area, usually for a specified period, and can be traumatising for the patient if not used appropriately. Therefore, seclusion and segregation should be used with caution and only as a last resort.

The following guidance is taken from the Mental Health Code of Practice (Department of Health, 2015) chapter on safe and therapeutic responses to disturbed behaviour:

- Seclusion refers to the supervised confinement and isolation of a patient, away from other patients, in an area from which the patient is prevented from leaving, where it is of immediate necessity for the purpose of the containment of severe behavioural disturbance which is likely to cause harm to others.
- If a patient is confined in any way that meets this definition, even if they have agreed to or requested such confinement, they have been secluded and the use of any local or alternative terms (such as 'therapeutic isolation') or the conditions of the immediate environment do not change the fact that the patient has been secluded. It is essential that they are afforded the procedural safeguards of the Code.
- Seclusion should only be undertaken in a room or suite of rooms that have been specifically designed and designated for the purposes of seclusion and which serves no other function on the ward. Seclusion does not include locking people in their rooms at night in accordance with the High Security Psychiatric Services (Arrangements for

Safety and Security) Directions (Department of Health, 2019).

- Seclusion should only be used in hospitals and in relation to patients detained under the Mental Health Act 1983. If an emergency situation arises involving an informal patient and, as a last resort, seclusion is necessary to prevent harm to others, then an assessment for an emergency application for detention under the Act should be undertaken immediately.
- Seclusion should not be used as a punishment or a threat or because of a shortage of staff. It should not form part of a treatment programme.
- Seclusion should never be used solely as a means of managing self-harming behaviour. Where the patient poses a risk of self-harm as well as harm to others, seclusion should be used only when the professionals involved are satisfied that the need to protect other people outweighs any increased risk to the patient's health or safety arising from their own self-harm and that any such risk can be properly managed.

The following factors should be considered in the design of rooms or areas where seclusion is to be carried out:

- The room should allow for communication with the patient when the patient is in the room and the door is locked (e.g. via an intercom).
- Rooms should include limited furnishings, including a bed, pillow, mattress and blanket or covering.
- There should be no apparent safety hazards.

(See NAPICU, 2016; Department of Health, 2015; Chapter 11, Section 2.)

Developed Activity and Engagement Programmes for Acute Disturbance

Developed activity and engagement programs can be an important part of managing acute behavioural disturbance, particularly for patients who are in seclusion or segregation. These programs aim to provide patients with structured and meaningful activities to occupy their time and help them to maintain their physical and mental well-being. Here are some examples of activity and engagement programs that have been used in the management of acute behavioural disturbance:

- **Music therapy**: Music therapy involves using music as a therapeutic tool to improve mood,

reduce anxiety and increase socialisation. Music therapists may work with patients one on one or in group sessions (Langhammer et al., 2019; Zadbagher et al., 2019; Ye et al., 2021).
- **Art therapy**: Art therapy involves using art as a therapeutic tool to express emotions, reduce stress and improve self-awareness. Patients may work on individual or group projects, and can use a variety of mediums, such as painting, drawing or sculpting (Inomjonovna, 2023).
- **Physical exercise**: Physical exercise can help to reduce stress, improve mood and increase physical well-being. Patients may participate in individual or group exercise programs, such as yoga, aerobics or strength training.
- **Mindfulness-based interventions**: Mindfulness-based interventions involve teaching patients techniques to improve their ability to focus and relax. This can include techniques such as breathing exercises, guided imagery and meditation (Fix and Fix, 2013).
- **Social skills training**: Social skills training involves teaching patients skills to help them to better interact with others. This may include communication skills, conflict resolution and problem-solving (Kolko et al., 1990).
- **Educational programmes**: Educational programmes can help patients to develop new skills and knowledge and can provide a sense of purpose and meaning. These programs may include classes on a variety of topics, such as language, history or job skills.

It is important to note that activity and engagement programs should be individualised to the patient's needs and preferences and should be developed in consultation with the patient and their care team. These programs can help to improve patient outcomes and reduce the need for restrictive interventions such as seclusion and segregation. (See Chapter 7 for further information.)

The Roles of the MDT, Levels of Training and Experience Mix Required for Effective Management of Acute Disturbance

A team approach involving professionals from different backgrounds such as psychiatrists, psychologists, social workers and occupational therapists can help to ensure that the individual receives comprehensive and coordinated care.

The skills mix of the MDT can have a significant impact on the management of acute behavioural disturbance. A team with a diverse range of skills and expertise can work together more effectively to manage the complex needs of patients with acute behavioural disturbance. An effective skills mix requires that each member of the team has the appropriate credentials and training for their role, as well as ongoing training and education to stay current on best practices and new interventions. Effective communication and collaboration among team members is also critical for successful management of acute behavioural disturbance.

Effective management of acute disturbance requires an MDT approach, with a mix of training and experience among team members. Here are some of the key roles and responsibilities within the team:

- **Psychiatric consultants**: Psychiatric consultants are usually certified psychiatrists who provide expert advice and guidance to the care team. They are responsible for conducting psychiatric evaluations, making treatment recommendations and prescribing medications when necessary. Psychiatrists can play a key role in providing accurate diagnosis and effective medication management for patients with acute behavioural disturbance.

- **Nurses**: Nurses play a critical role in the management of acute behavioural disturbance. They are responsible for monitoring the patient's vital signs, administering medications and implementing non-pharmacological interventions, such as de-escalation techniques and activity programs. Having experienced psychiatric nurses and nursing assistants who are trained in non-pharmacological interventions and de-escalation techniques can help to reduce the need for seclusion and restraint, which can have negative consequences for the patient.

- **Healthcare workers/nursing assistants/support workers/mental health workers**: Healthcare workers are often involved in the direct care of patients with acute behavioural disturbance. They may assist with patient care and monitoring, help to implement non-pharmacological interventions and provide support and supervision during seclusion or segregation.

- **Social workers**: Social workers can provide valuable support to patients and families during times of acute behavioural disturbance. They may assist with discharge planning, provide counselling and support services and connect patients with community resources. Social workers can help to address social and environmental factors that may be contributing to the patient's symptoms and may also provide support to family members and caregivers.

- **Occupational therapists**: Occupational therapists can play a key role in developing and implementing activity and engagement programs for patients with acute behavioural disturbance. They may also assist with assessments and interventions to improve the patient's daily functioning and independence. Having occupational therapists on the team who can develop and implement activity and engagement programs can help to reduce agitation and promote relaxation and positive coping strategies.

- **Psychologists**: Psychologists can conduct comprehensive assessments of the patient's mental health, including their psychological and emotional functioning. They can also provide a formal diagnosis to guide treatment approaches and provide a range of evidenced-based treatment approaches for acute behavioural disturbance such as individual and group therapy, cognitive-behavioural therapy and other psychotherapeutic interventions. They may also provide education and support to family members and caregivers, helping them to better understand the patient's condition and how to provide effective support.

- **Security personnel**: In some settings, security personnel may be involved in managing acute behavioural disturbance. They may assist with patient monitoring, the implementation of restrictive interventions and provide support and supervision as needed. They may also be required to provide secure transportation. Security personnel can help to ensure the safety of patients, staff and others in the environment, but it is important that their role is clearly defined and that they are trained in appropriate de-escalation techniques to avoid unnecessary use of force. This can also involve the police, who may be involved in admitting the patient due to the level of acute disturbance.

In terms of training and experience, each member of the team should have appropriate credentials and training for their role. For example, nurses should have specialised training in psychiatric and mental health nursing, while MHTs should have training in de-escalation techniques and crisis management.

In addition, team members should have experience working with patients with acute behavioural disturbance and should receive ongoing training and education to stay current on best practices and new interventions. Effective communication and collaboration among team members is also essential for successful management of acute behavioural disturbance.

Guidance has been produced for management within a pandemic and the reader is referred to *Managing Acute Disturbance in the Context of COVID-19* (NAPICU, 2020).

Conclusion

The management of acute behavioural disturbance requires a comprehensive and coordinated approach that involves an MDT with a diverse range of skills and expertise. Each member of the team has a specific role and responsibility in the assessment, management and treatment of patients with acute behavioural disturbance.

Effective communication and collaboration among team members, as well as ongoing training and education, are critical for success. Non-pharmacological interventions, such as de-escalation techniques, activity and engagement programs and social interventions, should be prioritised over restrictive interventions such as seclusion and restraint.

Ultimately, the goal of management is to provide safe and effective care that addresses the patient's individual needs and promotes recovery and well-being. This chapter has shown that there are many factors to the effective management of the acutely disturbed patient. It is essential that services are planned, resourced and supported to ensure the safety of the patients and staff in acute mental health services.

References

Alhaj,HA and Trist,A (2023) The Effects of Sensory Modulation on Patient's Distress and Use of Restrictive Interventions in Adult Inpatient Psychiatric Settings: A Critical Review. *Advances in Biomedical and Health Sciences* Ahead of print articles. www.abhsjournal.net/temp/AdvBiomedHealthSci000-5835674_161236.pdf.

Banerjee,S, Bingley,W and Murphy,E (1995) *Deaths of Detained Patients: A Review of Reports to the Mental Health Act Commission.* London: Mental Health Act Foundation.

Beer,MD, Pereira,SM and Paton,C (2008) Management of Acutely Disturbed Behaviour. In Beer,MD, Pereira,S and Paton,C (eds.), *Psychiatric Intensive Care.* pp. 12–24. Cambridge: Cambridge University Press.

Bowers,L (2014) Safewards: A New Model of Conflict and Containment on Psychiatric Wards. *Journal of Psychiatric and Mental Health Nursing* **21** (6) 499–508.

Bouchard,L, Montreuil,M and Gros,C (2010) Peer Support among Inpatients in an Adult Mental Health Setting. *Issues in Mental Health Nursing* **31** (9) 589–98.

Carr,A (2009) The Effectiveness of Family Therapy and Systemic Interventions for Adult Focused Problems. *Journal of Family Therapy* **31** (1) 46–74.

Cheung,T, Lee,PH and Yip,PSF (2017) Workplace Violence toward Physicians and Nurses: Prevalence and Correlates in Macau. *International Journal of Environmental Research and Public Health* **14**: 879.

Cockrell,JR and Folstein,MF (2002) Mini-Mental State Examination. In Abou-Saleh,MT, Katona,CLE and Anand, KA (eds.), *Principles and Practice of Geriatric Psychiatry.* New York: John Wiley & Sons. pp. 140–1.

Corrigan,P (2015) *Person Centered Care for Mental Illness: The Evolution of Adherence and Self-Determination.* Washington, DC: American Psychological Association.

Craswell,G, Dieleman,C and Ghanouni,P (2021) An Integrative Review of Sensory Approaches in Adult Inpatient Mental Health: Implications for Occupational Therapy in Prison-Based Mental Health Services. *Occupational Therapy in Mental Health* **37** (2) 130–57.

Department of Health (2015) *Mental Health Act 1983: Code of Practice.* London: Department of Health.

Department of Health and Social Care (2019) *High Security Psychiatric Services Directions 2019: Arrangements for Safety and Security.* London: Department of Health and Social Care. https://assets.publishing.service.gov.uk/government/uploads/system/uploads/attachment_data/file/810039/the-high-security-psychiatric-services-directions-2019.pdf.

Dyer,C (1996) Violence May Be Predicted Amongst Psychiatric Inpatients. *British Medical Journal* **313**: 318.

Ferri,P, Silvestri,M, Artoni,C and Di Lorenzo,R (2016) Workplace Violence in Different Settings and Among Various Health Professionals in an Italian General Hospital: A Cross-Sectional Study. *Psychology Research and Behavior Management* **9**: 263–75.

Fix,RL and Fix,ST (2013) The Effects of Mindfulness-Based Treatments for Aggression: A Critical Review. *Aggression and Violent Behavior* **18** (2) 219–27.

Flannery Jr,RB, Farley,EM, Rego,S and Walker,AP (2006) Characteristics of Staff Victims of Psychiatric Patient Assaults: Fifteen-Year Analysis of the Assaulted Staff Action Program (ASAP). *Psychiatric Quarterly* **78**: 25–37.

Flannery,RB, LeVitre,V, Rego,S and Walker,AP (2011) Characteristics of Staff Victims of Psychiatric Patient Assaults: 20-Year Analysis of the Assaulted Staff Action Program. *Psychiatric Quarterly* **82**: 11–21. DOI: https://doi-org.ezproxy.uwe.ac.uk/10.1007/s11126-010-9153-z.

Gilmartin,S, Martin,L, Kenny,S, Callanan,I and Salter,N (2020) Promoting Hot Debriefing in an Emergency Department. *BMJ Open Quality* **9**: e000913.

Hendricks,D (2010) Employment and Adults with Autism Spectrum Disorders: Challenges and Strategies for Success. *Journal of Vocational Rehabilitation* **32** (2) 125–34.

Inomjonovna,RI (2023) Factors of Working with Violent Children and Adults Using Art Therapy Technologies. *The Theory of Recent Scientific Research in the Field of Pedagogy* **1** (5) 80–8.

James,DV, Fineberg,NA, Shah,AK and Priest,RG (1990) An Increase in Violence on an Acute Psychiatric Ward: A Study of Associated Factors. *British Journal of Psychiatry* **156**: 846–52.

Jang,SJ, Son,YJ and Lee,H (2022) Prevalence, Associated Factors and Adverse Outcomes of Workplace Violence Towards Nurses in Psychiatric Settings: A Systematic Review. *International Journal of Mental health Nursing* **31** (3) 450–68.

Katz,P and Kirkland,FR (1990) Violence and Social Structure on Mental Hospital Wards. *Psychiatry* **53**: 262–77.

Kolko,DJ, Loar,LL and Sturnick,D (1990) Inpatient Social–Cognitive Skills Training Groups with Conduct Disordered and Attention Deficit Disordered Children. *Journal of Child Psychology and Psychiatry* **31** (5) 737–48.

Kustermans,J (2016) Boredom and Violence. In Gardiner,M and Haladyn,JJ (eds.), *Boredom Studies Reader*. London: Routledge. pp. 180–91.

Langhammer,B, Sagbakken,M, Kvaal,K, Ulstein,I, Nåden,D and Rognstad,MK (2019) Music Therapy and Physical Activity to Ease Anxiety, Restlessness, Irritability, and Aggression in Individuals with Dementia with Signs of Frontotemporal Lobe Degeneration. *Journal of Psychosocial Nursing and Mental Health Services* **57** (5) 29–37.

Laranjeira,C and Querido,A (2022) Hope-Inspiring Competence as a High-Quality Mental Health Nursing Care in Recovery-Oriented Practice. *European Psychiatry* **65** (S1) S872–3.

Lev-Ran,S, Nitzan,U and Fennig,S (2014) Examining the Ethical Boundaries of Harm Reduction: From Addictions to General Psychiatry. *Israel Journal of Psychiatry and Related Sciences* **51** (3) 175–81.

Lu,LI, Lok,K-I, Zhang,L, Hu,A, Ungvari,G, Bressington,D, et al. (2019) Prevalence of Verbal and Physical Workplace Violence against Nurses in Psychiatric Hospitals in China. *Archives of Psychiatric Nursing* **33** (5) 68–72.

McKenna,G, Jackson,N and Browne,C (2019) Trauma History in a High Secure Male Forensic Inpatient Population. *International Journal of Law and Psychiatry* **66**: 101475.

National Association of Psychiatric Intensive Care and Low Secure Units (NAPICU) (2014) *National Minimum Standards for Psychiatric Intensive Care in General Adult Services*. Glasgow: NAPICU. https://napicu.org.uk/wp-content/uploads/2014/12/NMS-2014-final.pdf.

National Association of Psychiatric Intensive Care and Low Secure Units (NAPICU) (2015) *National Minimum Standards for Psychiatric Intensive Care Units for Young People*. Glasgow: NAPICU. https://napicu.org.uk/wp-content/uploads/2014/08/CAMHS_PICU_NMS_final_Aug_2015_cx.pdf.

National Association of Psychiatric Intensive Care and Low Secure Units (NAPICU) (2016) *NAPICU Position on the Monitoring, Regulation and Recording of the Extra Care Area, Seclusion and Long-Term Segregation Use in the Context of the Mental Health Act 1983: Code of Practice (2015)*. Glasgow: NAPICU. https://napicu.org.uk/wp-content/uploads/2016/10/NAPICU-Seclusion-Position-Statement.pdf.

National Association of Psychiatric Intensive Care and Low Secure Units (NAPICU) (2020) *Managing Acute Disturbance in the Context of COVID-19*. Glasgow: NAPICU. https://napicu.org.uk/wp-content/uploads/2020/12/NAPICU-Guidance_rev5_15_Dec.pdf.

National Institute of Health and Care Excellence (NICE) (2011) *Self-Harm: Longer-Term Management in Adults, Children and Young People [Draft for Consultation]*. London: National Collaborating Centre for Mental Health.

National Institute of Health and Care Excellence (NICE) (2015) *Violence and Aggression: Short-Term Management in Mental Health, Health and Community Settings [NG10]*. London: NICE. www.nice.org.uk/guidance/ng10.

National Institute of Health and Care Excellence (NICE) (2017) *Violent and Aggressive Behaviours in People with Mental Health Problems [QS154]*. London: NICE.

National Institute of Health and Care Excellence (NICE) (2022) *Self-Harm: Assessment, Management and Preventing Recurrence [NG225]*. London: NICE.

Norcross,J (ed.) (2006) *Evidence-Based Practices in Mental Health: Debate and Dialogue on the Fundamental Questions*. Washington, DC: American Psychological Association. p. 435.

Olashore,AA, Akanni,OO and Ogundipe,RM (2018) Physical Violence against Health Staff by Mentally Ill Patients at a Psychiatric Hospital in Botswana. *BMC Health Services Research* **18**: 362.

Patel,MX, Sethi,FN, Barnes,TR, Dix,R, Dratcu,L, Fox,B, et al. (2018) Joint BAP NAPICU Evidence-Based Consensus

Guidelines for the Clinical Management of Acute Disturbance: De-escalation and Rapid Tranquillisation. *Journal of Psychopharmacology* **32** (6) 601–40.

Pereira,SM, Walker,LM, Dye,S and Alhaj,H (2021) National Survey of Psychiatric Intensive Care, Low Secure and Locked Rehabilitation Services: NHS Patient Characteristics. *Journal of Psychiatric Intensive Care* **17** (2) 79–88.

Reitz,S.M and Scaffa,ME (2020) Occupational Therapy in the Promotion of Health and Well-Being. *American Journal of Occupational Therapy* **74** (3) 7403420010–14.

Royal College of Psychiatrists (2023) *See Think Act*, 3rd ed. London: Royal College of Psychiatrists Quality Network for Forensic Health.

Ruben,B., Beneit,J and Jose,LG (2019) Violence in the Workplace: Some Critical Issues Looking at the Health Sector. *Heliyon* **5** (3) e01283.

Shugar,G and Rehaluk,R (1990) Continuous Observation for Psychiatric Inpatients: A Critical Evaluation. *Comprehensive Psychiatry* **30**: 48–55.

Stickley,T and Felton,A (2006) Promoting Recovery through Therapeutic Risk Taking. *Mental Health Practice* **9** (8) 26–30.

Sugarman M, Graham B, Langston,S, Nelmes,P and Matthews,J (2021) Implementation of the 'TAKE STOCK'

Hot Debrief Tool in the ED: A Quality Improvement Project. *Emergency Medicine Journal* **38**: 579–84.

Taylor,DM, Barnes,TR and Young,AH (2021) *The Maudsley Prescribing Guidelines in Psychiatry*. Chichester: John Wiley & Sons.

Teitelbaum,A, Lahad,A, Calfon,N, Gun-Usishkin,M, Lubin, G and Tsur,A (2016) Overcrowding in Psychiatric Wards is Associated with Increased Risk of Adverse Incidents. *Medical Care* **54** (3) 296–302.

UK Government (1983) Mental Health Act 1983. legislation.gov.UK. www.legislation.gov.uk/ukpga/1983/20/contents.

Ye,P, Huang,Z, Zhou,H, and Tang,Q (2021) Music-Based Intervention to Reduce Aggressive Behavior in Children and Adolescents: A Meta-Analysis. *Medicine* **100** (4) e23894.

Zadbagher Seighalani,M, Birashk,B, Hashemian,K and Mirhashemi,M (2019) The Effectiveness of Traditional Iranian Music Therapy on Depression, Anxiety, Aggression in PMS Patients. *Journal of Psychological Studies* **15** (3) 55–72.

Zeng,JY, An,FR, Xiang,YT, Qi,YK, Ungvari,GS, Newhouse,R, et al. (2013) Frequency and Risk Factors of Workplace Violence on Psychiatric Nurses and Its Impact on Their Quality of Life in China. *Psychiatry Research* **210**: 510–14.

Absconding

Roland Dix

Introduction

Absconding from mental health inpatient facilities is a long-standing and significant issue. Absconding is a core admission criterion for transfer to the psychiatric intensive care unit (PICU) (NAPICU, 2014). Defining absconding may be more difficult than one might expect.

Generally, the issue of 'absconding' can be thought of as most applicable to those who are detained in a hospital under legal authority (most often mental health legislation). That said, voluntary patients who leave hospital unexpectedly and/or without informing others can also raise significant worries, the response to which will have many similarities to those who are detained.

An argument could be advanced that absconding is not necessarily a concern in itself (for the patient) and that the worries are more associated with the consequences arising from absconding. These can be diverse, including potential serious risks for the patient or others. Equally, absconding can represent few risks with the decision to abscond taken simply to enact a desire to be out of hospital and in a different environment. For these reasons, absconding cannot be considered in isolation and must also encapsulate the secondary risks. Management of patients missing from the hospital is also a significant concern for people beyond the hospital and patients themselves. These include family members, significant others, the police and, at times, other agencies such as fire and rescue services.

What constitutes absconding also requires analysis. Some authors propose that there are three general domains within which a patient can be considered to have absented themselves from inpatient care that will be of concern to staff, the service and significant others (Exworthy and Wilson, 2010; Booth et al., 2021). These are:

- **Escape**: this is generally taken to represent those that transgress the building perimeter (i.e. through a window, over a fence or through a door) without agreement or authorisation from the hospital.
- **Absconding**: this is often taken to represent those who leave an escort while engaged in activity in or around the hospital or community.
- **Failure to return from leave**: many hospitals will operate programmes of unescorted leave where, for various periods of time, the patient is authorised to leave the ward or hospital. It is sometimes the case that the person fails to return at the agreed time (or at all) and therefore is considered absent.

Generally speaking, the hospital will be concerned about any patient who is not where they are expected to be and may be vulnerable, representing a risk to themselves or others. This concern is largely reserved for those patients detained under the UK Mental Health Act (MHA), although it can extend to voluntary patients as well. For the remainder of this chapter, the term 'abscond' will refer to the three domains outlined in the previous list.

Within the United Kingdom, 'Section 17 leave' (agreed time away from the hospital) is considered an important part of the legal framework and ethos underpinning inpatient care (Baily et al., 2017). Nurses and healthcare assistants on mental health wards typically manage 20–25 periods of leave a day (Baily et al., 2017). Furthermore, following the introduction of no-smoking policies, episodes of short leave have increased further in many hospitals.

Baily et al. (2017) reported that only 56% of those patients with unescorted leave returned on time. In addition, they showed that relatively simple steps such as having patients sign in and out and providing telephone reminders of time to return improved 'on-time return' by 50%.

This chapter considers the following questions:

- What factors are involved with a patient's decision to abscond?
- What is the applicable law associated with absconding?
- What measures reduce absconding?
- Which policies and procedures may be helpful in managing episodes of absconding?

Factors Involved with Absconding

Absconding from mental health facilities is a relatively well-researched area with a variety of studies and guidance documents produced. There have been several checklists and assessment tools proposed for identifying those at higher risk of absconding early on in the admission and at other times during the stay in hospital.

In a literature review, Bowers et al. (2002) proposed that those who abscond were more often young, male, from disadvantaged groups and suffering from schizophrenia, as compared to admissions generally. Roughly half of the absconding episodes had taken place whilst the patient was temporarily off the ward with permission. The remainder of patients used an assortment of means to make their exits.

Muir-Cochrane et al. (2013) concluded that patient perceptions that the unit was unsafe was a significant reason for absconding. Bowers et al. (1998) identified the following characteristics among those who had absconded from hospital.

- Needing to attend to unfinished business at home
- Experiencing an incident within the ward that caused subjective distress
- Receiving bad news while in hospital
- Acquiring alcohol or illicit substances
- Self-harming and/or suicidal behaviours.

Law

The UK MHA 1983, which was revised in 2007, includes various sections which allow for lawful detention of people presenting with a 'mental disorder' of a nature or to a degree that requires management in hospital. Other countries and jurisdictions will have variations on this theme, including authorities to prevent/manage absconding.

In terms of absconding, the UK MHA infers an authority for staff to 'retake an absconder'. The MHA does not specify what actions may be taken in order to prevent or return a person considered to have absconded from the hospital. The MHA Code of Practice (Department of Health, 2015) does acknowledge, however, that staff may at times employ 'restricted interventions' which include physical restraint and that this can be used to manage a variety of situations including, absconding.

In general terms, the law pertaining to the measures used to detain a person in hospital and/or to return those to hospital who have left without authority must be the minimum necessary to achieve the desired outcome and manage any associated risks. All actions are required to be proportionate in intensity and duration to the risk presented.

The MHA also affords authority to police officers as well as employees of the hospital to return a person to the hospital in which they were lawfully detained and from which they are considered to have absconded.

PICU and Absconding from General Adult Wards

Some patients who abscond from general adult wards may be referred to PICUs. PICU National Minimum Standards (NMS) (NAPICU, 2014) recommend the referral to PICU of detained patients for whom the consequences of persistent absconding are serious enough to warrant treatment in the PICU. For this reason, the extent to which absconding can be discouraged, prevented and managed within general adult acute wards is centrally important to the number of referrals and transfers to a PICU. Further, many of the measures known to be helpful in reducing and managing absconding from other inpatient environments will also be applicable to PICUs.

Reducing Absconding

Positive Ward Culture and Relationships

Good professional relationships have proven significant in maintaining security within mental health facilities and reducing incidents of absconding. It is important that there is a trusting relationship between staff and patients within which concerns and anxiety can be discussed and resolved (Gilburt et al., 2008).

An awareness of an individual patient's situation is also important to providing timely support which would likely reduce the probability of absconding. This can include being aware of bad news that may have been received and offering timely support.

Muir-Cochrane et al. (2013) stated that forming a therapeutic relationship with staff, familiarity with the unit, a comfortable environment and positive experiences with other patients all supported perceptions that the unit was safe, thus decreasing the likelihood of absconding. Findings extend existing work on the person–place encounter within psychiatric inpatient units and bring new knowledge about the reasons why people abscond.

Engagement and Activity Programmes

Positive engagement can be defined as a service approach designed to maximise motivation of inpatients to participate in treatment and promote positive outcomes. Positive engagement has long been accepted as a crucial, although often difficult to achieve (particularly for detained patients), facet of inpatient mental health care.

Meaningful activity within inpatient mental health services has been demonstrated to be important in improving treatment outcomes and diminishing the occurrence of a range of problematic behaviours (Foye et al., 2020), including aggressive responses, absconding, self-injury and more generalised disturbance.

Following incidents within inpatient facilities, it is important that a debrief takes place with fellow patients so that the ward atmosphere does not produce higher levels of anxiety which may lead to incidents of absconding.

Units which have access to vehicles can also play a useful role in assisting patients to return home with support to resolve any outstanding issues. Programmes of escorted and unescorted leave also serve to reduce frustration and build trust/confidence in the service. These measures will also likely have the effect of reducing probability of absconding.

Training

Training in absconding prevention and formalised security-enhancing tools are helpful in promoting a positive environment. Minimising absconding will occur within an overall framework of security involving physical security, supporting procedures and relational security. This has been represented within guidance documents and training such as 'See Think Act' generally used in the Secure Mental Health Estate (Markham, 2022).

Proactive Interventions

Bowers (2003) advocated for the identification of patients at higher risk of absconding with associated updating of care plans. Use of a signing in and out book for patients helps to clarify responsibilities and rules around leaving the ward. Careful and supportive breaking of bad news to patients (e.g. following refused requests for leave or a disappointing outcome of a mental health review tribunal) may decrease chances of a subsequent absconding attempt.

Also helpful are post-incident debriefings of patients following any aggressive or noisy altercation, with explanation and reassurance, especially at night. Targeted daily nursing time for patients perceived to be at high risk of absconding is important. This can provide opportunity for discussion of worries/concerns about home, family and other issues that can culminate in the motivation to abscond.

Summary of Specific Evidence-Based Absconding Reduction Measures

Bowers et al. (2005) proposed an anti-absconding intervention handbook for ward managers that suggests the following interventions to reduce absconding:

1. **Identification of patients at high risk of absconding** and associated updating of care plans.
2. **Use of a signing in and out book** for patients, thereby clarifying responsibilities and rules around leaving the ward.
3. **Careful and supportive breaking of bad news** to patients, for example, following refused requests for leave, or disappointing outcome of mental health review tribunals.
4. **Post ward incident debriefing** of patients following any aggressive or noisy altercation, with explanation and reassurance, especially at night.
5. **Targeted daily nursing time** for those at high risk of absconding for the discussion of worries/concerns about home, family and friends, followed by practical attempts to address those needs.
6. **Facilitated social contact** for those at high risk of absconding via phone contact, encouraging visiting or using all available resources to enable supervised temporary leave.

Helpful Post Absent Without Leave (AWOL) Intervention

- Discussion with the patient as to why they left the ward and how to prevent this from happening in the future
- Agreeing on therapeutic interventions to prevent further episodes and updating the patient's care plan
- Multidisciplinary review, usually but not necessarily within a ward assessment, of patients who had absconded more than once

The implementation of these interventions showed a reduction of absconding by at least 18% in one study (Bowers et al., 2003). Using the same interventions, a Public Health Agency for Northern Ireland report (2015) demonstrated an impressive 70% reduction in absconding over 6 months compared to the same period prior to the implementation.

Absconding Standard Operating Procedures

Most units will have a range of standard operating procedures (SOPs) for a variety of commonly experienced issues, including absconding. For prevention of absconding, the procedures associated with achieving an assessment of absconding risk on admission or at various points during hospital stay are helpful.

PICU and other inpatient environments should have policies/procedures for a number of absconding related scenarios. These include:

- Procedure for assessing absconding risk
- Steps to take when a person is discovered to be missing (AWOL policy)
- Steps to take when a patient with authorised leave is late to return
- Steps to take during escorting in the case of a patient's refusal to return.

Outline AWOL Procedure

Hospitals require a process for how they intend to manage episodes when a patient has gone missing. This process will involve several clear actions, detailing procedures to be undertaken at the point at which it is determined that a person is considered missing. These include:

- An attempt to establish the person's whereabouts, including contacting people who may have information and establishing the last known whereabouts of the individual
- Conducting ward and hospital searches
- Potentially, staff attending known possible locations
- Information to be given to the police, including the circumstances, appearance of the person, risk assessment and potential locations to be considered and so on.

Outline Escorting Procedure

SOPs supporting the use of communication systems are also an important part of absconding prevention and management policy. These procedures usually stipulate the minimum action to take in circumstances when a patient being escorted decides not to return to the hospital. An example of a common SOP for supporting escorted leave could include:

- Before leaving the unit, ensure that the shift coordinator is aware of the leave episode and expected destination/duration and that the communication system is taken and is working.

In the case the person refuses to return or attempts to absent themselves:

- Attempt to negotiate and agree upon action with the person
- If unsuccessful, follow at a safe distance
- Communicate and seek support from the hospital
- If an emergency or high-risk situation arises, call the police for assistance.

Systems of Communication

Communication systems such as mobile phones and/or handheld radios can be used by staff to speak with each other in the case of absconding attempts or when undertaking hospital or ground searches. These are also helpful in contacting relatives or significant others to try and establish the whereabouts of a person and/or to help with risk mitigation.

Physical Security and Absconding Reduction

Modern mental health inpatient facilities have several design and equipment features aimed at promoting security (including reducing absconding). PICU physical environment and design is dealt with in detail elsewhere in the volume. The following is confined to the common security measures aimed at reducing absconding, including an appraisal of the evidence (where available) for their effectiveness.

Locking Doors

In the United Kingdom, up until the early 2000s, many of the general adult inpatient facilities operated an open-door policy. Within the last decade, many mental health facilities have begun operating a locked-door policy with procedures for informal (not detained) patients to request to leave should they wish to do so.

Intuitively, locked doors may reasonably be thought to represent an obvious means of reducing absconding. The mental health inpatient estate operates three formal levels of physical security: high, medium and low. UK general adult PICUs are considered to operate physical security like that in low secure units (LSUs). Increasingly, many previous 'open' acute inpatient facilities within the United Kingdom operate some form of physical locked door security. However, this is not universally regulated or defined, as is the case for the three formal levels of security previously listed.

Locked versus Unlocked Wards and Absconding

Dickens and Campbell (2001) reviewed 148 AWOL incidents from mental health wards that occurred in a variety of circumstances. Patients from unlocked wards accounted for only 37.8% of the total patients who went AWOL. The majority of AWOL incidents (62.2%) involved patients from locked wards.

Bowers et al. (2008) completed a comprehensive study of the effects of locked doors in 128 general adult acute mental health wards. They concluded that locking the ward door reduces but does not eliminate absconding. Locking the door also had the effect of increasing feelings of social exclusion, stigmatisation and depression as well as being associated with increased rates of self-harm. It was also found that locking the ward door had no effect on the rate of use of alcohol or illicit drugs by inpatients.

Locked wards were associated with increased aggression and treatment refusal. This was underpinned by reported feelings of being trapped and confined with a lack of access to fresh air. Patients reported feeling like prisoners rather than patients and that they were mistrusted by staff. Open-door wards were not found to be associated with increased overall use of manual restraint to forcibly detain patients.

Possibly the largest and most robust study to date was undertaken by Huber et al. (2016) who analysed data from 21 German psychiatric inpatient hospitals over 15 years between 1998 and 2012. Aims of this study were to investigate any association between locked and open-door policies with numbers of suicides, suicide attempts and absconding. Of the 349,574 patients included in the study, 72,869 cases were matched as pairs according to patient characteristics and risk factors so that the researchers could directly compare the rates of suicide and absconding. Patients admitted to locked wards were more likely to be younger, male, to have a history of substance misuse and to have had previous suicide attempts than those in open wards. This robust study showed no difference in completed suicide or suicide attempts between hospitals with an open-door policy and those that locked hospital wards. Hospitals with open-door policies did not have higher rates of patients leaving without authorisation.

Quoting the lead author of the study Christian Huber, Mayer (2016) reported:

> These findings suggested that locked door policies may not help to improve the safety of patients in psychiatric hospitals and are not generally successful in preventing people from absconding.
>
> A locked door policy probably imposes a more oppressive atmosphere, which could reduce the effectiveness of treatments, resulting in longer stays in hospital . . . . The practice may even lend motivation for patients to abscond.

PICU 'Air Lock' Entrance Security

Design Guidance for Psychiatric Intensive Care Units (NAPICU, 2017) and *Standards for Psychiatric Intensive Care Units* (Royal College of Psychiatrists, 2020) recommend 'air lock' arrangements for main entrances of PICUs. An air lock system comprises two doors set opposite each other, one not being able to open until the other is closed. This is intended to make absconding very difficult.

In the case that electronic locks are used, there should be an emergency override to allow for situations in which many staff members need to enter or exit the PICU quickly.

Consideration should be given to the location of the PICU main air lock entrance. As far as possible, this entrance should be located away from the main communal area of the PICU. This is helpful to prevent absconding when the entrance is in use. It also helps to remove the focus from the main entrance, which is often the target of attempts to leave.

CCTV

CCTV monitoring of entrances and exits may be more useful in the managing of completed absconding rather than absconding prevention. CCTV allows for the retrieval of accurate images of the person leaving and can accurately define the specific time a person left and possibly the direction in which they went, depending on camera placement.

Some hospitals operate a policy of obtaining photographs of patients upon admission. This is often primarily done to assist in the reduction of medication errors, particularly by occasional or agency staff. However, it also can aid in managing episodes of absconding by informing others of the likeness of the person who is missing.

Conclusion

Within the general adult mental health estate, including the PICU, many patients will have committed no crime and will not have been involved with the criminal justice system. Their detention in hospital will have been solely because of their mental health condition and the need for treatment. The conditions to which a person is subject while receiving treatment in hospital are required to be the 'least restrictive' possible to manage any risks (Department of Health, 2015). In terms of reducing absconding, the first priority must be to promote an inpatient experience which is positive, engaging and innately creates an atmosphere likely to diminish the motivation to abscond. In contrast, it may be all too easy for clinicians and service managers to seek the seemingly common sense 'quick fix' of physical security to prevent absconding.

There is also good evidence that restrictive locked hospitals experience higher rates of dissatisfaction and aggression and may lend increased motivation to abscond. This is the opposite effect that the restrictions are intended to achieve.

PICUs are more challenging environments than general adult wards. It is important to recognise that most patients admitted to PICUs will have been referred from general adult wards, including for reasons of absconding with the associated secondary risks.

PICUs and other inpatient facilities require a holistic understanding of why people may be motivated to abscond. Units should invest in creating an environment in which those factors leading to absconding are proactively engaged and resolved. That said, attempts at and successful absconding episodes may be considered inevitable and therefore should be supported by a comprehensive range of policies and procedures to ensure that potential harm from absconding is as minimal as possible.

References

Bailey,J, Page,B, Ndimande,N, Connell,J and Vincent,C (2016) Absconding: Reducing Failure to Return in Adult Mental Health Wards. *BMJ Open Quality* 5: u209837.w5117. DOI: http://10.1136/bmjquality.u209837.w5117.

Booth,B, Michel,S, Baglole,S, Healey,L and Robertson,H (2021) Validation of the Booth Evaluation of Absconding Tool for Assessment of Absconding Risk. *Journal of the American Academy of Psychiatry and the Law* 49 (3) 339–49.

Bowers,L, Allan,T, Huglund,L, Mir-Cochrane,E, Nijman,H, Simpson,A, et al. (2008) *The City 128 Extension: Locked Doors in Acute Psychiatry, Outcome and Acceptability. Report for the National Co-ordinating Centre for NHS Service Delivery and Organisation, R&D (NCCSDO)*. London: HMSO.

Bowers,L and Jarrett,C (2002) Absconding: A Literature Review. *Journal of Psychiatric and Mental Health Nursing* 5 (5) 343–429.

Bowers,L, Simpson,A and Alexander,J (2005) Real World Application of an Intervention to Reduce Absconding. *Journal of Psychiatric and Mental Health Nursing* 12: 598–602.

Department of Health (2015) *Mental Health Act 1983: Code of Practice*. London: Department of Health.

Dickens,G, and Campbell,J (2001) Absconding of Patients from an Independent UK Psychiatric Hospital: A 3-Year Retrospective Analysis of Events and Characteristics of Absconders. *Journal of Psychiatric and Mental Health Nursing* 8 (6) 543–50.

Exworthy,T and Wilson,S (2010) Escapes and Absconds from Secure Psychiatric Units. *The Psychiatrist* 34 (3) 81–2 DOI: doi.org/10.1192/pb.bp.108.024372.

Foye,U. Li,Y, Birken,M. Parle,K and Simpson,A (2020) Activities on Acute Mental Health Inpatient Wards: A Narrative Synthesis of the Service Users' Perspective. *Journal of Psychiatric and Mental Health Nursing* 27 (4) 482–93.

Gilburt,H, Rose,D and Slade,M (2008) The Importance of Relationships in Mental Health Care: A Qualitative Study of Service Users' Experiences of Psychiatric Hospital Admission in the UK. *BMC Health Services Research* **8** (92) DOI: https://doi.org/10.1186/1472-6963-8-92.

HSC Public Health Agency (2015) *Pilot: Implementation of an Anti-Absconding Intervention South Eastern Health and Social Care Trust.* https://hscbusiness.hscni.net/pdf/Report_on_Absconding_PilotFinal_Doc.pdf.

Huber CG, Schneeberger,AR, Kowalinski,E, Frölich,D, von Felten,S, Walter,M, et al. (2016) Suicide Risk and Absconding in Psychiatric Hospitals with and without Open Door Policies: A 15 Year, Observational Study. *Lancet Psychiatry.* DOI: https://doi.org/10.1016/S2215-0366(16)30168-7.

Markham,S (2022) See Think Act: The Need to Rethink and Refocus on Relational Security. *Journal of Forensic Psychiatry & Psychology* **33** (2) 200–30. DOI: https://doi.org/10.1080/14789949.2022.2044068.

Muir-Cochrane,E, Oster,C, Grotto,J, Gerace,A and Jones,J (2013) The Inpatient Psychiatric Unit as Both a Safe and Unsafe Place: Implications for Absconding. *Journal of Mental Health Nursing* **22** (4) 304–12.

National Association of Psychiatric Intensive Care and Low Secure Units (NAPICU) (2017) *Design Guidance for Psychiatric Intensive Care Units.* Glasgow: NAPICU. https://napicu.org.uk/wp-content/uploads/2017/05/Design-Guidance-for-Psychiatric-Intensive-Care-Units-2017.pdf.

National Association of Psychiatric Intensive Care and Low Secure Units (NAPICU) (2014) *National Minimum Standards for Psychiatric Intensive Care in General Adult Services.* Glasgow: NAPICU. https://napicu.org.uk/wp-content/uploads/2014/12/NMS-2014-final.pdf.

Royal College of Psychiatrists (2020) *Standards for Psychiatric Intensive Care Units.* London: Royal College of Psychiatrists.

Substance Misuse

Lucy M. Walker and Stephen M. Pereira

In this chapter, we outline the scale of the problem of substance misuse in the context of psychiatric intensive care units (PICUs) and related services. Further, we discuss relevant health inequalities and how these impact on the issue. We also discuss the characteristics of dually diagnosed patients and illustrate how substance use commonly presents in clinical practice in PICUs, low secure units (LSUs) and locked rehabilitation units (LRUs).

We highlight risk factors and considerations relating to substance use, specifically drug-related deaths (DRDs). Finally, we examine why substance misuse is a major public health concern, considering responses from global, national and local perspectives, followed by a review of these approaches and suggestions for what frontline clinicians can do.

Prevalence

Substance use is a problem with far-reaching health and societal effects; prevalence is increasing year on year, with a recent report by the United Nations suggesting that 35 million people worldwide suffer from substance use-related disorders (UNODC, 2019).

The worst possible outcome of substance use/ misuse is drug-related death (DRD), which in the United Kingdom, Europe and globally is at an all-time high. In the United Kingdom, half of DRDs involve an opiate, with cocaine also being a significant problem, particularly for those aged 40–49 years (ONS, 2020; CDC, 2021). It is often substance-related harm and, sadly, death by overdose or complications of substance use that may present in clinical practice.

Impact of Inequalities in Health

The Marmot Review (2010) identified a social gradient in health: the less affluent the person, the worse their health. The review also provided evidence for reducing health inequalities.

Health inequalities are unfair and avoidable differences in health across the population and between different groups within society. They arise because of the conditions in which we are born, grow, live, work and age and influence our mental health, physical health and well-being (NHS England, 2021).

Dahlgren and Whitehead's (1991) 'rainbow' model of health inequalities illustrates how individual lifestyle factors, access to social and community networks, living and working conditions and general socio-economic factors may impact the rates of substance use (see Figure 9.1).

Men are more severely affected by DRD and accounted for two-thirds of DRDs in the United Kingdom in 2019 (ONS, 2020), a picture mirrored in the United States (CDC, 2021). However, it is unclear whether more men than women use drugs, whether men use at higher levels or whether men use drugs more hazardously.

Rates of DRD vary by location in the United Kingdom; North East England has significantly high rates of DRDs, which may be associated with levels of deprivation, as rates of DRD tend to be higher in more deprived areas of England and Wales when compared with less deprived areas (ONS, 2020). Rates of DRD are also higher in low-income households, specifically those with incomes less than £10,400 per annum (MoJ/PHE, 2017).

Sexuality can also be a risk factor. Those individuals who identify as LGBTQ+ are at greater risk of substance use and mental health issues (SAMHSA, 2016), a trend which is reflected in the authors' locality of Bristol, UK (BCC, 2020), and a trend consistently found within a large cohort of students in the United Kingdom (Pereira et al., 2019, 2000).

Substance use can be stigmatised within religious faiths, leading to under-reporting by service users and barriers to accessing substance misuse and/or mental health treatment in the community. Research has found that social pressures, domestic violence, language

The Main Determinants of Health

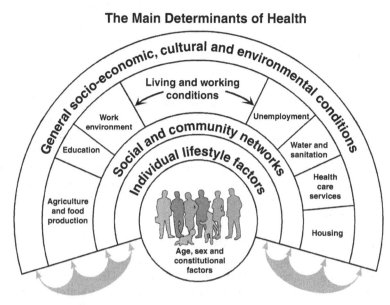

Figure 9.1 The main determinants of health
Source: Dahlgren and Whitehead, 1993

problems, racism and stereotyping amongst religious populations may result in substance misuse and/or self-harm (Khan, 2019).

Ethnicity and Drug Use

In the United Kingdom, recent statistics compiled by NHS Digital (2017) suggest that Black adults (11.7%) and White British adults (8.9%) were more likely to have used illicit drugs in the 12 months prior to survey compared with Asian adults (3.4%). Black women (9.7%), White British women (6.2%) and women from the White Other group (6.9%) were more likely to have used illicit drugs compared with Asian women (0.4%). White British men (11.8%) were more likely to have used illicit drugs compared with White British women (6.2%). Asian men (5.9%) were more likely to have used illicit drugs compared with Asian women (0.4%).

There were no meaningful differences between ethnic groups in the percentage of men using illicit drugs, which may explain the higher rates of DRD reported in this population. Unfortunately, this survey excluded those in institutional settings (hospitals, prisons), temporary housing and the homeless and the use of 'legal highs'. These results may explain why minoritised groups, particularly Black African males, are almost five times as likely to be detained under the Mental Health Act (MHA) (NHS Digital, 2022), perhaps due to their increased substance use,

but further research on substance misuse and ethnicity is warranted, particularly amongst PICU service users.

The situation is furthermore confounded by studies which report the highest levels of drug use amongst individuals of 'mixed ethnic' background (UKDPC, 2010) without further exploration of cultural issues associated with people who identify as such. What does 'mixed ethnic' actually mean? It is often poorly defined in research.

Children of parents who use substances are disproportionately exposed to chaotic households and parental drug use and may end up being carers for their intoxicated parents. They may also suffer neglect and live in fear, be exposed to criminality and disrupted education and live with the stigma of their parents using drugs (ACMD, 2010).

Children in these households have long been recognised as suffering from 'hidden harm' and are a priority for services. The risk of inability to parent should always be considered, even with those parents who just use alcohol, as often the harm is hidden under the guise of rationalisations such as 'nothing wrong with a drink because it's legal' or 'at least I'm not using drugs'. However, children and often partners of the substance user suffer neglect, harm or, sadly, more severe violence at the hands of alcohol-intoxicated parents/carers (ACMD, 2010).

Consequences and Impact of Substance Misuse

Physical health problems most common with drug use are cardiovascular and respiratory problems, injecting problems, abscesses and blood-borne viral infections. Hepatitis B and C viral infections are high (>75%) among drug users due to sharing of injecting equipment/paraphernalia. Hepatitis C can interact with alcohol consumption to accelerate liver damage. Poor dental health is associated with morbidity and mortality as well as cardiovascular and respiratory diseases. Drug users were found to engage in a higher incidence of sex work and suffer from sexually transmitted infections, accidental self-injury, trauma, overdose and DRD (Patton, 2013).

Psychological consequences of substance abuse include behavioural impulsivity, irritability, unpredictability and mood disturbances. These characteristics can often be observed in the PICU patient population. Many patients suffer with physical, psychological and social problems and present with complex needs such as homelessness/unstable housing. They may also have difficulties accessing benefits they are entitled to and face stigma for their substance use (AMCD, 2010; NICE, 2016).

Substance users' priorities become increasingly dominated by drugs and drug-seeking, leading to increasing debts, offending, acquisitive crime/fraud/prostitution/drug dealing, family breakdown, loss of employment, eviction and/or homelessness, possible incarceration and, sadly, often death, all of which damage the individual and their families, place pressure on public health and social care services and are harmful to their communities (ACMD, 2010; NICE, 2016). Drug-seeking behaviour can also be a major challenge to PICUs and other related inpatient services.

Studies of opiate users suggest 35% of offenders had committed a crime in the 24 months prior to starting treatment, had previously injected and were often homeless (MoJ/PHE, 2017). However, the relationship between crime and substance misuse is complex. Does substance use lead to offending? Or is offending committed whilst under the influence?

In the authors' experience of working with service users, offending may start with intoxication, leading to impulsive or reckless behaviour (i.e. violence and/or offending). However, offending usually results from an increasing need for substances due to physical dependence and increased tolerance levels and a subsequent need to commit crime to obtain funds to purchase more substances.

Dual Diagnosis

Many individuals who use substances often have co-existing mental health problems. UK studies suggest rates of comorbidity are high within statutory treatment services for substance misuse (75%), alcohol (85%) and community mental health teams (44%) (Weaver et al., 2003), psychiatric inpatients (43%) and secure mental health service users (56%) (Strathdee et al., 2002).

In their UK study, Isaac et al. (1995) reported that 71.3% of PICU patients were using cannabis. Those using cannabis were, in comparison to those abstaining, more severely ill and spent longer periods in the PICU; this scenario persists in the United Kingdom. Recently published repeats of national surveys of National Health Service (NHS) users show shocking increases in the prevalence of substance misuse in the last 10 years, suggesting that half of all PICU admissions have substance use identified as a complex need at the start (Pereira et al., 2021).

Table 9.1 presents previously unpublished national survey data relating to drugs reported on admission to PICUs, low secure units (LSUs) and locked rehabilitation units (LRUs).

Table 9.1 Substances found in positive urine drug screen on admission of UK NHS patients (NAPICU, 2021)

Drug	PICU % / (n)	LSU % / (n)	LRU % / (n)	Total
Cannabinoids	67.3 (109)	68.0 (17)	69.7 (23)	149
Stimulants	22.8 (37)	20.0 (5)	21.2 (7)	49
Ecstasy/MDMA	7.4 (12)	8.0 (2)	6.1 (2)	16
Hallucinogens	1.9 (3)	3.9 (1)	0 (0)	4
Opiates	0.6 (1)	0.1 (0)	3 (1)	2
Total	162	25	33	

The most used drugs found on admission were cannabis, followed by stimulants, ecstasy/MDMA, hallucinogens and opiates. Similar proportions of substances used across unit types were confirmed; there were no significant differences by unit type reported (x^2 = 3.479, P > 0.05), which suggests that similar substances are used by all patients regardless of unit type on admission.

Characteristics of the Dual Diagnosis Population

A meta-review of 18 UK studies of severe mental illness and substance misuse for the National Institute for Health and Care Excellence (NICE, 2016) reported the most common comorbid mental illness among substance users to be schizophrenia, with estimates ranging from 35.9% to 92.3%, followed by bipolar disorder ranging from 10.3% to 13% and substance-induced psychosis ranging from 37.5% to 48.7%.

Within service users of addiction services only, the most common mental health comorbidity was severe depression (73.1%). In terms of substances used, alcohol and cannabis were the most common (50.6%–84.6%), followed by cocaine/crack (9.7%–23.8%), stimulants (6.0%–20.8%), amphetamines (10.5%–12%) and opiates (0.9%–10%).

Substance Use and Clinical Effects on Mental Health Disorders

Substance use can have the following impact on the following mental health disorders:

- **Schizophrenia/schizoaffective disorder and bipolar disorder(s)** – Cannabis and stimulants such as crack cocaine and/or amphetamines can escalate destructive manic aggressive behaviour, leading to damage to property and threatened or actual violence to self and/or others, police involvement or detention via MHA Section 136 'Place of Safety', sometimes involving multiple police and hospital staff. This is also supported by Dyer (1996), who found that risk of violence in patients with substance use and psychotic disorder was increased fourfold.

- **Depression** – Intoxication can lessen positive resolve for continuing with life and disinhibit control of suicide/self-harm impulses which may end in death by misadventure. Toxicology reports frequently find that multiple substances, often alcohol, cocaine and heroin, are involved in DRDs. Deaths involving new psychoactive substances often called legal highs have also increased in recent years (PHE, 2014).

- **Personality disorder** – Studies have shown that individuals suffering with a personality disorder are at heightened risk of re-offending, especially those suffering with a substance use disorder (O'Driscoll, 2012). Cannabis and stimulants such as crack cocaine and amphetamines can make narcissistic/anti-social tendencies and psychopathic rage more severe and pronounced, leading to re-offending behaviour (Howard et al., 2013). In PICU settings, this may lead to fire-starting and episodes of self-harming or abusing self/others (Gintalaite-Bieliauskiene et al., 2020). In addition, illicit substance use may lessen resolve to abstain from sexual offending and/or lead to disinhibition and increased sexual arousal and thus further risk of offending/recidivism (Burca et al., 2013).

Substance use is present in the profiles of the majority of UK PICU, LSU and LRU admissions and this may be directly linked to circumstances surrounding hospital admission or offending behaviour. Box 9.1 lists common clinical presentations based on national survey patient characteristics (Pereira et al., 2021) and lived experience of PICU clinical practice.

Box 9.1 Common Clinical PICU/LSU Presentations

- **Drug-induced psychotic episode/breakdown/crisis** brought on by stimulants, such as crack cocaine, cocaine, MDMA, amphetamines and speed; hallucinogens, such as mushrooms, ketamine, spice (synthetic cannabis) and novel psychoactive drugs; high-strength cannabis; or skunk weed (Ham et al., 2017; Fiorentini et al., 2021).
- **Violent, aggressive, abusive or assaultive behaviour** (Anderson and Bukor, 2012) which may require high numbers of police, nursing or secure transport staff to manage safely.

Box 9.1 (cont.)

- **Crisis detentions** made via MHA Section 136 which may be closely located to the PICU (Laidlaw et al., 2009); service users are often found under the influence and picked up in community settings.
- **Recent sleep deprivation** which may cause hallucinations, visual and perceptual disturbances and/or manic or psychotic episodes (Petrovsky et al., 2014).
- **Suicide/self-harm attempts** (Gintalaite-Bieliauskiene et al., 2020) or **impulsive acts** whilst under the influence/intoxicated, particularly amongst women.
- **Accidental self-injury**, such as fractures and falls or trauma from intoxication (Rood et al., 2016).
- **Requiring detoxification on admission**; the person may deny use of alcohol/substances.
- **Sexual disinhibition** which may involve undressing, masturbation and/or trying to touch staff and/or other service users (Tarter et al., 2003).
- **Bizarre behaviour,** such as eating/smearing faeces and/or urinating in places other than the toilet (Haslam, 2012).
- **History of severe prolonged substance use**/preceding admission for psychosis (Fiorentini et al., 2021).
- **History of overdose**, whether accidental or intentional.
- **History of offending** *behaviour,* such as impulsive acts driven by emotional states; multiple/repeated offences for acquisitive crime, shoplifting, theft, burglary, prostitution, robbery and/or use of weapons to fund substance use, often seen in heroin and crack cocaine users (O'Driscoll, 2012; Burca et al., 2013)
- **Homelessness/unstable accommodation, comorbidity** and suicidal ideations/attempts (Trevedi et al., 2022).
- **High levels of physical health problems,** such as infections, injecting problems and sexually transmitted infections; cardiac problems related to bacterial infections, such as pericarditis and tricuspid value replacements; swollen legs/leg ulcers; groin sinuses from prolonged femoral artery access; skin breakdown around injection sites; infections and abscesses; bladder/urinary problems; blood-borne viruses such as hepatitis C; or deep vein thrombosis (Cornford and Close, 2016).
- **Admissions with existing opiate substitute treatment maintenance prescribing** and/or prescriptions for pregabalin, gabapentin, opiates and benzodiazepines, often associated with pain management (Cornford and Close, 2016).
- **Polypharmacy**
- **Escalating PRN requirement**

Clinical Testing and Assessment

Urinalysis

Urine testing should be performed on admission and on a regular or ad hoc basis depending on local protocols and procedures. Testing is often utilised following a period of Section 17 leave, when substance misuse has been an aggravating factor in illness or when substance misuse is suspected.

Most wards/units routinely test for presence of opiates, cocaine, amphetamines, benzodiazepines and cannabis (THC). Anecdotally, there is an increasing trend of ketamine use amongst young people, as it is easily available and cheap. With continued and prolonged chronic use, ketamine can cause serious genitourinary issues, such as irritation of the urethra leading to removal of the bladder and permanent catheterisation. This is due to the drug compound and its effects as it travels through the body. Often, ketamine use is missed/underreported because it requires a specialist urine test.

A specialist test is required to detect for Spice, an increasingly used drug amongst homeless and prison populations (HM Inspectorate, 2015), to monitor opiate substitution concordance and to check for buprenorphine use and methadone metabolites.

Adulteration of urine samples is commonplace in clinical practice, as are refusals and avoidance of testing. Having worked previously as a drug-treatment service clinician, this author has been provided with samples of green-coloured warm water (green to pass for methadone), old, cold urine (often someone else's urine) and apple juice. This author has also found evidence of concealments in condoms. These incidents highlight the importance of supervision of same-sex staff when collecting real-time specimens. Even still, concealments and adulteration practices are common.

Staff should not be alone if supervised urines are required. False positives and erroneous tests are also an issue, as there are many prescribed and over-the-counter formulations and food stuffs that will affect accuracy of results.

Breathalysers

Use of breathalysers depends on local protocols/procedures but is often not completed routinely unless the service user has returned from leave intoxicated or when alcohol use is suspected. Breathalysers should always be used if there are concerns regarding level of alcohol intoxication and medication administration.

The issue of consent to urine testing or a breathalyser raises difficulties for risk management. Patients have the right to refuse to provide a urine/breath specimen for analysis. If they refuse, this means that medications may not be able to be administered safely if overdose/over-sedation may be an issue. PICU nursing staff should automatically alert medical staff if a urinalysis is refused following an episode of suspected using. This author is aware of instances where sedating medication has been omitted for 24–48 hours by clinical teams because it is unclear what substances are in the patient's body and it may be negligent to administer the medication further, especially if it is a sedative.

This decision should not be taken in isolation, as it is complex and should be considered on an individualised case-by-case basis, with shared decision-making and risk managed across the whole team. Some trusts have policies that refusal of urinalysis is to be counted as a positive test, and each trust policy/protocol should be followed accordingly. Often, it is the case that refusal is due to not wanting to detect the extent of polydrug use but simply may be due to non-engagement on behalf of the service user.

Comprehensive Assessment

Comprehensive assessment of substance misuse should include questions about:

- Current drug/alcohol use, quantity and frequency
- Drug/alcohol history, including periods of abstinence and treatment, including detoxification
- Triggers for use/relapse
- Current medication
- Physical health assessment/needs, medical history and treatment
- Previous intravenous use, injecting practices and preferred routes; injection-related problems; and occurrence of any physical complications, such as ulceration, lumps, sinuses from groin injecting,

deep vein thrombosis and, in severe cases, leg amputation
- Risky sexual practices, such as sex work (consider safeguarding issues)

Chronic injecting drug users are frequently left with lifelong mobility problems. Individuals with dual diagnosis will frequently ignore infections at injecting sites and often present to accident and emergency or general practitioners, which may account for the higher prevalence of physical health problems disclosed by injecting drug and/or alcohol users in accident and emergency settings (Patton, 2013).

Clinicians should be mindful of the lack of venous access in injecting drug users. The expert on finding access will be the service user themselves.

Bloodborne Virus Risk

Testing for bloodborne viruses (BBVs) is important to enable early detection, prevention of transmission and occupational safety for staff. However, there is a stigma associated with testing, as it can be perceived as indication of high-risk behaviour or a lack of personal responsibility. This stigma can prevent individuals from seeking testing and treatment, which can lead to negative health outcomes and increased transmission of these viruses. Therefore, it is important to acknowledge and address this stigma in order to promote testing and reduce the spread of BBVs.

- Ask about sharing of any equipment, such as needles, barrels, filters, spoons, snorting tubes and so on.
- Ask about hepatitis B vaccinations.
- Many people with dual diagnosis may ignore the risk associated with sharing using equipment or high-risk sexual activities (i.e. unprotected sex with multiple partners), choosing to either deny or minimise that it is a problem. They are often too scared to hear what the outcome of any testing will mean for them and the possible effects on their life expectancy.
- It is good practice to make pre-testing counselling for BBV mandatory before performing any test.
- The actual effects of receiving a positive diagnosis should be fully explored with the individual, including what receiving a diagnosis means for them and what effects will it have on their life (work, relationships, family).
- Once the individual has had time to reflect on these points, only then should testing be arranged.

- Referral can be made to specialist hepatitis nurses and/or sexual health teams/clinics. Local variation in service provision will dictate how the clinician accesses this service for their patients locally.

Overdose Risk

Assessing overdose risk is an important step in preventing fatal overdoses and promoting the health and safety of individuals who use drugs. Some reasons why assessing overdose risk is important include early intervention, to prevent fatal overdoses and reduce stigma associated with drug, particularly IV and opiate, use. This stigma can prevent individuals from seeking help or disclosing their drug use to healthcare providers and from accessing harm reduction services, such as overdose prevention education or naloxone distribution programs, which in turn can increase their risk of overdose. A harm minimisation approach to enquiry should be adopted that prioritises the health and safety of individuals who use drugs.

- Ask about overdose history, if any. If the patient has experienced an overdose(s), ask about the number of incidents, when and where they occurred and whether they were intentional or accidental.
- Ask the individual how they use. Do they use to get high, relax, forget or blackout? Do they use on their own? With friends? Do they use only under certain circumstances?
- Ask if overdose, heavy use or polypharmacy was involved in their admission to hospital/index offence (crime committed which resulted in detention to hospital for treatment order – for forensic patients).
- Ask if they have ever taken too may substances before or lost track of how much they have taken.
- Ask if they have ever witnessed an overdose or been involved/around someone who has overdosed. Ask if they would know what to do in this case.
- Ask if they know about the recovery position.
- Ask if they heard of naloxone. Naloxone training can be conducted for staff. The focus of the intervention is to train other injecting drug users how to use 'emergency pens' to restore consciousness to a person who is overdosing. Lives can be saved. Often, service users can be directed to local drug agency charities who will provide the training and naloxone kits for free.
- Consider what the user will need upon discharge.

Psychological Health

In order to enable a holistic assessment, individuals should be asked about:

- Self-harm history
- Mental health history, including past and current contact with services
- Current mental health problems

Family and Social Situation

Holistic assessment should include questions about:

- Current domestic situation and relationships
- Accommodation
- Parental status. Is the user living with parent(s)? Is the parent(s) living with someone else? Is the parent(s) in a care facility?
- Possible pregnancy
- Parental and childhood history
- Education
- Major life events, including trauma
- Past relationships. Is there a history of domestic violence, abuse or alcohol/drug use?
- Alcohol/drug history in the family
- Financial issues
- Employment status

Legal Issues

Holistic assessment should address:

- Previous legal history
- Current and pending legal/criminal issues
- Significant offences
- History of violence, aggression or abuse (victim or perpetrator)

Risk of Ability to Parent

Often, children's needs are secondary to the parent's or caregiver's drug use. This is not always the case, but it is the exception to find children whose lives are not affected by parental substance use. Holistic assessment of parental drug use on ability to parent should address:

- Parental drug use, including amounts, route, frequency, when and where, exposure and so on.
- Where are the children when the parent is using?
- Where are the children when the parent goes 'to score' or use needle exchange?
- Where do they keep their drugs so that the children cannot access them?

- Where do they intend to keep their medicines/needles?
- Do they need any safe storage advice? Do they need a locked box? If so, contact local drug services who may be able to provide one free of charge.
- Is there anyone smoking tobacco around the children/in the household/in the car?
- Do they have/need any support with the children?
- Provision of basic needs, including food, warmth, affection. Is this a priority for the parent(s)/carer?
- How is substance use funded?
- Accommodation and home environment; include other users visiting the property, do they use there, are the children exposed to this, is the property being used for dealing?
- Safe disposal of sharps, risk of HIV/hepatitis C.
- Family/social network and support systems; include any non-users and if both parents are using and if they use together or separately.
- Driving. Does the client or any significant other take the children in the car under the influence of drugs and alcohol?
- Parent's perception of the impact of their use on their ability to parent.
- Presence of other carers, adequate care arrangements and level of cooperation with care-plans.

Risk Assessment Specific to Drug/Alcohol Misuse

Overdose

- Naïve drug user
- Recent loss of tolerance, detoxification or period of abstinence
- Regular injector
- High-level use
- Injected by others
- Uses alone
- Polydrug/alcohol use
- Seeking oblivion
- Previous accidental overdose
- Previous intentional overdose

Injecting Behaviour

- Regular injector
- Uses high-risk sites (e.g. neck/groin)

- Poor injecting practice
- Injects outside/in public places
- Shares (any) injecting equipment

Alcohol

- High-dose use
- Blackouts
- Frequent withdrawals
- Seizures/delirium tremens
- Frequent intoxication
- Liver damage (e.g. cirrhosis, hepatitis)

(North West Surrey Mental Health Partnership NHS Trust, 2008)

Procedural Considerations

Procedures are detailed in the PICU National Minimum Standards (NMS) (Pereira and Clinton, 2002; NAPICU, 2014). These include a policy for detection and management of substance misuse should it exist. Issues of contraband in the form of substances and concealments should be included as part of the search policy.

Escorting Patients

Issues with substance use can cause difficulties with using MHA Section 17 leave. Some patients may try to order alcoholic drinks in cafés, bars or shops. Individuals have also been caught shoplifting alcohol while on leave (both escorted and unescorted). Escorts need to remain vigilant whilst escorting patients on leave. The general public may even play a role, for instance, by offering drugs to a patient on leave when they are out in the community. Patients on leave may even encounter individuals openly using on the street. Open dialog can often be used in these instances to better understand the narrative about substance use.

Searching Patients

The search policy is designed to create and maintain a therapeutic environment in which treatment may take place and to ensure the security of the premises and the safety of patients, staff and the public. The authority to conduct a search of a person or their property is controlled by law, and it is important that hospital staff are aware of whether they have legal authority to carry out any such search. The policy may extend to routine and random searching without cause of detained patients, if necessary, without their consent, but only in exceptional circumstances. For example, such searches may be necessary if the patients detained in a particular unit tend to have dangerous or violent propensities, which means they create a self-evident, pressing need for additional security (MHCOP, 2015).

Searching on return from leave may involve a metal detector for weapons or other contraband. Many concealments go unnoticed due to the limitations on personal searches being confined to pat-downs. Searching should be proportionate to the identified risk and should involve the minimum possible intrusion into the individual's privacy. All searches will be undertaken with due regard to and respect for the person's dignity and privacy and with full consent of the patient (MHCOP, 2015).

Other ways substances find their way into clinical areas involve packages being delivered through and over fences, by people and drones, via takeaways or being left on the grounds and, sadly, from visitors. Article 8 of the European Convention on Human Rights (ECHR) requires public authorities to respect a person's right to a private life. Privacy, safety and dignity are important constituents of a therapeutic environment and staff should respect a patient's privacy as much as possible while maintaining safety. This includes enabling a patient to send and receive mail, including in electronic formats, without restriction. If restriction is deemed necessary, this should be clearly outlined in the patient's care plan by the clinical team. Respecting a patient's privacy encompasses the circumstances in which patients may meet or communicate with people of their choosing in private, including in their own rooms, as well as the protection of their private property.

Common Clinical Presentations of Substance Use within the Unit

Some common clinical presentations of substance use within the unit include:

- Service users returning from leave appearing to be intoxicated
- Patients staying up all night
- Service users appearing agitated, pacing and/or having red eyes or dilated pupils
- Actual violence due to disinhibiting effects of intoxication
- Strange smell in corridors and/or common areas
- Smoke in bedrooms and/or bathrooms

- Pill packets or small plastic 'baggies' found in bedrooms and/or hospital grounds
- Strange powders found in room searches
- Concealments or other contraband, such as lighters, found during room searches
- Substances being concealed and/or left on the grounds for pick up when the service user is on unescorted leave

When substances are found, Section 17 leave is often suspended to try and ensure that further contraband is not brought into the unit, as substances are often shared or sold with other service users, which can result in an extremely volatile and risky environment. It also raises a difficult issue for staff who must consider the extent of the usage for safe medication prescribing and administration.

Fortunately, many staff will experience that substance use within the clinical environment is usually time limited and often patient specific. Temporary suspension of Section 17 leave and intensive focused 1:1 intervention reduce the risk of reoccurrence.

Use of E-Cigarettes and Vaping

The literature regarding the use of e-cigarettes or vapes does suggest that they are less toxic than smoking cigarettes (Nutt, 2016), but their use is not without their own health risks (CDC, 2022).

Some vaping-related health incidents can be observed within PICUs, such as coughing, retching, spitting, complaining of palpitations and/or dizzy spells, vomiting, especially after eating, and sore throats, particularly when vape coils are burnt out and for whatever reason the service user chooses not to or is unable to replace them.

One case example involved an individual suffering with paranoid schizophrenia stating that the voices were worse after vaping. There have also been examples of vapes being used for potential absconding attempts by being used as tools/leverage to force open garden gates and larger heavier vapes being used as assault weapons. This risk can be minimised using disposable e-cigarettes.

Disposable e-cigarettes may offer some advantages over individual vapes, such as those just discussed, but this can be complicated if the service user has no access to money. Some units provide e-cigarettes or nicotine replacement therapy (NRT).

Whilst a blanket ban on smoking on hospital sites is an attempt at harm reduction, it has opened up wider issues of NRT implementation, including vaping. Practices may differ from unit to unit, with NRT provision being patchy and inconsistent. Caution is required to ensure that NRT is supplied with adequate support and follow-up from smoking cessation facilitators.

The seriousness of inconsistencies surrounding access to smoking preferences between units should not be underestimated. This was starkly illustrated by newspaper reports of the tragic premeditated killing of a mental healthcare support worker. The perpetrator had stated that the prospect of being moved to a non-smoking facility without Wi-Fi was part of his motivation for the fatal incident. On the day of the fatal stabbing, staff were preparing to escort the patient to a different facility (Smith, 2015).

Careful consideration needs to be given to local procedures/protocols and the effects of local policy on the mental state of patients. Many will recognise numerous flashpoints when new patient requests for smoking are denied or when vaping is encouraged instead. The least restrictive option should always be implemented when possible, and this could include approval of leave when requested with a view to reducing avoidable escalation and aggression.

Smoking remains legal in society, and it could be argued that patients should have the right to choose if they wish to smoke or not. This may need careful consideration in the often-restrictive environment of the PICU. Furthermore, such is the prevalence of smoking amongst mental health inpatients and the associated strong feelings that access to smoking facilities on transfer may require careful consideration. Further research in this area is likely to be helpful for future policy development.

Illicit Substance Use: Choice or a Disease?

Many substance misuse interventions are based on the assumption that using is an individual choice and that the individual has a right to make an unwise decision. That said, it is legitimate to question why an individual would choose to suffer serious harm or even die because of addictive behaviours. The simple paradigm of 'choice' may not be sufficient to explain some of the most severe consequences of substances use. These include:

- IV drug use leading to hepatitis C, leg ulcers, amputations or overdose revivals
- Alcohol use leading to pancreatitis, fatty/scarred liver, polydrug use and overdosing when intoxicated, accidental self-injury, Korsakoff's syndrome, bleeding oesophageal varices or liver failure
- Tobacco use leading to respiratory disorders associated with smoking such as lung and throat cancer.

Intervention

It is often not possible to 'stop' someone from using illicit substances by simply denying them access, although this is sometimes advanced as an option in the PICU. A more sophisticated approach is required to encourage a recovery journey, best described by the transtheoretical model (TTM) (Prochaska and DiClemente, 1983; Prochaska et al., 1992) (see Figure 9.2).

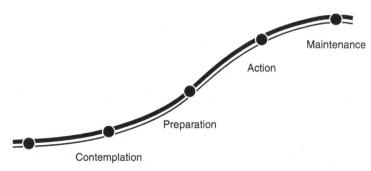

Figure 9.2 The transtheoretical model of behaviour change, reproduced with kind permission from Janet Prochaska, Pro-Change Behaviour Systems, Inc.

- Precontemplation – not intending to take action in the next 6 months
- Contemplation – intending to take action in the next 6 months
- Preparation – ready to take action in the next 30 days
- Action – has made overt lifestyle changes in the last 6 months
- Maintenance – doing a new behaviour more than 6 months

Stages of change lie at the heart of the TTM. Studies of change have found that people move through a series of stages when modifying behaviour. While the time a person can stay in each stage is variable, the tasks required to move to the next stage are not. Certain principles and processes of change work best at each stage to reduce resistance, facilitate progress and prevent relapse (Prochaska, 2022).

The model's basic premises include:

- Change is a matter of balance and people change their behaviour when there are more motivational forces in favour of change than in favour of the status quo.
- For the process of change to be effective, professionals must assess and work with the patient at the stage which the parent has reached in terms of their readiness to accept or deny the need to change.

There are also two blocks to change: pre-contemplation and relapse. There is also a theoretical distinction between 'lapse' and 'relapse'. A lapse is a short episode of use after which the person returns with motivation to continue their learning and behaviour change. A relapse is a longer period of using with no motivation from the person to learn from any control/reduction in use. Staff should look to discover the events leading up to a lapse/relapse collaboratively with the client and identify what needs to change in order for the next change attempt to be more successful.

Motivational Assessment

Motivation is a critical element of behaviour change that predicts client abstinence and reductions in substance use. Therefore, a motivational assessment is important for identifying reasons for change, assessing readiness to change and, if continually assessed during treatment, will aid with engagement and improve retention. Assessment questions could include:

- What was life like before you started using substances problematically?
- What problems is your current use causing you?
- What is good about your current use?
- What sort of help would be useful to you at this time? Why?
- What are your goals (immediate and long term) with respect to your substance use?
- What goals (immediate and long term) do you have in other areas of your life?
- What makes this the right time for you to be making these changes?
- What if anything has changed in your situation?
- What support do you have in place to help you make these changes?
- Where is the patient in the stage of change cycle and what help/support needs do they have to enable them to reach the next stage?

PICU clinicians should always maintain a shared optimism about change. Working with motivation to abstain is the focus of any intervention, as detention in locked units means attempts will be made to enforce abstinence from substances by the nature of the highly controlled environment. This may provide opportunity for intervention to be attempted as soon as is reasonably practical.

Problem drug use has many components, including genetics, early upbringing, mental health, personality and life events. No single approach will address everything simultaneously. Many different 'psychosocial' approaches to helping an individual control substance use have been described and shown to be effective in certain populations at certain times. These include:

- Motivational interviewing
- 12-step mutual self-help
- Cognitive behavioural therapy
- Contingency management
- Social/family interventions

It has often proved difficult to deliver any of these interventions in their entirety in a short-term PICU. Longer-term units may also be challenged by size of caseload or the limited availability of training or supervision (Day, 2013).

Questions regarding substance use are often mandatory in the admission assessment and can be a good starting point for opening up initial discussion about goals (see Table 9.2 for goals and associated interventions).

Table 9.2 Common approaches to substance misuse treatment and associated resources

Goals	Recommended approach	Resources
Unsure/ ambivalent	Motivational interviewing/Stage of change model (Transtheoretical approach TTM)	Miller, WR and Rollnick, S (2013) *Motivational Interviewing: Helping People to Change* (3rd ed.) New York: Guilford Press www.prochange.com/transtheoretical-model-of-behavior-change
To stop completely (abstinence)	Mutual help Narcotics Anonymous (NA) Alcoholic Anonymous (AA) UK Narcotics Anonymous 24/7 Narcotics Anonymous online meetings (Zoom)	https://na.org www.aa.org/ https://ukna.org/ (includes local meeting finder) Meeting ID: 4949 655 895 p/w: 1953
To reduce use (controlled use) To reduce harm	Cognitive behaviour therapy (CBT) Examine permission-giving beliefs and devise behavioural experiments regarding reducing use Harm reduction advice and intervention	SMART recovery https://smartrecovery.org.uk/ (includes local meeting finder) Mitcheson, L, Maslin, J, Meynen, T, Morrison, T, Hill, R and Wanigaratne, S (2010) *Applied Cognitive and Behavioural Approaches to the Treatment of Addiction: A Practical Treatment Guide.* Chichester: Wiley. www.drugwise.org.uk/harm-reduction-2/ www.talktofrank.com/

- Ask the person what they want to do, if anything, about their substance use.
- Request that they define their goals (abstinence or to control their use). The more non-judgemental the questioning, the better and more effective the intervention will be.

Understanding the patient's view here is crucial. Exploration of their perceptions of being able to control their using behaviour will determine what goals are attempted. It is not uncommon for patients to initially look to reduce the harm associated with using, then move to the goal of abstinence once they start to see the results and health benefits.

Many patients cannot tolerate the thought of never using again, as many of their permission-giving beliefs (Mitcheson et al., 2010) are tied into using to cope/soothe or as a reward to themselves. It can be useful to adopt a 'one day at a time' approach to abstinence or even seek to gain days of abstinence within periods of using.

- Assess the patient's motivation to change along with their confidence to do so. It is helpful to use rating scales of 0–10 to assess changes; 0 = no motivation/confidence and ≥10 = highly motivated/confident.
- Set SMART (specific, measurable, achievable, realistic and time-specific) goals.

Public Health England (Day, 2013) has published a 'For use by Clinicians' package to improve treatment

effectiveness derived from the International Treatment Effectiveness Project (ITEP).

Based on the common components of effective treatment described by Moos (2007) (see Figure 9.3), which uses the concept of node-link mapping, which is a series of visually represented counselling strategies in the form of templates to utilise with service users to support the delivery of these techniques in 'session-sized' chunks, commonly referred to as ITEP maps.

Whilst abstinence-orientated norms and models are contained with the maps, it is still possible to work within a harm-reduction framework with a goal of reducing substance use.

Helpful resources such as manuals and ITEP templates can be downloaded by PICU (and other inpatient) clinicians and used within the unit. Tools such as these are valuable resources for clinical practice, as they ask patients to rate each intervention. Each template includes a 1–10 rating scale for the client to provide feedback on the helpfulness of the session in order to plan for effective future sessions. It is recommended that clinicians remain aware of new developments in helpful tools which can be used at the unit level.

Figure 9.4 shows how a programme is designed to be delivered.

Substance Use and UK Initiatives and Law

Preventing DRDs using opioid substitution treatment (OST) is associated with markedly reduced risk of overdose death (Department of Health, 2017) and

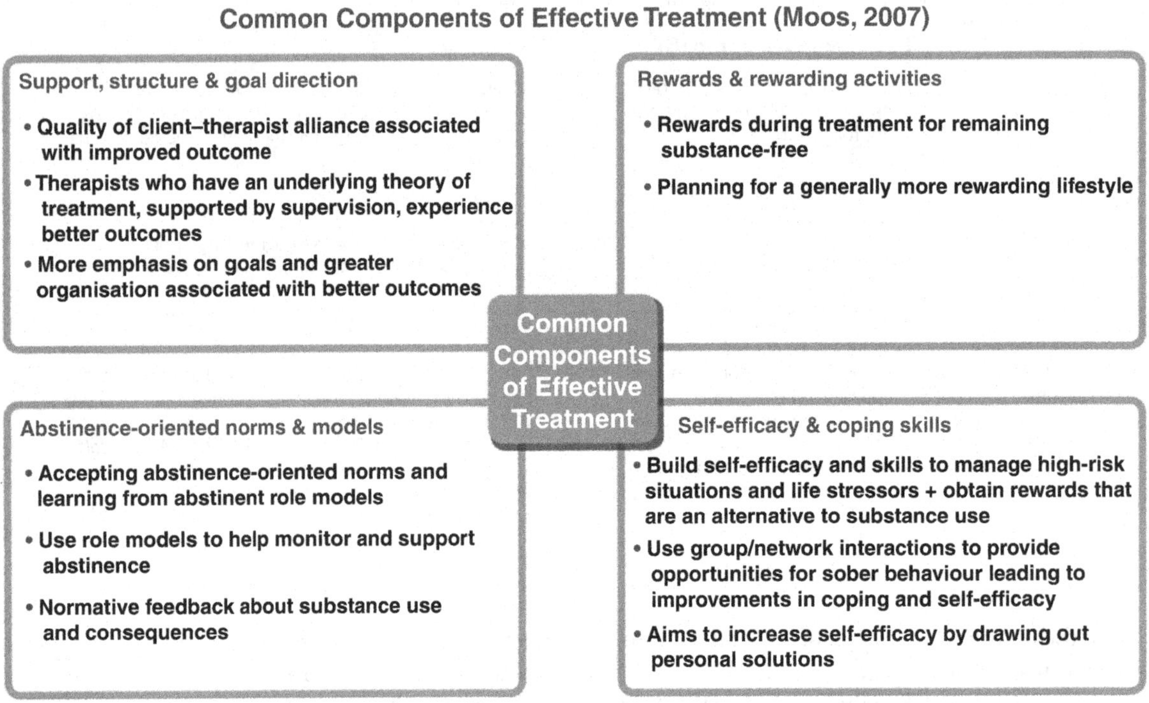

Common Components of Effective Treatment (Moos, 2007)

Figure 9.3 – Common components of effective treatment
Reproduced from Day (2013). Routes to recovery via the Community – A Mapping User Manual

behaviour change, with supporters calling for wider use in prisons and communities (Stone et al., 2021).

Naloxone, an opioid receptor antagonist which reverses the effects of overdose, was made more widely available by the Human Medicines (Amendment) (No. 3) Regulations 2015, thereby reducing harm to those most at risk of DRD (HM Government, 2015).

Other UK initiatives targeted at drug-related behaviour change are signposted via general practice surgeries, such as the Livewell Campaign (NHS, 2021a) and other general UK public information sites (FRANK, 2021).

Several new technologies are available, such as those designed to track progress and money saved, those that provide daily support and those used for relapse prevention, such as SoberTool (Apple, 2021). There are also better health campaigns designed to increase people's confidence to change their addictive behaviours along with apps to support behaviour change (NHS, 2021b).

UK and International Perspectives

In the United Kingdom, there is largely a prohibitionist and criminalising substance use policy (HM Government, 1971) as well as evidenced-based treatment service specifications, such as Models of Care (NTA, 2002), clinical guidelines from the Department of Health (Department of Health, 2017) and NICE guideline [NG58] (NICE, 2016).

International drug policy is also generally prohibitionist, which means it aims to prevent the production, supply and use of specific drugs and criminalises people who use them. This approach can prevent people who use drugs from accessing harm reduction services such as needle exchange programmes and medication-assisted treatment. This approach effectively bans the supply of controlled drugs for non-medical or research use in the form of the United Nations Conventions (UNODC, 1961, 1971, 1988). Opponents call for decriminalisation with a focus on prioritising a harm reduction approach which puts people's health first and aims to prevent the transmission of BBV (GCDP, 2021).

Decriminalisation of drug use and possession for personal use reduces the stigma and discrimination that hampers access to health care, harm reduction and legal services. In countries where drug use is decriminalised and comprehensive harm reduction is available, HIV prevalence and transmission tend to decrease sharply

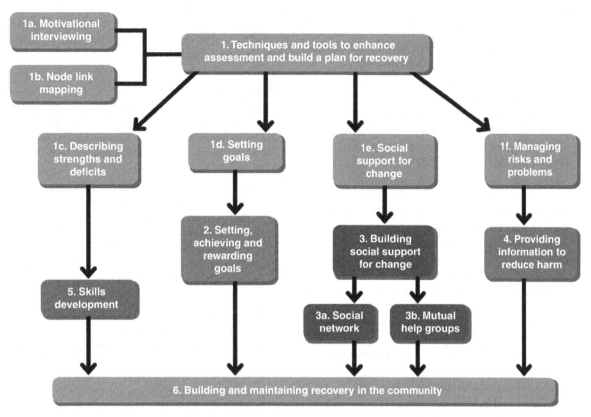

Figure 9.4 – International Treatment Effectiveness Project (ITEP) overview
Reproduced from Day (2013). Routes to Recovery via the Community – A Mapping User Manual

among people who use drugs, as do drug-related overdoses and deaths. The number of countries decriminalising drugs now stands at 25–30 countries; the Czech Republic, Netherlands and Switzerland have experienced these benefits (UNAIDS, 2020).

Other countries where drugs have been decriminalised are Antigua and Barbuda, Argentina, Armenia, Belize, Bolivia, Chile, Colombia, Costa Rica, Croatia, Czech Republic, Estonia, Germany, Italy, Jamaica, Mexico, Netherlands, Paraguay, Peru, Poland, Portugal, Russia, South Africa, Spain, Switzerland, Uruguay and the Virgin Islands (World Atlas, 2023).

The exact position on possession, production and supply varies among countries, with some retaining criminal charges if a person is found to possess large quantities (e.g. Czech Republic). In Germany, possession for personal use is decriminalised and people who want to deal in drugs can do so legally but only with a licence issued from the Federal Institute for Drugs and Medical Devices. Germany has also set up

drug-consumption rooms where people can use safely, access clean equipment and get immediate assistance in the event of an overdose.

International standards exist on drug use prevention that summarise the current available evidence, describe targeted interventions using a developmental approach in schools, with families and communities, and put forth policies, such as substitute prescribing, that result in positive outcomes via effective national systems (UNODC, 2020). There are also new global technologies, including 24/7 access to online, peer-led mutual aid meetings, which resulted from the global COVID lockdown, to reach those in need of help with their addiction (NA, 2021).

Safer injecting rooms exist in 12 countries; ending criminalisation, put people's health and safety first and reduce DRD (EMCDDA, 2018). Rooms exist in Germany (Townsend, 2019) and have recently been proposed to open in Glasgow, Scotland which is encouraging, but still remain prohibited in the rest of the UK.

Conclusion

PICU and other inpatient clinicians can make a significant, positive impact on illicit substance use and harm reduction. Key considerations include:

- Clinicians must recognise that every contact counts (PHE, 2018).
- Assessment should include capability of the person, the opportunities for success, motivation and willingness to abstain, and the person's behaviours (Michie et al., 2011).
- Engagement should involve a motivational interviewing style, exploring motivation, readiness and confidence to change and dealing with and acknowledging ambivalence (Prochaska and DiClemente, 1983; Norcross, 1992). Conceptualising where the individual is on the road to recovery can be helpful for both clinicians and clients. This may involve exploring barriers, perceived risks and benefits (Rosenstock, 1974), discussing previous attempts to stop/reduce use and providing positive feedback on any quit attempts to boost self-efficacy for future attempts (Bandura, 1997, 1998).
- Health inequalities should be considered (Dahlgren and Whitehead, 1991)
- Setting SMART goals (Specific, Measurable, Achievable, Realistic & with Timescales), such as progressing to the next stage of change.
- Always provide signposting to 24/7 mutual aid organisations and online resources and app technologies to provide maximum opportunities for behaviour change.

Sophisticated treatment provisions, such as OST and harm minimisation services, exist in the United Kingdom and elsewhere. However, significant international and UK policy reform may be indicated. This could include contentious issues such as detailed examination of criminalisation, reducing incarceration, protecting human rights, promoting public health and ensuring social justice, perhaps adopting a model of regulation based on risk assessment and harm minimisation (Transform, 2021b).

This approach would eliminate perceived barriers and threats to people changing addictive behaviours and, finally, in the authors' view, governments may need to recognise and accept the evidence emerging from around the globe for improving approaches to substance misuse. These may include difficult political conversations in many areas including safer-injecting /consumption rooms in all the United Kingdom and elsewhere to reduce DRDs to reduce the ever-increasing public health crisis of substance-related conditions and mortality rates.

References

Advisory Council on the Misuse of Drugs (2010) *Hidden Harm. Responding to the Needs of Children of Problem Drug Users.* https://assets.publishing.service.gov.uk/government/uploads/system/uploads/attachment_data/file/120620/hidden-harm-full.pdf.

Alcoholics Anonymous (AA) (2022) www.alcoholics-anonymous.org.uk/.

Anderson.PD and Bokor,G (2012) Forensic Aspects of Drug-Induced Violence. *Journal of Pharmacy Practice* **25** (1) 41–9. DOI: https://doi.org/10.1177/0897190011431150.

Apple Inc. (2021) SoberTool. Addiction Recovery. https://apps.apple.com/us/app/sobertool-addiction-recovery/id1078632750.

Bandura,A. (1997) *Self-Efficacy: The Exercise of Control.* New York: W.H. Freeman and Company.

Bandura,A (1998) Health Promotion from the Perspective of Social Cognitive Theory. *Psychology & Health.* **13** (4) 623–49. DOI: https://doi.org/10.1080/08870449808407422.

Bristol City Council (2020) Bristol Quality of Life Survey 2022/23. Bristol: Bristol City Council. www.bristol.gov.uk/files/documents/6332-quality-of-life-2022-23-final-report-with-appendix/file.

Burca,C, Miles,H and Vasquez,E (2013) Substance Use Amongst Mentally Disordered Offenders in Medium Security: Prevalence and Relationship to Offending Behaviour. *Journal of Forensic Practice* **15** (4) 259–68. DOI: https://doi.org/10.1108/JFP-08-2012-0010.

Centres for Disease Control. National Institute on Drug Abuse (2021) Overdose Death Rates. www.drugabuse.gov/drug-topics/trends-statistics/overdose-death-rates.

Cornford,C and Close,H (2016) The Physical Health of People Who Inject Drugs: Complexities, Challenges, and Continuity. *British Journal of General Practice* **66** (647) 286–7. DOI: https://10.3399/bjgp16X685333.

Dahlgren,G and Whitehead,M (1991) *Policies and Strategies to Promote Social Equity in Health.* Stockholm: Institute for Futures Studies.

Day,E (2013) *Routes to Recovery via the Community.* London: Public Health England.

Department of Health and Social Care (2017) *Clinical Guidelines on Drug Misuse and Dependence Update: UK Guidelines on Clinical Management.* London: Department of Health and Social Care. https://assets.publishing.service.gov.uk/government/uploads/system/uploads/attachment_data/file/673978/clinical_guidelines_2017.pdf.

Dyer,C (1996) Violence may be predicted amongst psychiatric inpatients. *British Medical Journal* **313**: 318.

European Monitoring Centre on Drugs and Drug Addiction (2018) Drug consumption Rooms: An Overview of Provision and Evidence. www.emcdda.europa.eu/topics/po ds/drug-consumption-rooms_en.

Fiorentini,A, Cantù,F, Crisanti,C, Cereda,G, Oldani,L, and Brambilla,P (2021) Substance-Induced Psychoses: An Updated Literature Review. *Front Psychiatry* **23** (1) 694863. DOI: https://10.3389/fpsyt.2021.694863.

FRANK (2021) Honest Information about Drugs. www.tal ktofrank.com/.

Gintalaite-Bieliauskiene,K, Dixon,R and Bennett,L (2020) A Retrospective Survey of Care Provided to Patients with Borderline Personality Disorder Admitted to a Female Psychiatric Intensive Care Unit. *Journal of Psychiatric Intensive Care* **16** (1) 35–42(8). DOI: https://doi.org/10.202 99/jpi.2020.002.

Global Commission on Drugs Policy (2021) The Five Pathways to Drug Policies That Work. www.globalcommis sionondrugs.org/the-five-pathways-to-drug-policies-that-work.

Ham,S, Kim,TK, Chung,S and Im,HI (2017) Drug Abuse and Psychosis: New Insights into Drug-Induced Psychosis. *Experimental Neurobiology* **26** (1) 11–24. DOI: https://10.5 607/en.2017.26.1.11.

Haslam,N (2012) Toilet Psychology. The British Psychological Society. www.bps.org.uk/volume-25/edition-6/toilet-psychology.

Health Education England (2018) Making Every Contact Count. www.hee.nhs.uk/our-work/population-health/mak ing-every-contact-count-mecc.

HM Government (1971) Misuse of Drugs Act. www.legisla tion.gov.uk/ukpga/1971/38/contents.

HM Government (2015). Human Medicines (Amendment) (No.3) Regulations 2015. www.legislation.gov.uk/uksi/201 5/1503/pdfs/uksiem_20151503_en.pdf#:~:text=3%29%20R EGULATIONS%202015%202015%20No.%201503%201.% 20This,of%20Her%20Majesty.%202.%20Purpose%20of%20 the%20instrument.

HM Inspectorate of Prisons (2015) *Changing Patterns of Substance Misuse in Adult Prisons and Service Responses.* London: Crown Copyright. www.justiceinspectorates.gov .uk/hmiprisons/wp-content/uploads/sites/4/2015/12/Substa nce-misuse-web-2015.pdf.

Howard,R, McCarthy,L, Huband,N and Duggan,C (2013) Re-Offending in Forensic Patients Released from Secure Care: The Role of Antisocial/Borderline Personality Disorder Co-morbidity, Substance Dependence and Severe Childhood Conduct Disorder. *Criminal Behaviour and Mental Health* **23** (3) 191–202. DOI: https://doi.org/10.100 2/cbm.1852.

Isaac,M, Isaac,M and Holloway,F (2005) Is Cannabis an Anti-psychotic? The Experience in Psychiatric Intensive Care. *Human Psychopharmacology* **20** (3) 207–10.

Joint United Nations Programme on HIV/AIDS (UNAIDS) (2020) Decriminalisation Works, but Too Few Countries are Taking the Bold Step. www.unaids.org/en/resources/pr esscentre/featurestories/2020/march/20200303_drugs.

Khan,H (2019) Exploring the Darkness: Self-Harm and Drug Use in Muslim Youth. Institute for Muslim Mental Health. https://muslimmentalhealth.com/exploring-the-da rkness-self-harm-and-drug-use-in-muslim-youth/.

Laidlaw,J, Pugh,D and Maplestone,H (2009) Section 136 and the Psychiatric Intensive Care Unit: Setting up a Health Based Place of Safety in Gloucestershire. *Journal of Psychiatric Intensive Care* **5** (2) 107–12. DOI: https://10.10 17/S1742646409990094.

Marmot,M (2010) *Fair Society, Healthy Lives: The Marmot Review.* Institute of Health Equality. www.instituteofheal thequity.org/resources-reports/fair-society-healthy-lives-th e-marmot-review.

Michie,S, van Stralen,MM and West,R (2011) The Behaviour Change Wheel: A New Method for Characterising and Designing Behaviour Change Interventions. *Implementation Science* **6** (42). DOI: https:// doi.org/10.1186/1748-5908-6-42.

Ministry of Justice and Public Health England (2017) *The Impact of Community-Based Drug and Alcohol Treatment on Re-offending.* https://assets.publishing.service.gov.uk/gov ernment/uploads/system/uploads/attachment_data/file/67 4858/PHE-MoJ-experimental-MoJ-publication-version. pdf.

Mitcheson,L, Maslin,J, Meynen,T, Morrison,T, Hill,R and Wanigaratne,S (2010) *Applied Cognitive and Behavioural Approaches to the Treatment of Addiction: A Practical Treatment Guide.* West Sussex: Wiley-Blackwell.

Moos,R (2007) Theory-Based Ingredients of Effective Treatments for Substance Use Disorders. *Drug and Alcohol Dependence* **88** (2–3) 109–21.

Narcotic Anonymous (NA) (2021) Meetings. https://vir tual-na.org/meetings/.

National Association of Psychiatric Intensive Care and Low Secure Units (NAPICU) (2014) *National Minimum Standards for Psychiatric Intensive Care in General Adult Services.* https://napicu.org.uk/wp-content/uploads/2014/ 12/NMS-2014-final.pdf.

National Association of Psychiatric Intensive Care and Low Secure Units (NAPICU) (2021) Unpublished data collected during benchmark for National Survey of PICU, Low Secure and Locked Rehabilitation.

National Health Service (NHS) (2021a) Drug Addiction: Getting Help. www.nhs.uk/live-well/healthy-body/drug-add iction-getting-help/.

National Health Service (NHS) (2021b) Quit Smoking. www.nhs.uk/better-health/quit-smoking/.

National Health Service (NHS) (2017) Ethnicity Facts and Figures. Illicit Drug Use. www.ethnicity-facts-figures.service.gov.uk/health/alcohol-smoking-and-drug-use/illicit-drug-use-among-adults/latest.

National Health Service (NHS) (2022) Ethnicity Facts and Figures. Detentions under the Mental Health Act. www.ethnicity-facts-figures.service.gov.uk/health/mental-health/detentions-under-the-mental-health-act/latest.

National Health Service (NHS) England (2021) Menu of Evidenced-Based Interventions and Approaches for Addressing and Reducing Health Inequalities. https://webarchive.nationalarchives.gov.uk/ukgwa/20211101142006/https://www.england.nhs.uk/ltphimenu/definitions-for-health-inequalities/.

National Institute for Health and Care Excellence (NICE) (2016) Coexisting Severe Mental Illness and Substance Misuse: Community and Healthcare Services. NICE Guideline [NG58]. www.nice.org.uk/guidance/ng58.

North West Surrey Mental Health Partnership NHS Trust (2008) Confidential Risk Screen. Risks Specific to Drug/Alcohol Use. Specialist Drug and Alcohol Services.

Nutt,D, Phillips,L, Balfour,D, Curran,VH, Dockrell,M Foulds,J, et al. (2016) E-Cigarettes Are Less Harmful than Smoking. *The Lancet* 387 (10024) 1160–2. DOI: https://doi.org/10.1016/S0140-6736(15)00253-6.

O'Driscoll,C, Larney,S, Indig,D and Basson,J (2012) The Impact of Personality Disorders, Substance Use and Other Mental Illness on Re-offending. *Journal of Forensic Psychiatry & Psychology* 23 (3) 382–91. DOI: https://doi.org/10.1080/14789949.2012.686623.

Office for National Statistics (2020a) Statistical Bulletin. Deaths Related to Drug-Poisoning in England and Wales: 2019 Registrations. Deaths related to drug poisoning in England and Wales from 1993 to 2019, by cause of death, sex, age and substances involved in the death. www.ons.gov.uk/peoplepopulationandcommunity/birthsdeathsandmarriages/deaths/bulletins/deathsrelatedtodrugpoisoninginenglandandwales/2019registrations.

Office for National Statistics (2020b) Drug Misuse in England and Wales; year ending March 2020. Data is from Crime Survey for England and Wales. www.ons.gov.uk/peoplepopulationandcommunity/healthandsocialcare/drugusealcoholandsmoking.

Office for National Statistics (2020c) *Statistical Bulletin. Deaths Related to Drug-Poisoning in England and Wales: 2019 Registrations.* Deaths related to drug poisoning in England and Wales from 1993 to 2019, by cause of death, sex, age and substances involved in the death. www.ons.gov.uk/peoplepopulationandcommunity/birthsdeathsandmarriages/deaths/bulletins/deathsrelatedtodrugpoisoninginenglandandwales/2019registrations.

Patton,R (2013) Identification and Management of Physical Health Problems Among an Injecting Drug Using Population. *Peer J Reprints.* DOI: https://doi.org/10.7287/peerj.preprints.108.

Pereira,SM and Clinton,C (2002) *Mental Health Policy Implementation Guide: National Minimum Standards for General Adult Services in Psychiatric Intensive Care Units (PICU) and Low Secure Environments.* London: Department of Health.

Pereira S, Reay,K, Bottell,J, Walker,LM, Dzikiti,C, Platt,C, et al. (2019) *University Student Mental Health Survey 2018: A Large Scale Study into the Prevalence of Student Mental Illness within UK Universities.* London: The Insight Network.

Pereira,S, Earley,N, Outar,L, Dimitrova,M, Walker,L, Dzikiti,C, et al. (2020) *University Student Mental Health Survey 2020: A Large Scale Study into the Prevalence of StudentMental Illness within UK Universities.* London: The Insight Network.

Pereira,SM, Walker,LM, Dye,S and Alhaj,H (2021) National Survey of Psychiatric Intensive Care, Low Secure and Locked Rehabilitation Services: NHS Patient Characteristics. *Journal of Psychiatric Intensive Care* 17 (2) 79–88. DOI: https://doi.org/10.20299/jpi.2021.004.

Petrovsky,N, Ettinger,U, Hill,A, Frenzel,L, Meyhofer,IM, Wagner,J, et al. (2014) Sleep Deprivation Disrupts Prepulse Inhibition and Induces Psychosis-Like Symptoms in Healthy Humans. *Journal of Neuroscience* 34 (27) 9134. DOI: https://doi.org/10.1523/JNEUROSCI.0904-14.2014.

Prochaska,J (2022) The Transtheoretical Model. An Integrative Model of Behaviour Change. www.prochange.com/transtheoretical-model-of-behavior-change.

Prochaska,JO and DiClemente,CC (1983) Stages and Processes of Self-Change of Smoking, Toward an Integrative Model of Change. *Journal of Consulting and Clinical Psychology* 51 (3) 390–5. DOI: https://psycnet.apa.org/doi/10.1037/0022-006X.51.3.390.

Prochaska,JO, DiClemente,CC and Norcross,JC (1992) In Search of How People Change: Applications to the Addictive Behaviors. *American Psychologist* 47 (9) 1102–14.

Public Health England (2014) Preventing Drug Related Death: Turning Evidence into Practice. www.gov.uk/government/publications/treating-substance-misuse-and-related-harm-turning-evidence-into-practice/preventing-drug-related-deaths-turning-evidence-into-practice.

Public Health England (2018) Making Every Contact Count. www.makingeverycontactcount.co.uk.

Rood,P, Haagsma,JM, Boersma,S, Tancica,A, Van Lieshout,E, Mulligan,T, et al. (2016) Psychoactive Substances (Drugs and Alcohol) use by Emergency Department Patients before Injury. *European Journal of Emergency Medicine* 23 (2) 147–54(8). DOI: https://doi.org/10.1097/MEJ.0000000000000186.

Rosenstock,IM (1974) The Health Belief Model and Preventive Health Behavior. *Health Education Monographs* **2** (4) 328–35.

Smith,J (2015) Paranoid schizophrenic who stabbed nurse to death so he wouldn't be sent to a no-smoking unit without Wi-Fi will never be released, judge tells him. Daily Mail. www.dailymail.co.uk/news/article-2903643/Paranoid-schizo phrenic-stabbed-nurse-death-wouldn-t-sent-no-smoking-u nit-without-wifi-never-released-judge-tells-him.html.

Medley,G, Lipari,RN and Bose,J (2016) *Sexual Orientation and Estimates of Adult Substance Use and Mental Health: Results from the 2015 National Survey on Drug Use and Health.* Rockville, MD: SAMHSA. www.samhsa.gov/data/sites/default/files/NSDUH-SexualOrientation-2015/NSD UH-SexualOrientation-2015/NSDUH-SexualOrientation-2015.htm

Strathdee,G, Manning,V, Best,DW, Keaney,F, Bhui,., Witton,J, et al. (2005) Dual Diagnosis in A Primary Care Group (PCG), (100,000 Population Locality): A Step-By-Step Epidemiological Needs Assessment and Design of a Training and Service Response Model. *Drugs* **12** (Supp 1) 119–23.

Tarter,R, Kirisci,L, Mezzich,A, Cornelius,J, Pajer,K, Vanyukov,M, et al. Neurobehavioral Disinhibition in Childhood Predicts Early Age at Onset of Substance Use Disorder. *American Journal of Psychiatry* 160 (6) 1078–85. DOI: https://doi.org/10.1176/appi.ajp.160.6.1078.

Townsend,M (2019) Safe Injecting Rooms are Key to Halting Risk in Drug Related Death – expert. The Guardian. www.theguardian.com/society/2019/aug/17/safe-injection-rooms-key-to-reducing-drug-deaths-home-office-opposition.

Transform Drug Policy Foundation (2021a) Drug Policy Fit for the 21st Century. 50 Years of the Misuse of Drugs Act. https://transformdrugs.org/mda-at–50.

Transform Drug Policy Foundation (2021b) Models of Regulation. Five Systems of Control. https://transform drugs.org/drug-policy/models-of-regulation.

Trevidi,C, Adnan,M, Shah,K, Manikkara,G, Mansuri,Z and Jain,S (2022) Psychiatric Disorders in Hospitalized Homeless Individuals: A Nationwide Study. Psychiatrist. com. www.psychiatrist.com/pcc/psychiatry/psychiatric-dis orders-hospitalized-homeless-individuals/.

UK Drug Policy Commission (2010) *Drugs & Diversity: Ethnic Minority Group. Learning from the Evidence. Policy Briefing Paper.* www.ukdpc.org.uk/wp-content/upl oads/Policy%20report%20-%20Drugs%20and%20diver sity_%20ethnic%20minority%20groups%20(policy%20bri efing).pdf.

United Nations Office on Drugs and Crime (2019) World Drug Report 2019. www.unodc.org/unodc/en/frontpage/2 019/June/world-drug-report-2019_-35-million-people-wor ldwide-suffer-from-drug-use-disorders-while-only-1-in-7-people-receive-treatment.html.

Weaver,T, Madden,P, Charles,V, Stimson,G, Renton,A, Tyrer,P, et al. (2003) Comorbidity of Substance Misuse and Mental Illness in Community Mental Health and Substance Misuse Services. *British Journal of Psychiatry* **183** (4) 304–13. DOI: 10.1192/bjp.183.4.304.

World Atlas (2023) Countries That Have Decriminalized Drugs. www.worldatlas.com/articles/countries-that-have-d ecriminalized-drugs.html.

Fire-Setting and Arson

Elliott Carthy, Bradley Hillier and Faisil Sethi

Introduction

There is an established association between fire-setting and mental disorder. However, the specific nature of this relationship has been complex and difficult to characterise, particularly for those within forensic and custodial settings. Compared to other areas of challenging behaviour, offending and mental health, there is very little research, despite many decades of evidence intimating a relationship. Following a rapid expansion of forensic psychiatric services in the United Kingdom during the 1980s to early 2000s, the non-forensic clinician may have not had as great an exposure to individuals in whom fire-setting is a prominent feature of presentation or history. However, as the expansion of the secure estate has plateaued, it is increasingly common for the non-forensic clinician to encounter fire-setting behaviour in patients either in their risk history or as part of the presentation leading to admission, or while an inpatient in non-secure services. Furthermore, this behaviour may or may not be a manifestation of an active mental disorder and may lead to legal proceedings through the criminal justice system coinciding with periods of assessment and treatment. It is therefore important that the needs of this group of patients, which may traditionally be more familiar to forensic clinicians, are borne in mind by all mental health professionals.

In this chapter, we define the terminological differences between the terms 'fire-setting', 'arson' and 'pyromania', including their place in current diagnostic manuals. We present an epidemiological perspective on fire-setting in those with mental disorder and describe classification systems and theories of fire-setting with prevailing conceptual models of fire-setting and mental disorder. We also discuss current approaches in the risk assessment of fire-setting and consider psychological and pharmacological interventions in fire-setting. Finally, we suggest a care pathway to guide clinical and risk assessment of

the patient with fire-setting as a feature of their behaviour or history.

Fire-Setting, Arson and Pyromania: Crime, Behaviour and Mental Disorder

Many professionals may understandably use the terms 'fire-setting', 'arson', and 'pyromania' interchangeably. However, these terms can have differing diagnostic, aetiological and legal implications (see Box 10.1, adapted from Dickens and Sugarman, 2011). Fire-setting is an act or a behaviour without inference of intent (indeed, fire-setting can be accidental), arson is a criminal offence and pyromania is a mental disorder. Since 1994, the UK Fire Rescue Service has classified fires at a high level into categories of primary, secondary, deliberate and accidental (see Box 10.2).

Within this chapter, we restrict our terminology as a default to 'fire-setting' and reserve the term 'arson' for a distinct sub-group of fire-setting that has attracted a conviction, or as is referred to in cited texts. The term pyromania was first coined by Marc in 1833 (Rix, 1994; Burton et al., 2012) and defined by Kraeplin as a type of impulsive insanity (Geller et al., 1986). Its classification as a diagnosis has varied over recent decades, with an arguable trend toward de-medicalisation and one of questionable relevance. It began as an obsessive-compulsive reaction in the first edition of the *Diagnostic and Statistical Manual of Mental Disorders* (*DSM*) before eventually being classified as an impulsive control disorder in the third edition (Johnson and Netherton, 2016). Today, pyromania continues to be defined as an impulse control disorder in the *International Classification of Diseases, 11th Edition* (ICD11) (World Health Organization, 2022) criteria. However, this does not fully align with the *DSM-5*, whereby pyromania has been reclassified from being a standalone disorder to being grouped as part of the

Box 10.1 Definitions

1. The Crime – Arson: The crime of arson is defined within Section 1 of the Criminal Damage Act 1971 c. 48. It relates to:
   (1) A person who without lawful excuse destroys or damages any property belonging to another intending to destroy or damage any such property or being reckless as to whether any such property would be destroyed or damaged shall be guilty of an offence.
   (2) A person who without lawful excuse destroys or damages any property, whether belonging to himself or another:
      (a) intending to destroy or damage any property or being reckless as to whether any property would be destroyed or damaged; and
      (b) intending by the destruction or damage to endanger the life of another or being reckless as to whether the life of another would be thereby endangered; shall be guilty of an offence.
   (3) An offence committed under this section by destroying or damaging property by fire shall be charged as arson. Thus 'arson' is the specific criminal act of destruction, comprising the specific criminal act of intention; an 'arsonist' has been convicted of the crime of arson.

2. **The Behavioural Phenotype – Fire-Setting**: A broad definition of fire-setting encompasses the behavioural phenotype consisting of deliberate setting of fires, which may or may not have been prosecuted for several reasons:

- Insufficiently severe to cause damage
- Fire not detected as deliberate
- Not possible to identify who has set the fire
- Insufficient evidence to secure a conviction
- Young age of the fire setter

3. **Pyromania**: According to the ICD11, pyromania (C670) is categorised as an impulse control disorder, also known as 'pathological fire-setting'.

- Pyromania is characterised by a recurrent failure to control strong impulses to set fires, resulting in multiple acts of, or attempts at, setting fire to property or other objects, in the absence of an apparent motive (e.g. monetary gain, revenge, sabotage, political statement, attracting attention or recognition).
- There is an increasing sense of tension or affective arousal prior to instances of fire setting, persistent fascination or preoccupation with fire and related stimuli (e.g. watching fires, building fires, fascination with firefighting equipment), and a sense of pleasure, excitement, relief or gratification during, and immediately after the act of setting the fire, witnessing its effects, or participating in its aftermath.
- The behaviour is not better explained by intellectual impairment, another mental and behavioural disorder, or substance intoxication.

NB: Pyromania in the DSM5 has been re-classified from being a distinct disorder in itself to being incorporated within the category of 'Impulse disorders not otherwise specified' (APA, 2013)

Box 10.2 Different Types of Fire

Primary fires are reportable fires in specific locations, including all fires in buildings, vehicles and outdoor structures, any fire involving casualties or rescues, or fires attended by five or more firefighting appliances. They are reported in detail.

Secondary fires are reportable fires constituting most outdoor fires not occurring in primary fire locations or meeting the criteria for primary fires; they are reported in less detail.

Accidental fires include those fires for which the cause is not known or is unspecified.

Deliberate fires include those fires for which deliberate ignition is merely suspected.

'impulse control disorders not otherwise specified' (American Psychiatric Association, 2013).

Ritchie and Huff (1999) found that only 0.1% of a sample of 283 individuals convicted of arson satisfied the diagnostic criteria for pyromania. This is a marked reduction from Lewis and Yarnell's (1951) seminal findings of 60% prevalence of pyromania among those convicted of arson. A 1967 study of 239 people convicted of arson found 23% to have underlying pyromania (Robbins and Robbins, 1967). Several other studies in the 1980s and 1990s found a prevalence of pyromania of less than 3.3% in those convicted of arson (Prins et al., 1985; Geller et al., 1986; Soltys, 1992; Lindberg et al., 2005). This highlights that the act of fire-setting can have different motivations and aetiological factors and should not be viewed as pathognomonic of an underlying mental disorder such as pyromania. While mental disorders more broadly are over-represented in those who have set fires, including those convicted of arson, the prevalence of pyromania is unknown and thus should be considered a rare disorder.

Epidemiology

The prevalence of fire-setting in the United Kingdom is difficult to estimate accurately. Triangulation of data from various sources, including fire service responses, criminal justice services and self-report research surveys and clinical studies provides a helpful proxy.

According to the Office for National Statistics (2023), the total number of fires attended by the Fire and Rescue Service in England decreased for about a decade from its peak in March 2004 (474,000 fires) to March 2013 (154,000 fires). Since then, the total number of fires has varied between approximately 150,000 to 183,000 up until March 2022. Furthermore, the number of fire-related fatalities in England has declined since the 1980s and the number of non-fatal causalities from fire setting has trended downward since the mid-1990s. The number of deliberate fires attended was more than 66,000 in the year ending September 2022, which has continued a downward trend since the peak of more than 320,000 deliberate fires attending in 2003–4. The total number of deliberate fires in healthcare settings fell in absolute numbers between 2001–2 and 2011–12, though the data since then remains unclear. These data may reasonably be expected to reflect, in part, patients whom we encounter in mental health services.

Fire-Setting in the General Population

The most comprehensive study of fire-setting outside of a forensic population can be found in the National Epidemiologic Study on Alcohol and Related Correlates (NESARC) from the United States (Blanco et al., 2010). More than 43,000 adults aged 18 years or older living in households were interviewed face-to-face by US Census workers between 2001 and 2002. Sociodemographic factors were collated as well as *DSM-IV* diagnoses using the Alcohol Use Disorder and Associated Disabilities Interview Schedule-DSM IV Version (AUDADIS-IV), a valid and reliable fully structured diagnostic interview designed for use by professional interviewers who are not clinicians. Diagnoses included in the AUDADIS-IV can be separated into three groups: substance use disorders (including any alcohol abuse/dependence, any drug abuse/dependence and any nicotine dependence); mood disorders (including major depressive disorder, dysthymia and bipolar disorder); and anxiety disorders (including panic disorder, social anxiety disorder, specific phobia and generalised anxiety disorder).

According to their results, the prevalence of lifetime fire-setting in the US population was 1.13 (95% CI [1.0, 1.3]). Fire-setting was strongly associated with deficits in impulse control, such as antisocial personality disorder (ASPD) (OR = 21.8; 95% CI [16.6, 28.5]), drug dependence (OR = 7.6; 95% CI [5.2, 10.9]), bipolar disorder (OR = 5.6; 95% CI [4.0, 7.9]) and pathological gambling (OR = 4.8; 95% CI [2.4, 9.5]). Associations between fire-setting and all antisocial behaviours were positive and significant. A lifetime history of fire-setting, even in the absence of ASPD diagnosis, was strongly associated with substantial rates of mental illness, history of antisocial behaviour, family history of other antisocial behaviours, decreased functioning and higher rates of treatment seeking. The researchers concluded that fire-setting may be best understood as a broader impulse control syndrome and part of the externalising spectrum of disorders.

In summary, NESARC demonstrated that a third of fire-setters had a diagnosable mental disorder and more than half were diagnosed with a psychiatric disorder and had a psychological motive during the time of reporting. Although there may be cultural and societal differences in translating this research to the UK population, the study by Blanco et al. (2010) is useful at providing an evidence base for the prevalence of fire-setting behaviour and its association with mental disorders in the general population outside of forensic and custodial settings.

Data on Criminal Justice System and Mentally Disordered Offenders

Most epidemiological data relating to mental disorders and fire-setting have traditionally been sourced from forensic populations, including those convicted of arson who are then referred for psychiatric assessment or populations within secure mental health settings.

It is less common for charges to lead to a successful conviction in cases of arson compared to other types of offending. Arson convictions are estimated to be between 7% and 28%. In comparison, 44% of convictions are for offences against the person, 86% are for homicides and 94% for drug offences (Averill, 2011). There have been several reasons postulated for this attrition, including an absence of witnesses and the deliberate classification made by the Fire and Rescue Service which prompts a criminal investigation that can be based on suspicion alone. It is therefore possible that the official statistics about the prevalence and impact of arson to individuals and society is an underestimation based on the manner in which the offence is dealt with by the criminal justice system (see Kelly et al., 2005 for more information).

There are several points in legal proceedings where an individual may require assessment and treatment for a mental disorder when arrested on suspicion of arson. Individuals may be diverted to non-secure services upon arrest but before being charged. They may require assessment and treatment in hospital either as unsentenced or sentenced prisoners. They may also be evaluated by independent expert witnesses for consideration of a hospital disposal. According to Tyler and Gannon (2012), 42 of the 1,407 adult arson offenders (3%) brought before the courts in England and Wales in 2009 received combined hospital orders and custodial sentence. The role of the psychiatric expert witness in arson proceedings has been well described elsewhere (Averill, 2011; Burton et al., 2012).

While there is a body of evidence to suggest that mental disorders are over-represented in those who have set fires, there does not appear to be any evidence to suggest that major mental illness directly *causes* fire-setting. Nonetheless, it is estimated that approximately one in 10 patients admitted to forensic psychiatry services has a history of fire setting (Repo et al., 1997; Coid et al., 2001; Fazel and Grann, 2002; Hollin et al., 2013).

In relation to quantifying the increased risk of mental disorder within a forensic psychiatric population convicted of arson, Anwar et al. (2011) carried out a case–control study using data from Swedish national registers for convictions and hospital discharge diagnoses. They calculated odds ratios for men and women with arson convictions having a schizophrenia diagnosis as 22.6 and 38.7, respectively, and for any other psychosis as 17.4 and 30.8, respectively, noting that this association is much higher than for most other types of violent offending. Arguably, given the prominence of psychotic illness in the inpatient environment, this study (in conjunction with Blanco et al., 2010) may provide one of the most helpful indicators of the attention that should be given to fire-setting screening, risk assessment and management in this group. Ritchie and Huff (1999) also found in a sample of 283 cases of arsonists in the United States, that 90% had recorded mental health histories, 36% satisfied diagnostic criteria for major mental illness such as schizophrenia or bipolar disorder, and 64% were abusing drugs or alcohol at the time of the index offence.

Rice and Harris (1991) examined the characteristics of 243 males convicted of arson within a maximum-security psychiatric facility in Canada. While only one subject had a diagnosis of pyromania, approximately half had a personality disorder and one-third had schizophrenia. Substance use disorders are also more common in both men and women convicted of arson (Enayati et al., 2008).

The prevalence of mental disorders in those convicted of arson has been shown to be greater than those convicted of homicide (Räsänen et al., 1995a, Räsänen et al., 1995b). There are also more frequent histories of suicide attempts (Burton et al., 2012). Yesavage (1983) found that 54% of those convicted of arson had a diagnosable mental illness, and that those who were also mentally ill set a greater number of total fires than those without a mental illness. Furthermore, it has been estimated that the prevalence of schizophrenia is anywhere from 4- to 20-fold greater in those convicted of arson compared to the general population (Yesavage et al., 1983, Räsänen et al., 1995b; Anwar et al., 2011).

Children and Fire-Setting

Although beyond the scope of this chapter, which focuses primarily on adult fire-setting behaviour, there is a significant body of research that investigates juvenile fire-setting, which may be encountered in the history of an adult admitted to the psychiatric intensive care unit (PICU). Counter-intuitively, epidemiological surveys among children and adolescents across different countries have consistently suggested that 'fire-interest' is common and may be the norm, but that this may decline with age (MacKay et al., 2009). However, Chen et al. (2003) identified several associations in adolescents which may suggest risk of a more deviant pattern of behaviour. These are detailed in Box 10.3.

Fire-setting in children is commonly found in children and adolescents with attention deficit hyperactivity disorder (ADHD) and conduct disorder as well as the phenomenon of curiosity fire setting (Johnson and Netherton, 2016). While there are case reports of those diagnosed with pyromania (Ceylan et al., 2011), the evidence base for this diagnosis in children and young people is extremely limited.

Classification and Explanatory Theories of Fire-Setting
Motive-Based Classifications
Lewis and Yarnell (1951) provided one of the earliest classification systems for fire-setters, including those who had set fires unintentionally through delusions,

for erotic pleasure and to acquire revenge. While distinguishing between these groups lacked validity and reliability, the researchers did provide a foundation for further study of motive-based classifications, which, in turn, aims to better understand why people intentionally start fires. There have been many such theories in the decades since. However, some have been criticised for conflating motive with individual characteristics, particularly among those with a possible mental disorder. Furthermore, many of the identified motives may not be mutually exclusive and may overlap with one another, which, combined with their subjectivity, can create inconsistencies and confusion in these classification systems (Geller, 1992; Gannon and Pina, 2010; Tyler and Gannon, 2021). Without clear and discrete categories, the explanatory value in these typologies has also been brought into question.

Canter and Fritzon (1998) developed a model that was notable for its theoretically informed development and incorporation of integrated action systems theory (Tyler and Gannon, 2021), which satisfies multiple criteria for evaluation of competing theories, including empirical adequacy, external consistency, unifying power, fertility and explanatory depth (Fritzon, 2011). Through their study of 175 arson cases dealt with by the courts, Canter and Fritzon (1998) identified two underlying axes upon which the motivation of fire-setting behaviour could be understood. The first axis related to the *target*, either people or objects, and the second related to the *purpose*, either instrumental (e.g. associated with theft or concealment of crime) or expressive in itself. Their classification subsequently proposed four typologies, as shown in Box 10.4.

Box 10.3 Associated Factors Indicating Risk of Persistent Fire-Setting Behaviour in Teenagers

- Male
- Young age
- Dysfunctional family background
- Stressful life events
- Low socio-economic status
- Academic or vocational difficulties

Box 10.4 Two-Axis Theory

		Object	
		Person	Object
Purpose	Instrumental	• Often arises from dispute • Often prior threats • Associated with discernible trigger • Serves a specific purpose, usually revenge • Fire set in attempt to restore emotional balance	• Associated with opportunistic fire-setting • Often to achieve criminal ends
	Expressive	• May be coupled with need for attention and deliberate endangerment of life	• Often involving serial offences • Public buildings, in particular

Source: Canter and Fritzon (1998)

Box 10.5 Harris and Rice Classification

- Psychotics: 33% with few previous incidents of fire setting
- Unassertives: 28% with little history of aggression and offending but considered to have revenge motivations
- Multi-fire-setters: 23% with disturbed childhoods who are younger with criminal versatility and high recidivism risk
- Criminals: 16% with disturbed backgrounds, likely to have personality disorder diagnosis, who are assertive and have a high risk of recidivism, including for new offences

Box 10.6 Jackson's Functional Analysis

1. Antecedents
   - Psychosocial disadvantage (mental illness, intellectual disability, social inadequacy)
   - Dissatisfaction with life and the self (low self-esteem, depression)
   - Social ineffectiveness (isolation, poor problem solving)
   - Specific stimuli (such as previous expose to fire)
   - Triggers (over which individual may be powerless)
2. Behaviour – Fire-setting behaviour
3. Consequences
   - Positive reinforcers (attention on the arsonist, financial or political gain)
   - Negative reinforcers (protection from stressors)
4. Factors indicating pathological fire-setting
   - Recidivism
   - Fire setting to property rather than person
   - Acting alone or repeatedly with an identified accomplice
   - Evidence of personality, psychiatric or emotional problems
   - Absence of financial or political gain

Source: Jackson et al. (1987)

Harris and Rice (1996) developed the first statistically derived typology by investigating a population of 243 male mentally disordered offenders with fire-setting history admitted to a high-security psychiatric setting. They recorded several variables as well as subsequent recidivism for fire-setting or other offences. Their analysis suggested four subtypes of offender, as shown in Box 10.5. Despite this nomenclature offering an alluring invitation to classify the motivation in simplistic terms, Gannon and Pina (2010) convincingly argued that this provides a two-dimensional picture and does not incorporate other elements, including, for example, personality factors and characteristics of the fires set, to provide unifying explanatory power.

A full history of typological classifications of fire-setting is provided by Dickens and Sugarman (2011) and Tyler and Gannon (2021) for the interested reader.

Explanatory Models

Dynamic Pathways – Dynamic pathway models are data-driven models to generate theory based on qualitative research focused on descriptive accounts of context, thoughts and feelings leading up to the behaviour (Tyler and Gannon, 2021). In turn, common subtypes or pathways to offending can be identified based on overlapping features. The first such pathway was developed by Tyler et al. (2013) who identified three common pathways to offending based on fire-related factors in childhood: the onset of a mental disorder, the level of planning of the fire and whether the individual stayed to watch the fire. These pathways have subsequently been validating in a prison cohort of people with a diagnosed mental disorder (Tyler and Gannon, 2017). While dynamic pathways provide detailed descriptions of how fire-

setting may occur, they are limited to single incidents and tend to be based on small sample sizes (Tyler and Gannon, 2021).

Functional Analysis: The Only Viable Option Theory – In this model, the 'Antecedent, Behaviour, Consequence' (ABC) analysis is applied to recidivistic arson. When antecedents and consequences of arson are such that certain criteria are met, then the behaviour will manifest as 'the only viable option' to resolve the situation, viewing it as an adaptive mechanism. Further, Jackson et al. (1987) described criteria describing a situation where arson has become pathological. Box 10.6 details the antecedents and consequences identified as well as the factors suggesting pathological fire-setting. Gannon and Pina (2010) again noted that although the theory is based in social learning theory, there is little empirical evidence to support it, and it lacks explanatory depth.

Box 10.7 Action System Model as Applied to Fire-Setting and Arson

Source of Action	Effect of Action	Mode	Characteristics
Internal	Internal	*Integrative*	e.g. internal distress resulting in fire-setting, self-directed, within own home with suicidal features; often remains at scene
Internal	External	*Expressive*	e.g. exercising power on the external environment, potentially associated with emotional acting out, vicarious attention, remains at scene, often serial offender
External	Internal	*Conservative*	e.g. acts that may arise from external events provoking desire for revenge, remove cause of internal distress, to redress emotional well-being, gain emotional relief, may have witness who may be the main source of distress
External	External	*Adaptive*	e.g. responding to external events and making adjustments to the environment, probably opportunistic, aim to gain or vandalise, cover up another crime

Source: Fritzon (2011)

Dynamic Behaviour Theory – Fineman's (1995) model develops Jackson et al.'s (1987) model of behavioural analysis to include a number of environmental contingencies, including characteristics of the fire, cognitive factors such as cognitive distortions and feelings before, during and after the fire, as well as triggering events. The model describes a sequence of events leading to the fire with its consequences in several domains.

The Action Systems Model – Fritzon (2011) applied systems theory to arson and created the 'Action Systems Model', which differentiates behaviour according to its origin (i.e. internal or external) and its desired locus of effect (internal or external). This model describes and develops the application of the four modes of functioning (expressive, conservative, integrative and adaptive) based on research in multiple studies (Almond et al., 2005). Box 10.7 describes these modes of functioning.

Miller and Fritzon (2007) also demonstrated concordance between the mode of functioning in relation to fire-setting behaviour and self-harming behaviour. Comparison has also been made with the more established and evidenced model for sexual offending (Fritzon, 2011). Overall, the Action Systems Model is evolving and gradually developing an evidence base to support a unifying explanatory theory for fire-setting behaviour that has the potential to incorporate findings from other models and typologies. In so doing, it also forms a basis on which to begin to assess risk and to identify and direct potential treatment modalities. We would encourage any clinician who encounters fire-setting behaviour and wishes to gain a greater understanding of the individual motivation to familiarise themselves with this model.

Multi-Trajectory Theory of Adult Fire-Setting (M-TTAF) – This theory by Gannon et al. extended the work of Fineman into a unified, two-tiered, multifactor theory (Gannon et al., 2012). This included an aetiological framework that considered how developmental factors can lead to psychological vulnerabilities that predispose an individual to fire-setting. It also considers the triggers and moderating factors and how these interact with psychological vulnerabilities to become critical risk factors that ultimately increase the risk of fire-setting. The M-TTAF then goes on to describe five subtypes or trajectories towards fire-setting based on the aforementioned characteristics: antisocial, grievance, fire interest, emotionally expressive/need for recognition and multifaceted. We direct readers to the work of Gannon et al. (2012) and Tyler and Gannon (2021) for further reading on this theory.

Clinical and Risk Assessment of Fire-Setting

The clinical and risk assessment of fire-setters is not straightforward due to a variety of reasons, not least of which is a lack of research and the absence of

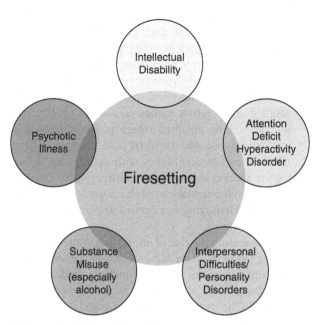

Figure 10.1 Mental health diagnoses associated with fire-setting behaviour

a structured, validated arson-specific risk assessment tool.

Diagnostic Considerations

As detailed earlier in this chapter, there is an emerging picture of fire-setting behaviour being associated with poor impulse control. Many mental disorders are associated with poor impulse control as a core feature of their psychopathology and behavioural disturbance. Psychosis, intellectual disability, autistic spectrum disorders, substance misuse disorder (especially alcohol) and personality disorders have been noted as having a stronger association with fire-setting within forensic populations (Figure 10.1). Specialist assessment of intellectual functioning or screening for autistic spectrum disorder may be less common in the general inpatient setting but should be borne in mind along the assessment pathway in those with fire-setting behaviours. There has been some association identified between fire-setting and ADHD in childhood (Johnson and Netherton, 2016). Although there is no data currently available for adults, given the association with impulsivity that is emerging in other avenues of fire-setting research, it may reasonably be speculated that adult ADHD may be similarly associated with this type of offending, as is becoming clear in other types of offending behaviour (Young and Thome, 2011).

Substance Misuse – Any individual who demonstrates fire-setting behaviour or risk factors should be carefully assessed for concomitant substance misuse problems. In particular, alcohol misuse has been found to have a high prevalence in several studies (Lindberg et al., 2005, Blanco et al., 2010) as well as in female fire-setters (Linaker, 2000). Consideration should be given to referring to a dual-diagnosis service or substance misuse liaison where available.

Personality Assessment – Concomitant assessment of personality using a semi-structured tool such as the International Personality Disorder Examination (IPDE) (Loranger et al., 1994) may provide helpful information, allowing further insight into the relational aspects of fire-setting behaviour in an individual in the context of their personality structure; for example, anti-social personality traits or disorder are known to be associated with increased risk of fire-setting (Blanco et al., 2010), and characteristics of self-harm behaviour in women with personality disorder may indicate the action systems type which may be manifest in a potential fire-setter. The importance of interpersonal inadequacy in the fire-setting population is well established (Lewis and Yarnell, 1951, Rix, 1994), and there has been considerable discussion of the role of individuals who are unable to effect change through socially acceptable means, using fire as a vehicle for this (Stewart, 1993).

Other Areas – Impulsivity, anger, psychopathy and cognitive distortions are areas which are considered by expert consensus to be relevant in the risk assessment of fire-setting, although as yet there remains little robust evidence (Doley and Watt, 2011). Impulsivity plays a role in various theories of antisocial behaviour but has not been specifically characterised in relation to fire-setting. In contrast, anger has been identified as a precursor to fire-setting, potentially as a disinhibiting factor as in its association with violence. Cognitive distortions describing offender relationships with antisocial attitudes and justifications for offending behaviour are well characterised in a diverse range of offending, particularly sexual offending, and have been postulated to impact on the employment of empathy. Psychopathy, however, reflecting amongst other things a stable combination of persistent irresponsible behaviour, lack of empathy and deceitful behaviour, has not shown significant differences between arsonists and non-arsonists in a high-secure population (Labree et al., 2010) nor have psychopathic traits been associated with fire-setting recidivism (Thomson et al., 2015).

Assessment of Risk of Fire-Setting in Mental Disorder

It may not be immediately obvious, or even known, if there is a history of fire-setting behaviour. It is clearly important in such patients to establish the presence or absence of a history from the outset. In this case, an initial approach may simply involve asking one or two questions to make an assessment. Questions investigating whether they have or have ever had any thoughts or history of using fire to harm themselves or others, or whether they have ever engaged in any fire-play as a teenager or adult, may be a starting point. Positive answers to questioning of this nature should prompt more in-depth inquiry as to the specific circumstances, motivations, emotions, number of incidents, consequences, criminal justice involvement and other factors previously described in obtaining a clear picture of the behaviour. If concerns are raised, these should be further investigated, as we discuss later in the chapter.

Some patients may present with an already known history of fire-setting behaviour or arson convictions. Such patients should immediately prompt a detailed past and recent history and mental state examination characterising the fire-setting behaviour. Similarly,

any known history of fire interest in the past, either in the community or during previous admissions, threats or behaviour forming part of the circumstances of the current admission, nursing staff noting some concerning behaviour relating to lighters or threats to burn others whilst on the ward indicates detailed investigation. Collateral sources of information should be obtained where possible, including from the police and criminal justice system where relevant, and in accordance with appropriate information sharing arrangements. History of fire interest from a developmental and adult perspective should be obtained, identifying any deviant or pathological patterns of concern.

In assessing the risk of fire-setting in the inpatient setting (and indeed other forms of violence), validated structured assessment tools should be used. At present, there is no specific tool to assess risk of fire-setting in the mentally disordered population. In the absence of such a tool, the inpatient clinician is directed to the HCR-20 (Guy et al., 2013), which is validated as a structured risk assessment tool in mentally disordered populations. The main clinical utility of this tool is to assist in forming an overall impression of risk in the criteria of 'low', 'moderate' and 'high' based on characterising static and dynamic risk factors (scored as absent, unknown, partially/possibly present or definitely present), allowing scenario planning to anticipate situations where risk may be increased and to identify strategies to reduce the risk. Clinicians should consider applying the concepts described in Box 10.7 when populating the risk assessment to allow identification and formulation of the patient's fire-setting behaviour in the context of the action systems framework. It is recommended that such an assessment be carried out in a multidisciplinary fashion by staff who have received appropriate training. There may be benefit in also obtaining a forensic psychiatric opinion for a variety of reasons, including to support the risk assessment, to provide a specialist opinion regarding care pathway and to advise on any outstanding medicolegal issues, for example.

There are several useful tools that may be employed for characterising a variety of factors relating to fire interests and fire attitudes in a patient. These are the Fire Interest Rating Scale (FIRS) and the Firesetting Assessment Schedule (FAS). The FIRS provides 14 descriptions of fire-related situations and the subject self-rates on a seven-point Likert scale how the scenario makes them feel, ranging from 'most upsetting' to 'very exciting'. The FAS provides 32 statements, 16 that relate to cognitions and feelings prior to a fire and 16 that relate to feelings post fire, that the person rates as 'never', 'sometimes', or 'usually'. These have also been used for individuals with an intellectual disability (Murphy and Clare, 1996). The Fire Attitude Scale is a 20-item task that examines the respondent's attitudes to fire in different contexts to provide an overall attitude score, whereby higher scores indicate more problematic attitudes towards fire-setting (Muckley, 1997).

Ó Ciardha et al. (2015a, 2015b) have since developed the Four Factor Fire Scales focusing on the concepts of identification with fire, serious fire interest, poor fire safety and fire-setting as normal. These scales have proven to be more effective than the aforementioned scoring systems in adequately discriminating between fire-setting and non-fire-setting individuals.

It also remains unclear as to what proportion of individuals will reoffend through fire-setting. A recent meta-analysis investigating this found that 57%–66% of fire-setters would reoffend in some way, with 20% engaging in deliberate fire-setting. The odds of future fire-setting were fivefold greater for those with a known history of fire-setting compared with other offenders (Sambrooks et al., 2021). However, there was significant variability and heterogeneity between samples, follow-up periods and definitions of reoffending, indicative of the urgent need for more research in this area.

Reporting of Threats or Fires

From a practical perspective, it is the authors' view that any incidents such as threats made by a patient to harm an individual or organisation through the use of fire or actual setting of fires on a ward should be taken extremely seriously and prompt a report to the police, who can take forward any criminal investigation as appropriate. As described earlier, the setting of fires in hospitals is not unknown, and attendance at psychiatric hospitals by the Fire Service as compared to general hospitals (one in three callouts to hospital) is disproportionately represented in terms of the number of beds (20% of all National Health Service [NHS] beds). There have also been a number of major fires in recent years at NHS and private hospitals which could have resulted in (although fortunately did not) loss of life (Grice, 2011).

Risk Management Strategies in Inpatient Settings

The risk management of those who set fires when presenting to an inpatient setting will, in many respects, be guided by the risk assessment and the types of concurrent risk behaviours with which the individual is presenting. Active mental disorder and associated behavioural disturbance should be managed on a case-by-case basis using established inpatient risk management and treatment modalities. Without providing an exhaustive list, these will include pharmacological treatment of any active mental disorder and behavioural disturbance, supportive nursing care, with consideration of low-stimulus environment, or extra-care areas (ECAs) where available. If behavioural disturbance is not responsive to de-escalation, then consideration should be given to the need for additional tranquilisation, including intramuscular medication and supervised confinement. However, the important principle to bear in mind is that the risk of fire-setting is elevated in such individuals, particularly in the context where impulsivity may be enhanced, such as following an

---

Box 10.8 Suggested Practical Risk Management Strategies Specific to Fire-Setting

- Ensure that there are clear procedures and rules regarding fire-setting threats and behaviours, and that boundaries are known to patients and are adhered to.
- Ensure fire detection and safety equipment and fire safety procedures are known to staff.
- Take any threats to make a fire seriously and consider this an opportunity to engage with a patient to obtain further information to inform the risk assessment.
- Pay close attention to the circulation of lighters or matches on the ward (count required), particularly at smoking times. Consider enhanced staff presence at these times.
- Be aware of accelerants being obtained or secreted (e.g. wax crayons, soap bars, tissue paper) and whether these are present on the ward.
- Consider whether 1:1 observations are appropriate if risk is escalating.
- Consider whether the physical, procedural and relational security of the ward is sufficient to manage the risk.

argument with staff or another patient, in the context of active psychosis or threats of self-harm. Specific risk management strategies can be used to reduce the risk of a fire occurring; many of these are common sense, and we outline some suggestions in Box 10.8.

The Treatment of Fire-Setters

At a fundamental level, given that fire-setting is not associated with a specific disorder, assessment and treatment of any underlying disorder should be the main thrust for patients presenting in an inpatient setting. Clearly, this will be dependent on the nature of the diagnosis reached in the first instance and the concomitant gathering of information obtained throughout the admission, including behaviour related to observed fire-setting. However, in terms of specific specialised fire-setting therapy, there is very little evidence-based intervention to offer beyond an educational approach.

Education

In the inpatient setting, there may be an opportunity to provide basic education concerning fire risk and enable the acquisition of fire safety skills. Although this may not be immediately feasible in the inpatient setting, it should be flagged and signposted along the care pathway for further development. Even a brief home visit by a firefighter may be of benefit. Evidence for the efficacy of this has come from juvenile populations (Hollin, 2011).

Group Work

There have been several statistically low-powered studies which have attempted to evaluate specific group therapy with mentally disordered offenders who set fires with evaluation using the FAS and FIRS. There is very little robust data to demonstrate efficacy, although the targets for development through this work include developing coping skills and self-esteem, increasing understanding of risks and developing personalised relapse prevention plans along a cognitive behavioural model.

Gannon et al. (2015) conducted a non-randomised trial of 54 male prisoners who had deliberately set fires and were enrolled in a standardised cognitive behavioural therapy group to specifically target this behaviour. This was shown to improve measures of problematic fire interest and associations with fire at three-month follow-up as measured through the Fire Factor Scale (Ó Ciardha et al., 2015a). While robust long-term outcome data remains to be seen, such specialist treatments may be of benefit to those with the most serious fire-setting behaviour.

Pharmacotherapy

The use of pharmacotherapy in treating fire-setting behaviour is extremely poorly understood. To our knowledge, there have been no clinical trials or other studies to evaluate the benefit (or harm) of specific pharmacological agents. Parks et al. (2005) reported a case study of pyromania in a homeless person responding to treatment with olanzapine; and given the emerging picture of impulse control being an important factor, medications that are known to have this effect in other forms of behaviour may be of benefit (Pallanti et al., 2002). Further research is urgently needed in this area.

Care Pathway Considerations

The care pathway for fire-setters in the inpatient (non-forensic) setting will depend upon several factors including, for example, the presence of active mental disorder, response to treatment with medication of underlying mental disorder, comorbidity of mental disorder or active substance misuse and severity of behavioural disturbance. The care pathway should be additionally informed from the structured risk assessment and assessment of personality.

Figure 10.2 shows a proposed process to guide the assessment of individuals admitted to hospital with an identified or known risk of fire-setting or arson. Owing to the absence of a clinically validated tool to assess arson risk, this is subject to individual clinical experience with working with this patient group and using clinical judgement incorporating the information obtained through assessment. Specialist support and assessment from a forensic psychiatrist should be considered at an early stage, and ongoing liaison maintained throughout the assessment and treatment, particularly where there are changes or escalation in presentation with relation to fire-setting behaviour. This may include threats made, actual fires set or the bringing of criminal charges.

Consideration of whether the level of security is appropriate should remain under constant review. The availability of appropriate treatment from a psychological perspective may not be available in the non-forensic setting, and this should be incorporated into care pathway decisions, again in consultation with forensic psychiatric services where such treatment is available. The involvement of the patient

Suggested Assessment and Care Pathway for Fire Setting in Inpatient Settings

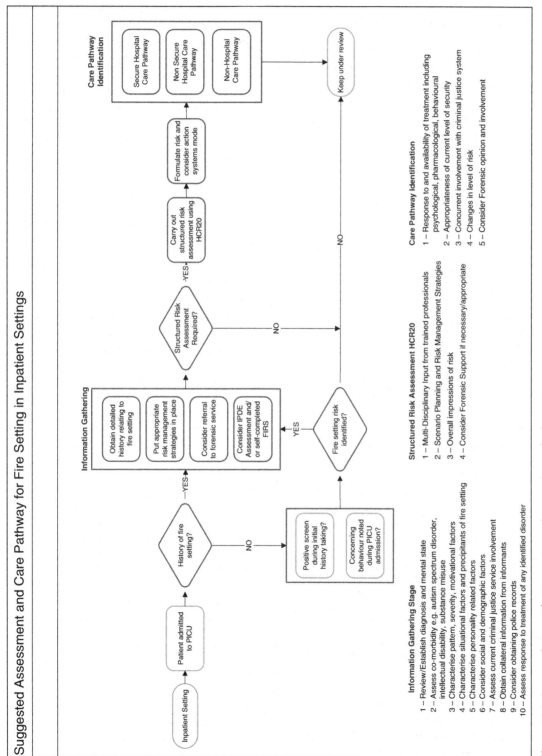

Figure 10.2 Suggested process for assessment and care pathways for fire-setting in inpatient units

with criminal justice or probation services may also be relevant, and this may be a care pathway through which access to treatment may be achieved, whether in a hospital, custodial or community setting, again informed by the risk assessment and broader clinical presentation.

Conclusion

In this chapter, we provided an overview of some of the core knowledge and clinical aspects which we consider to be of importance in the clinical and risk assessment of patients who present with fire-setting behaviour or histories. Key points for the busy clinician to use should they encounter fire-setting behaviour in their patient group include:

- Fire-setting behaviour in mental health populations is more common than in the general population, although a robust evidence base to quantify specific associations is not yet developed. It is likely that the inpatient clinician will encounter patients with fire-setting behaviour with some frequency.
- There is emerging evidence to suggest that poor impulse control may be associated with fire-setting behaviour in relation to mental disorder and mental illness. In forensic populations, there are associations between fire-setting and psychosis, autistic spectrum disorder, intellectual disability, substance misuse and interpersonal inadequacy.
- An emerging explanatory theory uses systems theory as applied to fire-setting to describe the source and effect of the behaviour.
- The risk of fire-setting should be taken seriously by any clinician. It is important to screen and, if identified, investigate in detail where evidence of historic or recent fire-setting behaviour or arson are found.
- Since there are no structured risk assessment tools currently available specifically for fire-setting, the use of the HCR-20 is recommended, with forensic input if considered appropriate. Even when fire-setting behaviour is not identified, this should be kept under review owing to the associations with mental disorder.
- Clinicians encountering fire-setting behaviour in patients should combine careful clinical diagnosis, response to treatment and risk assessment in the identification of an appropriate care pathway, and liaison with forensic services should occur where

more specialised treatment may be available. This may include greater therapeutic physical, procedural and relational security. We propose a care pathway to guide clinicians through this process.

- There is limited information on the effectiveness of psychological treatment interventions, which include cognitive behavioural therapy and educational individual and group work.
- The ground is fertile for clinicians to contribute to the evidence of fire-setting in the context of mental health in terms of epidemiology, diagnostic associations, response to pharmacological treatments and formulation of care pathways.

*This chapter originally appeared as a paper in the *Journal of Psychiatric Intensive Care* (Hillier et al., 2015). It has been updated and adapted for publication in this book.

References

Almond,L, Duggan,L, Shine,J and Canter,D (2005) Test of the Arson Action System Model in an Incarcerated Population. *Psychology, Crime & Law* 11 (1) 1–15.

American Psychiatric Association (APA) (2013) *Diagnostic and Statistical Manual of Mental Disorders, Fifth Edition*. Washington, DC: American Psychiatric Association.

Anwar,S, Långström,N, Grann,M and Fazel,S (2011) Is Arson the Crime Most Strongly Associated with Psychosis? – A National Case-Control Study of Arson Risk in Schizophrenia and Other Psychoses. *Schizophrenia Bulletin* 37 (3) 580–6.

Averill,S (2011) Legal Perspectives on Arson. In Dickens,G, Sugarman,P and Gannon,T (eds.), *Firesetting and Mental Health*. London: RCPsych Publications.

Blanco,C. Alegría,AA, Petry,NM, Grant,JE, Simpson,HB, Liu,SM, et al. (2010) Prevalence and Correlates of Fire-Setting in the United States: Results from the National Epidemiologic Survey on Alcohol and Related Conditions (NESARC). *Journal of Clinical Psychiatry* 71 (9) 1218–25.

Burton,PR, Mcniel,DE and Binder,RL (2012) Firesetting, Arson, Pyromania, and the Forensic Mental Health Expert. *Journal of the American Academy of Psychiatry and the Law* 40 (3) 355–65.

Canter,D and Fritzon,K (1998) Differentiating Arsonists: A Model of Firesetting Actions and Characteristics. *Legal and Criminological Psychology* 3 (1) 73–96.

Ceylan,MF, Durukan,I, Türkbay,T, Akca,OF and Kara,K (2011) Pyromania Associated with Escitalopram in a Child. *Journal of Child and Adolescent Psychopharmacology* 21 (4) 381–2.

Chen,YH, Arria,AM and Anthony,JC (2003) Firesetting in Adolescence and Being Aggressive, Shy, and Rejected by Peers: New Epidemiologic Evidence from a National Sample Survey. *Journal of the American Academy of Psychiatry and the Law* 3 (1) 44–52.

Coid,J, Kahatan,N, Gault,S, Cook,A and Jarman,B (2001) Medium Secure Forensic Psychiatry Services: Comparison of Seven English Health Regions. *British Journal of Psychiatry* 178 (1) 55–61.

Dickens,G and Sugarman,P (2011) *Adult Firesetters: Prevalence, Characteristics and Psychopathology*. In Dickens, G, Sugarman,P and Gannon,T (eds.), *Firesetting and Mental Health*. London: RCPsych Publications.

Doley,RM and Watt,BD (2011) *Assessment of Firesetters*. In Dickens,G, Sugarman,P and Gannon,T (eds.), *Firesetting and Mental Health*. London: RCPsych Publications.

Enayati,J, Grann,M, Lubbe,S and Fazel,S (2008) Psychiatric Morbidity in Arsonists Referred for Forensic Psychiatric Assessment in Sweden. *The Journal of Forensic Psychiatry & Psychology* 19 (2) 139–47.

Fazel,S and Grann,M (2002) Older Criminals: A Descriptive Study of Psychiatrically Examined Offenders in Sweden. *International Journal of Geriatric Psychiatry* 17 (10) 907–13.

Fineman,KR (1995) A Model for the Qualitative Analysis of Child and Adult Fire Deviant Behavior. *American Journal of Forensic Psychology* 13 (1) 31–60.

Fritzon,K (2011) *Theories on Arson: The Action Systems Model*. In Dickens,G, Sugarman,P and Gannon,T (eds.), *Firesetting and Mental Health*. London: RCPsych Publications.

Gannon,TA, Alleyne,E, Butler,H, Danby,H, Kapoor,A, Lovell,T, et al. (2015) Specialist Group Therapy for Psychological Factors Associated with Firesetting: Evidence of a Treatment Effect from a Non-Randomized Trial with Male Prisoners. *Behavior Research and Therapy* 73: 42–51.

Gannon,TA, Ó Ciardha,C, Doley,RM and Alleyne,E (2012) The Multi-Trajectory Theory of Adult Firesetting (M-TTAF). *Aggression and Violent Behavior* 17 (2) 107–21.

Gannon,TA and Pina,A (2010) Firesetting: Psychopathology, Theory and Treatment. *Aggression and Violent Behavior* 15 (3) 224–38.

Geller,JL (1992) Arson in Review: From Profit to Pathology. *Psychiatric Clinics of North America* 15 (3) 623–45.

Geller,JL, Erlen,J and Pinkus,RL (1986) A Historical Appraisal of America's Experience with "Pyromania" – A Diagnosis in Search of a Disorder. *International Journal of Law and Psychiatry* 9 (2) 201–29.

Grice,A (2011) *Fire Risk and Fire Safety in Psychiatric Care*. In Dickens,G, Sugarman,P and Gannon,T (eds.), *Firesetting and Mental Health*. London: RCPsych Publications.

Guy,LS, Wilson,CM, Douglas,KS, Hart,SD, Webster,CD and Belfrage,H (2013) *HCR-20 Version 3: Item-by-Item Summary of Violence Literature. HCR-20 Violence Risk Assessment White Paper Series, No. 3*. Burnaby, Canada: Mental Health, Law, and Policy Institute, Simon Fraser University.

Harris,GT and Rice,ME (1996) A Typology of Mentally Disordered Firesetters. *Journal of Interpersonal Violence* 11 (3) 351–63.

Hillier,B, Cherukuru,S and Sethi,F (2015) Care Pathway Process Proposal and Rationale for the Assessment and Management of Firesetting in the Inpatient Setting. *Journal of Psychiatric Intensive Care* 11 (2) 119–27.

Hollin,C (201) *Arson: Treatment and Interventions*. In Dickens,G, Sugarman,P and Gannon,T (eds.), *Firesetting and Mental Health*. London: RCPsych Publications.

Hollin,CR, Davies,S, Duggan,C, Huband,N, McCarthy,L and Clarke,M (2013) Patients with a History of Arson Admitted to Medium Security: Characteristics on Admission and Follow-up Postdischarge. *Medicine, Science and the Law* 53 (3) 154–60.

Jackson,HF, Glass,C and Hope,S (1987) A Functional Analysis of Recidivistic Arson. *British Journal of Clinical Psychology* 26 (3) 175–85.

Johnson,RS and Netherton,E (2016) Fire Setting and the Impulse-Control Disorder of Pyromania. *American Journal of Psychiatry Residents' Journal* 11 (7) 14–16.

Kelly,L, Lovett,J and Regan,L (2005) *A Gap or a Chasm? Attrition in Reported Rape Cases. Home Office Research Study 293*. London: Great Britain Home Office Research Development and Statistics.

Labree,W, Nijman,H, Van Marle,H and Rassin,E (2010) Backgrounds and Characteristics of Arsonists. *International Journal of Law and Psychiatry* 33 (3) 149–53.

Lewish,NOC and Yarnell,H (1951) *Pathological Firesetting (Pyromania)*. Nervous and Mental Disease Monograph Series. New York: Nervous and Mental Disease Monographs, no. 82.

Linaker,OM (2000) Dangerous Female Psychiatric Patients: Prevalences and Characteristics. *Acta Psychiatrica Scandinavica*, 101 (1) 67–72.

Lindberg,N, Holi,MM, Tani,P and Virkkunen,M (2005) Looking for Pyromania: Characteristics of a Consecutive Sample of Finnish Male Criminals with Histories of Recidivist Fire-Setting between 1973 and 1993. *BMC Psychiatry* 5: 47.

Loranger,AW, Sartorius,N, Andreoli,A, Berger,P, Buchheim,P, Channabasavanna,S., et al. 1994. The International Personality Disorder Examination. The World Health Organization/Alcohol, Drug Abuse, and Mental Health Administration International Pilot Study of Personality Disorders. *Archives of General Psychiatry* 51 (3) 215–24.

Miller,S and Fritzon,K (2007) Functional Consistency across Two Behavioural Modalities: Fire-Setting and

Self-Harm in Female Special Hospital Patients. *Criminal Behaviour and Mental Health* 17 (1) 31–44.

Muckley,A (1997) *Firesetting: Addressing Offending behaviour. A Resource and Training Manual.* UK Redcar and Cleveland Psychological Service.

Murphy,GH and Clare,ICH (1996) Analysis of Motivation in People with Mild Learning Disabilities (Mental Handicap) Who Set Fires. *Psychology, Crime & Law* 2 (3) 153–64.

Ó Ciardha,C, Barnoux,MFL, Alleyne,EKA, Tyler,N, Mozova,K. and Gannon,TA (2015a) Multiple Factors in the Assessment of Firesetters' Fire Interest and Attitudes. *Legal and Criminological Psychology* 20 (1) 37–47.

Ó Ciardha,C, Tyler,N and Gannon,TA (2015b) A Practical Guide to Assessing Adult Firesetters' Fire-Specific Treatment Needs Using the Four Factor Fire Scales. *Psychiatry* 78 (4) 293–304.

Office for National Statistics (2023) *Fire Statistics Data Tables.* UK Government. www.gov.uk/government/statis tical-data-sets/fire-statistics-data-tables.

Pallanti,S, Quercioli,L, Sood,E and Hollander,E (2002) Lithium and Valproate Treatment of Pathological Gambling: A Randomized Single-Blind Study. *Journal of Clinical Psychiatry* 63 (7) 559–64.

Parks,RW, Green,RD, Girgis,S, Hunter,MD, Woodruff,PW and Spence,SA (2005) Response of Pyromania to Biological Treatment in a Homeless Person. *Neuropsychiatric Disease and Treatment* 1 (3) 277–80.

Prins,H, Tennent,G and Trick,K (1985) Motives for Arson (Fire Raising). *Medicine, Science, and the Law* 25 (4) 275–8.

Räsänen,P, Hakko,H and Väisänen,E (1995a) Arson Trend Increasing – A Real Challenge to Psychiatry. *Journal of Forensic Sciences* 40 (6) 976–9.

Räsänen,P, Hakko,H and Väisänen,E (1995b) The Mental State of Arsonists as Determined by Forensic Psychiatric Examinations. *The Bulletin of the American Academy of Psychiatry and the Law* 23 (4) 547–53.

Repo,E, Virkkunen,M, Rawlings,R and Linnoila,M (1997) Criminal and Psychiatric Histories of Finnish Arsonists. *Acta Psychiatrica Scandinavica* 95 (4) 318–23.

Rice,ME and Harris,GT (1991) Firesetters Admitted to a Maximum Security Psychiatric Institution: Offenders and Offenses. *Journal of Interpersonal Violence* 6 (4) 461–75.

Ritchie,EC and Huff,TG (1999) Psychiatric Aspects of Arsonists. *Journal of Forensic Sciences* 44 (4) 733–40.

Rix,KJ (1994) A Psychiatric Study of Adult Arsonists. *Medicine, Science, and the Law* 34 (1) 21–34.

Robbins,E and Robbins,L (1967) Arson with Special Reference to Pyromania. *New York State Journal of Medicine* 67 (6) 795–8.

Sambrooks,K, Olver,ME, Pag,TE and Gannon,TA (2021) Firesetting Reoffending: A Meta-Analysis. *Criminal Justice and Behavior* 48 (11) 1634–1651.

Soltys,SM (1992) Pyromania and Firesetting Behaviors. *Psychiatric Annals* 22 (2) 79–83.

Stewart,LA (1993) Profile of Female Firesetters: Implications for Treatment. *The British Journal of Psychiatry* 163: 248–56.

Thomson,A, Tiihonen,J, Miettunen,J, Sailas,E, Virkkunen,M and Lindberg,N (2015) Psychopathic Traits among a Consecutive Sample of Finnish Pretrial Fire-Setting Offenders. *BMC Psychiatry* 15: 44.

Tyler,N and Gannon,TA (2012) Explanations of Firesetting in Mentally Disordered Offenders: A Review of the Literature. *Psychiatry* 75 (2) 150–66.

Tyler,N and Gannon,TA (2017) Pathways to Firesetting for Mentally Disordered Offenders: A Preliminary Examination. *International Journal of Offender Therapy and Comparative Criminology* 61 (8) 938–55.

Tyler,N and Gannon,TA (2021) The Classification of Deliberate Firesetting. *Aggression and Violent Behavior* 59: 101458.

Tyler,N, Gannon,TA, Lockerbie,L, King,T, Dickens,GL and De Burca,C (2013) A Firesetting Offense Chain for Mentally Disordered Offenders. *Criminal Justice and Behavior* 41 (4) 512–30.

World Health Organization (WHO) (2022) *International Classification of Diseases, 11th Revision.* World Health Organization.

Yesavage,JA, Benezech,M, Ceccaldi,P, Bourgeois,M and Addad M (1983) Arson in Mentally Ill and Criminal Populations. *Journal of Clinical Psychiatry* 44 (4) 128–30.

Young,S and Thome,J (2011) ADHD and Offenders. *World Journal of Biological Psychiatry* 12 (Suppl 1) 124–8.

Sexually Problematic Behaviour in Mental Health Inpatient Units

Roland Dix

Introduction

The interaction between mental illness, some personality disorders, psychological and developmental problems and sexual behaviour is a complex area. While some studies have suggested that most sex offenders do not have serious mental disorder (Narayanan et al., 2006), Moulden et al. (2022) argue that the relationship between mental disorder and problematic sexual behaviour could be related to the mechanisms through which symptoms confer risk, including problem-solving, sexual disinhibition and social/intimacy deficits. This was observed in psychosis, although it was most prevalent in brain injury. Sexual needs and behaviour amongst mental health inpatients is also a complex area presenting several clinical, ethical and legal challenges.

Similarly, sex offending has not been considered to be correlated either (Hanson and Bussiere, 1998; Stone et al., 2000; Gordon et al., 2004; Hanson and Morton-Bourgon, 2004). However, some large studies (n = 8495) have challenged this assertion by suggesting that there is a six-fold increase in a history of psychiatric hospitalisation for serious mental illness in sexual offenders compared to the general population (Fazel et al., 2007).

Some mental illness, learning disabilities and personality disorders have been reported as significant in problematic sexual behaviour (Gordon and Grubin, 2004). It may also be significant that many people with mental health problems will have themselves been the victims of sexual abuse (Spataro and Mullen, 2004). Therefore, when considering longer-term patients within mental health units, Welch et al. (1996) commented that expressions of sexuality should be considered a basic human need which should be understood and humanely considered by the staff.

This chapter focuses on sexually problematic behaviour (SPB) by adult patients in mental health inpatient settings. Some reports have suggested that 33% of female inpatients had been the recipients of unwanted sexual comments or molestation, although this very often went unreported at the time (Thomas et al., 1995). In other reports, as many as 56% of female inpatients said they had been sexually bothered by men, with 8% suggesting that they had experienced a sexual encounter against their will (Barlow and Wolfson, 1997).

The National Patient Safety Agency (2006) produced a report detailing concerns about sexual assaults on patients in National Health Service (NHS) mental health units. Sexual boundary issues have been considered in detail by the Royal College of Psychiatrists (2007) which also included useful policy guidance for psychiatric treatment settings. However, it appears that SPB has remained an enduring and serious concern. The UK regulator, the Care Quality Commission (2018), undertook an analysis of nearly 60,000 incident reports that took place on NHS trust mental health wards from April to June 2017. They found 1,120 sexual incidents involving patients, staff, visitors and others. About two-thirds (594) of the people affected were categorised as patients and one-third (301) were staff, with a small number (24) who were others, such as visitors to the ward. Females were more likely to be the persons affected (CQC, 2018).

Most professionals and patients would accept that hospitals or other mental health settings should have policies which aim to protect patients, staff and visitors from sexual harassments or assault.

Within the literature, reference to SPB as a reported feature within patients admitted to a variety of inpatient settings is not difficult to find (Coid, 1991; Muthkumaraswamy, 2008; Lawn and Mcdonald, 2009). Some studies have shown a prevalence of up to 15% for SPB in the low secure inpatient population (Beer et al., 2005). Specific characterisation of actual SPBs is more difficult to define based on clear evidence. The CQC's (2018) detailed examination of incident reports also provides some indication of incident type.

Concepts/Definitions

Sexualised behaviour considered as challenging within inpatient units or other mental health settings may often fall into one or a combination of the following categories:

- Sexualised comments that are unwelcome or inappropriate to the context of interactions with fellow patients, professional staff, visitors and the public
- Interpersonal sexually orientated physical contact including touching, brushing up against or other attempts to make uninvited physical sexual contact with another person
- Exposing sexual areas of the body
- Sexualised self-touching, masturbation or sexual gestures enacted to cause discomfort or distress in others
- More serious behaviours that would meet the definition of a sexual criminal offence including rape or forced sexually gratifying act

These behaviours can present significant challenges to an inpatient environment, community mental health setting and to the wider community. An additional layer of complexity is added when the SPB is more subtle or specifically targeted towards individuals, which may often fail to be observed by others. Approaches to managing and engaging in SPB may differ according to the specific motivation for and manifestation of the behaviour.

Sexually Problematic Behaviour Definition

SPB may be defined as interpersonal communication or behaviour with a sexual theme that has the potential to case discomfort, distress, humiliation or fear in others. Particular religions, cultures and subcultures often attach differing values and tolerances to acceptable sexual expression and behaviour. The important variable for defining SPB is the potential for it to have a significant negative impact upon others and generally overstepping the boundaries of sexual expression that would be considered the cultural norm.

The Sexual Offences Act 2003 describes the acts, behaviours and means of exploitation that constitute sexual criminal offending in England and Wales. This is a complex area of criminal law within which issues of consent and capacity to consent are central. In circumstances where a clear criminal sexual offence may have taken place, reports to the police are required.

Severe Sexually Problematic Behaviour and Offending: Is There a Difference?

Many of the SPBs previously listed have similarities with, and will often meet the criteria for, criminal offending. Moreover, if many of the SPBs often witnessed within modern-day psychiatric institutions were enacted in community or public settings, they may well attract the attention of the police.

Many practitioners and often patients may generally consider SPBs to be more frequent, although less severe than sexual offences for which an individual may face criminal prosecution.

While some patients exhibiting SPB could be regarded as in conflict with the law, their characterisation may be discrete from straight-forward sexual offending. The behaviours may have manifested because of acute symptoms or as part of a longer-term behavioural pattern in the context of poor mental health. This may differ from episodic criminal sexual offences in the absence of serious mental disorder.

The Role of the Criminal Justice System

NHS Protect (2017) developed a national partnership protocol between the police, Crown Prosecution Service and the NHS as to when and how the criminal justice system should be engaged for patients demonstrating challenging/offending behaviours.

Most public agencies accept that there are times when it may be necessary to involve the criminal justice system for the engagement of challenging/offending behaviour presented by a mental health inpatient. Also, for some patients who find themselves in police custody, a more collaborative approach between the criminal justice system and mental health services may be necessary, beyond that of simple transfer from one to the other.

For people experiencing acute symptoms, which are often the causation factors in any challenging or offending behaviour, it is appropriate to consider all treatment options and approaches before resorting to criminal justice system involvement. In terms of SPB, clear upper-level offences require engagement by the criminal justice system.

There are several reasons why it may be appropriate to report to or process a current inpatient through the criminal justice system. Table 11.1 lists important

Table 11.1 Important factors when considering the role of the criminal justice system in dealing with challenging/offending behaviour.

- A prosecution would be in the wider public interest.
- A victim has the right to make a complaint regarding an alleged offence and receive the protection of the law.
- The person has presented SPB in the form of a definable offence while engaged with treatment, and the offending behaviour is not assessed to be a result of their mental disorder.
- The assessment indicates that the person should be engaged by the criminal justice system and so doing would diminish the likelihood of repeat behaviour.
- In order for offences to be properly examined. This can be achieved by the collection of witness statements and consideration by the police.
- It is thought important that challenging/offending behaviour be reported so that a true 'forensic history' is recorded.
- To offer the person the proper protection of the law for alleged offences so that they may properly and legally defend themselves.
- So that the offence can be assigned a police incident number that may be necessary for future action (e.g. in order to pursue criminal compensation).

issues to bear in mind when considering the role of the criminal justice system in dealing with challenging/offending behaviour.

Considerations Important to the Successful Engagement of the Criminal Justice System

At the time that an alleged offence has occurred, and the multidisciplinary team (MDT) decides to involve the criminal justice system, the person who was the victim of the offence will need to be aware of their rights/responsibilities. This will often involve a willingness to provide the police with a witness statement detailing the events and nature of the complaint being made against the alleged perpetrator of the offence.

Some victims within mental health units may not be able to provide a statement or easily describe what happened. In these circumstances, other evidence, for example, statements from staff, CCTV footage, and so on, may be needed to assist the criminal justice process.

Patients Detained under the Mental Health Act?

Detention under the Mental Health Act (MHA) does not prevent a person being processed through the criminal justice system.

This is a complex area in which the interface between criminal law and mental health legislation can provide a confusing picture. If a patient, for example, is detained under a treatment order (e.g. Section 3 of the Mental Health Act), this is often a concern for the CPS or the police as an issue that

is likely to result in difficulty in achieving a satisfactory conviction. Whilst this a legitimate concern, it need not be resolved at the point of arrest or initial court appearance and may be tested much later within the legal and clinical framework.

Further considering the clinical engagement/management of SPB within an inpatient unit setting may be assisted by reference to a case vignette.

Case vignette

Bradley is a 34-year-old man with a history of protracted manic episodes. He had experienced multiple admissions to hospital with extended periods of elevated mood and thought disorder. His first admission was when he was only 16 years old. Over the years that he has received mental health services, he has experienced extended admissions to general adult psychiatric inpatient wards, a psychiatric intensive care unit (PICU and a low secure recovery unit as well as one episode of treatment within a medium secure setting. Bradley has a long history of substance and alcohol misuse with a preference for stimulants, particularly amphetamines. He also was a long-term daily cannabis user. At the current time, he had not consistently used alcohol or drugs for the past 3 years. He has, however, been in some form of institutional care during most of this time.

He is currently placed in an all-male (patient) low secure unit (LSU) which specialises in treatment and recovery of adult patients with mental health problems. He has been resident at the unit for one year of an expected two-year admission.

Forensic History

Bradley had been arrested several times in the past for several minor offences, mostly shop lifting and public order issues.

He had been arrested three times during the last 15 years for sexually inappropriate behaviour, including one occasion where it was reported that he had exposed himself to a 17-year-old female. On another occasion, he was arrested because of a rape allegation made by a fellow patient while they were both inpatients in a general adult facility.

It appeared that he was having a relationship with the alleged victim at the time of the allegation. None of the arrests led to conviction, although he was charged with indecent exposure. In all cases, he was diverted to the mental health system in preference to proceeding with prosecution.

Mental and Behavioural State

Bradley maintains a fixed delusional system that he has received significant military training and will be periodically called upon to perform missions. He also believes he is a talented musician who will soon be discovered for a major record deal. Overall, his delusional ideas are not immediately apparent, although they often emerge during extended conversations. His mood is often considered elevated. He is able to take part in escorted leave for unit activities including cycling, gym and badminton at the local leisure centre.

Assessment of Sexually Problematic Behaviour

SPBs become much more frequent and intense during periods of elevated mood and involve persistent sexualised comments and innuendoes to female members of staff. Periodic attempts to brush against females include opportunistic sexual touching of female staff member's breasts. During his admission to the LSU, Bradley was periodically caught masturbating in his bedroom when he knew he was being observed.

When less symptomatic, Bradley's specific SPB diminishes, although he often maintains a theme of more appropriate sexualised humour which is considered on the boundary of acceptable social norms in the unit.

When out of the unit and taking part in escorted leave, Bradley's SPB diminishes significantly. He often presents himself as somewhat shy or nervous in his interactions with females out of hospital.

Causes

Psychosexual History

Recording psychosexual history is an important aspect of assessment (Singh and Beck, 1997; Green 2009). Although the value of the psychosexual history is well recognised, it is very often an overlooked aspect of psychiatric assessment (Rele 2008; Gordon 2004). Within the assessment of causes for SPB, an accurate psychosexual history is important. The following headings are important for the assessment of Bradley's sexual history and development.

Age at which sexual awareness and interest first developed

Bradley reported that his first interest in sexuality was when he was around 12 years old. He reported having a 'crush' on several girls at school and stated that he started masturbating around this time.

Age and number of sexual relationships

Bradley said that he had his first girlfriend was when he was 15 years old and she was 16 years old. He reported losing his virginity at this time within the relationship which lasted approximately six months.

Ability to initiate and develop intimate relationships

Between the ages of 15 and 17 years, Bradley reported being relatively successful with developing sexual relationships with girls of a similar age. He recounted three sexual relationships with girlfriends and another casual sexual relationship by the age of 18 years.

Sexual and intimate relationships post adolescence

Following his first psychiatric admission at 16 years old, Bradley reported finding it increasingly difficult to initiate and sustain intimate relationships. He attributed this to frequent psychiatric admissions, losing many of his friends/peer group at this time and being considered by some girls as 'weird'.

Between the ages of 26 and 29 years, Bradley had one longer-term relationship with a 35-year-old woman whom he met while he was a psychiatric inpatient. She also was suffering with longer-term mental health problems. This was his last relationship, and he had been single for six years at the time of assessment.

Sexual interests

Bradley described his sexual interests as 'pretty normal'. He reported enjoying watching pornography whenever he gets the chance.

He also described the urge to masturbate regularly, especially following amphetamine use.

Insight into previous sexual problematic behaviour

Bradley denied ever sexually offending in the past. He said that he was once arrested for alleged sexual assaults while an inpatient, although he claimed that the relationship was reciprocal and that the allegation was only made because he had discontinued the relationship.

He denies exposing himself to the young girl and claimed that he was drunk at the time and was intending to go to the toilet outside when he was alleged to have exposed himself.

Clinical Assessment of Sexually Problematic Behaviour

There are several formalised assessment schedules concerned with risk of sexual offending. The Risk for Sexual Violence Protocol (Hart et al., 2003) is a specific instrument for assessing sexual violence applicable to those with mental disorder. Other approaches that may be useful are assessment formats aimed at determining the extent to which an individual understands sexual issues, sexual behaviour and its impact on others.

Many of these approaches have been developed for use with people with intellectual difficulties (Michie et al., 2007). These instruments can also add value to the assessment of people with mental health problems by increasing understanding of sexual knowledge, attitudes and insight into the impact of SPB.

Marshall (2004) proposed several areas of importance for assessing potential for sexual offending by adults against women. We outline this in the sections that follow.

Social Skills

Some studies have shown that sexual offenders have diminished social skills in comparison to those of the general population (Bradford, 2006). Important social skills include assertiveness, ability to build rapport and the ability to recognise social cues, particularly when another person may be uncomfortable or offended by comments or behaviours.

During assessment, Bradley can describe how he tends to use his perception of humour to initiate conversations. He is also observed to try to rationalise his behaviour as a joke when confronted or challenged. During assessment, he also volunteered that he believed that the rules are different while in hospital and that female staff should be used to and accepting of the behaviour of patients.

Cognitive Distortions

The tendency to reframe the impact of SPB as much less significant or denying its occurrence altogether has been reported (Bumby, 1996). Denial and minimisation are important areas of assessment which can also inform the type of interventions likely to be successful in improving insight into the nature of the SPB.

In Bradley's case, he often denied completely that a sexual comment was made when reported by the staff. He also tended to re-frame his masturbation displays as being the fault of the person who witnessed it. He also rationalised his brushing up against staff as sometimes being invited by the staff member, an accident or just a 'laugh'.

Empathy Deficits

It has long been recognised that sexual offenders experience difficulty in being able to empathise with their victims regarding the effects of their behaviour (Covell and Scalora 2002; Blake and Gannon, 2008).

During assessment, Bradley suggested that his behaviour was 'harmless' and that the staff were paid to tolerate difficult behaviour. He said that he did not believe that anything he had done was perceived as upsetting by others. He went on to say that he would not wish to upset any of the female staff and would feel remorseful if this had been the case.

Acute Symptoms

Elevated mood is often accompanied by disinhibited behaviours, including in Bradley's case. His mood is described as often slightly elevated which is generally characterised by him becoming very easily overly excitable with minimal stimulation.

Specific clinical management of SPB profile within an inpatient setting

In consultation with the unit psychologist, the named nurse created an assessment format requiring that all behaviours considered sexually problematic were noted over a four-week period. The assessment schedule required that the following be noted:

- Short description of SPB
- Time of occurrence
- Duration of episode
- Effect of behaviour on recipient/recipients
- Short description of any antecedents

- Short description of any immediate intervention employed
- Any circumstances in which SPBs were less likely

At the conclusion of the four-week assessment period, the specific SPBs were described and categorised. In Bradley's case they were as follows:

- Sexual comments during the course of otherwise appropriate one-to-one interaction referring to his genitals or comments related to the bodies of female staff
- Opportunistic comments during general socialising with others and periodically trying to encourage his peers to contribute or support (laugh) at his comments
- Seemingly timed periods of exposure or masturbation when he was aware that an observation by female staff or an engagement was likely to take place
- Invasion of personal space with female staff, including opportunist attempts to brush up against them, very often when not observed by others

The frequency and duration of these behaviours were also noted over a two-week period with the following results:

- Individual episodes tended to last between 10 seconds and 2 minutes
- Episodes were reported between twice and four times a week during the assessment period (average around three episodes weekly)
- The episodes were generally reported in the evening and night-time
- All of the exposure/masturbation behaviours occurred during routine night-time observation when it appeared that Bradley was aware that a female member of staff would be performing the observation or would be coming to his room for another reason
- SPBs were not observed outside the unit while on escorted leave or during engagements involving male staff

Effects of behaviour on the recipient
- Some staff reported finding the sexualised comments uncomfortable and distressing
- One member of staff reported feeling upset in relation to comments made regarding areas of her body
- Two members of staff reported feeling significantly threatened by the invasion of personal space with accompanying sexual overtones

Immediate interventions employed
Several, often different, interventions were recorded as attempted by staff during the assessment period. These included:

- Medication review aimed at better controlling acute manic symptoms

- Ignoring comments and immediately disengaging
- Verbal intervention from staff member stating the inappropriateness of behaviour and request that comments/behaviours desist
- Verbal distraction from SPB and attention directed towards other appropriate interaction

Formulation
The detailed information achieved within the assessment period provided a solid basis for case formulation of SPB.

At this point, an MDT meeting is required to present, discuss and arrive at a consistent view of the SPB based on the assessment data. It is often helpful to structure the general case formulation. In this example related to SPB, the axis headings offered in the *Diagnostic and Statistical Manual of Mental Disorders, Fifth Edition* (*DSM-5*) are used.

Clinical Psychiatric Factors
The mood elevation was noted within the context of a longstanding schizoaffective-type illness. The mood component was considered relevant to the SPB, although not causative.

Medical Conditions
There are several organic pathologies that can cause impulsivity and disinhibited behaviour. Conditions that affect the temporal lobe areas of the brain are of particular importance (Starkstein and Robinson, 1997). For individuals where SPB has emerged for the first time and is considered out of character, physical investigations should be performed to exclude organic pathology.

In the case of Bradley, his history personality structure and psychiatric/psychological clinical profile provided an adequate explanation for the SPB.

Personality Factors
It was acknowledged that Bradley had issues with personality development resulting from spending developmental milestones within institutions.

The extent of his experience with developing intimate relationships in adulthood was also judged to have affected his personality structure in his expressions of sexuality.

It was not concluded that the SPB originated from any specific disorder of personality.

Psychosocial and Environmental Factors

The sexual history highlighted several areas considered relevant to Bradley's SPB. This included him developing mania in late adolescence and spending long periods of time in hospital settings. He also reported losing many of his premorbid skills in developing intimate relations around this time.

He also presented several attitudes and perceptions of females, particularly staff, based on his interpretation of institutional culture. This was coupled with a lack of insight into the true impact of his SPB.

The diminished opportunities in the all-peer group LSU environment were also considered a significant factor in Bradley's SPB.

Medication

Sexual dysfunction is a well-recognised side effect of many antipsychotic medications (Gordon and Gruoin, 2004). One forensic psychiatrist has gone as far as to suggest that such medication may represent a means of involuntary castration (Stone, 1992). Historically, the butyrophenone benperidol was sometimes prescribed to reduce SPB in psychiatric patients (Sterkmans and Geerts, 1966). However, no reliable evidence has been advanced to support its efficacy and its use in contemporary practice is not recommended. Antilibidinal drugs such as cyproterone acetate have been used with recidivist sex offenders and other patients repeatedly exhibiting unacceptable or dangerous sexual behaviour (Xeniditis et al., 2001).

Some reports have suggested the potential value of selective serotonin reuptake inhibitors (SSRIs) in the treatment of paraphilia (Gordon and Gruoin, 2004). One hypothesis proposed for their efficacy is a reduction in obsessive–compulsive behaviour, thus reducing sexual preoccupation and intrusive sexual urges. The National Institute for Health and Care Excellence (NICE, 2015) considered the use of fluoxetine for hypersexuality. Some improvements were noted, although they were marginal and based on small studies.

A Cochrane review by Khan et al. (2015) presented some encouraging results for SSRIs, although the studies reviewed did not provide clear evidence of efficacy. Any treatment in line with these findings should be in collaboration with the patient based on informed consent.

Generally, the use of medication specifically for SPB has a poor evidence base. Reliable use of medication will be centred around trying to reduce active symptoms of mental illness, particularly elevated mood and delusions.

During the period of the four-week assessment activity and previously, Bradley's mood was generally more elevated than could be the case at other times. His medication regime included a mood stabiliser along with typical depot medication. PRN medication was also available, including additional antipsychotics.

Care plan

Having completed a detailed assessment of the nature, content and context of SPB, a care plan can be created defining specific interventions within a number of treatment/management paradigms.

Observation and exhibitionism

A plan was devised that included specific times within which night-time observation would be carried out, clearly identifying when masturbation could be performed unobserved. Male staff were assigned to night-time observation where ever possible.

Psychotherapeutic sessions

The named nurse and unit psychologist (one of whom is male) care planned to meet with Bradley twice weekly for up to an hour, to be reviewed in six weeks.

During the first of these sessions, the data from the four-week assessment period was fed back to Bradley, including the effect of his behaviour on some of the recipients, although no specific victim was named.

Empathy Training

Maletzky (1997) suggested empathy training as a useful intervention for lower-level SPD such as exhibitionism. The idea being that some perpetrators may diminish the potential effects of this type of behaviour as compared to more serious offences such as rape.

Important objectives in this type of training include that the subject be able to:

- Identify who is a victim from their behaviour
- Identify the victimising act
- Identify the harm done
- Understand the preceding by way of role reversal
- Develop empathy

A counselling approach was used in subsequent sessions centred around meeting these objectives.

Social Skills Awareness

The sessions within the care plan were also used to identify appropriate skills in relation to the use of humour and the appropriateness of interactions with females. Examples of behaviours that were considered appropriate, borderline or inappropriate were discussed. These were colour-coded into green, amber and red categories as suggested within the Reinforce Appropriate, Implode Disruptive (RAID) behavioural approach (Davis, 1993).

Behavioural

A behavioural context to the care plan was established following the principles of the RAID approach. This involved defining behaviours and establishing a set of responses ranging from ignoring the behaviour to the provision of additional incentives, such as extra periods of escorted leave for activities. The overall aim is to focus on and reward positive behaviours rather than the SPB.

Activities and Positive Reinforcements

A programme of specific activity was created and targeted toward the evenings. The activity included playing badminton in the unit gym with a male member of staff. Other elements included cooking and taking part in the future planning of activities during the week. Out-of-unit activities supported by escorted leave were also established.

Within this aspect of the care plan, clear definitions of positive behaviours were agreed and discussed during the psychotherapeutic sessions. Furthermore, the conditions within which incentives (additional escorted leave for activities) would be achieved as result of positive behaviours were also agreed upon.

Progress

During the first three weeks, Bradley was sometimes mildly hostile to some female members of staff saying that they were 'telling stories' about him. As a result of two episodes of SPB in the first three weeks, Bradley was not allowed to take advantage of three additional escorted leave activities and instead engaged in unit-based activity.

The sessions with his named nurse and the unit psychologist were initially difficult, with Bradley leaving early in the first two sessions.

After six weeks, Bradley seemed to develop a better understanding of the effects of his behaviour on others. The fact that all SPB behaviours had been recorded and fed back as an initial stage in the care plan significantly diminished the extent to which he felt they went unnoticed.

He started to work within the sessions on differentiating between appropriate and inappropriate comments and humour. The focus of the care plan was on reinforcing positive behaviours.

Within six weeks, it became apparent that Bradleys SPBs had significantly reduced. He continued to periodically engage in sexual humour, although this was considered to be much less problematic in terms of content and impact than previous behaviours.

Conclusion

SPB is a complex area of challenging behaviour, and the best management approach is likely to be multi-faceted. The management considered in the Bradley's case included medical, psychotherapeutic and behavioural approaches. Detailed assessment and carefully considered care planning are essential characteristics of clinical engagement and can include the use of structured tools where appropriate.

Generally, mood elevation has a common association with disinhibited behaviours which may often be associated with SPB (Torrey and Knable, 2005). Delusional beliefs, particularly those of a grandiose nature, can also be significant in SPB (Remien and Johnson, 2004)

The treatment in this domain will often involve medication, although other approaches can also be effective.

The effect of the institution in producing behaviours that would not otherwise occur outside of the institution has been long accepted (Goffman, 1961) In the case of SPB, Rowe and William (2007) reported on the specific effects of the institution on sexual behaviour and highlighted lack of privacy, gender-separated living environment, lack of sex education and lack of opportunity for sexual expression as major concerns. Moreover, they suggested that institutionalisation often set the conditions for sexual assault and exploitation.

Treatment factors in this domain include programmes of escorted leave and maximising the potential for patients to remain influenced by the social norms and expectations of behaviour associated with wider community living outside the institution.

Ford et al. (2003) identified loneliness and boredom as possible motivating factors for SPB. Well-developed, positive relationships between the staff and patients provide good opportunity for the promotion of empathy and understanding, which is also a major consideration for SPB.

Unit culture and regime should provide for high levels of engagement and activity. Unit regimes which have established activity programmes both within and outside the unit diminish the probability of challenging behaviours in the first place. In addition, they provide maximum opportunities for an incentive-based behavioural approach.

Although challenging and often uncomfortable, SPB requires specific and careful consideration supported by well-considered care plans. Wherever possible, tendencies towards diminishing the behaviour or (at the other extreme) punitive approaches should be avoided. It is important, however, that where there is evidence that behaviour meeting the criteria of a sexual offence, this should be reported with appropriate support given to the victim.

References

Barlow,F and Wolfson,P (1997) Safety and Security: A Survey of Female Psychiatric In-Patients. *Psychiatric Bulletin* **21** (5) 270.

Beer,MD, Turk,V, McGovern,P, Gravestock,S, Brooks,D, Barnett,L, et al. (2005) Characteristics of Patients Exhibiting Severe Challenging Behaviour in Low Secure Mental Health and Mild Learning Disability Units. *Journal of Psychiatric Intensive Care and Low Secure Units* **1** (1) 17–24.

Blake,E and Gannon,A (2008) Social Perception Deficits, Cognitive Distortions, and Empathy Deficits in Sex Offenders: A Brief Review. *Trauma, Violence, & Abuse* **9** (1) 34–55.

Bradford,J (2006) On Sexual Violence. *Current Opinion in Psychiatry* **19** (5) 527–32.

Bumby,KM (1996) Assessing the Cognitive Distortions of Child Molesters and Rapists: Development of the Molest and Rape Scales. *Sexual Abuse: A Journal of Research and Treatment* **8** (1) 37–57.

Care Quality Communion (CQC) (2018) Report on Sexual Safety on Mental Health Wards. CQC–421–092018.

Coid,JW (1991) A Survey of Patients from Five Health Districts Receiving Specialist Care in the Private Sector. *Psychiatric Bulletin* **15** (5) 257–62.

Covell,CN and Scalora,MJ (2002) Empathic Deficits in Sexual Offenders – An Integration of Affective, Social, and Cognitive Constructs. *Aggression and Violent Behavior* **7** (3) 251–70.

Davis,W (1993) The RAID Programme for Challenging Behaviour: Leicester Association for Psychological Therapies.

Fazel,S, Sjostedt,G, Langstrom,N and Grann,M (2007) Severe Mental Illness and Risk of Sexual Offending in Men: A Case-Control Study Based on Swedish National Registers. *The Journal of Clinical Psychiatry* **68** (4) 588-96.

Ford E, Rosenberg,M, Holsten,M and Boudreaux,T (2003) Managing Sexual Behaviour on Adult Acute Care Inpatient Psychiatric Units. *Psychiatric Services* **54** (3) 346–50.

Goffman,E (1961) *Asylums*. London: Penguin.

Gordon,H and Grubin,D (2004) Psychiatric Aspects of the Assessment and Treatment of Sex Offenders. *Advances in Psychiatric Treatment* **10** (1) 73–80.

Green,B (2009) *Problem-Based Psychiatry*, 2nd ed. Oxford: Radcliffe Publishing.

Hart,SD, Kropp,PR, Laws,DR, Klaver,J, Logan,C and Watt, KA (2003) *Risk for Sexual Violence Protocol (RSVP)*. British Columbia: Simon Fraser University, Mental Health, Law and Policy Institute.

Khan,O, Ferriter,M, Huband,N, Powney,M, Dennis,J and Duggan,C (2015) Pharmacological Interventions for Those Who Have Sexually Offended or Are at Risk of Offending. *Cochrane Database of Systematic Reviews* **2015** (2) CD007989. DOI: https://doi.org/10.1002/14651858.CD007989.pub2.

Lawn,T and Mcdonald,E (2009) Developing a Policy to Deal with Sexual Assault on Psychiatric In-Patient Wards. *The Psychiatrist* **33** (3) 108–11.

Maletzky,BM (1997) Exhibitionism Assessment and Treatment. In Laws,DR and O'Donohue,W (eds.), *Sexual Deviance Theory, Assessment, and Treatment*. pp.40–74. London: The Guildford Press.

Marshall,WL (2004) Adult Sexual Offenders Against Women. In Hollin,CR (ed.), *The Essential Handbook of Offender Assessment and Treatment*. pp. 147–62. Leicester: Wiley.

Michie,A, Lindsay,W, Martin,V and Grieve,A (2006) A Test of Counterfeit Deviance: A Comparison of Sexual Knowledge in Groups of Sex Offenders with Intellectual Disability and Controls. *Sexual Abuse: A journal of Research and Treatment* **18** (3) 271–8.

Moulden,HM, Myers,C, Lori,A and Chaimowitz,G (2022) The Relationship Between and Correlates of Problematic Sexual Behavior and Major Mental Illness. *Frontiers in Psychology* **12**: 719082. DOI: https://doi.org/10.3389/fpsyg.2021.719082.

Muthkumaraswamy,A, Beer,MD and Ratnajothy,K (2008) Aggression Patterns and Clinical Predictors of Inpatient Aggression in a Mental Health Low Secure Unit. *Journal of Psychiatric Intensive Care and Low Secure Units* **4** (1–2) 9–16.

Narayanan,P, Rotte,M and Khadivi,A (2006) Mentally Ill Sexual Offenders: A Descriptive Study. Presented at

American Academy of Psychiatry and Law Annual Meeting. Chicago.

National Health Service (NHS) Protect (2017) National Partnership Protocol for Managing Risk and Investigating Crime in Mental Health Settings.

National Institute of Health and Care Excellence (NICE) (2015) Hypersexuality: Fluoxetine: Evidence Summary (ESUOM46).

National Patient Safety Agency (2006) With Safety in Mind: Mental Health Services and Patient Safety. Patient Safety Observatory Report 2/July 2006. National Patient Safety Agency.

Rele,K (2008) Awareness and Management of Psychosexual and Relationship Problems in Mental Health Services. *The Psychiatrist* **32** (11) 436.

Remien,RH and Johnson,JG (2004) Psychiatric Disorders and Symptoms Associated with Sexual Risk Behavior. *Psychiatric Times* **XXI** (11).

Rowe,WS (2007) The Effects of Residential Institutions on Adult Sexual Adjustment. *Journal of Human Behaviour in the Social Environment* **15** (4) 81–92.

Royal College of Psychiatrists (2007) Sexual Boundary Issues in Psychiatric Settings. College Report CR145. London.

Singh,S and Beck,AJ (1997) 'No Sex Please, We're British': Taking a Sexual History from Psychiatric Inpatients. *Psychiatric Bulletin* **21** (2) 99–101.

Spataro,J and Mullen,P (2004) Impact of Child Sexual Abuse on Mental Health Prospective Study in Males and Females. *The British Journal of Psychiatry* **184**: 416–21.

Starkstein,SE and Robinson,R (1997) Mechanism of Disinhibition After Brain Lesions. *Journal of Nervous and Mental Disease* **185** (2) 108–14.

Sterkmans,P and Geerts,F (1966) Is Benperidol the Specific Drug for the Treatment of Excessive and Disinhibited Aexual Behaviour? *Acta Neurologica et Psychiatrica Belgica* **66**: 1030–40.

Stone,H (1992) Depot Neuroleptics: Involuntary Castration? *Journal of Forensic Psychiatry* **3** (1) 7–11.

Thomas,C, Bartlett,A and Mezey,GC (1995) The Extent and Effects of Violence among Psychiatric In-Patients. *Psychiatric Bulletin* **19** (10) 600–4.

Torrey,EF and Knable,MB (2005) *Surviving Manic Depression: A Manual on Bipolar Disorder for Patients.* New York: Basic Books.

Welch,SJ and Clements,GW (1996) Development of a Policy on Sexuality for Hospitalized Chronic Psychiatric Patients. *Canadian Journal of Psychiatry* **41** (5) 273–9.

Xeniditis,K, Russell,A and Murphy,D (2001) Management of People with Challenging Behaviour. *Advances in Psychiatric Treatment* **7** (2) 109–16.

Self-Harm and Personality Disorders in PICU

Reena Panchal and James Baker

Introduction

In this chapter, we focus on deliberate self-harm and borderline personality disorder. The evidence base for other personality disorders and severe mental illness likely to admitted to psychiatric intensive care units (PICUs) with deliberate self-harm (DSH), is generally scant. The clinical view is that inpatient admission for borderline personality population is probably best avoided. However, this approach is unrealistic in clinical practice, often due to patient presentations and risk deemed unmanageable in community or acute ward settings.; There are inevitable issues with such a patient profile in the PICU.

Definitions and Mental Disorders Associated with Self-Harm

There are various definitions offered for 'deliberate self-harm'. Understandably, there is often debate around whether a behaviour can categorically be described as self-harm, given the complexities associated with such presentations. Within literature and clinical practice, there are a range of terms synonymously used with 'deliberate self-harm' and these include 'self-mutilation, 'self-injury', 'parasuicide behaviour', 'self-wounding' and 'self-destructive behaviour'. Though there are a range of descriptions available to describe DSH, there is a commonality of distinguishing it from suicide. Intent and outcome are considered when delineating the two. For the scope of this chapter, DSH will be used to describe behaviour where there is a non-fatal outcome and the intent is to cause harm to self.

DSH is independently associated with serious mental illnesses such as schizophrenia, depression and bipolar affective disorder. It also occurs within the context of harmful substance misuse. However, stereotypically personality disorders, most frequently borderline personality disorder, are linked with self-harm, with the *International Classification of Diseases,*

Tenth Edition (ICD-10) (World Health Organization, 1993) criteria specifically referencing it as a symptom. Just as there are challenges in defining DSH, mental disorders associated with it are often not clear cut. The cases in which there is DSH that requires admission to a PICU are often complex with comorbidities of severe mental illness and personality disorders or traits. There is a considerable overlap of trauma, psychotic-like phenomena and personality dysfunction, which may prove difficult to disentangle, but all of which may influence the accompanying DSH.

Common Challenges with Personality Disorder in PICU Settings

The psychiatric intensive care model is based on rapid, targeted assessment and treatment with an aim to deliver specific intervention to acutely disturbed patients. There is an emphasis on mental illness, aggression towards others and compulsory admission; a PICU being an environment that is necessary to manage those who cannot be contained in the community or acute open wards. There is a lack of consensus regarding the suitability of inpatient admission to PICU for borderline personality disorder. In fact, guidance fails to address issues with inpatient admission of this population to any great degree (Paris, 2002; NICE, 2009; Ali and Findlay, 2016; NAPICU, 2016; Royal College of Psychiatrists, 2020; Royal College of Psychiatrists, 2023).

National guidance recommends that any inpatient admission for patients with personality disorder should be the last resort, and if it is necessary, it should be short term with a clear exit plan. 'Crisis admissions' should, in theory, be managed with a clear time-directed management plan with specific goals for the patient to achieve whilst being an inpatient. The patient and the multidisciplinary team (MDT) should be collaborating while upholding the autonomy of the patient in decisions. As far as possible, compulsory admissions under the Mental Health Act (MHA) should be avoided. Comparing the criteria for admission to PICU and the guidelines endorsed for management of personality disorder shows that there is a stark conflict from the outset. Adherence to a consistent approach is also varied (Fagin, 2004; Howard et al., 2006; Haw et al., 2017).

Should it be the case that a patient with personality disorder does require admission to a PICU, the narrative is often that they are 'inappropriately placed' or 'difficult to manage'. This is usually the weight carried by both the PICU team and the patient, which can lead to compromise of effective therapeutic relationships. There is risk of the patient feeling ostracised and out of place in a unit where the milieu is set to manage psychotic, aggressive patients who are often lacking capacity. Due to the relative silence of national bodies on the appropriate pathways for personality disorder, the PICU teams can often feel hopeless when formulating a care plan for these patients. There is poor evidence for acute interventions that work well for crisis presentations. This is compounded by the inconsistent practices across inpatient settings in the management of personality disorder. With more complex presentations, the default position is often to refer for an opinion from forensic services, which seem to be equally as varied in their approach. The uncertainty and unpredictable approach to management may be transferred to the patient, leading to them feeling uncontained. This, again, directly poses a contradiction the role of a PICU.

The very nature of borderline personality disorder poses a challenge to the PICU; individuals are highly distressed, emotionally unstable, may be in a state of regression and engage in serious DSH. Although aggression towards others may also be a feature, this may not be the main presentation. High levels of self-injurious behaviour, care-seeking behaviours and manifestation of dependency may occur, which can lead to team splitting and pushing of boundaries and have a significant impact on the daily interactions between staff and patient. It is important to recognise that one of the greatest challenges of working with patients with personality disorder is the range of feelings they may invoke in the staff group caring from them. These can range from anxiety, fear, guilt, helplessness and anger to perhaps a false sense of security.

The patient perspective on inpatient admissions often is tainted by victimisation and experience of trauma (Fallon, 2003). PICU interventions may include more restrictive measures such as seclusion, increasing observations, lack of privacy, room searches, use of anti-rip clothing and intramuscular medications. This may cause patients with borderline personality disorder to relive previous traumas leading to further de-stabilisation of their crisis state. This makes such interventions counterproductive and ineffective. In complex cases, increasing restrictions leads to patients escalating their maladaptive behaviours in order to deal with perceived instability. This can lead to protracted admissions and iatrogenic harm. The latter is characterised by patients resorting to more severe self-harm, new self-harm behaviours, aggression towards staff within the context of restraint and increasing dependency on staff, losing the ability to self-manage on and beyond an artificial ward setting, which perpetuates the admission. The result is often a burnt-out PICU team who opine the patient to be 'untreatable' and a patient who has become severely disordered with a heightened sense of poor containment and detachment from their community life. This situation, again, opposes the clinical practice that PICU is designed for. There is the notion that inpatient admission can lead to adverse outcomes for such patients (Bennett et al., 2013), though research on outcome measures is limited.

Short-Term Management in PICU for Borderline Personality Disorder and Self-Harm

The most likely scenario of a patient with a sole diagnosis of borderline personality being admitted to a PICU is for 'crisis presentations' or 'crisis management' (Oldham, 2004; Bennett et al., 2013; Oldham, 2019; Gintalaite-Bieliauskiene et al., 2020; Hong and Kasher, 2020). These terms incorporate a range of psychopathology, including disturbed behaviour, self-harm, impulsive aggression, psychotic symptoms, intense anxiety, depression and anger. PICUs are often viewed as the next option, particularly when strategies are perceived to have failed on open wards. A PICU that is low in stimulus, 'sterile' and intensely staffed is felt to be ideal in containing such acute states.

There is a lack of clinical guidance mapping out a specific approach to patients presenting with crisis in PICU and high levels of self-harm in the context of personality disorder (Mangall and Yurkovich, 2008). However, there are basic principles a general PICU team can utilise to achieve stability in these situations using input from all MDT members. The main aim for an approach in the short term is to enable the patient to reach stability, which in turn should lead to a decrease in their risk behaviour. The onset of a 'crisis' is associated with a precipitating event, so management strategies should focus on underlying issues rather than adopt a reactive stance.

Pharmacological Interventions

Rapid tranquilisation (RT) is commonly used when self-harm behaviour or aggressive behaviour has not responded to other interventions, often as a last resort. PICUs will have a policy offering guidance on the use of RT and which medications to use (Patel et al., 2018). Typical options include benzodiazepines or antipsychotics, or a combination of both, administered intramuscularly. As it stands, there is no licensed medication for borderline personality disorder, so any prescriptions will be off license (Paton and Okocha, 2006; Kendall et al., 2010). There is no evidence to suggest that higher doses lead to superior response, and polypharmacy should be avoided.

When considering the use of RT, clinicians should ensure that there is an appropriate legal status in place, the capacity and consent of the patient is sought and documented and that the intervention is proportionate to the risk posed. Any physical health conditions must also be factored in when deciding the prescription of RT, and robust monitoring must occur post administration.

Teams should be mindful of the patient's perspective when RT is used; the use of restraint, removal of clothing to expose site for injections and the presence of several staff may cause patients to relive traumatic experiences where similar interactions have occurred (i.e. sexual abuse, previous hospital admissions) or indeed lead to new traumatic memories being formed. This will compound existing crisis presentations.

Another pitfall with the use of RT is that patients may become accustomed to the entire intervention and seek it to gratify other deficits. For example, use of intramuscular injection may consolidate the sick role and the need for inpatient care and lack of responsibility, elicit care from a number of staff, reinforce behaviour and be a means of addressing sensory deficits. It is important to be aware of the

benefit a patient may be achieving from RT, particularly if there is a pattern of overuse or regular seeking behaviour. RT is a short-term measure with the aim to stabilise patients with borderline personality as safely and as quickly as possible so that they are able to engage with longer-term treatment. Therefore, the prescription should be regularly reviewed and used for the shortest time necessary.

Restrictive Practice

There is a challenge regarding managing self-harm in all inpatient settings, and PICUs are no exception. The perception by acute wards is that due to its greater restrictions, the PICU is better suited to manage DSH. Borderline personality disorder is associated with a wide repertoire of self-injurious behaviour, with patients often able to cause self-injury by inventive means. Head banging, ingesting and/or inserting objects, cutting, ligaturing, and friction burns are some examples of methods. The approach to managing self-harm is to acknowledge that this behaviour, like all behaviours, has a function. It is important to undertake functional behavioural analysis to understand what the patient is hoping to gain by engaging in self-harm and what it means to them. Once this is understood, professionals can proceed to encourage patients to take on other strategies to replace the self-injurious behaviour and still achieve a similar gain as they do from self-harm. This may take a significant amount of time to understand and consolidate due to complexities in this behaviour. To allow full understanding of behaviour and make strategies as effective as possible, it is ideal to gain the insight of the referring team and incorporate their observations and strategies (if possible) prior to admission to PICU.

There may be instances where a patient engages in severe DSH, to the point of significantly compromising their physical health. It is usually at this point where restraint, anti-rip clothing, intramuscular injection, limited access to items and enhanced nursing observations may be required. Mechanical restraint, such as use of the emergency restraint belt (ERB), although used in secure settings, has a role in PICUs that is contentious. As with other interventions, these should be care planned and time limited with regular reviews. There is a danger of placing increasing restrictions on a patient with no real exit plan, reaching a situation where the patient may counter this by engaging in progressively more severe self-harm to the point where the PICU has exhausted its management options and teams begin to feel that the patient can no longer be cared for safely. Associated with this is iatrogenic harm, with new ways of self-harm being sought out and learnt and the patient's feelings of lack of control, identity and dignity (due to invasive interventions) and hopelessness exemplified. Lack of autonomy can lead to dependency and institutionalisation. High restrictions can also be massively traumatising for patients or can regenerate past traumas. Of note, there is a group of patients with borderline personality who respond with violence towards staff in the context of being restrained or feeling that they are in an 'us vs them' (them being professionals) dynamic.

A balance ideally should be struck between teams exercising the necessary interventions to ensure that the patient is safe and not physically at risk and the patient having responsibility and autonomy (Crawford et al., 2021). Collaborative care and joint decision-making in respect of restraint care plans, RT and nursing observations should be practiced, with the aim of sharing responsibility for the patient's outcomes. Any restriction placed on the individual should be carefully assessed as being proportionate and with there being a viable exit plan in place to work towards with specified time scales (Georgeiva et al., 2010). If such measures do not work, then it may be that the PICU team considers alternative placements or external opinions. Positive reinforcement of maladaptive behaviour should be avoided to prevent or at least minimise the patient using self-harm to meet a need that could be otherwise achieved in a healthier way.

Psychological Interventions

Formulation of the patient's history and current difficulties is an essential starting point in understanding factors that have precipitated and that may be perpetuating their crisis state. It is also key in directing management plans and looking beyond 'behaviour' and the label of 'personality disorder'.

Positive behavioural support (PBS) plans play a pivotal role in managing behaviours associated with crisis. The PBS model looks to identify early warning signs of maladaptive behaviour and directs de-escalation and distraction techniques to prevent a crisis situation. Functional analysis of antecedents to self-harm provides collateral information to inform PBS plans. It is patient centred, collaboratively constructed and a 'live document' to be adapted and honed according to new information

and circumstances. It consists of primary prevention, secondary prevention and crisis management. The model strives to empower individuals in the management of their behaviours in a proactive manner.

Crisis Care Plans

When a patient is in an emotional crisis, symptoms and signs of this should be carefully collated, along with any triggers. Once stabilised, the patient and staff can collaboratively put together a crisis plan which identifies early warning signs and come up with a contingency plan including primary prevention (i.e. prevent the crisis occurring) and secondary prevention (if in crisis, to minimise the extent). An example may be: 'When I am in crisis I stop speaking to staff. However, when I am well, I utilise 1:1 sessions with staff. To help me speak to staff when I am in crisis, I will use flash cards to communicate my feelings. It would be helpful to me as well as make me feel understood if staff can offer me flash cards when they notice this.'

Approach to Incidents of Serious Violence

Unfortunately, due to the nature of the PICU population, many of the patients pose a risk of violence to others. Violence within the context of a personality disorder is usually within the situation of staff intervening to stop self-harm when restrictive measures are put in place (i.e. items removed from room) or there are interpersonal conflicts with peers. The risk incidents should be carefully logged with detail of the extent of violence. These reports can build a picture of the risk to others and allow staff to identify antecedents to the violent behaviour. The team may take the view to involve the criminal justice system to investigate such assaults; this may help reinforce the consequences of harmful actions. This process may require an opinion on capacity at the time of the assault and whether a patient is fit to be interviewed by the police. Advice from forensic services can be sought in cases where there are serious acts of instrumental violence to others. The risk of DSH in police custody and its implications may need to be explored. Of note, if serious violence to others occurs in the context of staff intervening when a patient is self-harming or being restricted in another way, the team may need to consider alternative interventions to manage self-harm.

Seclusion and long-term segregation should not be used solely for self-harm; however, such facilities may be justified if input from staff to manage self-harm leads to violence towards staff. If used, an exit plan should be formulated as soon as possible to avoid a situation in which progress becomes static and interventions focus only on risk incidents. There is also the difficulty of managing DSH while the patient is in seclusion. Concealed items, slower staff response to physical injury (due to the barriers of seclusion and risk of violence) and evolving and sophisticated methods of DSH while in the restricted environment of seclusion (head banging, choking using food, ligature with hair, self-biting) are all concerns. The decision to seclude a patient with such DSH repertoire would require input from a range of professional disciplines and a regular review of whether the risk to others outweighs the risk of DSH.

Longer-Term Strategies for Engagement and Management of Borderline Personality Disorder and Self-Harm in a PICU Setting

Sensory Needs

Patients with borderline personality may resort to DSH to regulate sensory deficits (Brown et al., 2009). Therefore, a sensory assessment may be important in informing interventions to minimise DSH. For example, certain sensations that result from DSH can be replaced by safer, more grounding sensory interventions such as weighted blankets, fidget gadgets, ice, soothe boxes, scents or lights. Patients may benefit from experimenting with a range of sensory items and find techniques that are likely to work for them when they are in a distressed state. A dedicated sensory room may be a helpful resource. Overall, it is important for teams to acknowledge that PICUs can cause hyperarousal and be overwhelming environments, and that this may be hindering recovery in cases complicated with past trauma (Sutton and Nicholson, 2011).

Psychological Therapies

There is a range of possible longer-term therapies that can be delivered once crisis states have improved; the suitability will depend on the main symptoms and formulation. Dialectical behavioural therapy (DBT) and mentalisation-based therapy are often considered. Patients may not meet criteria for intensive therapy, as there is a prerequisite for emotional stability, little or no risk incidents and an ability to tolerate and process trauma. However, there is scope for an adapted form of DBT or skills-based interventions that can provide patients with skills to deal with crisis behaviours and reduce the level of crisis (Hoch et al., 2006; Walsh-Harrington et al., 2020). This may be delivered individually or via ward-based groups. The only real necessity is that the patient should have some motivation to want to address their behaviours and lessen distress. A 'DBT-informed' PICU environment with staff consistently using and implementing techniques to support patients is also key.

Occupational Interventions

Occupational interventions and structured meaningful activities which have personal meaning to the individual can lead to a decrease in emotional instability, DSH and impulsivity. Creating a structured day allows for the individual to be involved in meaningful activity and distraction. Valued activities and achievement of vocational goals can improve a sense of self and help establish identity, the latter being a core trait of emotionally unstable personality disorder. Routine is important to increase the perception of control, which leads to increased feelings of safety. This in turn leads to a reduction in instability, chaos and DSH.

Pharmacological Options

While psychological treatments and occupational therapies are constructive interventions for the individual with borderline personality disorder on a PICU, they are of limited effectiveness if there is a lack of engagement and commitment. This may be due to severe symptoms causing a hindrance in functioning. Clozapine has been used by psychiatrists with a view to treat challenging symptoms which may be obstructing engagement. Studies have shown that clozapine can reduce aggressive behaviour and self-harm. In addition, there are qualitative findings of the drug improving mental health and well-being (Zarzar and McEvoy, 2013). There are no medications licensed for the treatment of borderline personality disorder; therefore, clozapine is prescribed off license. There is currently a randomised controlled trial in phase IV with objectives to investigate and gather evidence for the clinical effectiveness and cost effectiveness of clozapine (Crawford et al., 2022). Clozapine appears to be more readily used in secure settings (Ingehoven et al., 2009) and thus there may be a role for use of clozapine in PICUs.

A common finding in borderline personality disorder is the use of psychotropic medication at high doses, often over long durations. Antidepressants, mood stabilisers and antipsychotics are widely used, however, there is little evidence to suggest they improve mental health or social functioning.

A treatment algorithm for borderline personality disorder does not exist. It is more often the case that medication is used to address destructive behaviours and high levels of distress. A symptom-targeted approach may be of benefit.

It is recommended that if medication is used for personality disorder, it should be regularly reviewed and carefully monitored. The patient should also be aware why medication is prescribed and their consent and acknowledgement of it being off license should be clearly documented.

Clear Goals

As far as possible, a clear clinical goal should be identified when a patient is admitted to the PICU and a realistic time set to achieve this (i.e. SMART goals). Ideally, the patient should be involved in the care plan. If the goal is not met within the specified time, there should be a thorough review of what progress has been made and/or what are the barriers to progress. At this point, there may need to be decisions regarding changing approach, using new assessments, reformulating the care plan or re-evaluating whether the PICU is a suitable setting for further management.

Discharge can be a challenging time for patients with personality disorder; they are moving on from one staff group whom they are likely to have formed attachments with to an unfamiliar, uncertain place. They may feel abandoned or rejected by the PICU team and may 'act out' to sabotage progress. It is important in this situation to ensure that the discharge is appropriately paced (some may prefer a quick discharge or section 17 leave beforehand, whereas others may feel more comfortable with a slower transition). However, there needs to be a balance struck to avoid repeated breakdowns in discharge. Successful discharge plans usually require the patient to be invested and motivated to moving on, with supportive receiving teams and a consistent approach from the PICU team.

This is certainly a challenge within today's climate with current bed pressures; however, one has to bear in mind the clinical impact (and cost) of failed discharges when facing such dilemmas.

Collaborative Working

As far as possible, collaborative working with individuals with borderline personality disorder should be encouraged. Therapeutic relationships and investment in their care is an intervention in itself. Basic principles of respect, being shown dignity, honesty and trust should be practiced; this can assure individuals that they are in a safe space and can trust others and enable them to avoid feeling rejected or abandoned. Collaborative decision-making can avoid the scenario of the patient feeling like 'things are done to them' or 'things are taken away from them' and, instead, allow the patient to become invested, enabled and motivated to take steps towards recovery. This also avoids the toxic 'me vs them' dynamic.

Collaborative working is also essential among teams involved. To maximise assessment and management as well as achieve the objectives of PICU admission, ideally, a specific pathway with active involvement from the acute ward or community team who will take over care at discharge should be established. A model where community team members are present and partake in clinical decisions and interventions while the individual is an inpatient increases chances of forging therapeutic relationships, which would frame discharge positively. An example of this may be the community therapist delivering sessions on the PICU.

Extended Support for Professionals and Carers

The distress associated with these crisis states can ripple through those caring for the patient and those in their social support system. There may be situations where carers and professionals mirror feelings of distress, uncertainty, anger and anxiety as a result of transferred feelings. It is therefore important that crisis interventions and long-term plans include support for all individuals involved in the case. Transparent communication and joint working with carers can be useful to work through issues to help with clinical progress. 'The triangle of care' developed by the Carers Trust is a key framework to aid practice (Hannan, 2013).

Positive Risk Management

Suicidal thoughts and gestures are chronic features of emotionally unstable personality disorder. However, they can become the predominant presenting symptoms in crisis states. This can lead to teams reacting solely to these acts and becoming distracted from therapeutic goals. Over time, use of restrictive measures to contain self-injurious behaviour can lead to an increase in risk. Individuals can perceive this as a loss of control, so they try to regain control by escalating their behaviour and seeking out alternative ways to self-harm using methods that they may not have tried before. Such modifications in behaviour can be of greater risk than original presentation. There is also a false sense of security created with intense staff interventions which may also drive the individual to engage in higher levels of misadventure.

Positive risk-taking is identifying that there is a risk present and acknowledging that harm may occur but empowering the patient with an opportunity to manage the risk with support from the clinical team. This is an important aspect of treatment and recovery. Examples of positive risk management include reduction in observations, allowing leave off unit, access to personal belongings and timely discharge.

Accurate and detailed descriptions of risk behaviour, such as self-harm, will inform positive risk-taking strategies. By understanding the function of self-harm behaviours, staff are better equipped to address unmet needs and take positive risks based on a more holistically informed assessment (Ougrin et al., 2012).

Example of Positive Risk-Taking Approach to Ligature-Tying Behaviour

Ligature-tying behaviour is complex, and individuals engage in this method of self-harm for a diverse range of reasons. In whatever context, use of ligatures carries a serious risk of fatality and can cause great anxiety and uncertainty in how this can be managed in an inpatient setting. To inform a management strategy, each ligature incident should be analysed in detail (see Box 12.1.) (Panchal et al., 2019). Themes in the ligature-tying behaviour can build a picture of the nature of the individual risk and the function of the behaviour. This can be formulated in MDT meetings. Once there is a risk formulation, a detailed risk document of the ligature-tying behaviour (i.e. a 'ligature-tying profile') can be made and interventions can be based upon this. For example, if a patient is known to tie ligatures using socks or clothing only, it may be that taking a positive risk and enabling the individual to have access to headphones that may be useful for distraction can be justified.

It is important that positive risk-taking plans be regularly reviewed and collaboratively constructed with all professionals working with the individual as well as with the patient theirself.

Box 12.1 Ligature Assessment Tool

1. Were alarms activated?
2. Which area of the ward did ligature take place?
3. What item was used to ligature?
4. Was the item tied or held?
5. Were there any other additional items used in the ligature? Any knots? Any modifications?
6. How long (approximately) was the ligature on?
7. Was it a tight or loose ligature?
8. Was there any change in physical health of the patient whilst the ligature was on?
9. Was restraint involved?
10. Were ligature cutters used?
11. Was the ligature concealed in any way?
12. Were there any concerns with physical health after the ligature was removed? What, if any, physical observations were needed after ligature removal?
13. Were there any obstruction/resistance to removal?
14. Was this an actual or attempted ligature?
15. Was there any additional risk behaviour?

Common Challenges with Habitual Self-Harm in the PICU Setting

Habitual self-harm poses many difficulties for staff in a PICU setting, as incidents of self-harm are often impulsive with little or no observable antecedent. Staff who work with self-harm on a regular basis may experience numerous challenges. Staff may feel frustrated by the patient's lack of progress despite their intense input and investment in their treatment. Multiple interventions may have been tried yet failed to address the self-harm. This may lead to staff feeling hopeless and despondent. There is also the sense of inadequacy and an inability to fulfil their role. In addition, constant self-harm incidents equate to an increase in workload (increased observations, incident forms, responding to incidents, dealing with self-harm injuries, hospital escorts when referred out for physical treatment, updating risk assessments, etc.). Staff reactions to self-harm can vary from those who are overly reactive to those who may be de sensitised, which leads to team splitting and inconsistent approaches. Staff may also fear external scrutiny of their interventions or lack thereof. Self-harm acts can be perpetuated by staff focusing on the physical act rather than addressing the underlying function.

Regular self-harm incidents on a PICU not only effect the staff but also have a profound impact on the patient. In addition to physical injury, psychological harm can occur; the patient suffers ongoing distress, trauma, relives traumatic memories of past abuse (from self-harm or an abuser), feelings of hopelessness and low self-esteem. They may be receptive to staff's changing attitudes towards them because of their self-harm behaviour. Fractured therapeutic relationships can cause the patient to experience rejection and abandonment. This can seriously hinder recovery and lead to both parties feeling stagnated. There is also risk of patients coming to harm with overuse of medication, restrictive measures and restraint.

Strategies for Managing Impact of Self-Harming Behaviour upon PICUs

It is important for staff to be supported when they are responding to self-harm on a PICU. This can take various forms. Regular reflective sessions for staff facilitated by psychology staff not directly involved in the case is an important resource for staff to express their experiences and associated feelings in a safe space.

Training and education dedicated to understanding self-harm behaviour in the context of borderline personality disorder is important in ensuring staff are skilled in their approach to self-harm and are doing so in a consistent manner. As with other areas, PICU settings may benefit from a member of staff who has an interest in borderline personality disorder and self-harm (a 'personality disorder/self-harm champion') to specialise in this area and share their expertise among their colleagues. The stigma attached to self-harm and borderline personality disorder can also be addressed through acting in a consistent manner.

PICU principles have a focus on short stay, targeted assessment and treatment and management of risk. Self-harm can blur all of these, and the usual approaches may feel redundant. It is important to acknowledge this and accept that cases of borderline personality disorder are complex. Requesting second opinions and reviewing diagnostic formulations via these proposed strategies regularly allow PICU teams to consider new perspectives and new strategies in moving forward with a case. Advice from specialist personality disorder services in challenging cases is a valuable resource to access, particularly as these teams are well versed in dealing with such complex cases.

Conclusion

The very nature of personality disorder opposes the role of a PICU setting. It can lead to protracted admissions, unclear management plans, overuse of restrictive measures and potentially a long-stay patient in an environment that may no longer be therapeutic, leading to a counterproductive admission. It is important to acknowledge that complex patients who require PICU and exhibit DSH may have a range of comorbidities (both personality dysfunction and mood/psychotic disorders) and thus a robust formulation and holistic management strategies are essential. It should also be accepted that understanding DSH in such individuals is extremely complicated.

References

Ali,S and Findlay,C (2016) A Review of NICE Guidelines on the Management of Borderline Personality Disorder. *British Journal of Medical Practitioners* 9: 1.

Bennett,L Dixon,R and Gintalaite-Bieliauskiene,K (2013) Is Management of Borderline Personality Disorder in Female

Psychiatric Intensive Care Unit (PICU) Appropriate? *Abstracts of the 21st European Congress of Psychiatry* 28 1.

Brown,S, Shankar,R and Smith,K (2009) Borderline Personality Disorder and Sensory Processing Impairment. *Progress in Neurology and Psychiatry* 13(4) 10–16.

Crawford,MJ, Leeson,VC, Evans,R, Barrett,B, McQuaid,A, Cheshire,J, et al. (2022) The Clinical Effectiveness and Cost Effectiveness of Clozapine for Inpatients with Severe Borderline Personality Disorder (CALMED Study): A Randomised Placebo-Controlled Trial. *Therapeutic Advances in Psychopharmacology* 12: 20451253221090832.

Crawford,O, Khan,T and Zimbron,J (2021) Rethinking Risk Assessments in a Borderline Personality Disorder Unit: Patient and Staff Perspectives. *Cureus* 13 (2) e13557.

Fagin,L (2004) Management of Personality Disorders in Acute In-Patient Settings. Part 1: Borderline Personality Disorders. *Advances in Psychiatric Treatment* 10 (2) 93–9.

Fallon,P (2003) Travelling through the System: The Lived Experience of People with Borderline Personality Disorder in Contact with Psychiatric Services. *Journal of Psychiatric and Mental Health Nursing* 10 (4) 393–401.

Fowler,J, Clapp,J, Madan,A, Allen,J, Frueh,B, Fonagy,P, et al. (2018) A Naturalistic Longitudinal Study of Extended Inpatient Treatment for Adults with Borderline Personality Disorder: An Examination of Treatment Response, Remission and Deterioration. *Journal of Affective Disorders* 235: 323–31.

Georgieva,A, De Haan,G, Smith,W and Mulder,C (2010) Successful Reduction of Seclusion in a Newly Developed Psychiatric Intensive Care Unit. *Journal of Psychiatric Intensive Care* 6 (1) 31–8.

Gintalaite-Bieliauskiene,K, Dixon,R and Bennett,L (2020) A Retrospective Survey of Care Provided to Patients with Borderline Personality Disorder Admitted to a Female Psychiatric Intensive Care Unit. *Journal of Psychiatric Intensive Care* 16 (1) 35–42.

Hannan,R (2013) The Triangle of Care: Carers Included. *Journal of Public Mental Health* 12 (3) 171–2.

Haw,C, Kotterova,E and Otuwehinmi,O (2017) Out of Area Referrals to Two Independent Sector PICUs: Who, How, Why and When? *Journal of Psychiatric Intensive Care* 13 (1) 37–45.

Hayward,M, Slade,M and Moran PA (2006) Personality Disorders and Unmet Needs among Psychiatric Inpatients. *Psychiatric Services* 57: 538–43.

Hoch,J, O'Reilly,R. and Carscadden,J (2006) Best Practices: Relationship Management Therapy for Patients with Borderline Personality Disorder. *Psychiatric Services* 57 (2) 179–81.

Hong,V and Casher,M (2020) The Inpatient with Borderline Personality Disorder. In Casher,M and Bess,J (eds.), *Manual of Inpatient Psychiatry*. Cambridge: Cambridge University Press. pp. 82–105.

Ingenhoven,T, Lafay,P, Rinne,T, Passchier,J. and Duivenvoorden,H (2009) Effectiveness of Pharmacotherapy for Severe Personality Disorders. *The Journal of Clinical Psychiatry* 71 (01) 14–25.

Kendall,T, Burbeck,R and Bateman,A (2010) Pharmacotherapy for Borderline Personality Disorder: NICE Guideline. *British Journal of Psychiatry* 196 (2) 158–9.

Mangnall,J and Yurkovich,E (2008) A Literature Review of Deliberate Self-Harm. *Perspectives in Psychiatric Care.* 44 (3) 175–84.

National Association of Psychiatric Intensive Care and Low Secure Units (NAPICU) (2016) *Guidance for Commissioners of Psychiatric Intensive Care Units (PICU)*. Glasgow: NAPICU. https://napicu.org.uk/wp-content/uploads/2016/04/Commissioning_Guidance_Apr16.pdf.

National Institute for Health and Care Excellence (NICE) (2009) *Borderline Personality Disorder: Recognition and Management (clinical guideline [CG78])*. London: NICE. www.nice.org.uk/guidance/CG78.

Oldham,J (2004) Borderline Personality Disorder: The Treatment Dilemma. *Journal of Psychiatric Practice* 10 (3) 204–6.

Oldham,J (2019) Inpatient Treatment for Patients with Borderline Personality Disorder. *Journal of Psychiatric Practice* 25 (3) 177–8.

Ougrin,D, Tranah,T, Leigh,E, Taylor,L and Rosenbaum Asarnow,J (2012) Practitioner Review: Self-Harm in Adolescents. *Journal of Child Psychiatry* 53 (4) 337–50.

Panchal,R, Attard,S and Baker,J (2019) *Development of Ligature Assessment Tool. [Poster]*. Faculty of Forensic Psychiatry Annual Conference, The Royal College of Psychiatrists 6–8 March 2019. Vienna.

Paris,J (2002) Clinical Practice Guidelines for Borderline Personality Disorder. *Journal of Personality Disorders* 16 (2) 107–8.

Patel,M, Sethi,F, Barnes,T, Dix,R, Dratcu,L, Fox,B., et al. (2018) Joint BAP NAPICU Evidence-Based Consensus Guidelines for the Clinical Management of Acute Disturbance: De-escalation and Rapid Tranquillisation. *Journal of Psychopharmacology* 32 (6) 601–40.

Paton,C and Okocha,C (2006) Pharmacological Treatment of Borderline Personality Disorder. *Journal of Psychiatric Intensive Care* 1 (2) 105–16.

Royal College of Psychiatrists (2020) *Standards for Psychiatric Intensive Care Units*. London: Royal College of Psychiatrists. www.rcpsych.ac.uk/docs/default-source/improving-care/ccqi/quality-networks/picu/picu-qn-standards-qnpicu/qnpicu-standards-for-psychiatric-intensive-care-units-2020-(2nd-edition)-v2a38355b0f61d4b46ba68b586c46bdf1e.pdf?sfvrsn=e09e1ee8_2.

Royal College of Psychiatrists (2020) *PS01/20: Services for People Diagnosable with Personality Disorder*. London: Royal College of Psychiatrists. www.rcpsych.ac.uk/docs/de

fault-source/improving-care/better-mh-policy/position-statements/ps01_20.pdf?sfvrsn=85af7fbc_2.

Sutton,D and Nicholson,E (2011) *Sensory Modulation in Acute Mental Health Wards: A Qualitative Study of Staff and Service User Perspectives.* Auckland, NZ: The National Centre of Mental Health Research, Information and Workforce Development (Te Pou).

Walsh-Harrington,S, Corrigall,F and Elsegood,KJ (2020) Is it worthwhile to offer a daily 'bite-sized' recovery skills group to women on a psychiatric intensive care unit (PICU)?. *Journal of Psychiatric Intensive Care* **16** (1) 29–34.

World Health Organization (1993) *The ICD-10 Classification of Mental and Behavioural Disorders: Diagnostic Criteria for Research.* Geneva: World Health Organization.

Zarzar,T and McEvoy,J (2013) Clozapine for Self-Injurious Behavior in Individuals with Borderline Personality Disorder. *Therapeutic Advances in Psychopharmacology* **3** (5) 272–74.

Chapter 13

Activity and Positive Engagement within a PICU

Rebecca Davies, Robert Rathouse and Wendy Sherwood

Introduction

Human beings have an innate drive toward doing – actively engaging with the environment, using materials and objects, interacting with and doing with people. Through doing tasks, activities and occupations, human beings learn, develop knowledge, gain essential sensory, motor, cognitive, emotional and social stimulation, develop skills, express themselves and find meaning in their lives. To quote Hooper and Wood (2019, p. 46), 'in essence, humankind is occupational by nature'.

Being able to do activities is fundamental to the health, well-being and quality of life of every single one of us. Access to meaningful activity or occupation is a matter of justice; hence, deprivation of activity participation due to being inhibited by the environment is occupational injustice (Durocher et al., 2013) and a major concern for all psychiatric intensive care unit (PICU) multidisciplinary teams (MDTs).

Human beings have three universal needs which are essential to health and well-being, regardless of age, culture, gender or ethnicity. These needs are for autonomy, competence and relatedness (social belonging and connectedness) (Deci and Ryan, 1985, 2000, 2008). *Autonomy* refers to having choice and control over what one does and does not do. We all need to have *competence* in what we do so that our doing is successful, we experience mastery, develop abilities and self-esteem and gain satisfaction. We also need activities that involve people and enable us to *connect with and form relationships* with others. For people coming into the psychiatric intensive care setting, the meeting of these human needs is significantly affected and therefore the provision of meaningful and satisfying activity is as important for the PICU team to provide as any other intervention. Doing so has been found to increase patient engagement, enable their development and recovery of abilities, reduce problematic behaviours, improve ward atmosphere and the therapeutic environment, and increase staff–patient contact and staff job satisfaction. Hence, meeting patient needs for activity enhances positive engagement for patients and staff and has the potential to empower individuals to actively participate in their care as an aim of therapeutic engagement (Pereira and Wollaston, 2007). A focus on engagement should be a culture within inpatient psychiatry (NICE, 2015), and enhancing positive engagement through meeting needs for activity participation requires careful consideration in a PICU.

Given that all activity provision carries risks, it is understood that thorough risk assessment informs MDT decision-making in all individual and group-based activities.

Why Activities Are Important to Every Patient

The activities of our lives are a central part of our identity – when we meet someone new, one of the first and natural questions to ask is, 'what do you do?' Activities shape our daily lives, roles, responsibilities and the contribution we make to the lives of our friends, families, communities and society.

We need a balance in our activities in two main ways. First, we need a balance in broad categories of activities that shape day-to-day life. These include activities for personal management (self-care, domestic activities, managing home and second, personal affairs), productivity (work, study, hobbies, roles) and use of free time (recreation). Amongst these activities, we also need activities that enable social contact, interaction and relationships. We also need balance between activities that require adherence to socially defined norms, rules, standards and expectations, and activities that are freer, for fun and/or allow for self-expression. We require activities and roles to be organised into a routine, providing our lives with structure, purpose and meaning (Lilja and Hellzén, 2008, p. 282). On admission into a PICU, all these needs remain; however, when a person experiences acute psychiatric illness, ability to do meaningful activities is diminished. This is particularly so during acute psychosis, which due to disturbances in how an individual perceives theirself and the surrounding world, including the people, materials and objects involved in daily activities, there is a profound and devastating effect on a person's ability to engage in and do activities (Hitch et al., 2013). In dealing with the confusion of disturbed perceptions of reality, the unfamiliarity of everything around them can have a significant impact on individuals. A person admitted into a PICU is detached from their daily roles and the routine of activities and social interactions that make up their lives. Instead, patients are experiencing unfamiliar surroundings that can be confusing, leaving them feeling socially isolated, disconnected from people and without control over their lives (Wood and Alsawy, 2016). This contributes to the distressing experience of being a patient in a psychiatric ward (Wood and Alsawy, 2016).

It is important that the PICU team understand the potential impact on individuals of being unable to do meaningful activities for a length of time, which is likely to occur in PICUs. Occupational deprivation is 'a state of preclusion from engagement in occupations of necessity and/or meaning due to factors that stand outside the immediate control of the individual' (Whiteford, 2010, p. 201). Deprivation is unavoidable to a certain degree not only because individuals are detached from their usual activities, roles and routine but also because risk management means they are unable to access and use materials and objects that are essential for doing certain activities. This can make doing them unsatisfying or impossible, resulting in frustration, aggression, destructive behaviours and decline in mental and physical health and well-being. Deprivation can also occur because there is a lack of understanding about what is meaningful activity for individual patients. There is a complete lack of literature on the meaningfulness of activities in PICUs for patients from Black, Asian and minority ethnic (BAME) backgrounds. This is striking, given that BAME populations are disproportionally represented within inpatient mental health settings, particularly under detentions of the Mental Health Act (MHA) (Burki, 2018) and are more likely to undergo containment measures (Department of Health and Social Care, 2018).

Prolonged activity/occupational deprivation or lack of stimulation in inpatient psychiatric units often results in the dissatisfying and frustrating experience of boredom (Shepherd and Lavender, 1999; NICE, 2011; Taube-Schiff et al., 2016), which can be understood as an affective state (Marshall et al., 2020) – 'the aversive experience of wanting, but being unable to engage in satisfying activity' (Eastwood et al., 2012, p. 482). High levels of boredom negatively affect patients (Chervalier et al., 2018) and can be experienced as a chronic stressor (Eastwood et al., 2012), leading to depression and anxiety (Goldberg et al., 2011), overeating and binge eating (e.g. Stickney and Miltenberger, 1999). Furthermore, boredom due to a lack of satisfying activities can negatively affect the ward environment (Akther et al., 2019) and lead to an increase in unsafe behaviours (Royal College of Psychiatrists, 2011), such as self-harm (Molin et al., 2016), aggression (Lamanna et al., 2016) and violence (Chaplin et al., 2006), as well as interfere with recovery (Royal College of Psychiatrists, 2011; Molin et al., 2016). Hence, for these reasons and to minimise the trauma of a PICU admission, enabling individuals to engage in and do activities is part of everyone's role in a PICU service; it is as important as enabling patients to receive their medication (Royal College of Psychiatrists, 2011).

The National Institute for Health and Care Excellence (NICE, 2019, p. 30) outlines the need for patients in inpatient mental health services to access meaningful culturally appropriate activities. Their purpose is to 'help provide a structure to their day and reduce stress, frustration and boredom . . . help to increase their social interactions, relieve anxiety and improve well-being' (NICE, 2011, p. 43).

Benefits of Doing Activities

What daily activities we do is generally motivated by having an interest in them and/or valuing them for providing purpose and meaning to our lives in our socio-cultural contexts. Individuals with certain diagnoses can be negatively affected in terms of their motivation to engage in activities, for example, a decline in interest, motivation and sense of satisfaction from activity engagement is common with depression. It can, therefore, be significantly challenging to actively engage depressed individuals in activity and for them to perceive its therapeutic value. Conversely, mania can increase motivation to participate in activities and drive a need to do many activities for long periods of time, the benefits from which are somewhat difficult to define or predict. Equally, mania can result in individuals being too distracted to meaningfully participate at all. Although there are such challenges to activity engagement, it is important to provide activities and enable engagement as best we can while being sensitive and responsive to individual needs and stages of recovery.

We also occupy ourselves as a distraction from stressors, anxieties and worries, as being occupied with something else for a while can result in feeling more relaxed or alleviated by the respite. This is also true for many patients who find being distracted from disturbing symptoms beneficial (Bryant et al., 2016).

Significantly, we do activities because they pose us with challenges, which, if we can master, positively impacts self-esteem, confidence, sense of competence and development of knowledge, functional abilities and skills. This is an important point. The provision of activities in a PICU does not mean that patients will be motivated to do them; having activities of interest is not sufficient to satisfy human beings. We need to experience challenge, allowing our abilities to be used and stretched, and to experience mastery of challenges and acquisition of new skills (van der Reyden and Sherwood, 2019). Only providing activities that are either very easy to do or are beyond a person's capabilities is likely to result in patient boredom with negative consequences.

The following list provides insight into some of the benefits of doing activities:

- Meets fundamental human need 'to do'
- Connects the person with theirself and the surrounding world (human and non-human environment); orientation to surroundings and reality
- Enables maintenance of present level of motivation and functioning
- Enables the development or recovery of motivation, functional abilities and skills
- Provides opportunities to develop insight and understanding of mental illness
- Enables experience of pleasure and enjoyment (Cook and Chambers, 2009; Hitch, 2009)
- Elicits feelings of hope and purpose (Molin et al., 2016)
- Facilitates relaxation
- Facilitates self-expression

- Provides sense of purpose
- Enhances confidence, self-efficacy, self-worth and sense of self (e.g. that the patient can do things despite being unwell, promoting hope and ability to cope) (Hitch, 2009)
- Promotes choice, autonomy, sense of control and contributing to managing illness through doing
- Provides opportunities for social contact and relating to people
- Provides opportunities for taking on roles and responsibilities
- Provides respite from challenging aspects of the lived experience of mental illness (Hitch et al., 2013)

Activity for Treatment

Historically, enabling patients to participate in activities has been misunderstood as being solely the role of occupational therapists in mental health services. However, the provision of activity for the purpose of giving patients something meaningful and purposeful to do, reduce boredom and structure their day differs from the activity-based interventions provided by occupational therapists, psychologists and music and art therapists who use activity as a means of assessment, treatment and discharge planning (CCQI, 2017, p.9; Fitzgerald, 2016).

The overall aim of occupational therapy in a PICU is to enable patients to increase their level of functioning, skills and promote recovery (Sims, 2014), using activity (also termed occupation) as the primary assessment and treatment medium. Additionally, occupational therapists undertake specialised assessments of motivation, function and occupational needs, and provide targeted intervention/treatment that is graded to each individual's abilities, needs, goals and treatment aims. To this purpose, occupational therapy is identified to be a complex intervention (Pentland et al., 2018).

The therapeutic use of activity by occupational therapists is valued for enabling patients to manage their mental distress, develop or recover skills and function better in their daily lives (Curtis et al., 2007; Lim et al., 2007; Kennedy and Fortune, 2014), gain confidence in own abilities (Lim et al., 2007), gain respite from anxieties and the ward and prepare for discharge, as described by Lloyd and Williams (2010).

Occupational therapists have professional knowledge and skills that should support the PICU team in effectively providing activity to patients who differ greatly in motivation and abilities, whether on an individual or group basis, and when relatively stable or most acutely disturbed, including when in seclusion.

Assessing Suitability of Activity Provision

To identify what activities are likely to be beneficial to individual patients and how they are best structured and facilitated, the team needs to assess an individual's motivation and ability to engage in an activity or activities. Information on patients' interest in activities and ability for activity participation may be gained from their family or carers, in addition to that gained directly from the patient. However, motivation and ability fluctuate in response to changes in the individual's mental and physical state as well as changes in the environment, including people; therefore, dynamic risk assessment is essential.

Assessing the suitability of activity provision involves identifying what is interesting, meaningful (including culturally appropriate) and purposeful activity in order to stimulate and meet motivation. Plus, the mental, physical and social demands of activities and situations in relation to the patient's abilities must be considered. The complexity of this task can be underestimated, hence it is recommended that the PICU team includes an occupational therapist (NAPICU, 2014); however, all members of the PICU team can undertake and contribute to assessments. This will enable practitioners to work alongside patients to set personalised goals and treatment plans which are highly likely to include participation in activity-based opportunities as well as manage associated risks.

Challenges in assessing include the frequent fluctuation in patient motivation and ability to engage with staff, do activities and communicate. Subsequently, informal, non-standardised assessment is commonly used in a PICU environment, although occupational therapists may also use formal, specialised standardised assessment methods.

Informal observational assessment involves watching how the patient interacts with peers and staff on the ward and within small group situations. This involves close observation of ability to:

- understand the situation
- actively participate and engage with people, in activities and the situation

- manage the challenges that this poses to the individual in terms of mental, physical and social demands

The informality of staff doing activities alongside patients and having casual conversations with them can help to obtain important assessment information as well as build trust and therapeutic rapport. A simple conversation with someone can prompt them to open up about their interests. Taking individuals to the activity room to show them what is available affords the opportunity to observe what they immediately gravitate towards, such as art materials, indicating what is motivating in terms of interest and meaningfulness. The patient's understanding of activities and the materials and processes involved provides important information on their cognition, perception, sensory processing and other skills. Whether a patient can accurately judge whether they have the ability to do activities of interest provides valuable information on cognition (e.g. self-evaluation, judgement) and their insight into their mental state and abilities.

Occupational therapists can assess all these factors and relate them to information on the individual's past, present and future occupational needs in detail using theory-based assessments, including standardised tools provided by models of practice. For example, from the Model of Human Occupation (Taylor, 2016), tools include the Interest Checklist, the Model of Human Occupation Screening Tool (MOHOST) (Parkinson et al., 2006) and the Volitional Questionnaire (De las Heras et al., 2007), which may be used to inform use of the re-motivation process (De las Heras et al., 2019) as an intervention strategy. The Vona du Toit Model of Creative Ability (van der Reyden et al., 2019) enables the team to identify a patient's level of motivation and corresponding abilities, guiding all intervention with an individual, including enabling the patient to maintain activity participation within seclusion (Jeffries, 2021). Additionally, occupational therapists can assess specific cognitive, physical, social and sensory functioning for which there are a broad range of assessment tools, including specialised tools.

Risk Assessment and Management

Experienced PICU clinicians should be skilled in identifying and reducing risk in all areas of PICU practice and therapeutic activity is no exception. When considering risk in relation to activity, including therapeutic activity on a 1:1 or group basis, the general ward-based risk management procedures are a required starting point for planning the activity. An awareness of staffing levels, training in de-escalation skills and access to alarms are all relevant when planning a group or 1:1 activity. Dynamic risk assessment is essential, for example, considering how the patient is feeling just prior to activity and whether some 1:1 time with staff is needed before doing activities either individually or in a group.

When preparing for a group session that are several environmental factors to consider to keep risk to a minimum:

- Where is the most appropriate location for the group to take place?
- Is the room or space conducive to creating a therapeutic atmosphere?
- Does the space suit the needs of the session?
- Is it in an easily accessible area of the ward where support can reach you easily if necessary?

The maximum number of patients that can join a group is important when considering the size of the room/space. A higher-risk activity, such as cooking, will potentially have less participants than an exercise group to allow the group facilitator/s to be able to observe, identify and proactively reduce the likelihood of risk incidents occurring. The facilitator will also need to observe patient interaction with utensils and tools within the session and ensure they are used appropriately and not removed from the room. The number of participants in a group session can be dynamic from one week to the next and may vary depending on the specific risks associated with individuals and the acuity on the ward on a given day. In order to make these decisions, the facilitator should have an awareness and knowledge of each patient and, if possible, the personal dynamics between them.

Many activities such as cooking and art require the use of materials and tools. Seemingly innocuous items such as paint brushes, colouring pencils and glue can all become charged with risk if used inappropriately. There is the potential that they could be used as weapons against others or as tools for self-harm within a session or secreted to use later. Cupboards storing resources should be locked and risk items signed in and out by staff (e.g. count how many pens are put out and ensure the same number is returned to the cupboard before the end of the session). This is the responsibility of the session facilitator and observing staff members of patients on enhanced observation.

The ward occupational therapist typically creates generic risk assessments for ward therapeutic spaces such as the kitchen and activity room, including safe storage and use of equipment and the potential risks to self or others and how to reduce them. For each group that takes place in these spaces, there should be a group protocol and a risk assessment detailing the purpose and goals of the group and risk management. Depending on the needs of individual patients, it may be necessary to create personalised risk assessments or care plans for specific activities, resources and ward spaces as well as degree of support, observation and supervision required.

Positive Risk-Taking

Many patients have personal skills and interests that they would like to continue to pursue during a PICU admission. It may be possible to support patients to continue with these interests during admission with a view to helping them remain in touch with their typical roles and routines. The feasibility of such requests can be considered and care planned with potential for positive risk-taking which is perceived by psychiatric inpatients to promote recovery (Sustere and Tarpey, 2019). An example of positive risk-taking is allowing a PICU patient to use a personal sewing machine and guitar. In this case, each activity was discussed with the full MDT and all potential risks were considered. Care plans were drawn up in collaboration with the patient in which necessary regulations around use were established and agreed by all. Deviation from the care plan would lead to an MDT decision as to whether it was safe to continue with the activity on a longer-term basis. It was noted that patients greatly gained positive therapeutic benefit from their chosen activity, and that adverse incidents were extremely rare or non-existent when the risk management measures were adhered to.

Activity Engagement in the Management of Violence and Aggression

The use of activity can be highly effective for preventing, reducing and managing violence and aggression on inpatient psychiatric wards, reduce length of admission (Antonysamy, 2013) and help reduce levels of restraint (Wilson et al., 2018). As a preventative intervention, staff joining individuals in activity and engaging with them in the process can build rapport (Janner and Delaney, 2012; Hall et al., 2019) and trust and reduce an individual's feelings of anxiety. Staff taking time to provide and do activities is valued by patients (Hall et al., 2019) and can reduce the risk of aggression (Robinson et al., 1999; Janner and Delaney, 2012). Staff therapeutic engagement with patients helps with getting to know individuals in terms of their likes, dislikes, stressors and relaxants, informing how to minimise frustrations and triggers, mitigate agitation and react helpfully when it occurs (MacKay et al., 2005). For example, enabling 1:1 meaningful activity in a quiet space because the patient prefers this when they are agitated.

When a patient is under continuous observation by a staff member, patient agitation and frustration due to inability to perform usual activities could be reduced by staff doing activity with them, subsequently preventing aggressive incidents. For the management of violence and aggression, observation should be engagement-focused (NICE, 2015), informed by what is meaningful to the individual, such as helping them with their washing or playing a game (Pereira and Woolaston, 2007).

Another preventative strategy which is often overlooked is providing structure and routine, both of which are important to health and well-being. This not only prevents boredom, which can lead to agitation and aggression (Marshall et al., 2020), but also provides a structured environment for patients who find a chaotic environment destabilising. A framework can help these patients to feel more organised, in control and secure. Furthermore, routine and structure can reduce violence and aggression (Beer et al., 2008). As part of a framework, a structured therapeutic activity timetable can be enabling, build familiarity and offer patients an element of choice in what can otherwise be a limiting and restrictive environment. It is important to make patients aware of the ward layout and rules and keep them informed of ward structures and protocols as well as changes to activity programmes and opportunities in order to reduce their frustration with regulations and restrictions and minimise the potential for staff persecution down the line.

Combining risk assessment and de-escalation knowledge and skills with engaging individuals in meaningful activity can de-escalate situations and reduce the likelihood of violent incidents on wards (Kazi et al., 2008; Janner and Delaney, 2012). However, the team should take care that doing this routinely does not result in the embedding of violent or aggressive behaviours due to patients perceiving that negative behaviours achieve the gaining of staff attention or desired resources.

Planned Individual and Group-Based Activity and Engagement

What individual or group-based activity is meaningful to patients should be determined through consultation with patients (Department of Health, 2001). Such collaboration should not only improve patient engagement in the activities but also empower and give patients greater confidence (Sumsion and Law, 2006). Activity engagement requires that the service provides adequate space for activities, including specific spaces for activity-based therapy, in order to support quality of life on the ward and increase mental health (Csipke et al., 2016; NAPICU, 2014). Although space is commonly provided, whether it is adequate needs to be established in consultation with occupational therapists.

Individual Engagement Programmes

Although group work is a common and well-evidenced intervention on psychiatric wards, including psychiatric intensive care (Royal College of Psychiatrists, 2019), it should be noted that group-based intervention is not always conducive to positive patient care for all individuals at every stage of their recovery. It can be necessary to think outside the parameters of traditional patient care, which can be particularly relevant in a fast-paced, dynamic environment where the levels of acuity are high and often fluctuating.

Factors that influence decisions to work with individuals on a 1:1 basis as opposed to a group include their personal interests and goals, the likelihood that proximity to others will cause distress or anxiety, the level of acuity and the patient's mental state and functional ability. Regarding the latter, patients experiencing mania or psychosis may be restless, paranoid or delusional and find it challenging to sit still, interact, concentrate or apply cognitive skills to activity participation. Reducing demands by providing 1:1 activity can enable activity participation and, in the process, prepare the individual for engaging and working alongside others (Pentland et al., 2018). Such 1:1 intervention usually requires staff to provide encouragement and close supervision, facilitation and/or assistance. Supervision is overseeing the person's activity participation to ensure safety and a reasonably successful and satisfying outcome of activity participation and to keep them on task. Facilitation is the interaction required between the staff member and the individual to enable the person to initiate, do, maintain focus and complete the activity. Assistance is physically helping the individual, such as staff placing their hand over the patient's hand to physically move it for enabling participation or practically helping with parts of the activity. This should be accomplished without doing everything for the patient and thus enabling them to gain a sense of satisfaction from their own efforts. It is essential to have realistic expectations of a patient's abilities and not make activities too challenging and unachievable.

Sometimes patients can only manage 30 seconds of activity participation; therefore, having a broad range of activities and ideas is essential together with gaining support on grading activities, staff interaction and environments from occupational therapists. The benefits of this are illustrated by Jeffries (2021) who reported on enabling activity participation in seclusion. On a PICU, temporary risk management strategies such as segregation afford opportunity for patients to engage with activities and staff on a 1:1 basis. Activity choice will depend on the patient's interests and needs at the time, an assessment of risk and availability of resources. Art-based activities such as mindful colouring, painting and drawing, or accessing music and apps on a tablet, are potential activities for segregation, but there is opportunity to be creative in collaboration with the patient and the MDT.

More generally on the ward, some patients with improved mental state and functional abilities benefit from tailored 1:1 intervention because the ward group activities are usually targeting the needs of more acutely unwell patients. This may also be therapeutic for individuals with personality disorder who do not experience mania or psychosis but can manage longer and more complex activities than many other patients. Individual sessions could involve supporting a patient to write a curriculum vitae, develop skills for relaxation or managing anger or stress, pursue a new skill or utilise the ward kitchen for cooking sessions.

Group-Based Activity and Engagement

Group programmes are paramount in a PICU for providing a sense of order in what can be a chaotic environment, as well as meaningful activity, routine and structure for patients who find the concept of time difficult to manage (Poon et al., 2010).

The facilitation of the group programme on the ward is an MDT responsibility in which all disciplines can offer their varying skills (Cook et al., 2016). Activity coordinators and occupational therapists may facilitate or help to implement groups, but there is tremendous value in having diversity in the disciplines facilitating groups within the timetable. It is important to ensure that groups can be effectively facilitated by the staff members that are on hand at the time they are scheduled. This may mean that groups that can be implemented more easily or run on evening and weekends depending on the skills and the time available of individual staff members on shift, but also that all team members have an understanding of the importance of the therapeutic group programme and engagement in it. As NICE (2014, p. 27) suggests, it is the responsibility of staff to 'place emphasis on engagement rather than risk management'.

Programmes should offer a range of activities that are meaningful for a specific patient population that can be diverse in terms of ethnicity and culture; hence, it is preferable to co-produce programmes with patients to best ensure meaningfulness and engagement (Cole, 2014b). However, not all group-based activities are going to be suitable or beneficial to all patients, therefore the team needs to assess the suitability of group-based activities for each individual. This means that there will be times when staff are required to explain to individual patients that they cannot attend a group that they want to go to. This can be a difficult process but is important for preventing more unwell, chaotic patients from disrupting sessions for those further along in their recovery, as well as having a negative experience of activity participation for themselves. Equally, patients just starting to engage in activities can become demoralised and demotivated by seeing the achievements of higher-functioning patients within a group. Therefore, creating groups for patients at the same level of functioning can better enable patients to engage, have a satisfying experience and fulfil their potential (Carpenter et al., 2021; Murphy, 2021; Walker, 2021).

The benefits of group-based activity become apparent in some of the following discussion of specific activities, but the general benefits of doing activities as a group are that individuals can:

- build confidence
- develop a sense of identity and belonging (Cole, 2014b)

- improve social connectedness and feeling of inclusion (Hall et al., 2019)
- improve difficult dynamics with other patients – being engaged in the same activity and working towards the same goal can help resolve minor disputes or at least distract from them through staff promoting interaction and easing communication (Hutcheson et al., 2010)
- improve relationships with staff (Hall et al., 2019)

Critical tasks for staff are planning groups (Cole, 2014b), including developing protocols, risk assessments and plans. These identify the potential value and suitability of the group in a PICU and should mean facilitation and repetition of groups are safer and easier to implement than those that are unplanned or poorly planned and ensure consistency of delivery for new or unfamiliar group facilitators.

When creating a group timetable, some thought should be given to the length of sessions and the time of day they take place as well as ensuring that they are not limited to weekdays or 9–5 hours (Lim et al., 2007). Recurring groups and consistent start and end times can provide structure and routine as well as promote engagement.

Activity and Engagement Programmes for the Unit

As explained at the start of this chapter, people need a balance in activities; hence, activity programmes should include a wide variety of activity sessions including 'fun-based' activities (Pereira and Woollaston, 2007; NAPICU, 2014) and activities that resemble life in the community (Sustere and Tarpey, 2019). The programme should be flexible and informed by patients' needs and requests and resources available, including adequate spaces, staffing and material resources.

Physical Exercise

The evidence for the positive impact of physical activity on mental health has increased exponentially over the last 20 years (Harvey et al., 2018), and its importance is reflected by it being a duty of care for healthcare professionals to provide and encourage patient engagement in physical activities (NICE, 2014; NAPICU, 2016). There are many benefits to physical activity for people with mental illness, including its potential to address associated physical health issues (Alexandratos et al., 2011). For example, medication can lead to akathisia, weight gain and other side effects which can detrimentally effect sleep patterns, self-image and physical health. Physical activity can address many of these issues as well as improve cognition, help control substance misuse, reduce low mood and improve self-image (Cole, 2014a).

In a PICU, physical activity groups can be experienced as a shared activity with shared goals and a shared sense of achievement (Feighan and Roberts, 2017). Exercise-based groups or activities can take the form of competitive sports in which there can be a focus on team camaraderie, or exercise groups for which achieving goals such as keeping up with or completing an exercise routine can offer a sense of accomplishment or inclusion. For those less willing or able to participate in traditional sport/exercise activities, there is a myriad of physical activities that can be engaged in.

In PICUs, there are numerous barriers to patient participation in physical activities. Internal factors include limited motivation and impaired cognitive functioning hindering ability to follow instructions, maintain focus or get organised for exercise. Comorbidities are also common and must be considered, especially if the exercise is physically strenuous. Restricted access to equipment is an external barrier, as is the infeasibility of preferred physical and social environments in which to do physical activity, such as the choice between indoor or outdoor. Large outdoor spaces normally used for sport, and people to engage in sports or activities with, may be inaccessible. Lack of trained staff to facilitate specific physical activities is also a barrier. Such constraints can reduce the activity's meaning for the individual, negatively affecting motivation.

Despite barriers, there are also opportunities, such as:

- Timetabling and carefully structuring exercise groups or sports sessions, including planning staffing
- Tailoring 1:1 sessions to the individual's needs, abilities and motivation
- Capitalising on the physical aspects of other activities (e.g. physically demanding aspects of meal preparation such as whisking by hand, dancing, gardening, maintaining a ward allotment space or flower bed)
- Providing opportunities to sweep, mop, wipe tables (large movements)
- Creating a physical aspect to an activity (e.g. wall-based art work requiring standing, reaching, stretching, bending)

The key is for the individual to find activities meaningful, motivating and doable with the right amount of staff enthusiasm, encouragement and support.

Music

Music is recognised as a beneficial therapeutic medium (Lubner and Hinterberger, 2017; Hall et al., 2019), providing sensory stimulation which can be significantly therapeutic (see Sensory Interventions). Using music requires careful consideration, as it can alter mood, emotions, mental state (Lubner and Hinterberger, 2017) and subsequently the therapeutic environment. For example, listening to loud or fast-paced music can be overstimulating, while the opposite can be calming; certain songs can trigger memories and strong emotions resulting in distress and agitation, while some genres may promote anger, violence and aggression. Responses to music are individualistic; therefore, finding out about music preferences and identifying responses to music is essential, as is using music with care in communal areas.

In the authors' experience, music-based sessions such as listening/music appreciation sessions, including dancing to music, have been among the most popular and best-attended groups. Reasons for this include music's meaningfulness; music activities bring patients together and often lift mood and ward atmosphere (Hall et al., 2019). Sessions can be accessible to all at any level of acuity and are often most successful when patients are at their most unwell, as concentration, focus and many other skills are not required for this activity.

Dancing can be absorbing and both physically and psychologically relaxing (Froggett and Little, 2021). Sessions incorporating singing and playing musical instruments are also engaging and satisfying for many patients, but are best facilitated by staff (nurses, occupational therapists, music therapists) who are competent in coordinating/teaching singing and in the use of instruments with groups of acutely disturbed patients. This is important due to the complexity of the activity, especially on a group basis, and the risk of patients becoming more disturbed and/or the group becoming chaotic. Any music-based session can lead to increased agitation in patients and subsequently a more unsettled ward (Hall et al., 2019), therefore it should be carefully considered.

Use of Technology

Technology is a broad term and is used here to refer to electronic appliances, devices or apps, in particular those providing Internet accessibility, online media or stored content. Daily technology use has become the norm for most people and influences our lives in positive and negative ways (Nygard and Rosenberg, 2016; Carpenter-Song et al., 2018; Panova and Carbonell, 2018; Keles, et al., 2020). For individuals on a PICU, accessing and using technology has potential risks and benefits, as outlined in Table 13.1. It is essential that healthcare professionals make vulnerable individuals aware of risks associated with technology use.

Despite the risks, the use of technology as outlined can prove valuable for reducing boredom, enabling a sense of choice and autonomy, assisting patients to occupy themselves or take responsibility for self-management or reduce feelings of anxiety and stress, among many other benefits.

The PICU team has a responsibility to support patient use of technology and recognise it not only as something for social contact or leisure but also as an integral part of being independent for some patients. There is the potential for individuals to become deskilled or lose skills in technology use during an admission, therefore, care planning to support maintenance of skills can be important. This can be challenging considering the potential risks (Table 13.1), thus thorough risk assessment and care planning are vital. Supervised computer or technology access as well as regular capacity assessments to ensure appropriate usage are just some ways to mitigate risk when considering technology use in any inpatient environment.

Food-Based Activities

Cooking, food preparation and eating activities are commonly popular in PICUs, as they meet basic needs for food and sense of gratification which can be heightened during illness, and are activities which, for many, have significant meaning within day-to-day life. Food is a social facilitator; hence, preparing and eating together can encourage communication and well-being (Ruddock et al., 2019), contributing to the need for relatedness as previously mentioned. Patients usually experience the kitchen as a normal domestic environment where food-based activities enable practical and social skills to be regained (Birken and Bryant, 2019), and meaningful roles and routines can be upheld while in hospital.

Table 13.1 Risks and benefits of patients using technology in a PICU

Risks	Benefits
Disinhibition could lead to posting messages or images online that are regretted in the future, and when paired with preoccupation may lead to possible repetitive contact (via phone, e-mail, social media), resulting in harassment, even if unintentional.	Opportunity to study/learn in an environment which otherwise offers little or no access to conventional education.
Use of cameras on devices carries confidentiality risks, not only for a disinhibited patient but also for their peers.	Can compensate for poor organisation skills and support the patient's development/recovery (e.g. alarm clocks, 'to do' apps, diaries, personal management such as online banking, paying bills).
Risk of dependence on the use of technology which could affect engagement in other domains (Elhai et al., 2017)	Microwaves can simplify cooking whilst reducing risk, allowing more risk-prone individuals to engage in cooking.
Sleep may be detrimentally impacted (Gradisar et al., 2013)	Provides access to leisure activities (TV, film, music, console games, relaxation techniques) to occupy time, distract from distressing experiences/worries or promote socialisation.
Impulsivity could lead to overspending on online shopping sites.	Enables access to current affairs and news in order to stay orientated to one's wider environment whilst also offering diverse opinion and an element of choice that a single newspaper may not provide.
Vulnerability could put individuals at risk of cyber bullying, cybercrime and grooming or recruitment for illegal activities.	Enables individuals to keep in contact with their social environments and support networks through various means, including video calling, which is helpful when visits to the ward are not possible. Confidentiality and safeguarding issues relating to those involved should be scrutinised.
There is increased risk of suicide, self-harm, violence and aggression due to self-harming with glass screens and headphone wires.	Assists in the management of sensory experiences such as auditory hallucinations (Trygstad et al., 2002) (e.g. playing music or white noise on personal devices) and address sensory needs (e.g. noise-cancelling headphones and technology within ward sensory rooms).

In PICUs that have kitchens for patient use, a myriad of risk issues should be considered and continually monitored. These include food hygiene, storage and management of cleaning products, cleaning protocols, infection control, fire safety and risk of harm to self or others. A full and detailed generic risk assessment should be completed for the kitchen that covers all the domains of potential risk. This risk assessment should be reviewed regularly. Kitchens for therapy use are typically managed by the occupational therapy team who develop protocols and undertake risk assessments, but all ward staff should familiarise themselves with how to use the kitchen while following policy and procedures. Along with the generic risk assessment, careful consideration should be taken to identify and reduce dynamic risks associated with individual patients and groups of patients using the kitchen, informing decisions regarding the appropriateness of kitchen use and/or measures that can be put into place to allow sessions to proceed more safely, such as 2:1 staffing.

Due to the nature of a PICU, there may be times when it is not appropriate to facilitate a group in the kitchen, or it may be suitable to run a group in which as many patients as possible can participate. Conversely, it may be that the ward does not have its own kitchen. An occupational therapist approaches decisions around how to tailor a session to the needs of the patient by identifying the patient's current level of functioning. A lower-functioning patient at a more acute phase of their mental illness or a patient who has specific risk behaviours may be more able to engage in a simple food-based group in the communal ward environment. Light meals such as salads, sandwiches, wraps, dips or fruit salads can be prepared using plastic cutlery, or some food can be prepared using hands only. Some patients may only be able to contribute to certain aspects of the task, such as squirting sauce or stirring. This format can encourage and allow more patients and staff to participate in preparing food and eating together than when running a group in a kitchen. Open sessions are accessible to the acutely unwell patients who are not able to use the kitchen or whose current mental state would reduce their ability to prepare more complex meals. This style of group food preparation session promotes inclusion and wider participation.

It is important to recognise that patients whose functioning is significantly disturbed may benefit most from food-based activities that do not require any use of tools or equipment but can be engaged in with their hands only (van der Reyden et al., 2019). Examples are putting prepared ingredients (e.g. sliced tomato and cucumber, grated cheese) into a large tortilla wrap and pulling apart/manipulating lettuce, deli meats and other ingredients with their hands and squeezing bottles of sauce. When patients are acutely unwell and lack awareness of social norms or ability to comply with them, it should not matter that their engagement with food is messy or lacks social graces; the sensory and other therapeutic benefits gained from engagement is enough. Therefore, this type of activity should not include patients for whom recovering or improving ability to behave according to social norms is an aim.

Creative Activities and Self-Expression

Being creative does not require artistic flair or talent, which is the common perception. To create something is to bring something new into existence for the person creating it, and creativity is within every individual (Walters et al., 2014).

Creative activities that are constructive (i.e. aimed at making something through a defined process) can be therapeutic in terms of both the process of doing it and satisfaction gained from the end product. Constructive activities are particularly beneficial for:

- sense of autonomy (Birken and Bryant, 2019)
- maintaining/developing decision-making, cognition (e.g. planning, organising, sequencing, problem-solving)
- relaxation
- gaining self-confidence and esteem through achieving satisfying end products
- distraction, as being absorbed in activities allows for peaceful silence rather than experiencing anxiety about what to say in a group setting (Birken and Bryant, 2019)
- release of frustration and energy
- self-expression

Regarding self-expression, human beings need a balance between activities that are controlled and/or require norm compliance and those that enable self-expression. PICUs are restricted environments that exert a high degree of control over people therein, making it important to provide activities that can be undertaken freely with choice and allow for expression of oneself. It is important to note that due to the demands placed on one's functioning, creative activities are problematic for individuals who are exhausted, have difficulty concentrating and have low motivation (Csikszentmihalyi, 2013). Conversely, manic patients may have trouble curtailing their enthusiasm and self-expression and require support to remain grounded and focused. These problems are common in PICU patients; therefore, activities need to be graded to be achievable for patients with differing functional abilities and motivation levels.

Activities that are both constructive and enable self-expression will vary depending upon a person's age, gender and culture, but may include clay/play dough modelling, drawing, painting, photography, crafts, creative writing, poetry writing, mindfulness activities such as colouring, music listening, gardening, model-making, t-shirt printing, making music and dancing. Having a place to show patients' creations (if they wish them to be viewed) can provide opportunities to admire their creativity while also positively enhancing the milieu (Taube-Schiff, 2016). An activity commonly valued in a PICU is gardening, as it involves projects that patients can undertake together, mirrors processes of recovery such as building optimism and hope for the future (Leamy et al., 2011), provides space and time away from the ward when done outdoors and helps patients to manage problems associated with psychosis (Birken and Bryant, 2019).

Use of Activity in Seclusion

Seclusion rooms are designed to be de-escalating spaces for patients whose severe behavioural disturbance is likely to cause harm to others; hence, they are isolated from others and prevented from leaving the seclusion room (Department of Health, 2015). The seclusion environment is intentionally minimalistic, with plain walls and a mattress for the purpose of providing a low-stimulus environment that supports and encourages de-escalation.

Seclusion is not typically considered a place where activities are facilitated, but this can be challenged given the inherent need for all human beings 'to do' and the negative effects of occupational deprivation as previously explained. Patients in seclusion have

Box 13.1

Printed pages of mindful colouring, quizzes, word searches, sudoku and other puzzles. Crayons are the most risk-averse writing tool and can be easily washed off walls if used in this way.

- Printed reading material (e.g. poems, short stories)
- Paperback books (controversial)
- Listening to music through seclusion room speakers or a tablet or laptop outside the door
- Watching music/other videos on YouTube through a window
  Using sensory items (e.g. stress balls, scented tissues or fabrics oils, ear plugs)

reported they lacked activities such as being able to read a book or magazine, listening to music or physical exercise (Kontio et al., 2014), and patients have identified lack of meaningful activity as the most negative part of the seclusion experience, as it allows for rumination and boredom, causing increase in frustration (Swan, 2019).

In recent years, there have been various innovations aimed at making seclusion rooms more therapeutic whilst maintaining a low-stimulus environment as much as possible. The art and mental health charity Hospital Rooms transformed the seclusion room of a female PICU in London by installing calming and relaxing art works to the observation area of the seclusion space (Butler et al., 2020). The use of calming colours within the seclusion room is a move away from the traditional stark clinical white walls. Media walls (Department of Health, 2011) have also been installed in various seclusion rooms; this technology enables individuals to access games, movies and music of their choice. For some professionals, these innovations are controversial and viewed as being in direct opposition to the purpose and definition of seclusion. Conversely, these innovations are also considered as transforming and redefining modern seclusion care.

With thorough risk assessment and management, enabling activity participation that is suited to the individual and the environment has the potential to support recovery, prepare for return to the main ward area, enhance the quality of care and reduce the length of time in seclusion. In various settings, doing meaningful activity in seclusion that is tailored to individuals' values, interests and capabilities enables a break from rumination (Department of Health, 2015) and improves the quality of the seclusion experience while shortening length of seclusion (Maguire et al., 2011). Tully et al. (2016) assert that bespoke occupational therapy may lead to a more effective model of reducing seclusion in psychiatric settings.

Occupational therapists have tested many activities for their suitability in seclusion while attending to individual needs for meaningful activity (Jeffries, 2021). Activities in Box 13.1 are suggested activities, but decisions regarding their use should arise from MDT risk assessment, discussion and agreement. MDT support and involvement in making activity available is important.

Individuals requiring seclusion may be too manic or chaotic to be able to engage in sedate activities such as reading, quizzes or puzzles, and use of music should take into consideration the issues discussed earlier in the chapter.

Sensory Interventions

In terms of sensory experiences, it is recognised that many inpatient environments can present patients with excessive sensory stimulation (Carpenter et al., 2021) or cause sensory deprivation. The latter occurs due to clinically sterile environments, a lack of sensory-rich opportunities (i.e. movement, textures and touch, visual and auditory stimulation), lack of opportunities for touching other people and being touched, lack of a varied diet, control over heating and lighting and so on. The use of sensory methods in mental health settings is a relatively new development (Sutton and Nicholson, 2011; Novak et al., 2012; Sivak, 2012; Lloyd et al., 2014), and benefits within an acute mental health setting have been explored internationally in recent years as the evidence base for this innovative area of mental health practice gains momentum (Champagne and Stromberg, 2004; Sutton and Nicholson, 2011; Björkdahl et al. 2016; Wiglesworth and Farnworth, 2016).

Activities need to be considered for offering a wide variety of sensory opportunities. This is best informed by individual sensory assessments and specific plans for those with specific sensory needs. There is a range of sensory interventions that could be utilised in mental health settings if tailored to the type of the service and individual patient's needs. These can be categorised as environmental, individual sensory needs and sensory rooms.

Enhancing the Sensory Aspects of the Environment

A simple and beneficial sensory intervention in a PICU is the making of environmental adaptations throughout the ward, as aspects of the environment impact on people's senses and subsequently their mental state and sense of well-being. For example, use of music in communal areas can have a significant impact on the ward ambience and therapeutic atmosphere. Music can affect people in different ways (see Music), but relaxing or slow-paced music can create a calm atmosphere and is usually favoured in the busy and often chaotic PICU environment. The temperature of the ward, smells, furniture and décor all impact the senses, and it is beneficial to consider each of these environmental aspects. Incorporating visuals such as artwork and use of colour on the walls, similar to that described in the section on seclusion, can create a comfortable, homely feeling and offer visual stimulation that can be engaging and relaxing. Potential risks should be mitigated when making environmental changes and safety measures should be put in place, such as the use of tamper-proof screws and robust equipment that is designed to be PICU safe.

Individual Sensory Needs and Preferences

Each of us has individual responses to sensory stimulation and we usually have many opportunities to manage sources of sensory stimulation to suit our preferences, for example, avoiding spicey food, crowded or noisy places, or seeking high degrees of sensory input such as sky diving. Each patient will also have sensory preferences and may be experiencing sensory processing problems due to mental illness, however, without the degree of influence over everyday sensory stimulation that one usually has. Therefore, it is important to gain an understanding of individuals from a sensory perspective.

An individual may experience sensory hypo or hypersensitivities or sensory-seeking behaviours that require intervention, such as seeking out or making loud noises, covering their ears or eyes or avoiding busy communal areas or light. Such behaviours can occur for many different reasons.

Sensory processing difficulties can often be overlooked and therefore unidentified, which carries the risk of some behaviours being misinterpreted as signs of psychosis or disorder. The Sensory Profile (Brown and Dunn, 2002), Sensory Integration Inventory (Reisman and Hanschu, 1992 or the Adult Sensory History assessment (Spiral Foundation) can be useful to identify sensory needs, and are typically conducted by an occupational therapist, but can also be completed by psychologists or other MDT members. Results can be utilised to support the development of an individualised intervention plan to address sensory needs and support patients to optimise function.

Calm Down Methods is a Safewards (2021) intervention that involves having a box of items available for individuals to use at their request to help with remaining calm and reducing distress or agitation. Patients can be made aware of the Calm Down Box during community or planning meetings and by posters displayed around the ward. Items are usually signed out from the nursing office on a temporary basis for independent use or use with supervision. Examples of items are stress balls, letter-writing kits, ear plugs, face masks, essential oils dispensed onto tissues, positive affirmations or breathing exercise cards, herbal teas, iPods with relaxing music uploaded or fidget toys. Calm Down Boxes have been found to be successful and are a recommended and widely supported intervention in inpatient mental health settings (Dickens et al., 2020).

Sensory Rooms

In recent years, sensory rooms have become increasingly prevalent in mental health settings including PICUs (e.g. Bjorkdahl et al., 2016; Davies et al., 2019. Sensory rooms are therapeutic spaces designed to relax or stimulate the senses and provide an immersive environment to promote self-organisation and self-regulation and reduce levels of distress and agitation (Sutton and Nicholson, 2011). They provide a safe and comfortable space for an individual to explore their sensory needs in order to achieve the optimum level of arousal to function effectively (Larocci and McDonald, 2006).

PICU sensory rooms can be utilised as a proactive measure to reduce levels of violence and aggression on the ward (Sutton et al., 2013). Patients should have the option to request 1:1 time in the sensory room if they identify that they are beginning to feel agitated. Alternatively, a staff member might recommend that the patient has a 1:1 session in the sensory room if they observe that their agitation levels are rising. For patients who experience benefits from sensory rooms, their utilisation as a first-line method for de-escalation could be viewed as encouraging least coercive and restrictive methods of de-escalation and promoting the national agenda for reducing restrictive practices (NICE, 2015; Champagne and Stromberg, 2004).

Small group sessions for relaxation or yoga can also serve as a proactive means to prevent high levels of agitation and distress and are well suited to being held within a sensory room due to the ability to adapt the lighting, sounds and aromas within the space. Factors such as maximum numbers allowed in the room and personal dynamics between group members need consideration before facilitating a session in the sensory room.

Community-Based Activity

Leave within a PICU setting is a much under-researched area, perhaps due to its infrequent occurrence. Accessing leave is a conversation most patients understandably want to have throughout their admission (Schel et al., 2015), as it can have many therapeutic benefits that support recovery (Wright and Sugarman, 2009; Barlow and Dickens, 2018). Experiencing the freedom to walk away from the ward, even for short periods of time with a staff escort, can be empowering, key to recovery and a pertinent reminder of what a patient is working towards, as well as provide a break from the challenging ward environment. Being in one's community can have a normalising effect and being in familiar surroundings, even if only for a brief time, can offer a degree of reassurance and comfort (Hasselkus, 2002) as well as feelings of social inclusion and feeling connected to one's community-based life (Wood and Alsway, 2016). Seeing individuals outside of the ward environment can also contribute to the team developing a more accurate assessment of how the patient's recovery is progressing, their behaviours and functional abilities in relation to living in the community, readiness for discharge or step down to an acute ward and subsequently more fully understanding individuals' needs and abilities (Department of Health and Social Care, 2015).

Gaining leave is an important goal for most patients and is a significant motivating factor for engagement during an inpatient admission. An essential aspect of ensuring any episode of leave is successful and beneficial is establishing its purpose and meaning for the individual, as increase in purpose and meaning correlates to increase in focus on success by the individual (Kelly et al., 2010). Involving patients in planning leave is important (Department of Health and Social Care, 2015), but finding purpose for initial short-duration leave can prove difficult, as individuals may only get leave to a specific place within the hospital grounds and this may not hold much meaning for them. It is important to work with individuals on deciding where to go, for example, a café, chapel or safe outdoor space, with a view to an activity that can be safely carried out there, even if the activity is simply walking. Family or friends could be included to add meaning, but this, as with the choice of environment, must be risk assessed. Accessing one's community through technology via video links to people, education or services is under-researched but could arguably be a safe way to provide time away from the ward environment of some nature, particularly for high-risk individuals.

Healthcare professionals have a duty of care to ensure physical healthcare needs are treated alongside mental health (Department of Health and Social Care, 2015), and acquiring leave can be essential for accessing specialist physical health care, such as sexual and reproductive health, dentistry and specific needs pertaining to comorbidities. Before granting leave, it is essential that the MDT thoroughly risk assesses both the potential impact of an individual on their community environment and vice versa, including their vulnerability to risks or threats, whether physical or social. The balance of therapeutic benefit against risk should always be a consideration when discussing leave (Department of Health and Social Care, 2015).

Conclusion

The benefits to patients, staff and the PICU service of providing meaningful individual and group-based activities is considerable and has gained increasing recognition in recent years. However, providing and facilitating activities for therapeutic benefit and positive engagement is not a simple task. It requires consideration of the dynamic relationship between a person's motivation (what is meaningful and motivating), their mental, physical and social abilities, the demands of the activity, the environment and the associated risks.

Although this chapter has been able to draw upon some literature on the therapeutic use of activity in PICUs, there has been much necessary reliance on research in other mental health settings serving people experiencing acute disturbance. What constitutes meaningful and therapeutic activity, its link to health and well-being and how activity and environments can be graded for therapeutic benefit has been extensively investigated by the occupational therapy profession. However, there is a significant lack of research and publications for PICU MDTs to draw upon. This needs urgent attention in order to inform further developments in the use of activities in PICU services. Similarly, the relationship between activities, patients and the role of nurses remains unexplored (Chan et al., 2012), as does nurses' understanding of what makes activity meaningful to patients (Foye et al., 2020). Given the increase in understanding the importance of activity provision in PICUs in recent years, there is some urgency for undertaking such research, particularly research that explores the needs of the BAME patient population and actively involves patients in research design and as co-researchers.

References

Akther,S, Molyneaux,E, Stuart,R, Johnson,S, Simpson,A and Oram,S (2019) Patients' Experiences of Assessment and Detention Under Mental Health Legislation: Systematic Review and Qualitative Meta-Synthesis. *BJPsych Open* **5** (3) E37.

Alexandratos,K, Barnett,F and Thomas,Y (2011) The Impact of Exercise on the Mental Health and Quality of Life of People with Severe Mental Illness: A Critical Review. *British Journal of Occupational Therapy* **75** (2) 48–60.

Antonysamy,A (2013) How Can We Reduce Violence and Aggression in Psychiatric Inpatient Units? *BMJ Quality Improvement Reports* 2: u201366.w834. DOI: https://10.1136/bmjquality.u201366.w834.

Barlow,EM and Dickens,GL (2018) Systematic Review of Therapeutic Leave in Inpatient Mental Health Services. *Archives of Psychiatric Nursing* **32** (4) 638–49.

Beer,MD, Paton,C and Pereira,SM (2008) Management of Acutely Disturbed Behaviour. In Beer,MD, Pereira,SM and Paton,C (eds.), *Psychiatric Intensive Care*, 2nd ed. Cambridge: Cambridge University Press. pp. 12–23.

Birken,M and Bryant,W (2019) A Photovoice Study of User Experiences of an Occupational Therapy Department within an Acute Inpatient Mental Health Setting. *British Journal of Occupational Therapy* **82** (9) 532–43.

Björkdahl,A, Perseius,K, Samuelsson,M and Lindberg,MH (2016) Sensory Rooms in Psychiatric Inpatient Care: Staff Experiences. *International Journal of Mental Health Nursing* **25** (5) 472–79. DOI: https://doi.org/10.1111/inm.12205.

Brown,C and Dunn,W (2002) *Adolescent/Adult Sensory Profile Manual.* San Antonio, TX: Psychological Corporation.

Bryant,W, Cordingley,K, Sims,K, Dokal-Marandi,J, Pritcchard,H, Stannard,V, et al. (2016) Collaborative Research Exploring Mental Health Service User Perspectives on Acute Inpatient Occupational Therapy. *British Journal of Occupational Therapy* **79** (10) 607–13.

Burki,T (2018) Increase in Detentions in the UK under the Mental Health Act. *The Lancet Psychiatry* **5** (11) 878.

Butler,S, Adeduro,R, Davies,R, Nwankwo,O, White,N, Shaw,T, et al. (2020) Art and Mental Health in the Women's Psychiatric Intensive Care Unit. *Journal of Psychiatric Intensive Care* **16** (1) 15-22(8)

Carpenter,C, Jordan,S and Lawrence,J (2021) Application of the VdTMoCA to Occupational Therapy within a High Secure Mental Health Hospital. In Sherwood,W (ed.) (2021) *Perspectives on the Vona du Toit Model of Creative Ability: Practice, Theory and Philosophy.* Watford: International Creative Ability Network.

Carpenter-Song,E, Noel,VA, Acquilano,SC and Drake,RE (2018). Real World Technology Use Among People with Mental Illness: Qualitative Study. *JMIR Mental Health* **5** (4) e10652.

Chevalier,A, Ntala,E, Fung,C, Priebe,S and Bird,VJ (2018) Exploring the Initial Experience of Hospitalisation to an Acute Psychiatric Ward. *PLoS ONE* **13** (9) e0203457. DOI: https://doi.org/10.1371/journal.pone.0203457.

Champagne,T and Stromberg,N (2004) Sensory Approaches in Inpatient Psychiatric Settings: Innovative Alternatives to Seclusion and Restraint. *Journal of Psychosocial Nursing & Mental Health Services* **42** (9) 34–55.

Chan,Z, Wu,CM and Yip,CH and Yau,KK (2012) Getting Through the Day: Exploring Patients' Leisure Experiences in a Private Hospital. *Journal of Clinical Nursing* **21**(21–22) 3257–67.

Chaplin,R, McGeorge,M and Lelliott,P (2006) The National Audit of Violence: In-Patient Care for Adults of Working Age. *Psychiatric Bulletin* **30** (12) 444–6.

Cole,F (2014a) Physical Activity for Mental Health and Wellbeing. In Bryant,W, Fieldhouse,J and Bannigan,K (eds.), *Creek's Occupational Therapy and Mental Health.* Edinburgh: Elsevier. pp. 205–22.

Cole,MB (2014b) Client Centred Groups. In Bryant,W, Fieldhouse,J and Bannigan,K (eds.), *Creek's Occupational Therapy and Mental Health.* Edinburgh: Elsevier. pp. 241–58.

College Centre for Quality Improvement (CCQI) (2017) *Standards for Inpatient Mental Health Services.*

Cook,S and Chambers,E (2009) What Helps and Hinders People with Psychotic Conditions Doing What They Want in Their Daily Lives?. *British Journal of Occupational Therapy* **72** (6) 238–48.

Cook,S, Mundy,T, Killaspy,H (2016) Development of a Staff Training Intervention for Inpatient Mental Health Rehabilitation Units to Increase Service Users' Engagement in Activities. *British Journal of Occupational Therapy* **79** (3) 144–52.

Csikszentmihalyi,M (2013) *Creativity: Flow and the Psychology of Discovery and Invention.* New York: Harper Perennial.

Csipke, E, Papoulias, C, Vitoratou, S, Williams, P, Rose, D and Wykes, T (2016) Design in Mind: Eliciting Service User and Frontline Staff Perspectives on Psychiatric Ward Design through Participatory Methods. *Journal of Mental Health* **25** (2) 114–21.

Curtis,S, Gesler, W, Fabian, K, Francis, S and Priebe, S (2007) Therapeutic Landscapes in Hospital Design: A Qualitative Assessment by Staff and Service Users of the Design of a New Mental Health Inpatient Unit. *Environment and Planning C: Government and Policy* **25** (4) 591–610.

Davies,R, Murphy,K and Sethi,F (2020) Sensory Room in a Psychiatric Intensive Care Unit. *Journal of Psychiatric Intensive Care* **16** (1) 23–28(6).

De las Heras,C, Geist,R, Kielhofner,G, (2007) *Volitional Questionnaire.* Chicago, IL: MOHO Clearing House.

De las Heras,C, Llerena,V and Kielhofner,G (2019) *The Remotivation Process Version 2.* Chicago, IL: MOHO Clearing House.

Deci,EL and Ryan,RM (1985) *Intrinsic Motivation and Self-Determination in Human Behavior.* New York: Plenum Press.

Deci,EL and Ryan,RM (2000) The 'What' and 'Why' of Goal Pursuits: Human Needs and the Self-Determination of Behavior. *Psychological Inquiry* **11** (4) 227–68.

Deci,EL and Ryan,RM (2008) Self-Determination Theory: A Macrotheory of Human Motivation, Development, and Health. *Canadian Psychology* **49** (3) 182–85.

Department of Health (2001) *Mental Health Policy Implementation Guide.* London: Department of Health.

Department of Health (2011) *Environmental Design Guide: Medium Secure Services.* London: Department of Health.

Department of Health (2015) *The Mental Health Act 1983.* London: Department of Health. www.gov.uk/government/publications/code-of-practice-mental-health-act-1983.

Department of Health and Social Care (2015) *New Mental Health Act Code of Practice.* London: Department of Health. www.gov.uk/government/news/new-mental-health-act-code-of-practice.

Dickens,GL, Tabvuma,T and Frost,SA (2020) Safewards: Changes in Conflict, Containment, and Violence Prevention Climate during Implementation. *International Journal of Mental Health Nursing* **29** (6) 1230–40.

Durocher E, Gibson,B and Rappolt,S (2013) Occupational Justice: A Conceptual Review. *Journal of Occupational Science* **21** (4) 418–30.

Eastwood,JD, Frischen,A, Fenske,MJ and Smilek,D (2012) The Unengaged Mind: Defining Boredom in Terms of Attention. *Perspectives on Psychological Science* **7** (5) 482–95.

Elhai,JD, Dvorak,R, Levine,JC and Hall,B (2017) Problematic Smartphone Use: A Conceptual Overview and Systematic Review of Relations with Anxiety and Depression Psychopathology. *Journal of Affective Disorders* **207**: 251–59.

Feighan,M and Roberts,AE (2017) The Value of Cycling as a Meaningful and Therapeutic Occupation. *British Journal of Occupational Therapy* **80** (5) 319–26.

Fitzgerald,M (2016) The Potential Role of the Occupational Therapist in Acute Psychiatric Services: A Comparative Evaluation. *International Journal of Therapy and Rehabilitation* **23** (11) 514–18.

Foye,U, Li,Y, Birken,M, Parle,K and Simpson,A (2020) Activities on Acute Mental Health Inpatient Wards: A Narrative Synthesis of the Service Users' Perspective. *Journal of Psychiatric Mental Health Nursing* **27**: 482–93.

Froggett,L and Little,R (2012) Dance as a Complex Intervention in an Acute Mental Health Setting: A Place 'In-Between'. *British Journal of Occupational Therapy* **75** (2) 93–9.

Goldberg,Y, Eastwood,J, LaGuardia,J and Danckert,J (2011) Boredom: An Emotional Experience Distinct from Apathy, Anhedonia, or Depression. *Journal of Social and Clinical Psychology* **30** (6) 647–66.

Gradisar,M, Wolfson,AR, Harvey,AG, Hale,L, Rosenberg,R and Czeisler,C (2013) The Sleep and Technology Use of Americans: Findings from the National Sleep Foundation's 2011 Sleep in America Poll. *Journal of Clinical Sleep Medicine* **9** (12) 1291–9.

Haley,L and McKay,EL (2004) Baking Gives You Confidence: Users' Views in Engaging in the Occupation of Baking. *British Journal of Occupational Therapy* **67** (3) 125–8.

Hall,TL, Mullen,A, Plummer,J, et al. (2019) Sound Practice: Exploring the Benefits of Establishing a Music Group on an Acute Mental Health Inpatient Unit. *International Journal of Mental Health Nursing* **28** (3) 697–705.

Harvey,S, Øverland,S, Hatch,S, Wessely,S, Mykletun,A and Hotopf,M (2018) Exercise and the Prevention of Depression: Results of the HUNT Cohort Study. *American Journal of Psychiatry* **175** (1) 28–36.

Hasselkus,BR (2002) *The Meaning of Everyday Occupation.* Thorofare, NJ: Slack Incorporated.

Hitch,D (2009) Experiences of Engagement in Occupations and Assertive Outreach Services. *British Journal of Occupational Therapy* **72** (11) 482–90.

Hitch,D, Pepin,G and Stagnitti,K (2013) Engagement in Activities and Occupations by People Who Have Experienced Psychosis: A Metasynthesis of Lived Experience. *British Journal of Occupational Therapy* **76** (2) 77–86.

Hooper,B and Wood,W (2019) The Philosophy of Occupational Therapy: A Framework for Practice. In Schell, BAB and Gillen,G (eds.), *Willard and Spackman's Occupational Therapy*, 13th ed. Philadelphia: Lippincott Williams & Wilkins. pp. 43–55.

Hutcheson,C, Ferguson,H and Nish,G (2010). Promoting Mental Wellbeing through Activity in a Mental Health Hospital. *British Journal of Occupational Therapy* **73** (3) 121–28.

Janner,M and Delaney,KR (2012) Safety Issues on British Mental Health Wards. *Journal of the American Psychiatric Nurses Association* **18** (2) 104–11.

Jeffries,L (2021) Seclusion: The End of the Road for Occupational Therapy or a New Route with the Vona du Toit Model of Creative Ability? In Sherwood,W (ed.), *Perspectives on the Vona du Toit Model of Creative Ability: Practice, Theory and Philosophy*. Watford: International Creative Ability Network.

Kazi,F, Flood,B and Hooton,S (2008) Therapeutic Activities within Psychiatric Intensive Care and Low Secure Units. In Beer,MD, Pereira,SM and Paton,C (eds.), *Psychiatric Intensive Care*, 2nd ed. Cambridge: Cambridge University Press. pp. 149–60.

Keles,B, McCrae,N and Grealish,A (2020) A Systematic Review: The Influence of Social Media on Depression, Anxiety and Psychological Distress in Adolescents. *International Journal of Adolescence and Youth* **25** (1) 79–93.

Kelly,M, Lamont,S and Brunero,S (2010) An Occupational Perspective of the Recovery Journey in Mental Health. *British Journal of Occupational Therapy* **73** (3) 129–35.

Kennedy,J and Fortune,T (2014) Women's Experiences of Being on an Acute Psychiatric Unit. *British Journal of Occupational Therapy* **77** (6) 296–303.

Kontio,R, Anttila, M, Lantta, T, Kauppi,K, Joffe, G and Välimäkial, M (2014) Toward a Safer Working Environment on Psychiatric Wards: Service Users' Delayed Perspectives of Aggression and Violence-Related Situations and Development Ideas. *Perspectives in Psychiatric Care* **50** (4) 271–79.

Lamanna,D, Ninkovic,D, Vijayaratnam,V, et al. (2016) Aggression in Psychiatric Hospitalisations: A Qualitative Study of Patient and Provider Perspectives. *Journal of Mental Health* **25** (6) 536–42.

Larocci,G and McDonald,J (2006) Sensory Integration and the Perceptual Experience of Persons with Autism. *Journal of Autism and Developmental Disorders* **36** (1) 77–90.

Leamy, M, Bird, V, Le Boutillier,C, Williams, J and Slade, M (2011) A Conceptual Framework for Personal Recovery in Mental Health: Systematic Review and Narrative Synthesis. *British Journal of Psychiatry* **199** (6) 445–52.

Lim,KH, Morris,J and Craik,C (2007) Inpatients' Perspectives of Occupational Therapy in Acute Mental Health. *Australian Occupational Therapy Journal* **54** (1) 22–32.

Lloyd,C, King,R and Machingura,T (2014) An Investigation into the Effectiveness of Sensory Modulation in Reducing Seclusion within an Acute Mental Health Unit. *Advances in Mental Health* **12** (2) 93–100.

Lloyd,C and Williams,PL (2010) Occupational Therapy in the Modern Acute Mental Health Setting: A Review of Current Practice. *International Journal of Therapy and Rehabilitation* **17** (9) 436–42.

Lubner,D and Hinterberger,T (2017) Reviewing the Effectiveness of Music Interventions in Treating Depression. *Frontiers in Psychology* **8**: 1109.

MacKay,I, Paterson,B and Cassells,C (2005) Constant or Special Observations of Inpatients Presenting a Risk of Aggression or Violence: Nurses' Perception of the Rules of Engagement. *Journal of Psychiatric and Mental Health Nursing* **12** (4) 464–71.

Maguire,T, Young,R and Martin,T (2011) Seclusion Reduction in a Forensic Mental Health Setting. *Journal of Psychiatric and Mental Health Nursing* **19** (2) 97–106.

Marshall,CA, McIntosh,E, Sohrabi,A and Ami,A (2020) Boredom in Inpatient Mental Healthcare Settings: A Scoping Review. *British Journal of Occupational Therapy* **83** (1) 41–51.

Molin,J, Graneheim,UH and Lindgren,BM (2016) Quality of Interactions Influences Everyday Life in Psychiatric Inpatient Care – Patients' Perspectives. *International Journal of Qualitative Studies on Health and Well-Being* **11**: 29897.

Murphy,L (2021) Implementing the VdTMoCA on an Inpatient Mental Health Rehabilitation Ward for Clients with Complex Needs. In Sherwood,W (ed.), *Perspectives on the Vona du Toit Model of Creative Ability: Practice, Theory and Philosophy*. Watford: International Creative Ability Network.

National Association of Psychiatric Intensive Care and Low Secure Units (NAPICU) (2014) *National Minimum Standards for Psychiatric Intensive Care in General Adult Services.*

National Association of Psychiatric Intensive Care and Low Secure Units (NAPICU) (2016) *Guidance for Commissioners of Psychiatric Intensive Care Units (PICU)*. (online) https://napicu.org.uk/wp-content/uploads/2016/04/Commissioning_Guidance_Apr16.pdf.

National Institute for Health and Care Excellence (NICE) (2011) *Service User Experience in Adult Mental Health: Improving the Experience of Care for People Using Adult NHS Mental Health Services*.

National Institute for Health and Care Excellence (NICE) (2014) *Psychosis and Schizophrenia in Adults: Prevention and Management (NICE clinical guideline 178)*. (online) www.nice.org.uk/guidancecg178.

National Institute for Health and Care Excellence (NICE) (2015) *Violence and Aggression: Short-Term Management in Mental Health, Health and Community Settings (NICE clinical guideline 10)*. (online) www.nice.org.uk/guidanceng10.

National Institute for Health and Care Excellence (NICE) (2019) *Service User Experience in Adult Mental Health Services*. (online) www.nice.org.uk/guidance/cg136.

Novak,T, Scanlan,J, McCaul,D, MacDonald,N and Clarke,T (2012) Pilot Study of a Sensory Room in an Acute Inpatient Psychiatric Unit. *Australasian Psychiatry* **20** (5) 401–6.

Nygard,L and Rosenborg,L (2016) How Attention to Everyday Technology Could Contribute to Modern Occupational Therapy: A Focus Group Study. *British Journal of Occupational Therapy* **79** (8) 467–74.

Panova,T and Carbonell,X (2018) Is Smartphone Addiction Really an Addiction?. *Journal of Behavioural Addictions* **7** (2) 252–9.

Parkinson,S, Forsyth,K, Kielhofner,G (2006) *User's Manual for the Model of Human Occupation Screening Tool (MOHOST) (version 2.0)*. (online) http://moho.uic.edu/pdf/MohostManual.pdf.

Pentland,D, Kantartzis,S, Clausen,MG and Witemyre,K (2018) *Occupational Therapy and Complexity: Defining and Describing Practice*. (online) www.rcot.co.uk/sites/default/files/OT%20and%20complexity.pdf.

Pereira,S and Woollaston,K (2007) Therapeutic Engagement in Acute Psychiatric Inpatient Services. *Journal of Psychiatry Intensive Care* **3** (1) 3–11.

Poon,M, Siu,A and Ming,SY (2010) Outcome Analysis of Occupational Therapy Programme for Persons with Early Psychosis. *Work* **37** (1) 65–70.

Reisman,JE and Hanschu,B (1992) *Sensory Integration Inventory — Revised for Individuals with Developmental Disabilities*. Hugo, MN: PDP Press.

Robinson,L, Littrell,SH and Littrell,K (1999) Managing Aggression in Schizophrenia. *Journal of the American Psychiatric Nurses Association* **5** (2) 9–16.

Royal College of Psychiatrists (2011) *Do the Right Thing: How to Judge a Good Ward. Ten Standards for Adult In-Patient Mental Healthcare. OP79*. London: Royal College of Psychiatrists.

Royal College of Psychiatrists (2019) *Standards for Inpatient Mental Health Services*, 3rd ed. (online) www.rcpsych.ac.uk/docs/default-source/improving-care/ccqi/ccqi-resources/rcpsych_standards_in_2019_lr.pdf?sfvrsn=edd5f8d5_2.

Ruddock,HK, Brunstrom,JM, Vartanian,LR, et al. (2019) A Systematic Review and Meta-Analysis of the Social Facilitation of Eating. *American Journal of Clinical Nutrition* **110** (4) 842–61.

Safewards (2021) Calm Down Methods. www.safewards.net/interventions/calm-down-methods.

Schel,S, Bouman,Y and Bulten,B (2015) Quality of Life in Long-Term Forensic Psychiatric Care: Comparison of Self-Report and Proxy Assessments. *Archives of Psychiatric Nursing* **29** (3) 162–7.

Shepherd,M and Lavender,T (1999) Putting Aggression into Context: An Investigation into Contextual Factors Influencing the Rate of Aggressive Incidents in a Psychiatric Hospital. *Journal of Mental Health* **8** (2) 158–70.

Sims,KL (2014) The Acute Setting. In Bryant,W, Fieldhouse,J and Bannigan,K. (eds.), *Creek's Occupational Therapy and Mental Health*, 5th ed. London: Churchill Livingstone. pp. 346–58.

Sivak,K (2012) Implementation of Comfort Rooms: To Reduce Seclusion, Restraint Use, and Acting-Out Behaviors. *Journal of Psychosocial Nursing and Mental Health Services* **50** (2) 24–34.

Stickney,MI, Miltenberger,RG and Wolff,G (1999) A Descriptive Analysis of Factors Contributing to Binge Eating. *Journal of Behavior Therapy and Experimental Psychiatry* **30** (3) 177–89.

Sumsion,T and Law,M (2006) A Review of Evidence on the Conceptual Elements Informing Client-Centred Practice. *Canadian Journal of Occupational Therapy* **73** (3) 153–62.

Sustere,E and Tarpey,E (2019) Least Restrictive Practice: Its Role in Patient Independence and Recovery. *The Journal of Forensic Psychiatry & Psychology* **30** (5) 1–16.

Sutton,D and Nicholson,E (2011) *Sensory Modulation in Acute Mental Health Wards: A Qualitative Study of Staff and Service User Perspectives*. New Zealand: The National Centre of Mental Health Research, Information and Workforce Development (Te Pou).

Sutton,D, Wilson,M, Van Kessel,K and Vaderpyl,J (2013) Optimizing Arousal to Manage Aggression: A Pilot Study of Sensory Modulation. *International Journal of Mental Health Nursing* **22** (6) 500–11.

Swan,T (2019) *Understanding Peoples Experiences of Seclusion*. Lancashire Care Foundation Trust.

Taube-Schiff,M, Carroll,A and Flogen,S (2016) The Development of a Modification of Behavioural Activation as a Solution to Reduce Patient Boredom in a PICU: Overcoming Patient and Staff Challenges. *Journal of Psychiatric Intensive Care* **12** (2) 63–8.

Taylor,T (2016) *Kielhofner's Model of Human Occupation: Theory and Application*, 5th ed. Philadelphia: Lippincott, Williams and Wilkins.

Trygstad,L, Buccheri,R, Dowling,G, Zind,R, White,K, Griffin,JJ, et al. (2002) Behavioural Management of Persistent Auditory Hallucinations in Schizophrenia: Outcomes from a 10-Week Course. *Journal of the American Psychiatric Nurses Association* **8** (3) 84–91.

Tully,J, McSweeney,L, Harfield,K, Castle,C and Das,M (2016) Innovation and Pragmatism Required to Reduce Seclusion Practices. *CNS Spectrums*, **21** (6) 424–9.

Van der Reyden,D, Casteleijn,D, Sherwood,W and De Witt, P (eds.) (2019) *The Vona du Toit Model of Creative Ability: Origins, Constructs, Principles and Application in Occupational Therapy*. Pretoria: Vona and Marie du Toit Foundation.

van der Reyden,D and Sherwood,W (2019) The Vona du Toit Model of Creative Ability: Core Constructs and Concepts. In Van der Reyden,D, Casteleijn,D, Sherwood,W and De Witt,P (eds.), *The Vona du Toit Model of Creative Ability: Origins, Constructs, Principles and Application in Occupational Therapy*. Pretoria: Vona and Marie du Toit Foundation. pp. 58–105.

Walker,B (2021) Therapeutic Steps in Low Secure Services through an Occupational Therapy Pathway: A Ten-Week Process of Discovery and Development. In Sherwood,W (ed.), *Perspectives on the Vona du Toit Model of Creative Ability: Practice, Theory and Philosophy*. Watford: International Creative Ability Network.

Walters,JH, Sherwood,W and Mason,H (2014) Creative Activities. In Bryant,W and Fieldhouse,J (eds.), *Creek's Occupational Therapy and Mental Health*, 5th ed. Oxford: Churchill Livingston.

Whiteford,G (2010) When People Cannot Participate: Occupational Deprivation. In Christiansen,CH and Townsend,EA (eds.), *Introduction to Occupation: The Art and Science of Living*, 2nd ed. Upper Saddle Creek, NJ: Prentice Hall. pp. 303–28.

Wiglesworth,S and Farnworth,L (2016) An Exploration of the Use of a Sensory Room in a Forensic Mental Health Setting: Staff and Patient Perspectives. *Occupational Therapy International* **23**(3) 255–64.

Wilson,C, Rouse,L, Rae,S and Kar Ray,M (2018) Mental Health Inpatients' and Staff Members' Suggestions for Reducing Physical Restraint: A Qualitative Study. *Journal of Psychiatric and Mental Health Nursing* **25** (3) 188–200.

Wood,L and Alsawy,S (2016) Patient Experiences of Psychiatric Inpatient Care: A Systematic Review of Qualitative Evidence. *Journal of Psychiatric Intensive Care* **12** (1) 35–43.

Wright,R and Sugarman,L (2009) *Occupational Therapy and Life Course Development*. Chichester: Wiley-Blackwell.

De-escalation

Roland Dix and Mathew Page

Introduction

The ability to use communication skills to engage with someone to alleviate their distress and reduce agitation and hostility is an essential component of the skill set of any psychiatric intensive care unit (PICU) practitioner. Not only does this approach have a strong moral and ethical imperative but it is also associated with other core aspirations of good PICU culture, including reducing restrictive practice and achieving the best possible clinical outcome.

As in many other domains of health care, early intervention in a clinical issue will reduce acuity, chronicity, length of hospital stay, use of higher-dose treatment and myriad other issues which could be bad for the patient and costly for the healthcare system. To this end, de-escalation skills will be routinely deployed in a PICU, which by its nature receives people who are often in a profound state of 'escalation'.

De-escalation of Disturbed Behaviour

A comprehensive literature review undertaken by the National Association of Psychiatric Intensive Care and British Association of Psychopharmacology described guidelines for the clinical management of acute disturbance. The guidelines indicate that, in all instances, de-escalation is the first stage of a process which could include more restrictive interventions later on (Patel et al., 2018). Similarly, research has identified that practitioners tend to operate on a 'care-control' continuum which begins with de-escalation, moving through non-physical means of control to actual physical control (Price et al., 2018).

Stevenson (1991) defined de-escalation as a 'complex, interactive process in which a patient is redirected towards a calmer personal space'. Becoming competent in de-escalation is in itself a sophisticated activity requiring much more than just a theoretical understanding of aggression. It cannot be considered in purely academic terms. The practitioner must undertake a developmental process resulting in high self-awareness, enabling the skills of de-escalation to become instinctive. Put simply, the practitioner of de-escalation must use their own personality and sense of self to actively engage the person they wish to de-escalate.

The PICU has an unavoidable role in setting limits to disturbed behaviour and therefore requires team members to develop a high standard of de-escalation skills. Authors such as Boettcher (1983), Kaplan and Wheeler (1983), McHugh and West (1995) and Turnbull et al. (1990) have proposed models of de-escalation. These models have much to offer the PICU, although they do not specifically address the PICU patient.

While training and competence in de-escalation is essential, Johnston et al. (2022) point to essential related components which must also be in place:

- Collaborative antipsychotic prescribing
- Debriefing and de-escalation planning
- Modifications to the physical environment
- Ward manager role modelling of emotional vulnerability
- Therapeutic intimacy in nurse–patient relationships

Ward milieu will always be the context in which any potential de-escalation scenario emerges, hence it is vital to ensure this is proactively led at all times. Models such as Safewards have been found to have a positive impact on therapeutic relationships, cohesion, and ward atmosphere (Ward-Stockham et al., 2022).

The model described in this chapter was specifically designed for use in PICUs and was largely developed from practice experience in such facilities.

Experience in the PICU suggests three basic components for effective face-to-face de-escalation:

- Assessment of the immediate situation
- Communication skills designed to facilitate cooperation
- Tactics aimed at problem solving

This chapter examines these components and demonstrates their practical value within the context of the PICU. The model for de-escalation offered here is in daily use in several inpatient facilities and has shown good efficacy.

Component 1: Assessment of the Aggressive Incident

Before considering how best to assess an episode of aggression, it is essential that ward staff have a shared understanding of what constitutes aggressive or unacceptable behaviour. This is particularly important for services that operate 24 hours a day across several shifts. Failure to share an agreed definition of aggressive or unacceptable behaviour may result in an incident being responded to with humour by one shift and PRN medication by another. Rating scales such as the assaultive rating scale described by Lanza and Campbell (1991) provide a useful framework.

Assaultive Rating Scale (ARS)

1. Threat of assault but no physical contact
2. Physical contact but no physical injury
3. Mild soreness/surface abrasion/scratches/small bruises
4. Major soreness/cuts/large bruises
5. Severe lacerations/fractures/head injury
6. Loss of limb/permanent physical disability
7. Death

This scale helps to focus the minds of staff when considering the level of risk or actual aggression they are dealing with. Such scales are helpful in adding objectivity to potential or actual incidents of aggression.

Many studies have considered inpatient violence in terms of a behavioural expression of underlying psychopathology (Betempts et al., 1993). Correlations between aggression with symptom profiles, diagnosis and other demographic details have been suggested (Davis, 1991; Webster et al., 1997). An understanding of these factors is useful to the practitioner of de-escalation, but it does not provide the most practical theoretical framework. Situational analysis is a much more useful basis from

which to consider de-escalation. This line of reasoning is supported by Cheung et al. (1997), who concluded that 69.9% of inpatient assaults (n = 332) were precipitated by interaction with staff. There is also good evidence that issues such as administering medication, preventing absconding and setting limits, all of which are common in the PICU, are often the start of aggressive escalation (Blair 1991; Bensley et al., 1995; Pelto-Piri et al., 2020). The realities of inpatient life will provide many situations that can result in a sense of injustice, real or perceived provocation and reason for discharge of aggression.

Frude (1989) suggested a model for the situational analysis of an aggressive incident. The model describes a progression of five factors through which aggression can result (see Figure 14.1).

Within the context of the PICU, a common example of the model's application is discussed in the sections that follow.

Situation

A patient is informed about the restrictions on smoking within an inpatient setting and demands to either smoke on the ward or be allowed to leave to smoke elsewhere.

Appraisal

The patient considers this restriction a further infringement of their liberty having recently been detained under the Mental Health Act (MHA) (Department of Health, 1983). They consider the offer of nicotine replacement therapy (NRT) in the form of chewing gum as further control of their lifestyle choices and potentially a route by which medication could be covertly administered.

Anger

Frustration results from an inability to make choices and decisions on their own and a loss of control of their personal circumstances. The emotional result is a feeling of anger.

Inhibitions

The patient is suffering with mild manic symptoms resulting in a degree of grandiosity. They have poor tolerance to their needs not being immediately met. The patient is also suffering some effects from nicotine withdrawal.

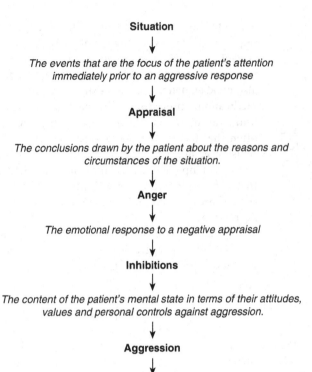

Situation
↓
*The events that are the focus of the patient's attention
immediately prior to an aggressive response*
↓
Appraisal
↓
*The conclusions drawn by the patient about the reasons and
circumstances of the situation.*
↓
Anger
↓
The emotional response to a negative appraisal
↓
Inhibitions
↓
*The content of the patient's mental state in terms of their attitudes,
values and personal controls against aggression.*
↓
Aggression
↓
The behavioural result of the progression to the model's other components.

Figure 14.1 A model for the situational analysis of an aggressive incident

Aggression

The patient is verbally abusive to the staff member and kicks the unit entrance several times.

The preceding is an example of the model's application to a common PICU scenario. It can also be applied to many other situations that occur in the PICU, for example, offering unwanted medication. When interacting with the potentially aggressive patient, the practitioner of de-escalation should attempt to make a rapid assessment of the incident's components.

During handovers and at other times when aggressive incidents are discussed, the incident in the example could have been simply described as 'the patient became aggressive because they weren't allowed to smoke'. The application of Frude's model allows this situation to be more thoroughly interrogated, resulting in a superior level of description. Through a comprehensive understanding of the incident, intervention may be applied at each point attempting to derail the journey from event to aggression. This may be achieved by using specific communication skills in combination with de-escalation tactics.

Component 2: Communication

It is not possible to set out a list of communication skills, the application of which will de-escalate an aggressive patient. The communication skills set out here are merely tools that are to be used by the practitioner and moulded by their individual style and personality. The content of communication with an aggressive patient needs to appear genuine and sincere and not just evidence of the theoretical aspects of the process. A successful de-escalation will be firmly based within the principles of the therapeutic relationship.

Non-Verbal Communication Principles

* Position your body so that you are communicating at an angle that is not confronting.
* Be aware of your body posture. Avoid postures that may appear authoritarian or defensive (e.g. folded arms or hands on hips).
* Attempt to communicate at the same height as the patient (i.e. standing or sitting). Being sat down during de-escalation is sometimes useful in appearing non-threatening. However, this may

place the staff member at increased risk if physical assault actually occurs.

- Be aware of your facial expression, ensuring that it reflects what you are saying verbally.
- Comfortable proximity between individuals during communication may be approximately one metre. This distance may need to be increased at least threefold in response to escalating verbal aggression (Lanza, 1988). As the intensity of the aggressive responses diminishes, then the distance can be reduced accordingly.
- Avoid the temptation to use reassuring touch early in the de-escalation process. As the situation calms, look for non-verbal and verbal cues suggesting permission to touch.
- Be aware of the use of eye contact. Maintain eye contact in the same way you would if you were communicating with a non-aggressive person. Avoid intimidating stares; appropriate use of eye contact will communicate genuineness and confidence.

Verbal Communication Principles

- Use a calm, warm and clear tone of voice. Voice tone may be altered as appropriate to reflect energy in the conversation (see 'mood matching').
- If a rapport is not already present, personalise yourself as quickly as possible (e.g. appropriate self-disclosure). This will help to increase inhibitions against assault.
- In the early phase of de-escalation, ask for specific acts which are relatively simple to agree on and do, and avoid long complicated statements (e.g. 'Let's sit down and discuss what you need').
- Avoid personal confrontation by remaining focused on the issues at hand, ignoring any personally directed attack.
- In the early phase of de-escalation, avoid being selective with your attention to the issues the patient is verbalising. Deal with what appears to be the main problem, even if this is uncomfortable.
- Avoid 'passing the buck'. Show yourself to be someone in a position to problem solve. Even if this means others are needed to resolve the issue after initial de-escalation.
- Avoid using jargon.

- Highlight the impact of the patient's behaviour, showing they are being listened to (e.g. 'You are scaring people with your shouting'). Statements like this can help to demonstrate that the patient is making an impact and thus diminish the need for further escalation.
- Reinforce your position as a helper rather than a restrictor.
- Keep the communication fluid and attentive to the content of the problem. Mood matching is useful in achieving this. This is where the energy in the discussion is temporarily matched by the staff member (e.g. by facial expression or raising the energy in your voice). (For further explanation, see Davis, 1989.)
- There are limits to what can be achieved verbally. Remain astute to the progress made towards de-escalation. It may not be possible to return the patient to a complete state of calm. If the expressed aggression has significantly reduced, then be prepared to disengage rather than risk re-escalation. Avoid the need to have the last word.

Component 3: De-escalation and Negotiation Tactics

In general terms, tactics can be defined as specific actions which aim to achieve specific results. Given the range of potential scenarios within a PICU, it is not possible to have an exhaustive list of tactics; however, developing one's understanding of a range of potential responses, which the practitioners feel comfortable using, is likely to be a firm foundation for any de-escalation event.

The Attitude and Behaviour Cycle

The attitude and behaviour cycle is sometimes referred to as the 'Betari Box'. Its origins are unknown and yet its logic is a base for many negotiating models across a range of sectors, including business and marketing. In the context of de-escalation within a PICU, the cycle has usefulness in reminding practitioners of the impact they can have and how their own psychology can affect that of the patient. Many staff within inpatient mental health settings across the full spectrum of services will have fixed attitudes towards institutional rules and patient behaviour. These attitudes may exist at a conscious or subconscious level. The attitudes will affect the practitioner's behaviour, which will subsequently affect the attitude of the patient and, in turn, their behaviour. Like all people with a range of positive and negative life experiences, patients too will approach situations with a range of attitudes that they carry with them.

This is illustrated in Figure 14.2.

In this example, it is the collective attitude of a group of staff which leads to a negative culture in the unit which patients may quite rightly feel is unjust, leading to unnecessary conflict. Much of the art of working in a setting where a level of routine and limit setting are essential is the ability to positively reframe. The quality of leadership in a unit can be considered by the way in which issues are articulated. For example, a large sign in stating 'THIS GYM IS LOCKED BETWEEN MIDDAY AND 9 AM' could be replaced by a nicely constructed poster stating, 'The Gym is open from 9 am until midday – do drop in and meet Sam our Sports Therapist'.

The Win Lose Equation

Many of the situations that may lead to aggression involve a perceived conflict of interests between the patient and staff member. A drama is often enacted where one party is left with a feeling of loss and frustration. This general issue has been tackled by management theorists and has been described by Le Poole (1987) as the win lose equation. In essence, a win-or-lose scenario is created. It is the objective of the de-escalator to, as far as it is possible, negotiate a win–win situation. Fig 14.3 illustrates this basic situation.

A common situation in which a PICU patient may enter the win-or-lose scenario is negotiating with a patient to accept unwanted medication. If the patient is given the medication against their will, they will feel as if they have lost and that the staff have won, which may lead to aggression. Through the process of negotiation, a win–win is sought. One method of achieving this during the process of

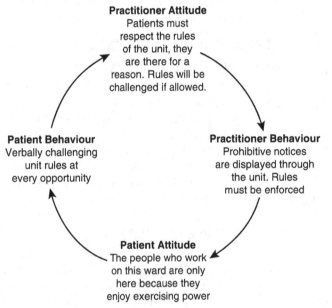

Figure 14.2 The attitude and behaviour cycle

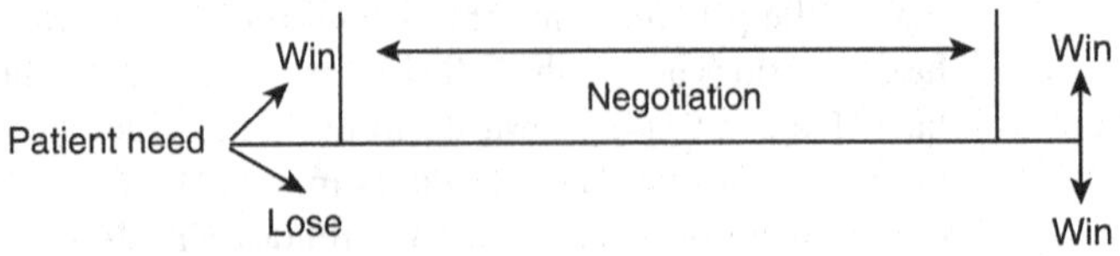

Figure 14.3 The win lose equation

negotiation is to offer the patient choices over which they have control. In the case of the unwanted medication, an example would be to offer the patient time to consider the benefits of medication and then to return to you with their decision. This is usually employed in the latter stages of de-escalation. The overall tactic is to create a feeling of empowerment (real or perceived) for the patient. Experience of using this tactic shows that in many cases the patient will return with a statement to the effect of, 'OK I will take it this time, but I want to speak to the doctor again before I take any more'.

Debunking

This is the process of debunking the need of the patient to make their point using aggression. This may be achieved by unconditionally accepting the content of the patient's grievance (Maier, 1996). For example, a patient makes that statement 'I am bloody sick of being locked up here, just let me go home'. A debunking response may be 'I don't blame you. I would feel frustrated too. Let's sit down and discuss what is needed for you to go home'. The general principle here is to shift the patient's focus from confrontation to discussion. This tactic is particularly usefully in the early stages of de-escalation as a means of grabbing the patient's attention and confidence.

Aligning Goals

A frequent precipitant to aggressive escalation is perceived as a state of affairs where the patient feels they have completely different goals than the staff do Examples of this include preventing a patient from leaving, the need to take medication and limit setting with disturbed behaviour. It is very easy to reinforce this perception by maintaining a linear focus on the issue of confrontation. If we look at the wider issues, there may be far more common ground than there first appears. For example, the patient wishing to leave may feel in confrontation with the staff who are preventing them from doing so. During the de-escalation the staff may align these goals by saying, 'I want you to go home too. Success for us is when you have no need for hospital. We have been working towards this since the day you were admitted'.

Transactional Analysis

The use of Berne's (1964) transactional analysis (TA) can be a useful strategy for de-escalating aggression

(Farrell and Grey, 1992). This involves a detailed understanding of three different contexts within which interaction takes place. These are defined by Berne as 'ego states', and during social intercourse, they are in the form of either the parent, adult or child. During the course of de-escalation, the principle is to ensure that the ego state within which the de-escalator is interacting is complementary to the patient's ego state. TA is a large area of study and courses in its use are recommended.

One related theory is that of the 'drama triangle' developed by Karpman (2011). In this model, a conflict situation can be considered with the protagonists being in one of three states of mind:

1. The Victim – the person who describes being and feeling at fault or blamed
2. The Rescuer – desperate to step in and fix everything but intolerant of other views
3. The Persecutor – the person who blames the victim through verbalising and behaviour

In a conflict, individuals may move between the different states as the drama unfolds. For the practitioner of de-escalation, this model can be helpful in being mindful not to behave as a persecutor (thus potentially reinforcing the role of a victim for the patient) and stepping in to be the rescuer. The preferred scenario is to try and step out of the triangle and encourage people to interact objectively and as equals.

Trauma-Informed Care

The concept of trauma-informed care (TIC) is becoming more widely used to underpin service models in mental healthcare systems, including the PICU. While TIC might more accurately be described as a philosophy or set of values, there are some aspects that warrant consideration and may be useful in the de-escalation scenario.

In the development of a TIC model, SAMHSA (2014) describes four key assumptions for services and practitioners:

1. Realising the impact of trauma
2. Recognising the signs and symptoms of trauma
3. Responding appropriately
4. Resisting re-traumatising

There are also six key considerations for successful application of the model:

1. Safety
2. Trustworthiness and transparency

3. Peer support
4. Collaboration and mutuality
5. Empowerment, voice and choice
6. Cultural, historical and gender issues

The wider concepts of TIC are likely to be relevant to any practitioner facing a distressed and possibly agitated person. Approaching a situation with empathy, compassion and a spirit of inquisitiveness as to understanding the root causes are more likely to lead to both an immediate and longer-term improvement in relationships.

While TIC has an inherent and obvious validity in mental health settings, the complexity of fully implementing this model in an institutional setting, which by its nature is restrictive, cannot be underestimated and requires clinical and strategic consideration (Wilson et al., 2020).

Adapting Tools and Techniques from Other Arenas

The de-escalation practitioner should constantly be vigilant for techniques or theories which they can add to their personal toolbox or use with others to help to understand and resolve conflict. Management and leadership training often contain a range of communication models which are aimed at achieving desired objectives. Some of these may have equal value in the urgency of the clinical situation. For example, the 'outward mindset' is often taught as a means of improving personnel management and yet its model of encouraging people to not be inward looking (focussed on their own results) but rather outward looking (focussed on shared results) contains helpful insights into seeing other people as collaborators rather than objects which can be used or are in the way (Lazan, 2016).

The practice of de-escalation is not solely a scientific or a technical skill but is highly reliant one one's own use of self and, as such, practitioners should not feel limited to one specific way of doing things but rather to treat de-escalation as a craft which is improved over time based on knowledge and experience.

Conclusion

The model of de-escalation offered here comprises three separate but interdependent components: assessment, communication and tactics (ACT). The ACT model should be considered as cyclic and dynamic, requiring the de-escalator to remain fluid during de-escalation. During de-escalation, it is necessary to continually revisit each component and ensure they remain complementary to each other. This is illustrated in Figure 14.4.

Under each of the headings, tools that have shown to be effective in the PICU setting are suggested. The list is by no means exhaustive, and each practitioner can modify the suggested tools to suit their own individual styles. In this chapter, the focus of de-escalation has been on the content of situations rather than the psychopathology of the patient. There is good evidence that many aggressive responses are indeed precipitated by situations rather than driven by purely psychiatric symptoms (Poyner and Warne, 1986; Whittington and Patterson, 1996). In many situations, psychotic and

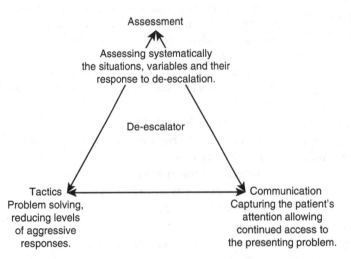

Figure 14.4 A model of de-escalation

other psychiatric phenomena no doubt play a part in the aggressive responses of patients. However, in many cases, these can be considered as some of many variables that need to be incorporated into the ACT model of de-escalation.

The PICU context, if unchecked, can become an environment in which conflict is the norm. The fact that most patients will have had their liberty removed and be detained against their will coupled with the potential for poor leadership culture can easily lead to disagreement, aggression and, potentially, violence.

PICU practitioners should view the desire to minimise conflict as a primary purpose of their work extending way beyond the immediacy of a critical incident into a much longer-term perspective of ensuring a therapeutic environment with time spent investing in therapeutic relationships.

References

Bensley,L, Nelson,N, Kaufman,J, Silverstein,B and Shield,J (1995) Patient and Staff Views of Factors Influencing Assaults on Psychiatric Hospital Employees. *Issues in Mental Health Nursing* **16** (5) 433–46.

Berne,E (1964) *Games People Play: The Psychology of Human Relationships*. Harmondsworth: Penguin.

Betempts,E, Somoza,E and Buncher,C (1993) Hospital Characteristics, Diagnoses, and Staff Reasons Associated with the Use of Seclusion and Restraint. *Hospital and Community Psychiatry* **44** (4) 367–71.

Blair,D (1991) Assaultive Behaviour: Does Provocation Begin in the Front Office?. *Journal of Psychosocial Nursing and Mental Health Services* **29** (5) 21–6.

Boettcher,E (1983) Preventing Violent Behaviour: An Integrated Theoretical Model for Nursing. *Perspectives in Psychiatric Care* **21** (2) 54–8.

Cheung,P, Schweitzer,I, Tuckwell,V and Crowley,K (1997) A Prospective Study of Assaults on Staff by Psychiatric In-Patients. *Medicine, Science and the Law* **37** (1) 46–52.

Davis,S (1991) Violence by Psychiatric In-Patients: A Review. *Hospital and Community Psychiatry* **42** (6) 585–9.

Davis,W (1989) The Prevention of Assault on Professional Helpers. In Howells,K and Hollin,C (eds.), *Clinical Approaches to Violence*. Chichester: Wiley. pp. 311–28.

Department of Health (2015) *The Mental Health Act 1983*. London: Department of Health. www.gov.uk/government/publications/code-of-practice-mental-health-act-1983.

Farrell, G and Gray,C (1992) *Aggression: A Nurse's Guide to Therapeutic Management*. London: Scutari Press.

Frude,N (1989) The Physical Abuse of Children. In Howells, K and Hollin,C (eds.), *Clinical Approaches to Violence*. Chichester: Wiley. pp. 155–81.

Johnston,I, Price,O, McPherson,P, Armitage,CJ, Brooks,H, Bee,P, et al. (2022) De-escalation of Conflict in Forensic Mental Health Inpatient Settings: A Theoretical Domains Framework-Informed Qualitative Investigation of Staff and Patient Perspectives. *BMC Psychology* **10** (1) 30.

Kaplan,S and Wheeler,E (1983) Survival Skills for Working With Potentially Violent Clients. *Social Casework* **64** (6) 339–46.

Karpman,SB (2011) Fairy Tales and Script Drama Analysis. *Group Facilitation* (11) 49–52.

Lanza,M (1988) Factors Relevant to Patient Assault. *Issues in Mental Health Nursing* **9** (3) 259–70.

Lanza,M and Campbell,R (1991) Patient Assault: A Comparison of Reporting Measures. *Quality Assurance* **5** (4) 60–8.

Lazan,M (2016) Changing Mindset to Improve Results. *Industrial and Commercial Training* **48** (5) 231–3.

Le Poole,S (1987) *Never Take No for an Answer: A Guide to Successful Negotiation*. London: Kogan Page.

Maier,G (1996) Managing Threatening Behaviour. The Role of Talk Down and Talk Up. *Journal of Psychosocial Nursing* **34** (6) 25–30.

McHugh,I and West,M (1995) Handle With Care. *Nursing Times* **91** (6) 62–3.

Nyberg-Coles,M (2005) Promoting Safer and Therapeutic Services. *Mental Health Practice* **8** (7) 16–17.

Patel,MX, Sethi,FN, Barnes,TRE, Dix,R, Dractu,L, Fox,B, et al. (2018) Joint BAP NAPICU Evidence-Based Consensus Guidelines for the Clinical Management of Acute Disturbance: De-escalation and Rapid Tranquillisation. *Journal of Psychopharmacology* **32** (6) 601–40.

Pelto-Piri,V, Warg,LE and Kjellin,L (2020) Violence and Aggression in Psychiatric In-Patient Care in Sweden: A Critical Incident Technique Analysis of Staff Descriptions. *BMC Health Services Research* **20** (1) 362.

Poyner,B and Warne,C (1986) *Violence to Staff: A Basis for Assessment and Intervention*. London: HMSO.

Price,O, Baker,J, Bee,P and Lovell,K (2018) The Support-Control Continuum: An Investigation of Staff Perspectives on Factors Influencing the Success or Failure of De-escalation Techniques for the Management of Violence and Aggression in Mental Health Settings. *International Journal of Nursing Studies* **77**: 197–206.

Stevenson,S (1991) Heading Off Violence with Verbal De-escalation. *Journal of Psychosocial Nursing and Mental Health Services* **29** (9) 6–10.

Substance Abuse and Mental Health Services Administration (SAMHSA) (2014) *SAMHSA's Concept of Trauma and*

Guidance for a Trauma-Informed Approach. https://ncsacw.a cf.hhs.gov/userfiles/files/SAMHSA_Trauma.pdf.

Turnbull,J Aiken,I, Black,L and Patterson,B (1990) Turn it Around Short-Term Management for Aggression and Anger. *Journal of Psychosocial Nursing* **28** (6) 7–10.

Ward-Stockham,K, Kapp,S, Jarden,R, Gerdtz,M and Daniel,C (2022) Effect of Safewards on Reducing Conflict and Containment and the Experiences of Staff and Consumers: A Mixed-Methods Systematic Review. *International Journal of Mental Health Nursing* **31** (1) 199–221.

Webster,CD, Douglas,KS, Eaves,D and Hart,SD (1997) *HCR-20 Assessing Risk of Violence, Version 2.* Burnaby:

Simon Fraser University and Forensic Psychiatric Services Commission of British Columbia.

Whittington,R and Patterson,P (1996) Verbal and Non-Verbal Behaviour Immediately Prior to Aggression by Mentally Disordered People: Enhancing Assessment of Risk. *Journal of Psychiatric and Mental Health Nursing* **3** (1) 47–54.

Wilson,A, Hurley,J, Hutchinson,M and Lakeman,R (2021) 'Can Mental Health Nurses Working in Acute Mental Health Units Really Be Trauma-Informed ?' An Integrative Review of the Literature. *Journal of Psychiatric and Mental Health Nursing* **28** (5) 900–23.

Chapter 15

Psychological Approaches to the Acute Patient in PICUs

Marc Jonathon Kingsley

Introduction

This chapter highlights some important features of psychological work within the context of acute psychiatric services. The specific focus is on psychological work within psychiatric intensive care unit (PICU) settings. The content offers an important opportunity to expand on the growing literature on multidisciplinary team (MDT) activities and holistic biopsychosocial conceptualisations within such contexts.

PICU treatment offers a short-term, multidisciplinary intensive treatment plan for patients admitted from a number of referring wards. An important feature of this treatment is the inclusion of psychological work. The role of the psychologist on PICUs may vary, and differences in treatment approaches may be expected. The National Association of Psychiatric Intensive Care and Low Secure Units (NAPICU) note in their National Minimum Standards (NAPICU, 2014) that all interventions should, however, be directed towards rapidly reducing acute symptoms whilst promoting self-management and recovery. This falls in line with broader literature written on the recovery, stepped-care approach to psychological therapy within acute psychiatric settings (Durrant et al., 2007; BPS, 2012; Paterson et al., 2018; Sweeney, 2018). According to this model, an inpatient admission highlights the point at which patients require the highest level of mental health care for the complexity of their presentations (BPS, 2012). Clinical psychologists are well trained to support the patient, their families and staff in consideration of the acute and longer-standing psychological triggers and vulnerabilities linked to relapse and admission (BPS, 2012).

The revised National Minimum Standards state that patients should have access to a range of psychological services. This includes access to a qualified clinical psychologist for a minimum of one day

(eight hours) per week per PICU unit, as well as low-intensity psychological provision by a range of MDT members, as a standard aspect of treatment. Hanna (2006) has noted how National Institute for Health and Care Excellence (NICE) recommendations prioritising psychological therapy for patients whose distress is persistent with high risk of relapse is a clear indication of the need for psychology within acute inpatient settings.

Evidence related to accessibility of psychology within UK PICUs remains limited. Literature is usually broader and applied to acute psychiatric wards in general. What literature is presented indicates the continued limited access to qualified clinical psychologists, with disparity in UK inpatient service provision (Small et al., 2018; Wood et al., 2018). This is despite national recommendations, such as those of the Royal College of Psychiatrists (2017) and NICE (2016), that the mental health acute care pathway should have direct access to qualified clinical psychologists who have the specialist psychological skills to lead on access to psychological interventions. A survey of inpatient experience of psychology on six acute wards, for example, found medical and nursing staff frustration over the lack of NICE-recommended, evidence-based psychological provision in the wards surveyed (The Regulation and Quality Improvement Authority, 2014–15). For patients, the quality of psychiatric inpatient care in the United Kingdom is reported as largely variable, often with concerns raised about lack of direct therapeutic and psychological activity on the ward (MIND, 2017).

A psychological perspective on patient admissions in PICU settings offers a valuable opportunity for mental health professions to investigate the holistic experience of ward culture and patient treatment on such wards. Such a holistic approach is important for the overall management of patients admitted to acute psychiatric services and is in line with preferred practice outlined in clinical governance. Clinical governance has been defined as a 'Framework to ensure that all NHS organisations have proper processes for monitoring and improving clinical quality' (Dewar, 1999). It is within this contextual framework that some important functions the psychologist may offer will be highlighted.

The role of the psychologist within a PICU may include several functions:

- Providing a psychological assessment of patients (Box 15.1):
  - delineating the link between the patient's current admission and their life history
  - forming a developmental history of the patient
  - providing a description of the underlying personality structure of the patient
- Contributing towards risk assessment and providing psychometric assessments when necessary
- Providing psychotherapeutic input to patients
- Providing carers' support
- Providing staff support (supervision and training)
- Contributing to ward activities (ward rounds, staff groups)
- Research studies

Box 15.1 Providing a psychological assessment of the patient

Patients admitted to acute psychiatric wards and PICU settings have a multitude of diagnoses and symptom presentations. The inability for such wards to have a homogeneous group of patients will result in patients with several different reasons for admission. A crucial aim of the psychologist in this setting is to offer a psychological formulation of the patient's difficulties. The major impetus to such formulations is to offer the MDT a glimpse into the patient's emotional world and the psychological triggers that may have contributed to the current episode and admission. On acute ward admissions, the focus may be narrowed to the symptom presentation and medication review, and the rich depth of emotional antecedents may be lost.

One of the key elements through which such psychological formulations are achieved is the provision of a psychological assessment; the format may vary, but the following points offer some preliminary outline of the assessment.

Attempting to Delineate the Link between the Patient's Current Admission and Life History

The significance of a patient's links between admission and life history can help the team gain a broader and more detailed recognition of underlying psychological factors that have contributed to the current presentation. Such historical links may be overlooked when patients present with overriding symptom descriptions. A case example illustrates this point.

Case History

A 30-year-old woman presented to a PICU with symptoms of agitation and mood lability. The psychiatric history of the patient was extensive and included a family history of bipolar affective disorder. The patient's life history was presented to the ward in short discharge summaries, but little was known of her developmental years. A psychological assessment gauged that the patient had lost her mother to suicide at the age of 5 years. She was cared for by her older sister who became a maternal figure. The patient functioned well until the time of her sister's marriage, shortly after which the patient had her first episode of depression. The patient described feeling like she had 'lost' a mother again. The psychological assessment gathered evidence of times in which the patient relapsed; a common theme seemed to be the patient's experience of loss or abandonment and her regression to an earlier emotional state.

This case example recognises the importance of an extensive developmental history for the team (Wallace, 1983). An investigation into the patient's significant life events and developmental milestones can offer the psychologist (and thus the ward team) the opportunity to formulate an outline of the patient's emotional life and personality structure. A detailed developmental history does not need to be performed exclusively for the psychologist but can be used by all team members to expand on the holistic understanding of the patient. For a detailed description of developmental history-taking see Wallace (1983). However, some important pointers to consider when taking a developmental history include (see Box 15.2):

- A patient's life history is integral to the understanding of their subjective experience (Wallace, 1983; Gabbard, 1994).

- A developmental approach recognises the significance of developmental milestones in the course of life maturity.
- Significant life stages include infancy, early childhood, middle childhood, adolescence and adulthood.
- The developmental history will attempt to track the patient's experiences throughout the different life stages.
- Detailed recognition will be given to situations in which the patient has been adversely affected emotionally (sometimes termed emotional deprivation).
- The links between such adverse life experiences and later personality development will be traced.
- It must be recognised that, for many psychiatric patients, their life history is a history of emotional deprivation, neglect, loss and abuse (Wallace, 1983).

Providing a Description of the Patient's Underlying Personality Structure

An important feature to investigate in the psychological assessment is the personality structure of the patient (Kernberg, 1975). The recognition of how the underlying personality structure of the patient makes them more vulnerable to admission will be outlined. An important aspect of this work is to differentiate those patients whose personality has been an integral and long-standing factor in their admissions from other patients for whom recovery from episodes of psychiatric illness leaves them reasonably intact (Gabbard, 1994). It may be difficult to fully assess the patients underlying personality structure during the period of admission on a PICU, as a person may be in the midst of an acute relapse in their mental health. The clinical team may need to rely on collateral from others or wait for a patient to recover from an acute episode to obtain a clearer understanding of their emotional functioning from their developmental histories.

The idea of personality structure has been investigated and outlined by several theorists and clinicians (e.g. Kernberg, 1975). The outline of such models of personality is beyond the scope of this chapter (see Wallace, 1983 for more detail). The basic outline, however, is for the psychologist to give the ward a basic formulation of the patient's ego functioning. Ego functioning can be broadly defined as that area of the person's personality that is primarily involved in adapting to internal drives as well as external environmental demands (Kaplan et al., 1994). Basic pointers that indicate weakened ego functioning (Kernberg, 1975) include:

- Poor control of basic impulses (sexual and aggressive)
- Difficulties with tolerating frustration or emotional pressure
- Maladaptive coping mechanisms (defences) in the event of stress and anxiety
- Poor/diffuse emotional boundaries
- Poor 'object-constancy', constantly changing experiences of both self and others (Kernberg, 1975)

The impact of psychiatric illness can often result in weakened ego functioning and the observation of these features. However, in some patients, such defects in ego functioning are an aspect of their underlying personality structure and are found even in the absence of psychiatric illness (Kernberg, 1975). It can be of use to the team treating the patient to have a clearer understanding of the long-standing ego functioning of patients on the ward. This is particularly important in their management and treatment. Those patients for whom longstanding ego weakness remains an integral part of their personality structure have particular therapeutic needs that will be described later.

Providing an Assessment of the Patient's Family and Social Dynamics

Providing a psychological profile of the patient should include addressing broader sociocultural issues that have an impact on patient admission and care. An important area is that of family dynamics. Much literature has been written on the role of the family in the lives of psychiatric patients (e.g. Faddon et al., 1987; Ostman et al., 2005). Mental health policies and guidelines suggest family, friend or carer involvement in patients' mental health care (Carers Trust Professionals, 2015), and the benefits of a family therapy approach have been noted, including relapse prevention and reduced hospital stays (Dirik et al., 2017). Innovative family and social systems approaches have developed, such as the Finnish-based Open Dialogue Approach, and its adapted Peer-Supported variant (Razzaque and Stockmann, 2016). Razzaque and Stockmann (2016, p. 348) have defined this approach as one ' . . . in which all staff receive training in family, systems and related methodologies, and treatment is largely carried out via whole-system/network meetings that include the patient'. Open Dialogue approaches to acute psychiatric work are a significant area of further therapeutic growth and innovation, and the reader is recommended to explore this area in further detail.

The Experience of the Admission to Hospital for the Patient's Family

Admission to a PICU is an emotional experience for both the patient and their close contacts. Coming to terms with the reality of a psychiatric illness can be an important aspect of the patient's stay on the PICU. This is equally an issue of concern for the patient's family and friends. The need for family members to have the opportunity to engage with staff members about this situation cannot be underestimated. The role of the psychologist on the ward is to guide the team within this area of treatment.

For many family members, having to face an illness of a loved one is a difficult and painful process to bear (Mervis, 1999). This applies to mental illness as much as to physical illness. The feelings associated with such a process can be complex and depend on the unique history of each family. However, overall, the experience can often be described as a grieving process in which loss can be a central aspect (Mervis, 1999). The team must be aware of the potential for the family to experience loss or, in certain cases, to defend against feelings of loss when the patient becomes ill or is admitted to the hospital. Understanding these feelings can assist the team to cope with the emerging dynamics and reactions experienced when dealing with families (Mervis, 1999).

Case History

A 30-year-old woman was admitted to a PICU. The ward soon began to receive phone calls from the patient's mother who was angry and demanding. Letters of complaint often arrived about the quality of care on the ward. Staff members felt defensive and angry in the mother's presence. A psychological formulation uncovered how the patient had experienced a steady decline in emotional functioning from early adulthood. Prior to the first admission, the patient had been a high achiever and successful. The psychological formulation helped to shed light on how painful the process was for the mother to watch her daughter steadily declining in mental health. The mother's anger helped her avoid feelings of underlying sadness and grief. Furthermore, the projection of 'poor care' on to the ward could have been linked to the mother's own feelings of guilt and her anxieties of not having offered sufficient emotional nourishment for her child.

This vignette offers an example of how important it is for the ward to be aware of the family's reactions to facing the psychiatric illness of the patient. The case is also found where, rather than loss being the overriding feeling for the family, it may be that feelings of fear and avoidance are prominent. When the family experiences a patient in the grips of acute mental illness this can have a lasting effect on carers. Often, family members witness bizarre or violent behaviour, and are left with feelings that need to be worked through. Without an opportunity for the family to face these feelings, 'acting out' by family members can occur, such as avoidance of the patient, with missed or short visits.

Family Dynamics 'Spilling Over' onto the Ward

It may be important for underlying family dynamics to be assessed so as to be aware of such dynamics if they are lived out on the ward. Staff may gain insight into the functioning of the family through observation of various interactions as they unfold on the ward. For example, it is important for staff to assess the patient's mental state following interactions with family or friends. A psychologist may be able to comment on some of the emotional effects on the patients and carers following family interactions, such as in ward rounds.

Case History

A 37-year-old man with a diagnosis of paranoid schizophrenia was admitted to a PICU. The patient spent most of his time isolated from the staff and fellow patients. He seemed suspicious and guarded. From the onset of his admission to the unit, the patient refused to eat hospital food. Staff queried whether this was due to his diagnosis of paranoia. However, it later unfolded that the patient would eat after cookery groups and preferred his mother's cooking. The family continually brought in food to the ward, spoke for the patient in the ward rounds and made decisions on his behalf. An examination of his home life indicated that the patient spent most of his time in his room, being brought meals by his mother and making minimal independent decisions. The team considered that there was evidence of an enmeshed family with poor boundaries, and it became apparent that this family dynamic was being replayed on the unit. This was particularly evident in the patient's resistance to making decisions and living independently without his family's constant supervision in ward affairs and activities.

The Provision of Psychotherapy for Patients

A core role of the psychologist on the PICU is to be involved in the provision of psychotherapy for patients. The evidence base for the effectiveness of psychological therapies, such as cognitive behavioural therapy (CBT) continues to be systematically documented (Radcliffe and Bird, 2016). The need to improve access to evidence-based psychological interventions for patients using acute inpatient mental health services is hence well documented.

NICE (2016) has endorsed and recommended low-intensity and high-intensity psychological treatments as an essential part of standard mental health care, including within acute psychiatric settings. Similarly, the Royal College of Psychiatrists' College Centre for Quality Improvement (2017) has developed standards for inpatient wards, which include recommendations for access to both low-intensity therapeutic activities and high-intensity, evidence-based psychological interventions. Similarly, NAPICU National Minimum Standards emphasise at least once-weekly access to a clinical psychologist (NAPICU, 2014).

Many people who use mental health services state a preference for talking therapies, or a combination of therapy and medication, over medication alone (Hanna, 2006). Small et al. (2018) emphasise the psychologist's need to be flexible and adaptable in delivering therapy in acute psychiatric settings, due to the patient's distress levels and the environmental constraints of the acute inpatient environment. Researchers have demonstrated the benefits of having a varied therapeutic programme on acute wards, including individual and group psychological interventions (Radcliffe and Bird, 2016). Radcliffe and Bird (2016) note, however, that inpatient groups may be particularly challenging and disruptive to run due to the nature of wards, with high patient turnover and unsettled mental state of participants.

The effectiveness of psychological therapies for those receiving acute adult mental health inpatient care remains unclear, partly due to the difficulty in conducting randomized controlled trials (RCTs) in such settings (Paterson et al., 2018). Similarly, the evidence base for the outcome of psychological therapies, including inpatient groups is limited due to the heterogeneous nature of ward treatments, with several possible variables impacting on outcome (Radcliffe and Bird, 2016). Paterson et al.'s (2018) systematic review and meta-analysis of controlled trials does appear to suggest, however, that brief psychological therapy on inpatient wards may be associated with reduced emotional distress, improvement in mental health symptoms and readmissions. The authors recommended that trials with both high internal and external validity were now required to establish the broader characteristics of effective brief psychological therapy with sustained benefits (Paterson et al., 2018).

The Therapeutic Relationship

It is well documented that the therapeutic relationship between patient and therapist in mental health care is one of the most important treatment factors which goes beyond the type of therapy type or treatment model (Theodoridou et al., 2012; Sweeney, 2018).

Psychologists will often differ in the type of therapy they offer. This will vary in technique and style. This chapter outlines the use of a particular therapeutic approach. The primary basis of such an approach is that of a relational and developmental model, which was outlined by Winnicott (1971) and later developed by Casement (1985), Gabbard (1994) and Wallace (1983). The core features of such an approach are:

- Recognition of how the provision of psychotherapy needs to address the level of emotional development in the patient
- Adjustment of therapeutic technique according to the developmental level of the patient

The importance of the clinician taking into account the level of emotional development of the patient was addressed by Winnicott (1971), who described how, for certain patients, the provision of a different experience to that of traditional psycho-analytic therapy was more effective. He termed this *therapeutic management*. These ideas have been expanded upon by Gabbard (1994) and Wallace (1983), who describe the importance of adapting the therapeutic technique to the level of ego development in the patient. This would include those patients whose fragility in ego strength is due to their present psychiatric illness. In terms of what this means for clinical work, the team will need to recognise certain key factors that may be applicable to a psychiatric intensive care setting:

- Psychotherapy should be more *supportive* (Wallace, 1983), in the sense of supporting the building up of ego resources in the patient.
- The therapist should be cautious not to unravel the fragile defences the patient is employing, and hence contribute to the patient regressing. (Regression is a term employed to describe a defence mechanism in which, in the face of anxiety, a person returns to an early level of emotional functioning.) (See Wallace, 1983 for more detail.)
- The emotional needs of the patient should be taken into account. Some of these needs may not be consciously recognised (Casement, 1985). One of the key emotional needs that has been outlined in work with such patients is the need for *containment*. This will be outlined in more detail later in the chapter.

In terms of the preceding descriptions, an important aspect of the therapeutic work is to keep the notion of *emotional vulnerability* in mind (Gabbard, 1994). In a short-term setting, this will assist the therapist to formulate a therapeutic strategy that will be meaningful for the patient. Patients may feel more contained if they have a sense of how long they will be working therapeutically and that sessions are more directive and structured. It could also be useful for therapists to encourage patients to openly address if they feel the therapeutic material is too emotionally painful or stressful.

Difficulties with forming a therapeutic rapport are part of the challenge for the therapist working with patients on the unit. Many of the difficulties found in therapeutic work in the psychiatric setting are highlighted in Chapter 7. It may be useful to expand on some other concerns that occupy the therapist working on the intensive care unit.

The Involuntary Patient

Patients admitted on to the PICU should have been detained under powers of the Mental Health Act (MHA) or equivalent legislation. Szasz (1998) described how the essence of the process of detention included ' ... the legal and/or physical ability to restrict another'. Compulsory actions, such as involuntary admission onto PICUs, and provision of regular psychotropic medication without choice, appear to increase the risk that patients will perceive their care as coercive (Theodoridou et al., 2012). Hence, it is important for the psychologist to consider the patient's subjective experience of the involuntary acute psychiatric admission and how much control and choice they feel they have over their psychological treatment. Procedural justice theory can be useful to consider in this respect, as it has been used to understand variations in compliance, such as between people with serious mental health difficulties and legal authorities (Watson and Angell, 2013). The nuance of this concept is that the more fairly a person feels they have been treated within a context outside of their control, the greater their cooperation with those providing treatment or management (Watson and Angell, 2013). It can similarly be applied to the relationship between mental health professionals in authority (such as psychologists) and patients who are involuntary detained (Theodoridou et al., 2012. Sweeney et al (2018) investigated the associations between patients' perceived coercion and the therapeutic relationship. Their study found that higher perceived coercion and less procedural justice was consistently related to a more negative patient–therapist relationship, as rated by the patient. This was particularly challenging in those patients with a history of previous involuntary admissions, as well as those with increased severity of illness.

Patients may appear resistant to making emotional contact with the therapist. There may be refusal to attend sessions or little initiative taken in therapy. The initial reaction of the therapist may be to see this as linked to the severity of the patient's mental illness. However, it is also important for the therapist to consider one explanation for the patient's withholding in sessions as being a possible reaction to the involuntary basis of the treatment. In a sense, the therapist's difficulty with engaging the patient in treatment may be the patient's only sense of control in treatment within which they feel disempowered. The patient may also fear that, in revealing these feelings, their stay on the unit may be prolonged. The therapist may need to spend time within the sessions addressing these issues with the patient and attempting in the process to build therapeutic rapport.

It thus would appear vital to consider the theme of perceived coercion in psychological therapy on PICUs, as this is generally a key feature of the patient experience and could adversely impact on the development and maintenance of a therapeutic relationship with the clinician.

Containment

Patients may need the physical holding inherent in the secure environment of the unit. This may leave patients with a belief that their anxieties or inner emotional states are unmanageable by themselves and those around them and that this is the reason for their admission to the unit. Patients may experience the involuntary basis of the treatment as a 'locking away' due to their inner sense of chaos or external behaviour. One important aim in psychotherapeutic work is to recognise that, for certain patients, a difficulty in making emotional contact may be due to the patient's deep sense of believing that they cannot be contained (Docker-Drysdale, 1991). A central role in psychotherapy would be to offer the patient the emotional space in which they may begin to experience their feelings and emotional states as bearable and tolerated by the therapist (Winnicott, 1971; Casement, 1985; Docker-Drysdale, 1991). Casement (1985) has provided a significant understanding of the therapists need to 'survive' highly charged emotional responses from patients without reacting too swiftly. He describes this further in the concept of 'analytic holding': 'Patients have taught me that when I allow myself to feel (even be invaded by) the patient's own unbearable feelings, and I can experience this (paradoxically) as both

unbearable and yet bearable, so that I am still able to find some way of going on, I can begin to 'defuse' the dread in a patient's most difficult feelings' (Casement, 1985, pp. 154–5).

The Violent Patient

Violence occurs frequently in psychiatric intensive care settings, particularly since risk and history of aggression within an acute psychiatric disturbance are key reasons for referral. Violent behaviour combined with severe mental health problems complicate the treatment of many mental health patients, particularly those with a forensic presentation (Fosse et al., 2021). Violence has a significant impact on patients, staff and teams, and hence a multidimensional approach to managing violence is vital on PICUs. This is explored in detail throughout this book.

Violent patients may pose a considerable challenge to the team on the intensive care unit. The psychologist working psychotherapeutically with these patients forms an integral role in their treatment. Violence may be the by-product of severe mental illness that will need particular pharmacological action. However, the psychologist may be able to point out to the team some of the *psychological* factors involved in patients' proneness to violence. Many patients who have admissions to acute psychiatric services have long-standing difficulties with regulating and containing their own feelings, which are hence turned into some form of action outside themselves. This action may include aggressive and violent behaviour.

From a developmental perspective, an understanding of this would include the idea that, since early development, the patient has given up in despair of believing that their emotional states could be understood or managed by the environment around them (Docker-Drysdale, 1991). This breakdown in feeling, as well as the concrete expression of feelings through actions, is important for the therapist to consider in the treatment of such patients. Another key aspect developmentally would be for the psychologist to consider the patient's (and their broader systems) capacity for boundary setting and management. In this regard, managing violence on the ward is thus intrinsically linked to the patient's need and capacity for containment. If this need for containment and boundaries is provided in too much of a physical manner (i.e. through restraint or seclusion), or by dulling emotions via sedation, a key opportunity is lost to help the patient to recognise that their emotional distress and anger can be managed and contained through the therapeutic environment of the ward and the development of their own emotional regulation strategies (Sweeney et al., 2016; Cusack et al., 2018; Sweeney et al., 2018).

Another important element of the psychological approach to the management of violent or aggressive patients is to understand their underlying feelings, which may include feelings such as rage and anger (Bradshaw, 1991). An investigation of the developmental history of the patient may give an indication of some of the antecedent features in the person's life that have left them feeling so angry and enraged. Such an approach recognises that the manifestation of violence constitutes a long-term building up of feelings that have their origin in some form of environmental failure and/or abusive experience (Winnicott, 1975; Miller, 1987, 1995). This approach could possibly help offer alternative considerations to the patient's violent behaviour so that the aggression is not just viewed as a manifestation and by-product of mental illness (Karatzias et al., 2019). In the last decade, there has been an increase in evidence pointing towards the important role of traumatic early emotional experiences, such as childhood abuse and neglect, in the later development of violent behaviour (Braga et al., 2018; Fosse et al., 2021). Recent clinical studies confirm, for example, that in people with a diagnosis of serious mental illness, those exposed to severe childhood abuse have an increased propensity of later being violent toward other people (Witt et al., 2013; Oakley et al., 2016; Hachtel et al., 2018; Buchanan et al., 2019).

Psychologists may utilise several psychological techniques to contain the patient and prevent the emergence of violence (see Chapter 7). An important element in the employment of interventions to assist patients with the management of violence is to give patients the opportunity to find ways to manage their own feelings and urges. The significance of this is to strengthen patients' coping skills, provide ways in which to enhance emotional regulation, as well as help patients to develop a growing sense of internal capacities and resilience. This is specifically linked to an attempt to reduce impulsivity in those patients with histories of impulsive aggression (Dawson et al., 2003). Specifically, certain behavioural techniques, such as anger and anxiety charts, may prove effective in such cases (Chaudhry et al., 2006).

It should be recognised, however, that the effectiveness of such psychological intervention is dependent partly upon the patient's capacity and willingness to use these interventions (Dawson et al., 2005). An example of this would be the patient's willingness to consider managing their own violent urges rather than relying on external containment such as drugs or physical measures of containment to manage their violence. For those patients who lack the abstract cognitive capacities to think about this, or who may on a deeper emotional level fear their own unmanageable feelings too much, the request by staff to use such techniques may be premature.

An important aspect of the role of a psychologist working on a PICU is to consider the emotional impact on staff who are regularly exposed to ward violence or the threat of patient aggression. Staff should feel supported and safe enough when expected to undertake this work, and the constant consideration of factors impacting adversely on staff safety should be regularly monitored and considered. This includes a recognition that staff on inpatient mental health units who rely on seclusion and restraint to manage aggression may themselves be traumatised by such practices or become demoralised in their work role and identity(Sweeney, 2018; Knight, 2015). There has been a recent move within the NHS to place work place well-being as a central component of the wider health service vision(Health and Wellbeing Framework, 2018; NHS England, 2021) and, as such, there is a growing recognition of the relationship between workplace violence, work stress and quality of life (e.g. Knight, 2015; Itzhaki et al., 2018). A vital role for a psychologist on the PICU would thus be to support staff on the PICU to consider the psychological impact of acute violence and long-standing risk of violence on their own well-being.

Suicide and Self-Harm

Many admissions to PICUs include patients who are actively suicidal or remain at high risk of suicide. A full understanding of suicidal behaviour remains challenging given its complexity and variability (Grandison et al., 2020; Zortea, et al., 2020), but there is a wide recognition of the central role that psychological factors may play in the development of suicidal distress (O'Connor et al., 2020). In a review of psychological autopsy studies for example, Foster (2011) found that at least one adverse life event was identified in the year preceding suicide in up to 91% of suicide deaths. There is a high concordance of suicide attempts with traumatic life experiences and repeated or pervasive exposure to traumatic events, such as childhood trauma, are known to further increase suicide risk (Angelakis et al., 2019). A psychological approach to suicide and self-harm on acute wards is hence a vital component of a more extensive biopsychosocial approach.

PICUs formulate effective and structured treatment plans in the assessment and management of the suicidal patient. This may include the implementation of high levels of observation and the consistent monitoring of patients' behaviour and mental state. An important aspect is the psychological assessment and management of suicide/self-harming.

In recent years, there has been a growth in evidence for psychosocial assessment interventions that are effective in reducing suicidal thoughts and behaviours (Zortea et al., 2020; Nuij et al., 2021). Zortea et al (2020) identified common elements across these varied psychological interventions. These include the vital need to undertake clinical assessments to provide crisis and safety planning and ensure that follow-up contact is available post discharge. Nuij et al. (2021) similarly conducted a meta-analysis of studies and found that safety planning-type interventions (SPTIs) are effective in reducing suicidal behaviour and should be included in clinical guidelines and treatment planning for suicide prevention.

There has, however, been a shift in the consideration of the value and benefit of psychiatric inpatient admissions for suicidal patients, especially when under an involuntary basis. Priebe (2019) linked the risk of loss of dignity in the forced admission of patients suffering with long-standing chronic and deeply entrenched suicidal despair. Borecky et al. (2019) similarly noted that more attention and research is needed to consider the potential harm resulting from the use of coercion and the loss of autonomy in managing suicidal despair and intent through involuntary admission. With this dilemma related to coercion versus dignity preservation in mind, if an alternative to involuntary admission cannot be safely found, it is vital to consider how it may be possible to provide a *therapeutic setting* for patients who experience suicidal despair and, as a result, are admitted to a PICU.

Addressing Hopelessness and Reasons for Living

An essential feature in the assessment and management of suicidal ideation and intent, independent of diagnosis, is to closely monitor the degree of hope/hopelessness patients may experience about their life and future (Department of Health, 2002). Hopelessness is greater in psychiatric patients who have a history of suicidal behaviour, both during and between episodes (Szanto et al., 1998; Mann et al., 1999), and is closely associated with whether individuals feel they have any reasons for living (Linehan et al., 1983; Mann et al., 1999; Malone et al., 2000).

Hopelessness is not only a potent predictor of suicidal intent in the short term. For example, Beck et al. (1985, 1989, 1990) have shown hopelessness to be a significant predictor of completed suicides up to 10 years later. Furthermore, hopelessness can increase depression and suicidal intent within self-harm populations (Wetzel et al., 1980; Salter and Platt, 1990). It has also been found to predict repetition of self-harming over varying follow-up intervals (Petrie et al., 1988; Sidley et al., 1999).

Hopelessness has traditionally been treated as a monolithic entity (Heisel and Marnin, 2004). However, researchers have begun exploring the dimensions of hopelessness in order to clarify the association between hopelessness and psychopathology (Flett and Hewitt, 1994; Hewitt et al., 1998; Heisel et al., 2003). Psychological examination of the dimensions of hopelessness, especially anticipated positive and negative future experiences and life events, can be greatly beneficial and is an important component to the psychological work with suicidal patients (MacLeod et al., 2005). It is important to consider the multidimensional components of hopelessness and, particularly, to consider domain-specific dimensions of hopelessness, such as social hopelessness (Hewitt et al. 1998; Heisel and Marnin, 2004). Social hopelessness is described as an interpersonal form of hopelessness in which negative, pessimistic expectancies regarding the prospect of experiencing satisfying interpersonal relationships is at the fore (Heisel and Marnin, 2004). Regarding this, Seager (2006, p. 7) notes that the risk of suicide sharply increases where people, ' . . . have lost all current meaningful psychological and social connections'. For people who have lost or failed to develop or maintain meaningful connections, the emergence of feelings of defeat and entrapment may add to the risk presentation (O'Connor and Portzky, 2018). O'Connor's Integrated Motivational-Volitional model and the role of defeat and entrapment in the development of suicidal ideation are helpful to consider in this respect (O'Connor and Kirtley, 2018).

As mentioned earlier, patients who are admitted within acute psychiatry often have long histories of destructive relationships, including being the victims of emotional neglect and abuse from early life (Wallace, 1983; Grandison et al., 2020). In terms of psychological work with PICU patients, the importance of considering the role that problematic, failed and or abusive relationships have had on the formation of hopelessness and feelings of defeat about the future is significant. Furthermore, re-enactment can occur within the relationship between staff and the patient, particularly with patients who present with challenging behaviour or are seen as 'manipulative' or 'attention-seeking' (Hinshelwood, 1999,). This may result in patients re-experiencing negative interactions with staff, such as that ranging from neglect to abusive experiences. This may intensify the sense of hopelessness the person may feel about their interpersonal relating or trust in others. The toxicity of such destructive relationships and environments is outlined by Seager (2006) in his conceptualisation of psychological safety in mental health services.

Psychologists working on PICUs can help implement psychological mindedness on the ward, in which concepts such as transference, negative countertransference/feelings in staff and an awareness and management of *malignant alienation* (Watts and Morgan, 1994), the potentially lethal distancing of patients from staff and other patients, are considered. It is thus important for psychologically minded ideas about the hospital and ward to be at the forefront of staff awareness. As Seager (2006, p. 6) notes, 'a hospital is much more than a place where an illness gets treated. It is a place where new attachments are sought out and even resisted, where the hope of being listened to, understood, contained and 'reached' is both restimulated and defended against. It is a place where new experience can repeat, reinforce or challenge old experiences.' Winnicott (1975) describes this eloquently in terms of the patient's unconscious hope for a return to a period of life predating emotional deprivation, in which good-enough attachments and experiences were held.

Seager (2006) reiterates the significant role that the hospital, wards and staff working with patients can offer in terms of 'hopeful attachments' and how detrimental 'ruptures of containment and attachment' in staff–patient relationships can be for patients. Work within this area is highly significant clinically, as patients who can begin to experience meaningful, consistent relationships may find their feelings of hopelessness about social relationships beginning to shift. A key area in which this can begin to be established is within the *therapeutic alliance* with staff. Hence, the overall attempt by staff to facilitate and develop supportive 'good enough' relationships with patients (Seager, 2006) is a crucial buffer against feelings of social isolation and consequent social hopelessness.

Suicide/Self-Harm Management and Staff Containment

As with suicidal patients, patients with presentations of self-harming can require complex management (Hawton et al., 2000; Harriss and Hawton, 2005; Leather et al., 2020). A key challenge for clinicians is in the categorisation of the self- harm as either being suicidal or non-suicidal in nature (Zortea et al., 2020). Zortea et al. (2020) note that reality is that self-harm behaviours often span both categories and can change in nature over time. We do know that for an individual who has engaged in self-harm, the risk of dying by suicide is significantly higher than for the general population (Hawton and Fagg, 1988; Owens et al., 2002; Leather et al., 2020), especially during the first 12 months following self-harm (Hawton et al., 2000). Repetition of self-harming increases the risk of further self-harm (Owens et al., 1994; Zahl and Hawton, 2004) and eventual suicide (Hawton and Fagg, 1988). Studies indicate, furthermore, that patients who have engaged in multiple (more than two) episodes of self-harm are at significantly greater risk of suicide (Zahl and Hawton, 2004). Hence, the importance of offering a therapeutic management plan for this patient group is an essential aspect of their stay on a PICU. It is vital for staff to be trained in the implementation of national guidelines on the assessment and management of self-harm, which is not always found in day-to-day clinical work. Leather et al. (2020), for example, have found in their recent study that fewer than 50% of their sample of healthcare professionals utilised national guidelines for self-harm, and less than 3% of their sample had used self-harm risk screening tools. Furthermore, as with suicidal patients, the therapeutic management of patients with self-harming behaviour can be challenging for staff (Watts and Morgan, 1994; Hinshelwood, 1999). The highly stressful nature of this form of patient treatment for the MDT is recognised by many staff (Watts and Morgan, 1994). Many such patients have had numerous hospital admissions and may evoke a range of emotions in the staff who manage their care (Hinshelwood, 1999; Chapter 7). The ability of staff members to feel able to recognise and manage the feelings that the suicidal/self-harming patient evoke will influence the overall treatment of such patients. Generally, these emotions may include negative feelings and a move towards moral judgement (Hinshelwood, 1999). The capacity to offer such patients a meaningful and therapeutic stay on the ward is challenged by their often difficult-to-manage behaviour.

Ongoing staff discussions and feedback about these patients are essential in considering the interpersonal effect such patients have on staff and fellow patients. It is often the role of the psychologist to help monitor the psychological effect such patients may have on the staff working with them and fellow patients on the ward. It is important, then, that staff working with suicidal/self-harming patients are given the opportunity to share their experiences and feelings about this work (Hinshelwood, 1999; Sweeney, 2018). Psychologists can offer support to staff in the form of support groups, post-incident debriefs or one-to-one supervision sessions. This offers staff the opportunity to talk about the emotional impact that such patients evoke and can hopefully have a containing function for the staff member, who then may feel more able to manage another shift and session with the patient. This can also help manage staff acting out, such as in negative counter-transference reactions to patients, and vicarious traumatisation and, even in certain cases, reduce high staff turnover via resignations from the unit (Hinshelwood, 1999; Sweeney, 2018). It can be helpful when staff experience 'iatrogenic trauma' (Cheng, 2021) on the ward. This is when staff may experience the nature of their work, including taking part in containing distressed patients, as potentially creating harm for patients, even if this is unintentional (Cheng, 2021).

Psychologists wanting to include such staff support groups on the ward need to recognise the possibility of the ambivalence that some staff members may feel about joining such groups (Hinshelwood, 1999).

The necessity for some staff to maintain a particular 'professional' image in front of peers and the fear that staff may experience feelings of becoming too vulnerable in a group should be considered. Furthermore, for those psychologists actively involved on the unit, the capacity to take on such a leadership role in the group may be seen as a possible boundary impingement. As such, outside facilitation may become a viable option.

Furthermore, the amount of time needed to work with such complex presentations may require a longer period of treatment than a short stay on a PICU. Ongoing support and professional contact with patients vulnerable to suicidal ideation/self-harming is necessary, and an investigation into the longer-term support available for such patients is important (Hawton et al., 2000). A key feature of the psychologist's role in the treatment of patients with suicide/self-harming is to address the possibility of referrals for psychotherapy post discharge, though this may be very difficult due to staff shortages and long waiting lists. It is also important for the MDT to be aware of the psychological dangers and risks of patients being discharged without ongoing containment and support from health professionals (Seager, 2006). Hence, it is essential for staff who meet at patient ward rounds and treatment reviews to consider psychosocial aspects of care, which MDT members may implement in the ongoing treatment plan post discharge from the PICU.

Reasons for Living

Patients who struggle with suicidal urges or feelings may describe reasons for living which help them resist these suicidal feelings (Malone et al., 2000). Addressing *protective factors* or buffers which may set in when patients contemplate suicide is as crucial as addressing the risk issues linked to the suicidal potential in the patient. Treatment strategies that increase awareness of reasons for living and meaningful purpose in life are seen as crucial in psychological work with patients presenting to the PICU. At such a vulnerable point in people's lives, strategies which could strengthen meaning and help patients to keep in mind reasons for living are crucial elements of a psychosocial approach on the PICU.

The work of Linehan et al. (1983) is crucial in this respect. The Reasons for Living Scale (Linehan et al., 1983) can help identify the factors associated with reasons for living. It can be used as an assessment technique in the suicide risk battery as well as a tool to guide the shorter-term therapeutic work on the PICU. This strategy is advised, independent of diagnosis, and is focused on helping staff to assess potential buffers and protective factors which may 'kick in' when suicidal ideation becomes prominent. The Reasons for Living Scale is a 48-item self-report measure that assesses the beliefs and expectations for not committing suicide. The scale consists of six subscales and a total scale. The subscales include Survival and Coping Beliefs (24 items), Responsibility to Family (7 items), Child-Related Concerns (3 items), Fear of Suicide (7 items), Fear of Social Disapproval (3 items) and Moral Objections (4 items). The subscales and total scale are scored by summing the items and dividing by the number of items. The overall objectives are: (1) to measure and assess whether the total score is above or below the cut-off point and (2) to assess the scores of each of the subscales and whether they fall above or below the cut-off point for that factor. The Survival and Coping subscale has been noted, in particular, to be an important shield to hopelessness and suicidal ideation, when strengthened. The essential feature of this subscale is the ability to utilise effective coping mechanisms and find effective solutions to problems when despair or hopelessness sets in. Helping patients to strengthen existing and/or find new adaptive coping mechanisms is an essential therapeutic intervention and is closely linked to therapeutic work on problem-solving. Problem-solving deficits are closely associated with hopelessness and increased risk of suicide/self-harming (Townsend et al., 2001), especially in patients with histories of suicide attempts and or self-harming. Hence, helping patients to adaptively find problem-solving techniques as well as strengthen protective buffers (i.e. reasons for living) is a crucial aspect of the brief therapeutic work that can be undertaken on the PICU. An integral element of this may be to help patients to draw up 'crisis cards' (Sutherby et al., 1999), in which they list their most significant reasons for living. These cards can be effective in times of emotional distress/crisis when it may be more difficult for the person to hold in mind the various reasons for living. It thus becomes an external reminder of those internal factors and, at times, may help buffer impulsive acts. However, the efficacy of such crisis cards in reducing overall repetition rates has in certain studies been found not to be effective (Evans et al., 1999). Psychologists can help with the training of the MDT in utilising this assessment tool as well as drawing up crisis cards. This can become an effective element of PICU interventions, ranging from nursing keyworker sessions to ward rounds.

Coming to Terms with Admission and Illness

As described in the section on 'Providing an assessment of the patient's family and social dynamics', the emotional impact of facing mental illness is crucial for the psychologist to address. For the person admitted on to the unit, the reality of facing a psychiatric diagnosis and admission to a locked ward can evoke an array of feelings. The psychologist needs to consider the psychological impact of the admission on the individual patient. *This becomes important in terms of how much the patient is able to accept the reality of their mental illness.* Patients may differ in this respect, and an integral role for the psychologist in individual sessions could be to assess the level of this acceptance of the illness. Some reactions the patient may experience in the struggle to come to terms with the diagnosis and treatment can be important to consider in the management of the patient on the intensive care unit and in referral back to the referring ward.

The MDT may be faced with patients who seem to have *poor insight* into their condition. They may deny the presence of mental illness or minimise the extent to which they are ill. This lack of insight may be seen by the team to be a by-product of the illness; the psychological approach would be to consider the possibilities of *denial* and *avoidance*. The patient may utilise defences such as these and it is important to consider how emotionally painful and frightening it can be to face the reality of such an illness. The psychologist may help uncover some underlying reasons for this reaction by the patient, such as the role which social stigma may play (Szasz, 1998). For patients, such as those who had high levels of social and occupational functioning, the label of psychiatric patient may be very difficult to acknowledge. An important aspect in facing this label may be the experiencing of feelings of self-loathing or shame. Bradshaw (1991) described shame as linked to a person's sense of feeling that there is something defective about themselves. The aim for the psychologist may be to examine such feelings and the impact of the mental illness on self-esteem.

Some patients may go through a period of low mood following admission to the unit and coming to terms with the reality of the mental illness. Rather than denying the extent of the illness, these patients may experience feeling emotionally 'stuck' and unable to move forward. They may be left with a sense of loss and hopelessness (Mervis, 1999). The psychologist may need to help the MDT become aware of this form of reactive depression, which may at times be confused with the initial presentation and hence overlooked in the management of the patient.

In other cases, admission to the unit may be one of several psychiatric admissions to acute psychiatric services (Wallace, 1983). Patients may respond well to acute management but may become more vulnerable when the recognition sets in of having been so ill again. This may be a crucial time for psychological work when the patient is particularly emotionally vulnerable. Patients may feel unable to bear living with another relapse. This is often found in the cases of patients with good premorbid functioning and in those patients who had assumed that they would not become ill again (Mervis, 1999). Patients may have the insight to recognise how much their functioning has declined and how different they may feel from those around them. The ability for the intensive care unit to offer psychological treatment, in which these issues can be addressed and worked with, is crucial. Patients may be able to do this in their individual therapy sessions as well as in group therapy sessions. It is also important for the referring wards who have admitted the patient to the unit to have an idea of how best to continue this psychological work after discharge from the intensive care unit.

Conclusion

This chapter highlighted some important features of psychological work in PICU settings. It outlined the psychological factors inherent in the process of patient care that the MDT must recognise. The essential aspect of this outline is the recognition of how patients admitted to and treated on the unit have an emotional experience and reaction to their illness and care. The aim of the psychological work is to bring these features to the fore and to address them with both the patient and the MDT. The psychological work begun on the unit is ideally continued once the patient is back in the referring ward so that the patient has a sense of continuity in terms of psychological care.

Appendix: Anger Management Group (example)
Khadija Chaudhry

Introduction
The anger management group (Chaudhry et al., 2006) comprises 12 weekly sessions lasting 40 minutes each, during which particular aspects of anger are examined. Due to variable lengths of stay and frequently changing group membership, sessions are designed to be self-contained and 'stand-alone', each focusing on a small number of key points.

Philosophy
Aggressive and violent behaviour coexist with a multitude of major psychiatric illnesses. Such behaviour tends to be more persistent in patients admitted to PICUs. These patients often have long-standing difficulties with managing their anger. The focus of an anger management group is to help the patients deal with their anger more appropriately and effectively, as well as to gain better understanding of some of the causes of their aggression and deeper feelings underlying the anger, such as hurt, resentment and disappointment.

Aims and Objectives
The main aims and objectives of an anger management group are as follows:

Psychoeducation
- To educate patients regarding the negative effects, both internal (mental health) and external (consequences), of poorly expressed anger
- To increase understanding about anger as a normal human emotion

Strategies and Skills
- To empower patients with the choice to control their anger
- To explore strategies allowing patients to cope more easily with angry feelings (e.g. relaxation exercises)
- To teach practical skills in assertive behaviour and problem-solving

Multidisciplinary Management

- To provide a regular and consistent information source for multidisciplinary treatment and management.

Methods and Theoretical Basis

- The programme utilises an integrative approach to problems of anger and aggression. This includes psycho-educational, cognitive behavioural, psychodynamic and group counselling models.
- The MDT, through ward rounds, refers patients to the group. Suitability of referred members is finalised in shift handover on the day of the group.
- The group is run with two assistant psychologist facilitators.
- The methods used in the group are:
- discussions
- role plays
- flip chart exercises
- picture exercises

Members are encouraged as much as possible to participate in all the different segments of the sessions. An effort is made to make the sessions as interactive and enjoyable as possible.

Group Boundaries

The importance of group boundaries cannot be overestimated. Considering the patient population of the PICU, it is particularly important to have consistent group boundaries which aid in the communication, containment and focus of the group (Nitsun, 1996). The group boundaries are presented to the group members at the start of each session and members are reminded about them if at any point in time the boundary is in danger of being broken.

Difficulties

Running an inpatient group can be quite a challenging task due to the heterogeneity and mental state of the patients. On a PICU, due to a short length of stay, the composition of the group constantly changes, adding to the difficulty. Some of the other difficulties that can occur in the anger management group include:

- The involuntary status of most PICU patients and the locked ward environment may produce feelings of frustration and resentment among the members. This could lead to the formation of the 'anti-group', which are the disruptive and destructive elements in the group (Nitsun, 1996). The limited group cohesiveness can allow destructive anti-group processes to manifest themselves in a variety of ways, ranging from deliberate disruption of the group to excessive dropout. The hostile, angry feelings that can be evoked during group sessions can place a strain on the facilitators and threaten the integrity of the group. In short, managing anti-group processes is a potentially challenging task for the facilitators, who must utilise alternative management strategies to strengthen the therapeutic process in the group.

- Facilitators need to be aware of their own emotional responses (counter-transference) to negative and hostile acting out in the group. Facilitators not addressing such counter-transference responses can lead to their potentially acting out and/or the emergence of feelings of burnout and amotivation.

- Often it is difficult for members to establish a therapeutic relationship in the group because of their short length of stay on the unit. As group members become more settled in the group and get to know other members and facilitators/staff better, they are transferred back to the ward from where they were referred. This adds to difficulties with group cohesiveness and group identity formation.

- For some members, behaving aggressively and violently may be an intrinsic part of their culture and identity (Robin and Novaco, 1999). For example, some members may have learned that aggression seems to be the only way to prevent violence being directed towards them. Furthermore, some members may feel that to show destructive aggression is a part of their being and they may consider anger management a direct threat to their sense of self or may simply consider that the group is not suitable for them.

- Gender issues may need to be considered in anger management. For example, many traditional views of masculinity assert that aggression (fights, verbal abuse/threats) is an acceptable and necessary part of daily life (Bem, 1981). Members may feel that to show anger and aggression is to show their power and, if an attempt is made to shift this behaviour, they may feel disempowered and less dominant. This feeling may be more prevalent among the male members. As a result, resistance to attend the group may be evident in such a situation. However, the reason for this resistance may need to be untangled. Other social and personal reasons for resistance to group attendance and change should also be considered, such as social class, cultural ethnicity issues as well as intrapsychic and other personal reasons.

In summary, the anger management group provides a psycho-educational and interactive experience for the members with an emphasis on understanding and dealing with anger and aggression in an appropriate way. The difficulties inherent in running such a group within a PICU setting need to be borne in mind. Particularly important is that facilitators recognise and work with patient resistance as well as their own emotional responses to the group.

References

Angelakis,I, Gillespie,EL and Panagioti,M (2019) Childhood Maltreatment and Adult Suicidality: A Comprehensive Systematic Review with Meta-Analysis. *Psychological Medicine* **49** (7) 1057–78.

Beck,AT, Brown,G, Berchick,RJ, Stewart,BL and Steer, RA (1990) Relationship between Hopelessness and Ultimate Suicide: A Replication with Psychiatric Outpatients. *American Journal of Psychiatry* **147** (2) 190–5.

Beck,AT, Brown,G and Steer,RA (1989) Prediction of Eventual Suicide in Psychiatric Inpatients by Clinical Ratings of Hopelessness. *Journal of Consulting and Clinical Psychology* **57** (2) 309–10.

Beck,AT, Steer,RA, Kovacs,M and Garrison,B (1985) Hopelessness and Eventual Suicide: a 10-year Prospective Study of Patients Hospitalized with Suicidal Ideation. *American Journal of Psychiatry* **142** (5) 559–63.

Bem,SL. (1981) Gender Schema Theory: A Cognitive Account of Sex Typing. *Psychological Review* **88** (4) 354–64.

Borecky,A, Thomsen,C and Dubov,A (2019) Reweighing the Ethical Tradeoffs in the Involuntary Hospitalization of Suicidal Patients. *American Journal of Bioethics* **19** (10) 71–83. DOI: https://10.1080/15265161.2019.1654557.

Bradshaw,J (1991) *Homecoming*. New York: Piatkus.

Braga,T, Cunha,O and Maia,A (2018) The Enduring Effect of Maltreatment on Antisocial Behavior: A Meta-Analysis of Longitudinal Studies. *Aggression and Violent Behavior* **40**: 91–100.

British Psychological Society (BPS) (2012) *Commissioning and Delivering Clinical Psychology in Acute Adult Mental Health Care*.

Buchanan,A, Sint,K, Swanson,J and Rosenheck,R (2019) Correlates of Future Violence in People Being Treated for Schizophrenia. *American Journal of Psychiatry* **176** (9) 694–701. DOI: https://doi.org/10.1176/appi.ajp.2019.18080909.

Carers Trust Professionals (2015) Triangle of Care Toolkit – A Resource for Mental Health Service Providers. (online) https://www.carers.org/resources/all-resources/60-the-triangle-of-care-toolkit-a-a-resource-for-mental-health-service-providers-introduction.

Casement,P (1985) *On Learning from the Patient*. London: Routledge.

Chaudhry,K, Kingsley,M and Ghafur,S (2006) The Anger Management Group at Pathways PICU. National Association of Psychiatric Intensive Care Units Bulletin **4**: 19–21.

Cheng,E (2021) Iatrogenic Trauma – What is It? Beyond the Cycle of Trauma Institute. www.beyond-the-cycle-of-trauma.org/for-physicians-and-nurses/iatrogenic-trauma-what-is-it.

Clinton,C (2000) Pathways PICU. [Unpublished survey] Goodmayes Hospital, Essex.

Cusack,P, Cusack,FP, McAndrew,S, McKeown,M and Duxbury,J (2018) An Integrative Review Exploring the Physical and Psychological Harm Inherent in Using Restraint in Mental Health Inpatient Settings. *International Journal of Mental Health Nursing* **27** (3) 1162–76. DOI: https://doi.org/10.1111/inm.12432.

Dawson,P, Galis,A, Hughes,L and O'Shaughnessy,M (2003) Development of an Anger Management Group Programme in PICU [Unpublished manuscript]. Pathways PICU. Goodmayes Hospital, Essex.

Dawson,P, Kingsley,M and Pereira,S (2005) Violent Patients within Psychiatric Intensive Care Units: Treatment Approaches, Resistance and the Impact Upon Staff. *Journal of Psychiatric Intensive Care* **1** (1) 45–53.

Department of Health (2002) *The National Suicide Prevention Strategy for England*. London: Department of Health.

Dewar,S (1999) *Clinical Governance Under Construction*. London: Kings Fund.

Dirik,A, Sandhu,S, Giacco,D, Barrett,K, Bennison,G, Collinson,S, et al. (2017) Why Involve Families in Acute Mental Healthcare? A Collaborative Conceptual Review. *BMJ Open* **7** (9) e017680. DOI: https://10.1136/bmjopen-2017-017680.

Docker-Drysdale,B (1991) *The Provision of Primary Experience: Winnicottian Work with Children and Adolescents*. New Jersey: Jason Aronson.

Durrant,C, Clarke,I, Tolland,A and Wilson,H (2007) Designing a CBT Service for an Acute Inpatient Setting: A Pilot Evaluation Study. *Clinical Psychology and Psychotherapy* **14** (2) 117–25.

Evans,M, Morgan,HG, Hayward,A and Gunnell,DJ (1999) Crisis Telephone Consultation for Deliberate Self-Harm Patients: Effects on Repetition. *British Journal of Psychiatry* **175**: 23–7.

Faddon,G, Bebbington,P and Kuipers,L (1987) The Burden of Care: The Impact of Functional Psychiatric Illness on the Patient's Family. *British Journal of Psychiatry* **150**: 285–92.

Flett,GL and Hewitt,PL (eds.) (1994) *Perfectionism: Theory, Research and Treatment*. Washington DC: American Psychological Association.

Fosse,R, Eidhammer,G, Selmer,LE, Knutzen,M and Bjørkly, S (2021) Strong Associations Between Childhood Victimization and Community Violence in Male Forensic Mental Health Patients. *Frontiers in Psychiatry* **11**: 628734. DOI: https://doi.org/10.3389/fpsyt.2020.628734.

Foster,T (2011) Adverse Life Events Proximal to Adult Suicide: A Synthesis of Findings from Psychological Autopsy Studies. *Archives of Suicide Research* **15** (1) 1–15.

Gabbard,GO (1994) *Psychodynamic Psychiatry in Clinical Practice*. Washington, DC: American Psychiatric Press.

Goldstein,MJ (1999) Psychological Approaches to Management of Violence. Paper delivered at King George Hospital, Goodmayes, Essex.

Grandison,G, Karatzias,T, Fyvie,C, Hyland,P, O'Connor, RC and Dickson,A (2020) Suicidal Histories in Adults Experiencing Psychological Trauma: Exploring Vulnerability and Protective Factors. *Archives of Suicide Research* **26** (1) 1–14. DOI: https://doi.org/10.1080/13811118.2020.1758262.

Hachtel,H, Harries,C, Luebbers,S and Ogloff,JR (2018) Violent Offending in Schizophrenia Spectrum Disorders Preceding and Following Diagnosis. *The Australian and New Zealand Journal of Psychiatry* **52** (8) 782–92. DOI: https://doi.org/10.1177/0004867418763103.

Hanna,J (2006) Psychology on the Wards. Star Wards. www.starwards.org.uk/psychology-on-the-wards.

Harriss,L and Hawton,K (2005) Suicidal Intent in Deliberate Self-Harm and the Risk of Suicide: The Predictive Power of the Suicide Intent Scale. *Journal of Affective Disorders* **86** (2) 225–33.

Hawton,K and Fagg,J (1988) Suicide, and Other Causes of death, Following Attempted Suicide. *British Journal of Psychiatry* **152**: 359–66.

Hawton,K, Townsend,E, Arensman,E, Gunnell,P, House,K and van Heeringen,K (2000) Psychosocial and Pharmacological Treatments for Deliberate Self-Harm. *Cochrane Database of Systematic Reviews* (2): CD001764.

Heisel,MJ, Flett,GL and Hewitt,PL (2003) Social Hopelessness and College Student Suicide Ideation. Arch Suicide Res 7 (3) 221–35.

Heisel,MJ and Marnin,J (2004) Suicide Ideation in the Elderly. *Psychiatric Times* **21** (3).

Hewitt,PL, Norton,GR, Flett,GL, Callander,L and Cowan,T (1998) Dimensions of Perfectionism, Hopelessness, and Attempted Suicide in a Sample of Alcoholics. *Suicide & Life-Threatening Behavior* **28** (4) 395–406.

Hinshelwood,RD (1999) The Difficult Patient. The Role of 'Scientific Psychiatry' in Understanding Patients with Chronic Schizophrenia or Severe Personality Disorder. *British Journal of Psychiatry* **174**: 187–90.

Itzhaki,M, Bluvstein,A, Bortz,P, Kostistky,H, Bar Noy,D, Filshtinsky,V, et al. (2018) Mental Health Nurse's Exposure to Workplace Violence Leads to Job Stress, Which Leads to Reduced Professional Quality of Life. *Frontiers in Psychiatry* **9**: 59. DOI: https://doi.org/10.3389/fpsyt.2018.00059/.

Kaplan,HI, Sadock,B and Grebb,J (1994) *Synopsis of Psychiatry*, 7th ed. Baltimore, MD: Williams and Wilkins.

Karatzias,T, Hyland,P, Bradley,A, Cloitre,M, Roberts,NP, Bisson,JI, et al. (2019) Risk Factors and Comorbidity of *ICD-11* PTSD and Complex PTSD: Findings from a Trauma-Exposed Community Sample of Adults in the United Kingdom. *Depression and Anxiety* **36** (9) 887–94. DOI: https://doi.org/10.1002/da.22934.

Kernberg,OF (1975) *Borderline Conditions and Pathological Narcissism*. New Jersey: Jason Aronson.

The Kings Fund (2015) *Patients' Experience of Using Hospital Services: An Analysis of Trends in Inpatient Surveys in NHS Acute Trusts in England 2005–13*. (online) www.kingsfund.org.uk/sites/default/files/field/field_publication_file/Patients-experience-Kings-Fund-Dec-2015.pdf.

Knight,C (2015) Trauma-Informed Social Work Practice: Practice Considerations and Challenges. *Clinical Social Work Journal* **43**: 25–37.

Leather,JZ, O'Connor,RC, Quinlivan,L, Kapur,N, Campbell,S and Armitage,CJ (2020) Healthcare Professionals' Implementation of National Guidelines with Patients Who Self-Harm. *Journal of Psychiatric Research* **130**: 405–11. DOI: https://doi.org/10.1016/j.jpsychires.2020.08.031.

Linehan,MM, Goodstein,JL, Nielsen,SL and Chiles,JA (1983) Reasons for Staying Alive When You are Thinking of Killing Yourself: The Reasons for Living Inventory. *Journal of Consulting and Clinical Psychology* **51** (2) 276–86.

MacLeod,AK, Tata,P, Tyrer,P, Schmidt,U, Davidson,K and Thompson,S (2005) Hopelessness and Positive and Negative Future Thinking in Parasuicide. *British Journal of Clinical Psychology* **44** (4): 495–504.

Malone,KM, Oquendo,MA, Haas,GL, Ellis,SP, Li,S and Mann,JJ (2000) Protective Factors against Suicidal Acts in Major Depression: Reasons for Living. *American Journal of Psychiatry* **157** (7) 1084–8.

Mann,JJ, Waternaux,C, Haas,GL and Malone,KM (1999) Toward a Clinical Model of Suicidal Behaviour in Psychiatric Patients. *American Journal of Psychiatry* **156** (2): 181–9.

Mervis,J (1999) Workshop on Loss and Grief. Presented to Mental Health Professionals at Tara Hospital. Gauteng, South Africa.

Miller,A (1987) *For Your Own Good.* London: Virago.

Miller,A (1995) *The Drama of Being a Child: The Search for the True Self.* London: Virago.

Milnes,D, Owens,D and Blenkiron,P (2002) Problems Reported by Self-Harm Patients: Perception, Hopelessness, and Suicidal Intent. *Journal of Psychosomatic Research* **53** (3) 819–22.

Mind (2017) *Ward Watch: Mind's Campaign to Improve Hospital Conditions for Mental Health Patients.* Mind: London.

National Association of Psychiatric Intensive Care and Low Secure Units (NAPICU) (2014) *National Minimum Standards for Psychiatric Intensive Care in General Adult Services.* (online) https://napicu.org.uk/wp-content/uploads/2014/12/NMS-2014-final.pdf.

National Institute for Health and Clinical Excellence (NICE) (2016) Transition between Inpatient Mental Health Settings and Community or Care Home Settings. National guideline [NG53]. (online) www.nice.org.uk/guidance/ng53.

NHS Employers (2018) NHS Health and Well-Being Framework. (online) www.nhsemployers.org/case-studies-and-resources/2018/05/nhs-health-and-wellbeing-framework/.

NHS England (2021) 2021/22 Priorities and Operational Planning Guidance. (online) www.england.nhs.uk/publication/2021-22-priorities-and-operational-planning-guidance/.

Nitsun,M (1996) *The Anti-Group: Destructive Forces in the Group and their Creative Potential.* London: Routledge.

Nuij,C, van Ballegooijen,W, Juniar,D, Erlangsen,A, Portzky, G, O'Connor,RC, et al. (2021) Safety Planning-type Interventions for Suicide Prevention: Meta-Analysis. *British Journal of Psychiatry* **219** (2) 419–26.

O'Connor,RC and Kirtley,OJ (2018) The Integrated Motivational-Volitional Model of Suicidal Behaviour. *Philosophical Transactions of the Royal Society of London* **373**(1754) 20170268. DOI: https://doi.org/10.1098/rstb.2017.0268.

O'Connor,RC and Portzky, G (2018) The Relationship between Entrapment and Suicidal Behavior through the Lens of the Integrated Motivational–Volitional Model of Suicidal Behavior. *Current Opinion in Psychology* **22**: 12–17. DOI: https://doi.org/10.1016/j.copsyc.2017.07.021.

O'Connor,DB, Gartland,N and O'Connor,RC (2020) Stress, Cortisol and Suicide Risk. *International Review of Neurobiology* **152**: 101–30.

Oakley,C, Harris,S, Fahy,T, Murphy,D and Picchioni,M (2016) Childhood Adversity and Conduct Disorder: A Developmental Pathway to Violence in Schizophrenia. *Schizophrenia Research* **172** (1–3) 54–9. DOI: https://doi.org/10.1016/j.schres.2016.01.047.

Ostman,T and Wallsten,KL (2005) Family Burden and Relatives' Participation in Psychiatric Care: Are the Patient's Diagnosis and the Relation to the Patient of Importance? *International Journal of Social Psychiatry* **51**(4): 291–301.

Owens,D, Dennis,M, Read,S and Davis,N (1994) Outcome of Deliberate Self-Poisoning. An Examination of Risk Factors for Repetition. *British Journal of Psychiatry* **165** (6) 797–801.

Owens,D, Horrocks,J and House,A (2002) Fatal and Non-fatal Repetition of Self-Harm: Systematic Review. *British Journal of Psychiatry* **181**: 193–9.

Paterson,C, Karatzias,T, Harper,S, Dougall,N, Dickson,A and Hutton,P (2018) A Feasibility Study of a Cross-Diagnostic, CBT-Based Psychological Intervention for Acute Mental Health Inpatients: Results, Challenges, and Methodological Implications. *British Journal of Clinical Psychology* **58** (2) 211–30.

Petrie,K, Chamberlain,K and Clarke,D (1988) Psychological Predictors of Future Suicidal Behaviour in Hospitalized Suicide Attempters. British Journal of Clinical Psychology **27** (3) 247–58.

Priebe,S (2019) Involuntary Hospitalization of Suicidal Patients: Time for New Answers to Basic Questions?. American journal of Bioethics **19** (10) 90–2. DOI: https://10.1080/15265161.2019.1654033.

Radcliffe,J and Bird,L (2016) Talking Therapy Groups on Acute Psychiatric Wards: Patients' Experience of Two Structured Group Formats. *BJPsych Bulletin* **40**(4) 187–91.

Razzaque,R and Stockmann,T (2016) An Introduction to Peer-supported Open Dialogue In Mental Healthcare. *Advances In Psychiatry Treatment* **22** (5): 348–56.

The Regulation and Quality Improvement Authority (2014–15) *A Review of Acute Mental Health Inpatient Access to Psychological Interventions and Therapies.* (online) www.rqia.org.uk/RQIA/files/aa/aaa0a727-0801-4e30-9947-313acef111a1.pdf.

Robin,S and Novaco,RW (1999) Systems Conceptualisation and Treatment of Anger. *Journal of Clinical Psychology* **55** (3) 325–37.

Royal College of Psychiatrists (2017) Standards for Inpatient Mental Health Services. (online) www.rcpsych.ac.uk›default-source›ccqi›quality-networks›aims/.

Salter,D and Platt,S (1990) Suicidal Intent, Hopelessness and Depression in a Parasuicide Population: The Influence of Social Desirability and Elapsed Time. *British Journal of Clinical Psychology* **29** (4) 361–71.

Seager,M (2006) The Concept of 'Psychological Safety' – A Psychoanalytically Informed Contribution Towards 'Safe, Sound & Supportive' Mental Health Services. *Psychoanalytic Psychotherapy* **20** (4) 266–80.

Sidley,GL, Callam,R, Wells,A, Hughes,T and Whitaker,K (1999) The Prediction of Parasuicide Repetition in a High risk Group. *British Journal of Clinical Psychology* **38** (4) 375–86.

Sinclair,J and Hawton,K (2004) Suicide and Deliberate Self-Harm. In Guthrie,E (ed.), *Handbook of Liaison Psychiatry.* Cambridge: Cambridge University Press.

Small,C, Huddy,V and Williams.,C (2018) Individual Psychological Therapy in an Acute Inpatient Setting: Service User and Psychologist Perspectives. *Psychology and Psychotherapy* **91** (4) 417–33.

Sutherby,K, Szmukler,GI, Halpern,A, Alexander,G, Thornicroft,G, Johnson,C, et al. (1999) A Study of 'Crisis Cards' in a Community Psychiatric Service. *Acta Psychiatrica Scandinavica* **100** (1) 56–61.

Sweeney,A, Clement,S, Filson,B and Kennedy,A (2016) Trauma-Informed Mental Healthcare in the UK: What Is It and How Can We Further its Development? *Mental Health Review Journal* **21** (3) 174–92.

Sweeney,A, Filson,B, Kennedy,A, Collinson,L and Gillard,S (2018) A Paradigm Shift: Relationships in Trauma-Informed Mental Health Services. *BJPsych Advances* **24** (5) 319–33. DOI: https://doi.org/10.1192/bja.2018.29.

Szanto,K, Reynolds,CF, Conwell,Y, Begley,AE and Houck,P (1998) High Levels of Hopelessness Persist in Geriatric Patients with Remitted Depression and a History of Suicide Attempt. *Journal of the American Geriatric Society* **46** (11) 1401–6.

Szasz,T (1998) The Involuntary Patient. *British Journal of Psychiatry* **15**: 216–25.

Theodoridou,A, Schlatter,F, Ajdacic,V, Rössler,W and Jäger,M (2012) Therapeutic relationship in the context of perceived coercion in a psychiatric population. *Psychiatry Research* **200** (2–3) 939–44. DOI: https://10.1016/j .psychres.2012.04.012.

Townsend,E, Hawton,K, Altman,DG, Arensman,E, Gunnell,D, Hazell,P, et al. (2001) The Efficacy of Problem-Solving Treatments after Deliberate Self-Harm: Meta-Analysis of Randomised Controlled Trials with Respect to Depression, Hopelessness and Improvement in Problems. *Psychological Medicine* **31** (6) 979–88.

Wallace,ER (1983) *Dynamic Psychiatry in Theory and Practice.* Philadelphia: Lea & Febiger.

Watson,AC and Angell,B (2013) The Role of Stigma and Uncertainty in Moderating the Effect of Procedural Justice on Cooperation and Resistance in Police Encounters with Persons with Mental Illnesses. *Psychology, Public Policy, and Law* **19** (1) 30–9. DOI: h ttps://doi:10.1037/a0027931.

Watts,D and Morgan,G (1994) Malignant Alienation: Dangers for Patients Who Are Hard to Like. *British Journal of Psychiatry* **164** (1) 11–15.

Wetzel,RD, Margulies,T, Davis,R and Karam,EI (1980) Hopelessness, Depression, and Suicidal Intent. *Journal of Clinical Psychiatry* **41** (5) 159–60.

Winnicott,DW (1971) *Playing and Reality.* New York: Basic Books.

Winnicott,DW (1975) *Through Paediatrics to PsychoAnalysis.* New York: Basic Books.

Winnicott,DW (1984) The Antisocial Tendency. In Winnicott,C, Shepherd,R and Davis,M (eds.), *Deprivation and Delinquency.* London: Tavistock Publications. pp. 120–31.

Witt,K, van Dorn,R and Fazel,S (2013) Risk Factors for Violence in Psychosis: Systematic Review and Meta-Regression Analysis of 110 Studies. *PLoS ONE* **8** (2) e55942. DOI: https://doi.org/10.1371/journal .pone.0055942.

Wood,L, Williams,C, Billings,J and Johnson,S (2018) The Role of Psychology in a Multidisciplinary Psychiatric Inpatient Setting: Perspective from the Multidisciplinary Team. *Psychology and Psychotherapy* **92** 4 554–64). DOI: https://europepmc.org/article/MED/29345801.

Zahl,D and Hawton,K (2004) Repetition of Deliberate Self-Harm and Subsequent Suicide Risk: Long-Term Follow-up Study of 11583 Patients. *British Journal of Psychiatry* **185**: 70–5.

Zortea,TC, Cleare,S, Melson,AJ, Wetherall,K and O'Connor, RC (2020) Understanding and Managing Suicide Risk. *British Medical Bulletin* **134** (1) 73–84. DOI: https://doi .org/10.1093/bmb/ldaa013.

Chapter 16

A Social Behaviour Theory Approach to Challenging Behaviours in Psychosis

Brian Malcolm McKenzie

Introduction

Defining the Model

This chapter presents an understandable and robust framework that a treating team can use in the face of challenging behaviour, even if team members come from differing theoretical positions. The model presented is based on functional analysis (Mace, 1994) while accepting that the challenging individual has historically determined distortions of internal cognitions which lead to a misappraisal of the ward social situation. The model also holds that the contextual features (the ward context and actions of the team) will determine patient perception and maintain behaviour.

Functional analysis arose out of instrumental or operant conditioning models (Skinner, 1957) and holds that behaviours followed by satisfying outcomes will be repeated (Thorndike's law of effect). This remains the core of the model proposed. The model draws from developments in behavioural and cognitive therapies (Beck and Freeman, 1990; Linehan, 1993), in particular cognitive behavioural therapy (CBT) for psychosis in which it is understood that the satisfying outcome of the behaviour may be an internal one, often the reduction of aversive emotional states associated with distorted cognitions (Garety et al., 2001) The work developed by trauma-informed approaches (Han et al., 2021) and the understanding of social context in determining behavioural outcomes (Byrt, 1999; Ackerman et al., 2018) are also incorporated.

Challenging behaviour may simply be defined as a pattern of behaviour that poses a risk, physically, psychologically or socially to self or others. More complex definitions exist; Shepherd (1999) defines the 'challenging behaviour group' as having 'a combination of severe and intractable clinical symptoms, a range of behavioural problems and profound social dislocation'. For the purposes of this chapter, complexity will be eschewed and challenging behaviour will be viewed as a pattern of behaviour that poses the risk described previously. For example, there exists a significant risk association between head injury and challenging behaviour (Brown et al., 2019). Behaviours such as medication non-compliance or drug use are also clearly risk associated. However, they will not be taken up in this chapter, but the model should be sufficiently elastic to incorporate these as functional factors.

Furthermore, the behaviour will be seen as primarily a ward-based problem insofar as the behaviour is contextual. The subjective appraisal of 'social–emotional' meaning of the ward situation will determine behaviour and choices of the challenging individual (Byrt 1999). In turn, this behaviour will be subject to interpretations and 'social reinforcements' from both the individual and staff group who ultimately determine the overall pattern of risk behaviour.

Difficult behaviour posed to the treating team will be seen as linked to psychosis, although the latter term is held purposefully loose. Ultimately, within this framework, psychosis becomes a connection of disturbed social transference, disturbed and disorganised perception of the social context, disinhibition and dysregulation of behaviour and, finally, distorted appraisal of reinforcing events. The more all these factors deviate from the norm, the more psychotic they are. It may be felt that a reality is being avoided and the chapter is adopting a social relativism, however, the reader should rest assured that psychological disturbance is associated with and determines psychotic conditions (Bental, 2004).

Psychosis and Risk

We know that psychosis is not invariably connected to patterns of severe risk behaviours but that an association exists. In the case of paranoid psychotic conditions, risk of harm to others is elevated. In a Danish birth cohort of more than 358,000 people, the risk for violent offending for men with schizophrenia was 4.6 times greater than that of the general population, even after controlling for the potentially confounding factor of low socioeconomic status (SES). For women, the risk was 23.2 times greater (Brennan et al., 2000).

In a meta review, the factor of psychosis being associated with inpatient violence was determined to be at least of moderate effect size and comparable to other risk factors such as substance misuse and personality disorder, leading to a 50%–70% increase in the odds ratio for violence over the general population (Douglas et al., 2009).

The relationship between psychosis and self-harm is even more pronounced. The rates of self-harm/suicide attempts in psychotic patients are up to 50% (Fedyszyn et al., 2016). After first-episode psychosis, patients are 12 times more likely to complete suicide than the general population (Challis et al., 2013). While the greatest risk period is during the first year after presentation, studies have noted that the risk of self-harm or a serious suicide attempt remains in more advanced stages of the disorder (Challis et al., 2013).

The link between psychosis and substance addiction is even more profound. It is generally a trick question to trap the unwary student, but the factor most associated with psychosis is smoking. It is estimated that up to 95% of individuals with schizophrenia have a nicotine addiction. While it has a secondary character in that substance misuse might not be severe risk behaviour in itself, the link between substance misuse and violence in inpatient settings is clear.

A review conducted by Fazel et al. (2009) found the odds of violence to increase at least fourfold in individuals with severe mental illness who abuse substances as compared to non-substance abusing individuals with the same disorders.

The Challenge Facing Inpatient Teams

Once all these risks have accumulated and are carried over into the inpatient setting, the clinician and frontline team have a clear potential challenge. They need to develop robust strategies because these disturbed behaviours pose a risk to their primary goal, which is the safe treatment and fostering of recovery in the group.

In this sense, maintaining the ward social setting is equally a consideration. We are all (via direct experience or anecdotally) aware of the impact one or two aggressive patients might have on the entire ward atmosphere with increased disturbed behaviour in the patient group at large and secondary impacts such as staff illness. Keeping the ward environment safe and with requisite emotional space to embark on rehabilitation becomes a priority in care planning.

The intensive aspect of patient care is therefore often more about the psychological and behavioural management of all these challenging behaviours than the direct treatment of psychotic symptoms, although there is an interactional effect.

In a discussion with Dr Beer (the original editor of this book), I lamented the chaotic and dangerous quality of the ward. Always the historian, he referenced that such qualities were inherent to psychiatric ward life and originated with the Bethlem, a psychiatric hospital in London. Nevertheless, he enthusiastically supported the addressing of these chaotic dangerous aspects with patients in a group setting and embarking on a process of repairing their internal conceptions of their relationship with staff, leading to a spectacular decrease in violent incidents. This approach was not fundamentally different from that espoused by the Henderson Hospital at the time with personality disorder but was more cautious in assuming a curative aspect.

Understanding Challenging Behaviour

Links between Psychosis and Challenging Behaviour

It is always useful to start with basic functional analysis of any patterns of problematic behaviour (See Figure 16.1). The basic model adopted by the chapter is modified by cognitive psychology. The model holds *that in any given situation (A) as perceived by the actor, the behaviour (B) achieves an immediate positive consequence (C) as appraised by the actor.* The model proposes that the (challenging) behaviour is at least perceived as subjectively rational by the individual.

Although a direct relationship between the A, B and C elements are often obscure, the processes as set out in functional analysis of ordinary behaviour

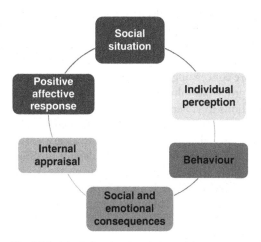

Fig. 16.1 A basic functional analysis model

underlie patterns of disturbed behaviours in individuals with psychosis. Put simply, it is in the area of distorted appraisal of the situation and distorted internal appraisal of the outcome of the behaviour, as well as disinhibition of the behaviour, that 'psychosis' exists. Looking specifically at violence committed by psychotic inpatients, this is a position largely forwarded by Douglas et al. (2009). They argue that if psychosis is a contributing cause to violence, there are three major roles it may potentially play:

- **A role in focusing (organising) decisions and behaviour**, giving individuals a clear motivation for violence. Behaviour and acts are complex, organised and goal oriented, even if appearing illogical to outside observers. This has been described aptly as the '**principle of rationality within irrationality**'.
- **A role in destabilising (disorganising) perception**, emotions and behaviour, interfering with the ability of individuals to manage interpersonal conflicts.
- A **disinhibiting** role in violence.

The authors examined several reports of inpatient violence. All models explained variance, but the model *Paranoid thoughts> anger > violence* (**rationality within irrationality**) explained most of the variance. *Anger > paranoid thoughts> violence* (**disorganising**) and *Anger >disinhibition > violence* (**disinhibiting**) were less explanatory.

The model of rationality within irrationality held in most situations, suggesting angry affective state arose out of distorted beliefs (delusional or paranoid thinking). Within the context of distorted cognitions, the behaviour was driven by subjective beliefs and, to that extent, was logical.

Central to any model of challenging behaviour must be distorted beliefs. In the case of patients with psychosis, these are often 'threat-driven beliefs' (i.e. paranoid beliefs that others wish to harm the self physically or psychologically). In reference to the proposed model, these distorted beliefs drive both the appraisal of the situation and the appraisal of outcome.

Trauma and the Development of Distorted Beliefs

While the functional analysis is not based on a historical understanding of the individual, psychosis is undergoing a sea change in its understanding as traumatic in origin. The understanding of the origins of psychosis being trauma driven has emerged from cognitive psychology conceptions of the development of psychosis. This is particularly formulated in the in the Power Threat Meaning Framework (PTMF) (Johntsone et al., 2018).

Whilst acknowledging biological and neurological changes, increasing understanding of the role of trauma in psychosis has begun to develop (Moskowitz et al., 2008). We are now in a much better position to understand that patients with psychosis are likely to have a history of trauma. Morgan and Murray (2020) show comprehensively through their meta-analysis that abusive experiences in childhood radically increase the chances of developing psychosis, especially if repeated and experienced as psychological abuse.

Wright et. al. (2020) show that these experiences are associated with 'psychotic phenotypes' (e.g. a clustering of 'soft' delusional ideation or hallucinations), which have phenomenological similarities to clinical psychosis. The authors also draw the link in the literature between childhood adversity and increased stress sensitivity in psychotic phenotypes.

It is highly likely that the individual struggling with patterns of self-harm has also experienced adversity. There are extremely clear links between the experience of attachment trauma and self-harm (Farber, 2008), sexual abuse and depression with self-harm (Gladstone et al., 2004).

This group may not only have powerful thoughts driving anxiety states but also negative emotions of self-worth. The links between hopelessness, self-harm, suicide and negative cognitions about self fit this model. Fixed negative cognitions or beliefs leading to depression and hopelessness have been identified as the strongest predictors of suicidal behaviour. This remained the case even where other psychotic symptoms such as voices or self-referential conditions pertained (Penn et al., 2003).

Trauma and 'Social Transference' on the Ward

The experience of trauma is likely to lead to strong beliefs about the threats (including staff) others pose. This original trauma may to be to physical integrity of the child or, even worse, the psychological integrity of the child, as shown in Table 16.1. It appears that severe psychological abuse makes the individual 20 times more at risk of developing psychosis. If a child's deepest fears are realised, this will indelibly leave a residue of anxiety and disturb perceptions of reality. The capacity to evaluate and discount future experiences as posing a threat (real or imagined) will also be impaired.

A pervasive underlying sense of traumatic experience can be generalised to the social context of the actor. Thinking is inherently social and emotional. The understanding of problematic behaviour as being driven through trauma-coloured misperception of context and appraisal of outcome is developed by Ackerman et al. (2018). The authors argue that an appraisal of a situation will frequently be based on 'social identification', which might carry with it a negative appraisal of other identification groups. Coloured judgments of 'social grouping' of individuals in the immediate environment of the actor can easily develop; hence, the 'us and them' situation is frequently found.

Table 16.1 Impact of abusive experience on chances of developing psychosis. Morgan and Murray (2020)

Odds Ratio for Developing Psychosis		
Type of Abuse	Less Severe	Severe Abuse
Bullying	1.43	3.64
Household discord	1.68	2.31
Physical abuse	2.28	9.98
Sexual abuse	2.58	8.54
Psychological abuse	3.95	21.36

This can inherently lead to distortions and the devaluation of other groups. This thinking in terms of 'groups' can lead to polarised or black-and-white thinking and allows for rapid distorting of appraisals. Even more concerning, it may lead to the devaluation of other groups as inhuman with consequent erosion of inhibitions to violent acts.

Under the influence of past trauma and social identifications, distorted beliefs of threat are easily developed. They are likely to be the default position of individuals with psychosis arriving on the ward. Staff will therefore be seen as threatening, aggressive and demeaning even in the most benign of teams.

Emotional Arousal

While these distorted beliefs must be seen as the well springs of challenging behaviour, it is really only states of high or disturbed emotion that will drive behaviour. Experiences of childhood trauma or adversity are associated with stress sensitivity (Wright et al., 2020). Stress has shown to be associated with paranoid thinking (Lincoln et al., 2010). Stress is also associated with subsequent impairments in emotion regulation and behavioural expression of this dysregulation (Lavi et.al., 2019). The heightened states of emotional and behavioural dysregulation are sufficient to lead to challenging patterns of behaviour. These high states of emotions lead to disturbed levels of arousal and, in turn, undermine any capacity for balanced appraisal.

High states of emotions are a necessary mediator between belief and action. Several factors may further disinhibit a belief-driven, disturbed emotional state. We might think of affective disorders, neurological disorder or substance misuse. This pathway is supported in a review of the literature on violence in psychotic patients with an antisocial background, where the authors stress the role of other factors in addition to distorted beliefs (Fazel et. Al., 2009).

'Social' Maintaining Factors

If the principles of operant conditioning hold, the outcome of the challenging behaviour, internally or externally, must be seen as positive by the actor. The consequence might be relatively simple, such as the reduction of anxiety or unwanted feelings or relief of frustration. It could also be a much more complex and obscure outcome. However, in order to stay theoretically coherent, it must be linked at least to the temporary obviation of anxieties inherent in the original appraised situation.

The social transference an individual displays on a ward will largely be historical in origin but may be emotionally tempered by appraisal of recent experience. There will be an interactional effect with the experienced perception of staff behaviour. A careful analysis of ward team responses and the impact on the individual should be made. It is worth noting that professionals are subject to the same operant principles and are capable of anxiety (and other emotion)-driven distortion.

However, once the patient and staff have developed expectations and predictions, both groups will have 'payoff matrices' and principles of normal game theory (e.g. prisoners dilemma; Leyton-Brown and Yoav, 2008) will apply. For example, the act of seclusion may lead to a sense of safety in both patient and staff. This is not to arrive at a negative judgment (it might be the best all round) but to point out that the reduction in paranoid anxiety might reinforce the behaviour. There will always be two operant models at work in a ward: that for the patient group and that for the staff group. In fact, each 'identification group'

will have its own cycle, so one might get different, seemingly contradictory, reactions from different staff groupings. This is often conceptualised as splits, but to avoid the pejorative connation of this, we should talk about different appraisals and responses to outcome.

A Model of Challenging Behaviour

We are now able to propose a basic model to understand challenging behaviour in psychosis. Despite the lopsided circularity of this functional analysis, it can serve as a basic model for understanding most challenging behaviours (Figure 16.2). You may note a connector line going from the positive appraisal of behavioural consequences straight back to disturbed appraisals. A subjective 'positive outcome' is likely to reinforce beliefs and appraisals, cutting out the historical or even any objective analysis on the situation on the ward and getting into a rapid cycle of challenging behaviour.

You might also note no reference to psychosis is made in the model. Effectively, psychosis in this model boils down to a combination of biased schema leading to disturbed appraisals and

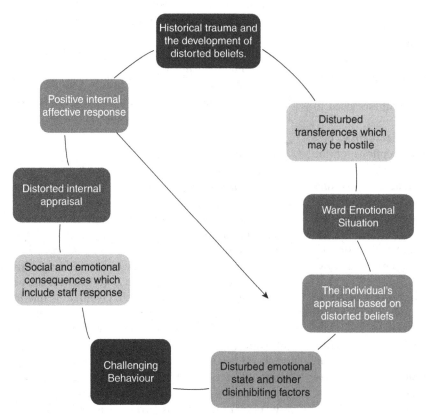

Fig 16.2 A functional analysis model of challenging behaviour in psychosis

conclusions, poor capacity to self-reflect or express and consequent disinhibited emotions. However, a psychiatric nomenclature of delusional thinking, perceptual disturbance and lack of insight is not that distant.

Making the Model Operational

Formulating

The previously describe A-B-C model might be expressed in a more complex formula:

A [history. transference. emotional situation. cognitive appraisal] x B [emotional arousal. dysregulation. behaviour] x C [social response. internal appraisal] = Pattern of challenging behaviour.

The model is in modern parlance a formulation; certainly, it will function as one once all the factors subsumed in the brackets are understood.

Observing

In many cases, however, we may only have the situation, the behaviour of the patient and behaviour of the professionals to go on with little direct explication from the patient. There may even be active disguise of the patient's perceptions and appraisals. It is the rare occasion that the clinician is handed something on a plate. In most situations, robust hypotheses need to be made for most of the elements to establish a functional formulation. These hypotheses need to be repeatedly examined.

We need to gain a view of this antecedent as best we can without the distorting perceptions of the patient or staff. Unfortunately, this is not always clear, and accounts from professionals can be rather bland and concrete. Peculiarly, it is frequently the original 'emotional situation' which staff teams find hard to identify and, to make matters worse, the situation might also be quite distant with short circuiting shown in the model above. Two techniques might be helpful.

Emotional chaining: It is worth tracking details of past events, emotional responses and behaviours until a commonality of situation is discovered.

Emotional classification: This is an inexact science, but a rough categorisation of the emotional event might be helpful. We might think of situations of loss, conflict, non-validation, frustration, rejection, derogation and so on.

Closely associated in understanding the distorted appraisal of the situation, it is often worth trying to understand or classify the anxiety present in the situation. For a patient admitted under the Mental Health Act (MHA) or transferred from prison, the original anxiety might be the prospect of unfair and endless incarceration. The legitimacy of staff to enforce medication, give behavioural injunction, prevent drug use or prevent the patient from leaving is often far from established in the patient's mind. It worth noting that in working with patients who move to the community, all these issues reappear. The behavioural problems then return in the community, leading to a revolving door (Shepherd, 1999).

As noted, the patient is likely to bring historical trauma and transferences to authority. These 'soft paranoid distortions' in the stress of ward life might rapidly become a hard distorting belief maintaining a pattern of disturbed behaviour. As already noted, the individual struggling with patterns of self-harm will have powerful punitive negative emotions of self-worth and a tendency to interpret staff behaviour as reinforcing these emotions.

These issues often set the 'reward structure' of the social context of the ward and, though little has been said to date, game theory will often apply. This is inherent in the functional analysis model, but often the 'wins' are determined with respect to these perceived points of conflict, perceived criticisms and the social approval of the patient group. The repeated bringing of drugs onto the ward might bring with it financial reward, status and triumph over staff.

Treatment

If a successful formulation is achieved, this should identify treatment needs. Let us start with a relatively simple table of examples (Table 16.2).

The table sets out key goals rather than specific treatment modalities. By definition, at least in the model outlined, the issue needs to be addressed at a systemic level rather than one to one, although this is a useful adjunct and in certain circumstances can be decisive. However, the approach 'favoured' is one in which the problem is identified with the patient as a social one and individual work is firmly anchored in this context.

It will require a coordinated approach across the team with responses from the front-line and secondary teams, as well as the authority of a cohering team. I would argue for this group that the ward and

Table 16.2 Potential treatments

Area of concern	Markers	Intervention
Negative transference	Anxiety when interacting Avoidance Expressions of hostility	Identifying and naming of social anxiety Identifying key concerns about detention and treatment, often during ward group discussion Developing a preferred plan with the patient for contact Developing a trauma-informed working model for staff Psychological work on historical trauma Exploring identifications
Distorted appraisals of situations	Heightened emotions	Identifying underlying schema
Heightened emotions	Arousal Anxiety Anger Lowered mood Disinhibition	Regulation emotions Developing a preferred management plan for high emotion with patient Developing anxiety and anger management strategies

Problematic
  behaviour
		Ignoring where possible
		Reinforcing appropriate behaviours
		Developing preferred management plan for de-escalation with patient,
		   but avoiding overt reinforcement by introducing other safe
		   management strategies

community treating teams are an important social reference. This type of approach is set out in the case studies that follow.

Case Studies

CASE #1 arrived after being nursed on her previous ward under two-to-one observation for six months because of frequent attacks on the nursing team. The patient was thought to be disordered and would express, rather alarmingly, thoughts seemingly disconnected to the current conversation. In particular, she expressed her preoccupying perception of the previous team in lurid religious terms as if they were all possessed by the devil.

Nevertheless, the team engaged with her in a positive and polite way, creating a daily routine that she approved of, including visits to her grandmother. The aggressive behaviour never re-emerged.

At face value, this is not a case of challenging behaviour but rather a situation quite frequently observed that points to a contextual basis for the aggression. This is a vital point, as patients can gain a reputation for being 'bad', when, in reality, the situation might be more complex. Further, in deconstructing why there was a difference across the wards, it was clear that in the patient's mind, the former team was 'bad' and personally negatively disposed towards her. This may arise out of a wish not to have been there originally. Regardless, this was clearly a 'psychotic

transference' which coloured the patient's perceptions of the previous team's actions and led to retaliatory aggression.

The case illustrates the importance of the relationship and the transference that the patient develops with the team. All the factors that accumulated within interaction between the patient and previous team would never become clear, but the history pointed to repeated rejection of the patient by her mother. An analysis of the history may give clues to what painful experiences might be writ large in the patient's mind.

CASE #2 is not one of psychosis per se but sets out principles of not reinforcing the problematic behaviour. The author, when working in a chaotic remand prison setting, noticed repeated return of younger prisoners to the segregation unit. They were referred to the mental health inreach services, as mental illness was suspected, but were not particularly dangerous nor were they overtly mentally unwell. On observation, the prisoners shared the characteristics of hyperactivity, cognitive disorganisation, paranoid thoughts, poor problem-solving and emotional dysregulation. On being placed in segregation, their behaviour calmed markedly.

On return to the wing, they tended to become more rapidly disturbed and come into conflict with wing officers. They repeatedly spoke of wing officers as 'bullies', although evidence for this was scant and conflict seemed largely around enforcing established rules and the prisoner's inability to tolerate frustration of gratification. The wing was quite chaotic with fights between prisoners and some objective instances of bullying. Drugs were available at inflated prices and drug debts easily accrued with negative consequences.

A simple approach was adopted to the formulation of a patient in this group. He was known to have suffered physical and emotional neglect with a history of failed foster placements. However, accessing a frank account of anxieties seemed difficult in one-to-one sessions. On return to the wing, he would become involved in disruptive behaviour, banging on his cell door and being verbally abusive to staff. He might, if given the chance, light small fires. If out on the wing, he might not return to his cell. He provoked anger from other prisoners trying to sleep and verbal retaliation from officers.

It was formulated that being placed on a wing provoked significant anxieties around being neglected or, conversely, physically or psychologically abused either by staff or other prisoners. The patient viewed his placement on the segregation wing as a positive outcome, as it allowed for him to have routine contact with a small number of relatively consistent staff who had developed a relationship with him, even if through a door, and time-limited outings.

A management program was developed where three identified staff would approach the patient at least once daily when he was not being disruptive. This was aimed at developing trust and allowing him to explore staff responses to his behaviour. If these interactions became disruptive, staff would politely remove themselves stating they would return. Staff enquired as to offence, his background and offered cups of tea when the patient engaged.

The disruptive behaviours were ignored. The most dangerous behaviour, fire lighting, was controlled by removal of lighters. The cell regime had its own behaviour program, including earning access to television, gym and football training. These were set as goals to make his stay more comfortable. After some hesitancy, the patient engaged with staff and became more settled.

The key issues here were to engage with staff to ameliorate their anxieties about the patient's mental health. They were then encouraged to search for a different outcome than sending him to segregation. It was agreed that they could try to adopt a pattern of behaviour aimed at reducing the patient's anxieties and, in classical behavioural terms, reinforce more

productive behaviours while ignoring or ruling out the reinforcement of dysfunctional behaviour.

CASE #3 had become very aroused with staff, leading to his restraint and seclusion. It was reported that he banged aggressively on the door to the nursing station, demanding (seemingly irrationally) a change of room. He only became more aroused the more this was queried, leading to the seemingly adverse outcome of seclusion.

Some days later, he described that he had misplaced his room key. He had started to walk down to the nursing station to report this when he heard laughter on the ward among other residents. He immediately thought they had taken the key. This led to the view that he was in danger at night when other residents would use the key to enter. The only answer was to change his room. The anxiety generated by this thought made him emotionally aroused and the 'hesitation' of staff was putting him in danger and, even more sinisterly, in collusion with the other patients. This is the 'whole emotional situation'. In this scenario, we can then see powerful paranoid schema distorting the appraisal of the situation.

The patient's high levels of arousal and behaviour, plus a history of aggression, made it entirely logical for staff to perceive this as a very threatening situation. Seclusion achieved a degree of security and was reinforcing to staff and reflects the reinforcement of the outcome from the staff side. As it worked out, the patient was quite amenable to CBT for psychosis and began to reappraise his assessment of the situation.

CASE #4 had a history of acute psychotic states within a borderline condition. She had made several severe self-injuries which were traumatising and disrupting to staff, often leading to long periods of one-to-one nursing. There would be a recovery period with increasing trust redeveloping and periods of leave. This would then be followed by a serious incident of self-harm.

It was difficult to establish a pattern, but over time it became clear that the most severe events followed a return to the ward after leave, but not inevitably. They appeared to occur after visits to her mother, highly desired by the patient, but again not invariably so. The patient professed that her mood declined because she did not want to return to hospital. In this context, the behaviour seemed entirely self-defeating, both in terms of being given leave to see her mother and making progress in leaving hospital.

It was also difficult to explain why loss did not always trigger self-harm.

The analysis went back to basics, working backwards from the self-harm incident using emotional chaining. It was clear that a return to the ward from the family could be associated with significant lowered mood in the context of conflict with the family and 'emotional loss'. Digging deeper, it seemed leaving her mother with her sister being present triggered feelings of exclusion and not being preferred. In fact, it appeared the patient's sister might even provoke a situation where there would be conflict and the patient would leave with mixed feelings of anger and rejection. These became intense on return to the ward and was redolent of her being placed in foster care while her sister remained with their mother.

Self-harm in part was an attempt to obviate the feelings and, to the author at least, contained a real suicidal element which felt dangerous to the patient. Being placed on one-to-one observations gave her a feeling of safety and therefore was appraised as positive. In this case, acknowledging the deep hurt provoked in this situation seemed the only right thing to do and helping with emotional tolerance and debriefing (essentially dialectical behaviour therapy [DBT] skills) by staff on duty was made the first response.

The patient was given the control to say when she felt that she could safely re-enter communal living. Staff were given a checklist to run through with the patient as a failsafe, for example, avoidance of eye contact was seen as a warning sign that she was not ready.

In this case, because of the high stakes, the 'positive outcome' was seen as harm reduction in terms of reducing self-harm by using emotional and verbal expression and shortening the periods of one-to-one nursing. The A-B-C cycle was not halted but modified.

CASE #5 had a history of auditory hallucinations which were experienced as well-formed 'voices'. Acting under the influences of the voices had gotten her into trouble with the law, and these types of difficulties continued. She would frequently become verbally threatening and destructive to property, requiring nursing intervention and, at times, restraint. She would then indicate she was acting under the influence of the voices.

A preliminary discussion indicated that these behaviours largely followed instances of frustration, such as being refused leave, being 'told off' or being asked to follow rules. The behaviours would not be immediate but would possibly occur one to three hours later. The patient acknowledged feeling anger but struggling with voices that criticised her when she returned to her room and advised her to confront staff. On occasion, she would give over to their injunctions. The verbal outbursts, throwing chairs and possible restraint would relieve the patient of the derogatory voices and struggling with her anger, hence the reinforcement of the behaviour.

Playing the 'voices card' gave her a degree of 'diplomatic immunity', as they were seen as out of her control. However, it was clear she needed to take responsibility for her anger, and the team implemented a debrief procedure in which her anger was verbalised. She also engaged in CBT for psychosis, challenging the legitimacy and authority of the voices. This approach was shared across the team, allowing all staff to reinforce her efforts to change behaviour.

CASE #6 struggled with a treatment-resistant psychosis that she did not want to explicate. She had made a serious suicide attempt in the past after the loss of a relationship. Reading her history might give a clue to the 'situation' being one of 'loss' and to the depth and severity of her impulses to self-harm. A serious incident of physical aggression occurred when she threw a chair at the doctor explaining that hospital care was not improving her state and she was about to be discharged. This resulted in her being transferred to another ward and an extension of her stay.

A pattern emerged where the patient would become highly emotional and angry over a relatively minor frustration of ward life. Staff would attend and that would calm her. She would apologise, and a genuinely positive interaction would ensue and the patient would return to her room. Sometime later, she would emerge in a furious and abusive state, forcing intervention from the nursing team, often leading to physical restraint.

The intense violence of her presentation after a positive exchange was puzzling to the team. As the patient developed trust, she began to explain that on her initial return to her room she would develop a sense of hopelessness followed by intense impulses to kill herself. In this rapidly deteriorated state of mind, staff were to blame for isolating her and leaving her to her thoughts.

The conflict with staff took her away from the feelings, relieved anger and resulted in close attention, all of which required close consideration and finding alternative ways of expression.

Discussion

The task of addressing challenging behaviour is frequently made more difficult by the fact that many other dimensions of the patient's functioning show significant challenges and impairment (Shepherd, 1999). Not least among these are hostility and denial, which prevent access to the patient's thoughts and motivations and preclude measured discussion. It is of note that there are few examples where the client openly gives an account of their thinking and motivations.

Within this context, the model has several significant advantages in allowing for a useful discourse to begin in the team; one is to move the understanding of the behaviour into a social contextual framework. There is significant theoretical and experimental evidence to show that behaviour is determined by the accumulation of social transactions within a specific context (Needs and Adair-Stanital, 2017). This gives a context for understanding the behaviour (i.e. the detention in hospital, the experience of control, the chaos of ward life, the experience of help and so on).

There is little doubt that developmental experiences of trauma are implicated in the latter manifestations of thoughts and behaviours which are seen as psychotic. Childhood adversity is much more than simply a 'risk factor' but contributes profoundly to the presentation of the patient when arriving on the ward (Rossiter et al., 2015). This gives a trauma-informed view for understanding the approach of the patient to the treating team. Alongside this is the understanding that the team's actions will play a role in maintaining the behaviour. Finally, there is the understanding that the patient's behaviour, whether driven by anger or anxiety, is often preferable to the alternative state of mind.

We therefore have a template around which a team discourse can take place in which the formulation and understanding of the patient and challenging behaviour can begin. It is accepted that this might initially be hypothetical but will always be inevitable in situations of incomplete information. Largely, this formulation must be jointly agreed upon and treatment responses must interconnect the medical, nursing and social interventions if any success is to be achieved.

References

Akerman,G, Needs,A and Bainbridge,C (eds.) (2018) *Transforming Environments and Rehabilitation*. London: Routledge.

Beck,A and Freeman,A (1990) *Cognitive Therapy of Personality Disorders*. New York: Guilford Press.

Bentall,R (2004) *Madness Explained: Psychosis and Human Nature*. London: Penguin Books.

Brennan,P, Mednick,S and Hodgins,S (2000) Major Mental Disorders and Criminal Violence in a Danish Birth Cohort. *Archives of Psychiatry* 57 (5) 494–500.

Brown,S, O' Rourke,S and Schwannauer,M (2019) Risk Factors for Inpatient Violence and Self-Harm in Forensic Psychiatry: The Role of Head Injury, Schizophrenia and Substance Misuse. *Brain Injury* 33 (3) 313–21.

Byrt,R (1999) Nursing: The Importance of the Psychosocial Environment. In Campling,P and Haig,R (eds.), *Therapeutic Communities: Past, Present and Future*. London: Jessica Kingsley.

Challis,S, Nielssen,O, Harris,A and Large,M (2013) Systematic Meta-Analysis of the Risk Factors for Deliberate Self-Harm Before and After Treatment for First-Episode Psychosis. *Acta Psychiatrica Scandanavia* 127 (6) 442–54.

Douglas,K, Guy,L and Hart,S (2009) Psychosis as a Risk Factor for Violence to Others: A Meta-Analysis. *Psychological Bulletin* 135 (5) 679–706.

Farber,S (2008) Dissociation, Traumatic Attachments, and Self-Harm: Eating Disorders and Self-Mutilation *Clinical Social Work Journal* 36 (1) 63–72.

Fazel,S, Gulati,G, Linsell,L, Geddess,JR and Grann,M (2009) Schizophrenia and Violence: Systematic Review and Meta-Analysis. *PLoS Medicine* 6 (8) e1000120.

Fedyszyn,I, Erlangsen,A, Hjorthøj,C, Madsen,T and Nordentoft,M (2016) Repeated Suicide Attempts and Suicide Among Individuals with a First Emergency Department Contact for Attempted Suicide: A Prospective, Nationwide, Danish Register-Based Study. *Journal of Clinical Psychiatry* 77 (6) 832–40.

Fonagy,P, Gergely,G, Jurist,E and Target,M (2004) *Affect Regulation, Mentalisation and the Development of the Self*. London: Karnac.

Garety,PA, Kuipers,E, Fowler,D, Freeman,D and Bebbington,P (2001) A Cognitive Model of the Positive Symptoms of Psychosis. *Psychological Medicine* 31 (2) 189–95.

Gladstone,G, Parker,G, Mitchell,P, Malhi,G, Wilhelm,K and Austin,M (2004) Implications of Childhood Trauma for Depressed Women: An Analysis of Pathways from Childhood Sexual Abuse to Deliberate Self-Harm and Revictimization. *American Journal of Psychiatry* 161 (8) 1417–25.

Han,H, Miller,H, Nkimbeng,M, Budhathoki,C, Mikhael,T, Rivers,E et al. (2021) Trauma Informed Interventions: A Systematic Review. *PLoS ONE* **16** (6) e0252747.

Johnstone,L and Boyle,M (2018) *The Power Threat Meaning Framework: Towards the Identification of Patterns in Emotional Distress, Unusual Experiences and Troubled or Troubling Behaviour, as an Alternative to Functional Psychiatric Diagnosis.* Leicester: British Psychological Society.

Lavi,I, Katz,LF, Ozer,EJ and Gross,JJ (2019) Emotion Reactivity and Regulation in Maltreated Children: A Meta-Analysis. *Child Development* **90** (5) 1503–24.

Leyton–Brown,K and Shoham,Y (2008) *Essentials of Game Theory: A Concise Multidisciplinary Introduction.* Williston: Morgan & Claypool Publishers.

Lincoln,T, Lange,J, Burau,J, Exner,C and Moritz,S (2010) The Effect of State Anxiety on Paranoid Ideation and Jumping to Conclusions: An Experimental Investigation. *Schizophrenia Bulletin* **36** (6) 1140–8.

Linehan,M (1993) *Cognitive Behavioural Treatment of Borderline Personality Disorder.* New York: Guilford Press.

Mace,FC (1994) The Significance and Future of Functional Analysis Methodologies. *Journal of Applied Behavior Analysis.* **27** (2) 385–92.

Morgan,C and Murray,R (2020) A Systematic Review on Mediators between Adversity and Psychosis: Potential Targets for Treatment. *Psychological Medicine* **50** (12) 1966–76.

Moskowitz,A, Schäfer,I, and Dorahy,M (2008) *Psychosis, Trauma and Dissociation: Emerging Perspectives on Severe Psychopathology.* New York: Wiley Blackwell.

Needs,A and Adair-Stantiall,A (2017) The Social Context of Transition and Rehabilitation. In Akerman,G, Needs,A and Bainbridge,C (eds.), *Transforming Environments and Rehabilitation.* London: Routledge.

Penn,J, Esposito,C, Schaeffer,L, Fritz,K and Spirito,A (2003) Suicide Attempts and Self-Mutilative Behavior in a Juvenile Correctional Facility. *Journal of the American Academy of Child and Adolescent Psychiatry* **42** (7) 762–9.

Rossiter,A, Byrne,F and Hallahan,B (2015) Childhood Trauma Levels in Individuals Attending Adult Mental Health Services: An Evaluation of Clinical Records and Structured Measurement of Childhood Trauma. *Child Abuse & Neglect* **44**: 36–45.

Schore,A (2003) *Affect Regulation and the Repair of the Self.* New Jersey: Lawrence Erlbaum.

Shepherd,G (1999) Social Functioning and Challenging Behaviour. In Meuser,KT and Terrier,N (eds.), *Handbook of Social Functioning and Schizophrenia.* Massachusetts: Allyn and Bacon.

Skinner,BF (1957) *Verbal Behavior.* New York: Appleton-Century-Crofts.

Wright,A, Coman,D, Deng,W, Farabaugh,A, Terechina,O, Cather,C, et al. (2020) The Impact of Childhood Trauma, Hallucinations, and Emotional Reactivity on Delusional Ideation. *Shizophrenia Bulletin* **1** (1) sgaa021.

17 Pharmacological Therapy

Chike I. Okocha and Jules Haste

Introduction

In psychiatric intensive care, treatment goals are generally short term, although, where appropriate, long-term goals can also be set. These goals are to reduce symptoms, build an alliance for long-term management and educate the patient and their families about the illness, its treatment and its course (treated and untreated). Diagnosis of the illness can be useful, but in most cases the main treatment goal is to treat the symptoms. Diagnoses can be dual or even multiple, therefore the long-term goals of treatment and use of evidence-based medicines should be considered for each of the conditions.

In the longer term, the primary goals of treatment are to aid return to premorbid levels of functioning and prevent relapse, as relapse results in symptom exacerbation as well as impairment in social and occupational functioning. In patients where benefits of continuing long-term medication outweigh risks, it is important to aim for the minimal effective dose while continuously monitoring adverse effects and life circumstances. It is also beneficial to maintain contact with families and carers to maximise adherence and reduce the burden of living with someone with a chronic psychiatric illness.

When prescribing in psychiatric intensive care, there may be a need for the addition of rapid tranquilisation (RT), oral pro re nata (PRN) or pre-RT medication. When already prescribed with regular medicines, this increases the risk of polypharmacy with added risk of side effects. Therefore, regular review of prescribing should be carried out by the multidisciplinary team (MDT) to ensure that the risk of 'high-dose' antipsychotic treatment is reduced and prescribing is rationalised. This chapter explores the medicines commonly used in psychiatric intensive care,

considers the evidence-based, best practice and national guidance for their use, and discusses side effects and monitoring of physical health.

History and Developments of Psychopharmacological Interventions for Acute Mental Illness

Treatment of Psychosis

The modern era of treating psychosis and acute anxiety with medication began in the 1950s with the introduction of chlorpromazine. Since that serendipitous discovery, several other medications have also been introduced. The terms 'major tranquillisers' or 'neuroleptics' were originally used to describe medications that had the capacity to alter neuronal activity, almost exclusively to describe medications with antipsychotic potency. However, with the advent of newer medications with different receptor sites of action the term has become obsolete.

Antipsychotics are classified into two groups: first-generation antipsychotics (FGAs) or second-generation antipsychotics (SGAs). All the older or so-called classical, conventional or typical antipsychotics are classified as FGAs, and any antipsychotics introduced since 1990 are classified as SGAs, with the exclusion of clozapine and olanzapine, which were both introduced prior to 1990. The main difference between the FGAs and SGAs is their propensity to produce adverse effects, with FGAs having higher propensity to produce extrapyramidal symptoms (EPS) and SGAs having a notably higher propensity to cause metabolic effects.

Due to the antipsychotics differing vastly in their licensed indication and ability to produce adverse effects, it is widely believed that the use of the neuroscience-based nomenclature (Nutt and Blier, 2016) is the most accurate way to describe the antipsychotics.

Rapid Tranquillisation (RT), Oral pro re nata (PRN) or Pre-RT

Early identification and management of an acutely disturbed patient is crucial in ensuring the safety and dignity of patients, visitors and staff. RT is the use of parenteral medication to treat acute disturbance when other non-medication strategies or oral medication has failed. RT does not rapidly 'treat' the underlying cause of acute disturbance; therefore, longer-term treatment should be considered. The use of oral medication defined as oral PRN or pre-RT may be given to reduce the need to administer by pre-emptively addressing the acute disturbance.

The most common medications used for RT, oral PRN and pre-RT include antipsychotics, benzodiazepines and antihistamines. The use of RT and oral PRN or pre-RT is discussed further in Chapter 18, including best practice evidence, administration, side effects and the monitoring required.

Treatment of Affective Disorders

Patients with a diagnosis of bipolar disorder will often have psychotic symptoms, and manic patients can present with delusions, irritability, agitation or aggressive and violent behaviour.

Mood stabilisers have been the main pharmacological treatment for bipolar disorder with the introduction of lithium in the 1940s and then the increasing use of antiepileptics. More recently, the role of SGAs in the treatment of bipolar disorder and severe depressive disorder with psychosis has become well established. However, all antipsychotics have very different licenses and evidence for their use and therefore should be considered individually.

Antidepressants have a long history with the introduction of monoamine oxidase inhibitors (MAOIs) and tricyclics in the 1950s. Since then, newer antidepressants with difficult receptor profiles have been introduced, and their adverse effects profiles differ greatly.

Treatment of Anxiety Disorder

'Minor tranquillisers' were first used in the 1950s and 1960s with the introduction of barbiturates to treat anxiety, seizures and sleep disorders, but their long action, risk of addiction and toxicity in overdose led to the arrival of benzodiazepines and Z-drugs. Low-dose antipsychotics were also used to treat acute anxiety, with sedative properties particularly useful in patients who are likely to be dependent on benzodiazepines. Currently, treatment of anxiety disorders is psychological therapy with the use of the anxiolytic medication, especially selective serotonin reuptake inhibitor (SSRI) antidepressants as second-line treatment.

Evidence Base and How to Include It in Practice

In the United Kingdom, the National Institute for Health and Care Excellence (NICE) and the British Association of Psychopharmacology (BAP) produce guidance relating to schizophrenia (Barnes et al., 2020), bipolar disorder (Goodwin et al., 2016), depression (Cleare et al., 2015), anxiety (Baldwin et al., 2014) and RT (Patel and Sethi, 2018). These consensus guidelines should be consulted to form the basis of prescribing in psychiatric intensive care units (PICUs). There are also other important documents relating to the prescribing of high-dose antipsychotic medication (Royal College of Psychiatrists, 2014) and the use of unlicensed medications (Royal College of Psychiatrists Psychopharmacology Committee, 2017).

Outline of Pharmacological Interventions Used in Inpatient Mental Health Setting

Antipsychotics

The use of antipsychotic medications in the treatment of acute psychosis aims to alleviate psychotic symptoms and shorten the acute episode of illness. The antipsychotic potency of the typical antipsychotics was thought to depend entirely on dopamine-2 (D_2) receptor blockade in the mesolimbic and cortical areas of the brain. The newer SGAs, however, do not have such a high affinity for D_2 receptors but appear to have affinity for other receptor types, particularly serotonin receptors. They all share a high 5-HT_{2A}: striatal D_2 receptor blockade ratio (Kapur and Remington, 2000).

Irrespective of the different pharmacodynamics, there is no convincing evidence that any antipsychotic, except clozapine, is more effective than another (Jones et al., 2006, Lieberman et al., 2005). Therefore, the choice of antipsychotic is determined largely by adverse effects, especially EPS and metabolic effects. Other factors of importance are patient preference, diagnosis, relevant medical history, the clinician's knowledge of available medications and dosage forms.

Considering the prevalence of adverse effects in patients prescribed antipsychotics, it is important that these are discussed and monitored. Adverse effects can cause long-term distress and function and contribute to chronic physical health complications and poor adherence to medication. Antipsychotics should be initiated at the lower end of the licensed dosage range (Barnes et al., 2020) and titrated accordingly.

Maintenance Treatment in Psychosis

Use of antipsychotics in maintenance treatment of psychosis is aimed at the prevention of relapse or any worsening of psychotic symptoms and disability. A meta-analysis (Leucht et al., 2012) reported that the one-year relapse percentage for those patients whose antipsychotic medication had been stopped (64%) was more than double that of those who had continued on medication (27%). National guidance (NICE, 2014c and Barnes et al., 2020) recommend that maintenance treatment with antipsychotic medication at a standard dose will substantially reduce the risk of relapse for at least two years.

However, maintenance treatment is associated with long-term risks of adverse effects. Therefore, regular reviews of the potential benefits and risks of treatment as well as assessment of adherence of medication should be carried out with patients at every review, combined with appropriate psycho-socio-educational strategies to achieve maximum benefits (Bellack and Mueser, 1993; Mortimer, 1997).

While studies comparing FGAs and SGAs (Leiberman et al., 2005; Jones et al., 2006) have found there were no significant differences in therapeutic efficacy, discontinuation over 12 months was significantly more common in patients assigned to low-dose haloperidol than in those treated with SGAs, with the lowest discontinuation occurring with olanzapine (Kahn et al., 2008; Boter et al., 2009).

The use of orodispersible agents does not reduce the time to peak plasma level or absorption but can ensure adherence (Hartley et al., 2019). Clozapine and long-acting (depot/injectable) antipsychotic medications are associated with the highest rates of prevention of relapse in schizophrenia when compared with no medication use. The risk of re-hospitalisation was about 20% to 30% lower during depot/LAI antipsychotic treatment compared with equivalent oral formulations (Tiihonen et al., 2017).

Depot or long-acting injectable antipsychotic (LAI) preparations are associated with a reduction in hospitalisations of 15% compared with oral antipsychotic medication despite greater illness severity in those patients receiving the depot/LAI preparations (Kishimoto et al., 2018). A key advantage of depot/LAI preparations is that non-adherence will be apparent with non-acceptance of the injection. The subsequent long half-life will allow time for prompt interventions/discussions with the patient before significant relapse may occur. Depots/LAIs should be considered for all patients early in treatment and not reserved for non-adherent patients due to the known reduction in relapse and rehospitalisation.

A main disadvantage with depot/LAI preparations is the long time to steady state, which can lead to a delay in effective treatment. Consequently, when switching from an oral drug to an LAI form, it is good practice to continue with the oral antipsychotic for the length of time required to establish the effective, best-tolerated dose before switching to the LAI form (Llorca et al., 2013).

Treatment-Resistant Schizophrenia (TRS)

About one-third of patients with schizophrenia do not respond adequately to antipsychotics. Treatment-resistant schizophrenia (TRS) is 'lack of satisfactory clinical improvement despite the use of adequate doses of at least two different antipsychotic agents, including an atypical antipsychotic agent, prescribed for adequate duration' (Britannia, 2020).

It remains uncertain whether TRS should be considered simply as the more severe end of the illness spectrum or as a distinct subtype of schizophrenia for which neurobiological correlates of treatment resistance should be explored (Gillespie et al., 2017).

Therefore, strategies for management of treatment resistance should also include ensuring compliance (with an LAI), dosage adjustment, change of antipsychotics and augmentation with other medications or treatment methods (Daniel and Whitcomb, 1998).

Of the antipsychotics, clozapine is the only medicine licensed in TRS; a response to clozapine has been found in 30%–70% of people with schizophrenia who have failed to respond to other antipsychotic medications (Barnes et al., 2020; Kane et al., 1988)

Mood Stabilisers

Mood stabilisers are medications that lower and maintain mood to euthymic levels in patients with mania or hypomania; they may also sustain euthymic mood in patients with bipolar depression. Mood stabilisers used in the treatment of patients with bipolar affective disorder include lithium, carbamazepine, lamotrigine and sodium valproate.

In addition to their antipsychotic potency, clinical trials and open label studies show that some antipsychotics are also effective for the treatment of mania, in some cases of bipolar depression and the long-term treatment of bipolar disorder (Goodwin et al., 2016).

However, not all mood stabilisers are equal in effectiveness, particularly in their ability to treat the manic phase, depressive phase or the long-term treatment of bipolar and each has its own licensed indications (see the Summary of Product Characteristics (SmPC) or British National Formulary (BNF) for more details).

Anxiolytics

Anxiety is frequently comorbid with other mental disorders; estimated rates vary. Between 68% and 93% of generalised anxiety disorder is in combination with another mental health disorder (Carter et al., 2001; Hunt et al., 2002), which further complicates the presentation. The treatment of anxiety disorders depends on the type and severity of the disorder as well as other associated factors, which will be evident from the assessment of the patient.

Treatment guidelines such as those produced by BAP and NICE recommend psychological treatments as a first-line approach. For a significant number of patients with anxiety disorder, medication may be indicated initially before the patient can participate effectively in psychological treatment, especially when depression is present.

When pharmacological therapy is required, antidepressants are licensed for the treatment of particular disorders. Once a good effect has been achieved, antidepressant treatment should be continued for about 6–8 months and then tapered to minimise the likelihood of symptom recurrence on withdrawal.

Benzodiazepines should be avoided, and, if prescribed, only for short term use. The tolerability profile of antipsychotic drugs is such that they should generally be reserved for treatment after nonresponse to other interventions (NICE, 2011).

Personality Disorders

Borderline personality disorder is common amongst psychiatric inpatients with a prevalence rate of 15% (Winston, 2000) and a suicide rate of 10% (Paris, 2000). Many of these patients are referred to the intensive care unit because of their challenging behaviour.

Pharmacological interventions should not generally be used for the treatment of personality disorders or the individual symptoms or behaviours associated with the disorders; however, medications are often used to treat comorbid disorders (NICE, 2009a). When considering pharmacological interventions for comorbid mental disorders, in particular depression and anxiety, treatment should be in line with recommendations in the relevant NICE and BAP clinical guidelines. Particular attention should be paid to issues of adherence and the risks of misuse or overdose.

Psychotropic medications are often prescribed off license for these patients, mostly for the control of three common symptom clusters: transient psychotic symptoms, affective instability and impulsivity. In reviewing the evidence that underpins the use of psychotropic medications, Paton and Okocha (2005) found that polypharmacy is likely to be high due to a high initial placebo response that is often short-lived.

Framework and Guidance for Developing Policy for the Use of Education within a PICU Setting

Almost all patients admitted to PICUs receive pharmacological interventions, and medications are often the major treatment intervention. PICU professional staff need to ensure that medication is used safely. Organisational policies that are especially relevant to the PICU are those regarding information management, confidentiality, prevention and management of violence and aggression, seclusion policy, Mental Health Act 1983 policies (DOH, 2015), RT and high-dose medication policies (NAPICU, 2014).

Alongside these policies, PICU professional staff should educate themselves on the licensed indications, doses and adverse effects of commonly used medications. A defined and well-understood procedure should be available for recognising and closely monitoring any side effects from prescribed medication.

Information on medicines should be clearly communicated to patients in a format suitable for their needs. Useful information tools can be found on the Choice and Medication website (www.choiceandmedication.org/) and on the Mind website (www.mind.org.uk/information-support/drugs-and-treatments/).

General Description of the Medication Types and Considerations for Use in the PICU Setting

Antipsychotics

Many of the antipsychotics have different formulations, including oral, orodispersible, short acting intramuscular (IM) injections and long-acting IM injections for selection according to prescriber and patient choice.

First-Generation Antipsychotics (FGAs)

Due to their higher receptor occupancy at D2 receptors, FGAs are more likely to cause EPS and hyperprolactinemia (Kapur and Remington, 2000)

FGAs include:

- phenothiazine derivatives (chlorpromazine hydrochloride, fluphenazine decanoate, levomepromazine, prochlorperazine, promazine hydrochloride, and trifluoperazine)
- butyrophenones (benperidol and haloperidol)
- thioxanthenes (flupentixol and zuclopenthixol)
- diphenylbutylpiperidines (pimozide)
- substituted benzamides (sulpiride)

Second-Generation Antipsychotics (SGAs)

SGAs act on a range of receptors in comparison to FGAs and are generally associated with a lower risk for EPS and tardive dyskinesia, although the extent varies between individual drugs. However, SGAs are associated with other adverse effects, especially metabolic side effects due to their action on histamine, 5HT and other receptors (Correll, 2010).

Amisulpride is a substituted benzamide that is effective against negative symptoms when used in low doses, such as 100 mg a day (Boyer et al., 1995; Loo et al., 1997). However, its main use is to augment clozapine (Assion et al., 2008). It results in a lower rate of weight gain compared with other SGAs (Leucht et al., 2013; Huhn et al., 2019) but causes significant dose-related hyperprolactinemia (Taylor et al., 2018).

Aripiprazole is a partial agonist effective against both positive and negative symptoms of schizophrenia with lower rates of adverse effects including EPS, weight gain and increased prolactin, glucose and lipids (Leucht et al., 2009a). Aripiprazole has also been shown to be affective in mania (Yildiz et al., 2011) and the mixed states (Muralidharan et al., 2013) of bipolar disorder. It has evidence as an adjunct to treat antipsychotic-induced hyperprolactinemia (Esteves et al., 2015) and augmentation for clozapine, especially with respect to reduction of clozapine-induced weight gain and lipid reduction (Srisurapanont et al., 2015). Nausea seems to be the most problematic adverse effect (Goodnick and Jerry, 2002). Aripiprazole is also available as an LAI (Otsuka, 2020).

Asenapine is only licensed for the treatment of mania (Organon Pharma, 2021), but its use is limited due to its method of administration (sublingual) and consensual bioavailability being less than 2% if swallowed.

Cariprazine is licensed in the United Kingdom for the treatment of schizophrenia and has shown effectiveness; it may have additional benefits to treat negative symptoms (Garnock-Jones, 2017). Although unlicensed for other conditions in the United Kingdom, it has shown to be effective in mania (Yildiz et al., 2011) and has some evidence for the treatment of bipolar depression (Durgam et al., 2015, 2016).

Clozapine is the only antipsychotic licensed for TRS (Britannia, 2020). A good response is more likely when the plasma level is greater than 350 ng/ml (Perry et al., 1991; Taylor and Duncan 1995; Cooper 1996). Clozapine causes agranulocytosis in up to 1% of patients, with most of these cases occurring between one and five months into therapy (Atkin et al., 1996). Weekly blood counts are required in the first 18 weeks of treatment, followed by two weekly counts until one year and then four weekly checks thereafter

(Britannia, 2020). Clozapine causes sedation, sialorrhoea and postural hypotension, therefore it should be initiated at low doses and increased slowly. It can lower seizure threshold (Wilson and Claussen, 1994), especially in doses greater than 600 mg a day, for which the risk of seizure is 4.4% (Devinsky et al., 1991). Clozapine has been associated with varying degrees of impairment of intestinal peristalsis; this effect can range from constipation, which is very common, to very rare intestinal obstruction, faecal impaction and paralytic ileus (MHRA, 2017). Particular care should be exercised in patients receiving other drugs known to cause constipation (especially anticholinergics) and any constipation should be actively treated as soon as possible.

Lurasidone is licensed in the United Kingdom for schizophrenia and has demonstrated efficacy for the treatment of acute schizophrenia (Meltzer et al., 2011) and long-term maintenance (Loebel et al., 2013a, b). Although not licensed in the United Kingdom, studies of lurasidone for bipolar depression, as monotherapy and as an add-on to lithium or valproate, have shown effectiveness (Loebel et al., 2014a, 2014b). Lurasidone has a low subjective adverse reactions burden and produces minimal changes in weight, blood lipids and glycaemic control. The commonest reported adverse reactions are akathisia and somnolence.

Olanzapine, in several studies, has shown it is at least as effective as haloperidol in a range of doses and causes a similar frequency of EPS as placebo (Beasley et al., 1996a, 1996b, 1997; Tollefson et al., 1997). Olanzapine has also been shown to be effective in acute mania (Yildiz et al., 2011), mixed states with predominant manic symptoms (Muralidharan et al., 2013) and in the long-term treatment of bipolar disorder (Vieta et al., 2001). Common adverse effects are drowsiness and weight gain, which can be significant. Others are anticholinergic effects such as dry mouth and constipation, dizziness, peripheral oedema and postural hypotension. Olanzapine formulations include a short-acting IM injection and an LAI.

Paliperidone is the metabolite of risperidone, 9-hydroxyrisperidone; it has been shown to reduce psychotic symptoms (Kane et al., 2006; Davidson et al., 2007) with adverse effects occurring in 2% or more patients. Paliperidone is available as a monthly or thrice-monthly LAI (Janssen-Cilag, 2018a, 2019).

Quetiapine has proven to be as effective as conventional antipsychotics in the treatment of schizophrenia in several double-blind, randomised trials (Hirsch et al. 1996; Markowitz et al., 1999). However, quetiapine has the most convincing short-term efficacy and relapse prevention profile for bipolar depression (Goodwin et al., 2016); trials have shown that the incidence of EPS in patients taking quetiapine was similar to those taking placebo across the full dosage range.

Risperidone appears to be at least equivalent and possibly superior to haloperidol in decreasing positive and negative symptoms (Castelao et al., 1989; Claus et al., 1992; Chouinard et al., 1993; Marder and Meibach, 1994). Because it causes hyperprolactinaemia, EPS at higher doses (Marder and Meibach, 1994) and has a somewhat inconsistent benefit in negative symptoms, some have disputed its place as an SGA (Cardoni, 1995). Common adverse effects of risperidone are insomnia, anxiety, agitation, sedation, dizziness, rhinitis, hypotension, weight gain and menstrual disturbances. Risperidone is available in an injectable form administered every two weeks (Janssen-Cilag, 2018b).

Adverse Effects

Extrapyramidal Symptoms (EPS)

Acute dystonia develops within 1–2 days and affects approximately 10% of patients. It usually affects the tongue, lips and jaw, although the trunk and limbs can also be affected. Treatment is by parenteral anticholinergic medication.

Akathisia is a subjective sense of restlessness accompanied by ceaseless movements of the hands or feet with repeated standing or pacing. It occurs in 20%–25% of patients taking antipsychotic medications and can be mistaken for increasing agitation and has been associated with aggression. Benzodiazepines and propranolol may provide relief. Anticholinergic medications are not particularly beneficial.

Parkinsonism is the most common EPS and ranges from bradykinesia to akinesia with rigidity, festinating gait, crouched posture, coarse tremor and hypersalivation. It is more common in women and the elderly. Its onset is usually in the first month of treatment and it tends to lessen with time, after dose reduction or anticholinergic medication administration.

Tardive dystonia and dyskinesia are long-term EPS of antipsychotic use. Tardive dystonia is relatively rare, with a prevalence of about 2%, which increases to 15%–25% or more after many years of treatment. It presents as choreoathetoid movements of the mouth and face, but the trunk and limbs can also be affected. The treatment of tardive dyskinesia is difficult, and strategies include dose reduction, benzodiazepines such as clonazepam as muscle relaxants, tetrabenazine (a dopamine depleting agent), vitamin E (a free radical scavenger) and clozapine.

Neuroleptic Malignant Syndrome (NMS)

Neuroleptic Malignant Syndrome (NMS) is the most dangerous neuromuscular adverse effect of antipsychotics and is fatal in up to 20% of patients. Although associated with FGAs, there are case reports with SGAs. The incidence in antipsychotic-treated patients is in the range of 0.2%–1%, often displayed in early treatment, high doses and/or rapid dose titration.

For more information about clinical features and treatment, see Rapid Tranquillisation.

Serotonin Syndrome (SS)

Serotonin syndrome (SS) is a syndrome that has many clinical features similar to those of NMS. It is due to increased amounts of serotonin after treatment with antidepressants; occasionally SGAs are causative (especially when switching over). For more information, see Rapid Tranquillisation.

Metabolic Syndrome

Metabolic syndrome is indicated by the presence of three or more of the following cardiometabolic risk factors: central obesity, hypertension, raised fasting glucose and dyslipidaemia. The risk of weight gain differs between antipsychotics; it is relatively common with SGAs. The greatest risk of weight gain occurs with olanzapine and clozapine. Quetiapine and risperidone confer an intermediate risk of weight gain, whereas aripiprazole confers a minimal risk of weight gain. (Leucht et al., 2009b; Cooper et al., 2016). Importantly, weight gain can be distressing for patients and can lead to discontinuation of treatment.

The mechanism of weight gain is multifactorial with affinity for the 5-HT2$_C$ receptor, which is involved in the modulation of hunger and satiety, but other mechanisms implicated include the histamine receptor and the polypeptide hormone leptin, which modulates eating behaviour and energy metabolism.

Hyperprolactinemia

Increased serum prolactin is also an important adverse effect of antipsychotic medication, which can lead to problems such as menstrual abnormalities, galactorrhea and sexual dysfunction, and in the longer term to reduced bone mineral density (Haddad and Wieck, 2004). When hyperprolactinemia is diagnosed, consider lowering the dose, switching to a less potent D2 blocker (some SGAs) or adding low-dose aripiprazole (Taylor et al., 2018).

Other Adverse Effects of Antipsychotics

- Sedation, which varies between medications
- Anticholinergic effects (e.g. blurred vision, dry mouth, constipation and urinary retention)
- Postural hypotension, reflex tachycardia and delayed ejaculation result from α_1-adrenergic antagonism
- Cardiac irregularities, including QTc prolongation
- Lowering of epileptic fit threshold

Use of 'High-Dose' Antipsychotics

High-dose antipsychotic treatment can be defined as the use of a total daily dose that exceeds the upper limit recommended by the SmPC or BNF, or a total daily dose of two or more antipsychotics that exceeds the SmPC or BNF maximum using the percentage method (Royal College of Psychiatrists, 2014). The use of high-dose antipsychotics increases the risk of the side effect burden, including EPS, hyperprolactinemia, sedation, anticholinergic effects, weight gain, lowering seizure threshold, NMS, QTc prolongation and sudden death. There is little convincing evidence that high doses have a therapeutic advantage and, when it is considered appropriate, prescribing should be within a time-limited trial with distinct treatment targets, clinical reviews and appropriate safety monitoring (Royal College of Psychiatrists, 2014).

Lithium

Lithium has also been shown to markedly reduce the risk of recurrence of manic and depressive episodes in patients with bipolar affective disorder (Baastrup et al., 1970; Coppen et al., 1971; Fieve et al., 1976). In adherent patients, lithium is still considered to be the first-line choice for long-term treatment (NICE, 2014b; Goodwin et al., 2016).

Plasma levels need to be monitored 12 hours after the last dose; levels between 0.4 and 1.0 mmol/l should be aimed for, with levels greater than 1.5 mmol/l leading to lithium toxicity. Adverse effects are worse with higher plasma levels. Before commencing lithium, thyroid and kidney function should be tested.

Reversible ECG changes due to the displacement of potassium in the myocardium have been described. Lithium interacts with several medications including nonsteroidal anti-inflammatory drugs (NSAIDS), angiotensin-converting-enzyme (ACE) inhibitors and diuretics.

Patients should be counselled on the toxic side effects of lithium, including coarsening tremor, nausea, vomiting and dizziness, ataxia, dysarthria, drowsiness, confusion, epileptic fits and coma.

Carbamazepine

Carbamazepine is a less effective maintenance treatment for bipolar than lithium but should be considered if lithium is ineffective (Goodwin et al., 2016). It appears to be almost exclusively effective against manic relapse. Carbamazepine induces liver enzymes and can reduce the effectiveness of co-prescribed medications including antipsychotics, antidepressants and oral contraceptives.

Carbamazepine has a number of adverse effects, for example, drowsiness, ataxia and diplopia, which develop when the plasma concentrations are too high. Others are erythematous rash, water retention, hepatitis and leucopenia or other blood dyscrasias.

Valproate

Sodium valproate or semisodium valproate (licenced for mania) has been shown in well-designed studies to be effective in the treatment of manic patients (Emrich et al., 1985; Pope et al., 1991; Freeman et al., 1992). However, it has been shown to be inferior to both lithium monotherapy and valproate/lithium combination in terms of total relapses (Geddes et al., 2010). Combination treatment carries a greater risk of medication adverse effects.

The common adverse effects of valproate are gastrointestinal disturbance, sedation and weight gain. Thrombocytopenia, tremor and impairment of liver function tests occur occasionally.

Valproate is a major teratogen and must not be used in any person able to have children unless they have a pregnancy prevention programme (PPP) in place. Any person capable of getting pregnant who is prescribed valproate should be reviewed yearly with assurance they are on a PPP (MHRA, 2018).

Lamotrigine

Lamotrigine has established acute efficacy for bipolar depression both as a monotherapy and in combination with lithium and quetiapine (Goodwin et al., 2016). However, the slow titration of dose due to the risk of Stevens-Johnson syndrome (GlaxoSmithKline, 2021) may limit its benefit for acute use. Other side effects include rash, dizziness, sedation, tremors and gastrointestinal effects.

Antidepressants

The main groups of antidepressants include the SSRIs, mirtazapine, serotonin–norepinephrine reuptake inhibitors (SNRIs), tricyclics and monoamine oxidase inhibitors (MAOIs). Antidepressant drugs have a similar efficacy in first-line use for the majority of patients with depression (NICE, 2009b; Cleare, 2015). In has been shown that mirtazapine, escitalopram, venlafaxine and sertraline appear to be marginally more effective than other SSRIs (Cipriani et al., 2009). In psychotic depression, a combination of an antidepressant with an antipsychotic is preferred to treating with an antidepressant alone or an antipsychotic alone (Cleare, 2015).

The choice of antidepressant drug should be assessed according to the needs of the patient, with SSRIs being the first line. They are often better tolerated and safer in overdose when compared to tricyclics, although some deaths have been attributed to citalopram (Ostrom et al., 1996). For SSRIs, the common adverse effects are nausea, headache, agitation and sexual dysfunction. All SSRIs have been used in the treatment of depression and various anxiety disorders. However, they are not all licensed for all conditions.

Benzodiazepines

Benzodiazepines are effective in the treatment of acute disturbance (Patel and Sethi et al., 2018) and are used for pre-RT (see Chapter 18). They are also effective anxiolytics and were for many years the mainstay of treatment. The risk of dependence has now greatly limited their use. Benzodiazepines all have the same pharmacological action with the difference being in their pharmacokinetics. Whenever possible, intermittent use of benzodiazepines, rather than regular use, must be encouraged and the risk of dependence discussed with patients before and during use. Adverse effects include postural hypotension, sedation, amnesia and respiratory depression. Respiratory depression can be reversed by flumazenil, and where benzodiazepines are used flumazenil should be made available (Patel et al., 2018) Disinhibition can also occur with benzodiazepines, although this is probably uncommon (Paton, 2002).

Monitoring and Auditing of Medication Use within the PICU Setting

When any medication is administered, the patient should be monitored for any immediate side effects such as postural hypotension, tachycardia, respiratory depression or sedation using a validated system (e.g. NEWS 2) (Royal College of Physicians, 2017). All relevant monitoring equipment and medicines to manage any adverse effects should be readily available.

Patients with a diagnosis of severe mental illness (SMI) have a greater risk of poor physical health as well as adverse effects of the medication. Physical health monitoring should occur yearly as a minimum, including weight/BMI, blood pressure, fasting blood glucose, HbA1 c, lipid profile and prolactin levels. Healthy eating, weight management and smoking cessation should all be explored and offered (NICE, 2014c).

Audits should be carried out to ensure the prescribing, administration, monitoring and review of medication is carried out. The Prescribing Observatory for Mental Health (POMH-UK) is a programme in which POMH-UK members take part in audit-based Quality Improvement Programmes (QIPs), which focus on specific topics within mental health prescribing.

The PICU should keep, maintain and update skills required to implement evidence-based, validated side effect assessment scales (NAPICU, 2014), including the Liverpool University Neuroleptic Side Effect Rating Scale (LUNSERS) (Day et al., 1995) and the Glasgow Antipsychotic Side-Effect Scale (GASS) (Waddell and Taylor, 2008).

Adherence

About 50% of people with schizophrenia and schizophreniform disorder are believed to be non-adherent to their medication (Nose et al., 2003). It is estimated that non-adherence to medication leads to higher relapse rates, repeated hospital admissions, and therefore increased economic and social burden for the service users themselves as well as for mental health services (Robinson

et al., 1999; Gray et al., 2006). Adherence should be investigated at each clinical review.

Policy Framework for Introducing Latest Evidence for Pharmacological Interventions

The National Association of Psychiatric Intensive Care Units and Low Secure Units (NAPICU) has produced National Minimum Standards for Psychiatric Intensive Care in General Adult Services (NAPICU, 2014) which are multidisciplinary and patient focussed. They ensure high-quality care of patients and should be consulted to advise on the minimum standards expected in a PICU unit.

Policies can change and situations can develop where rapid changes need to be evaluated. In 2020, the World Health Organization (WHO) declared a pandemic in response to a severe acute respiratory syndrome, COVID-19. Due to the high risk of illness with COVID-19, including subsequent risk of increased side effects with medication, guidance in managing acute disturbance in the context of COVID-19 (NAPICU, 2020) was produced, including the use of medication in this challenging situation. Many of the recommendations will be useful in the context of choice of medication in the longer term when there are complex needs due to COVID-19.

References

Assion,HJ, Reinbold,H, Lemanski,S, Basilowski,M and Juckel,G (2008) Amisulpride Augmentation in Patients with Schizophrenia Partially Responsive or Unresponsive to Clozapine. A Randomized, Double-Blind, Placebo-Controlled Trial. *Pharmacopsychiatry* **41** (1) 24–8.

Atkin,K, Kendall,F and Gould,D (1996) Neutropenia and Agranulocytosis in Patients Receiving Clozapine in the UK and Ireland. *British Journal of Psychiatry* **169** (4) 483–8.

Baastrup,PC, Paulsen,JC, Schou,M, Thomsen,K and Amidsen,A (1970) Prophylactic Lithium: Double-Blind Discontinuation in Manic-Depressive and Recurrent Depressive Disorders. *Lancet* **2** (7668) 326–30.

Baldwin,DS, Anderson,IM, Nutt,DJ, Allgulander,C, Bandelow,B, den Boer,JA, et al. (2014) Evidence-Based Pharmacological Treatment of Anxiety Disorders, Post-Traumatic Stress Disorder and Obsessive-Compulsive Disorder: A Revision of the 2005 Guidelines from the British Association for Psychopharmacology. *Journal of Psychopharmacology* **28** (5) 403–39.

Barnes,TR, Drake,R, Paton,C, Cooper,SJ, Deakin,B, Ferrier, IN, et al. (2020) Evidence-Based Guidelines for the Pharmacological Treatment of Schizophrenia: Updated Recommendations from the British Association for Psychopharmacology. *Journal of Psychopharmacology* **34** (1) 3–78.

Beasley Jr,CM Hamilton,SH and Crawford,AM (1997) Olanzapine versus Haloperidol: Acute Phase Results of the International Double-Blind Olanzapine Trial. *European Neuropsychopharmacology* **7** (2) 125–37.

Beasley Jr,CM, Sanger,T, and Satterlee,W (1996b) Olanzapine versus Placebo: Results of a Double-Blind, Fixed-Dose Olanzapine Trial. *Psychopharmacology* **124** (1–2) 159–67.

Beasley Jr,CM, Tollefson,G and Tran,P (1996a) Olanzapine versus Placebo and Haloperidol: Acute Phase Results of the North American Double-Blind Olanzapine Trial. *Neuropsychopharmacology* **14** (2) 111–23.

Bellack,AS and Mueser,KT (1993) Psychosocial Treatment for Schizophrenia. *Schizophrenia Bulletin* **19** (2) 317–36.

Boter,H, Peuskens,J, Libiger,J, Fleischhacker,WW, Davidson,M, Galderisi,S, et al. (2009) Effectiveness of Antipsychotics in First Episode Schizophrenia and Schizophreniform Disorder on Response and Remission: An Open Randomized Clinical Trial (EUFEST). *Schizophrenia Research* **115** (1–2) 97–103.

Boyer,P, Lecrucibier,Y and Puech,AJ (1995) Treatment of Negative Symptoms of Schizophrenia with Amisulpride. *British Journal of Psychiatry* **166** (1) 68–72.

Britannia (2020) *Summary of Product Characteristics – Denzapine 100 mg tablets (clozapine)*. Reading: Britannia Pharmaceuticals Ltd. www.medicines.org.uk/emc/product/6120/smpc.

Cardoni,AA (1995) Risperidone: Review and Assessment of Its Role in the Treatment of Schizophrenia. *Annals of Pharmacotherapy* **29** (6) 610–18.

Carter,RM, Wittchen,HU, Pfister,H and Kessler,RC (2001) One-Year Prevalence of Subthreshold and Threshold DSM-IV Generalized Anxiety Disorder in a Nationally Representative Sample. *Depression and Anxiety* **13** (2) 78–88.

Castelao,JF, Ferrerira,L, Gelders,YG and Heylen,SLE (1989) The Efficacy of the D2 and 5HT2 Antagonist Risperidone in the Treatment of Chronic Psychoses. An Open Dose Finding Study. *Schizophrenia Research* **2** (4–5) 411–15.

Chouinard,G, Jones,B and Remington,G (1993) A Canadian Multicenter Placebo-Controlled Study of Fixed Doses of Risperidone and Haloperidol in the Treatment of Chronic Schizophrenic Patients. *Journal of Clinical Psychopharmacology* **13** (1) 35–40.

Cipriani,A, Furukawa,TA, Salanti,G, Geddes,JR, Higgins,JP, Churchill,R, et al. (2009) Comparative Efficacy and Acceptability of 12 New-Generation Antidepressants: A Multiple Treatments Meta-Analysis. *Lancet* **373** (9665) 746–58.

Citrome,L, Cucchiaro,J, Sarma,K, Phillips,D, Silva,R, Tsuchiya,S, et al. (2012) Long-Term Safety and Tolerability of Lurasidone in Schizophrenia: A 12-Month, Double-Blind, Active-Controlled study. *International Clinical Psychopharmacology* **27** (3) 165–76.

Claus,A, Bollen,J and de Cuyper,H (1992) Risperidone versus Haloperidol in the Treatment of Chronic Schizophrenic Inpatient: A Multi-Centre Double-Blind Comparative Study. *Acta Psychiatrica Scandanavia* **85** (4) 295–305.

Cleare,A, Pariante,CM, Young,AH, Anderson,IM, Christmas,D, Cowen,PJ, et al. (2015) Evidence-Based Guidelines for Treating Depressive Disorders with Antidepressants: A Revision of the 2008 British Association for Psychopharmacology Guidelines. *Journal of Psychopharmacology* **29** (5) 459–525.

Cooper,SJ, Reynolds,GP, Barnes,TRE, England,E, Haddad, PM, Heald,A, et al. (2016) BAP Guidelines on the Management of Weight Gain and Metabolic Disturbances and Cardiovascular Risk Associated with Psychosis and Antipsychotic Drug Treatment. *Journal of Psychopharmacology* **30** (8) 717–48.

Cooper,T (1996) Clozapine Plasma Level Monitoring: Current Status. *Psychiatric Quarterly* **67** (4) 297–311.

Coppen,A, Noguera R and Bailey,J (1971) Prophylactic Lithium in Affective Disorders: A Controlled Trial. *Lancet* **2** (7719) 275–9.

Correll,CU (2010) From Receptor Pharmacology to Improved Outcomes: Individualising the Selection, Dosing, and Switching of Antipsychotics. *European Psychiatry* **25** (Suppl 2) S12–21.

Daniel,DG and Whitcomb SR (1998) Treatment of the Refractory Schizophrenic Patient. *Journal of Clinical Psychiatry* **59** (Suppl 1) 13–19.

Davidson,M, Emsley,R, Kramer,M, Ford,L, Pan,G, Lim,P, et al (2007) Efficacy, Safety, and Early Response of Paliperidone Extended-Release Tablets (Paliperidone ER): Results of a 6-Week, Randomised, Placebo-Controlled Study. *Schizophrenia Research* **93** (1–3) 117–30.

Day,JC, Wood,G, Dewey,M and Bentall,RP (1995) A Self-Rating Scale for Measuring Neuroleptic Side-Effects: Validation in a Group of Schizophrenic Patients. *British Journal of Psychiatry* **166** (5) 650–3.

Department of Health (2015) *Mental Health Act 1983: Code of Practice*. London: TSO.

Devinsky,O, Honigfield,G and Patin,J (1991) Clozapine-Related Seizures. *Neurology* **41** (3) 369–71.

Durgam,S, Earley,W, Lipschitz,A, Guo,H, Laszlovszky,I, Nemeth,G, et al. (2016) An 8-Week Randomized, Double-Blind, Placebo-Controlled Evaluation of the Safety and Efficacy of Cariprazine in Patients with Bipolar I Depression. *American Journal of Psychiatry* **173** (3) 271–81.

Durgam,S, Starace,A, Li,D, Migliore,R, Ruth,A, Nemeth,G, et al (2015) The Efficacy and Tolerability of Cariprazine in Acute Mania Associated with Bipolar I Disorder: A Phase II Trial. *Bipolar Disorder* **17** (1) 63–75.

Emrich,HM, Dose,M and von Serssen,D (1985) The Use of Sodium Valproate and Oxcarbazepine in Patients with Affective Disorders. *Journal of Affective Disorders* **8** (3) 243–50.

Esteves,P, Mota,D, Cerejeira,J and Mendes,F (2015). Low Doses of Adjunctive Aripiprazole as Treatment for Antipsychotic-induced Hyperprolactinemia: a Literature Review. *European Psychiatry* **30** (Suppl 1) 393.

Fieve,RR, Kumbaraci,T and Dunner,DL (1976) Lithium Prophylaxis of Depression in Bipolar I, Bipolar II, and Unipolar Patients. *American Journal of Psychiatry* **133** (8) 925–30.

Freeman,TW, Clothier,JL, Passaglia,P and Lesem,MD (1992) A Double-Blind Comparison of VPA and LI in the Treatment of Acute Mania. *American Journal of Psychiatry* **149** (1) 108–11.

Garnock-Jones,KP (2017) Cariprazine: A Review in Schizophrenia. *CNS Drugs* **31** (6) 513–25.

Geddes,JR, Goodwin,GM, Rendell,J, Azorin,JM, Cipriani,A, Ostacher,MJ, et al. (2010) Lithium Plus Valproate Combination Therapy Versus Monotherapy for Relapse Prevention in Bipolar I Disorder (BALANCE): A Randomized Open-Label Trial. *Lancet* **375** (9712) 385–95.

Gillespie,AL, Samanaite,R, Mill,J, Egerton,A and MacCabe, JH (2017) Is Treatment-Resistant Schizophrenia Categorically Distinct from Treatment-Responsive Schizophrenia? A Systematic Review. *BMC Psychiatry* **17** (1) 12.

GlaxoSmithKline UK (2021) *Summary of Product Characteristics – Lamictal Tablets (Lamotrigine)*. Middlesex; GlaxoSmithKline UK. www.medicines.org.uk/emc/product/8052/smpc.

Goodnick,PJ and Jerry,JM (2002) Aripiprazole: Profile on Efficacy and Safety. *Expert Opinion on Pharmacotherapy* **3** (12) 1773–81.

Goodwin,GM, Haddad,PM, Ferrier,IN, Aronson,JK, Barnes,TRE, Cipriani,A, et al. (2016) Evidence-Based Guidelines for Treating Bipolar Disorder: Revised Third Edition Recommendations from the British Association for Psychopharmacology. *Journal of Psychopharmacology* **30** (6) 495–553.

Gray,R, Leese,M, Bindman,J, Becker,T, Burti,L, David,A, et al. (2006) Adherence Therapy for People with Schizophrenia: European Multicentre Randomised Controlled Trial. *British Journal of Psychiatry* **189** (6) 508–14.

Haddad,PM and Wieck,A (2004) Antipsychotic-Induced Hyperprolactinaemia: Mechanisms, Clinical Features and Management. *Drugs* **64** (20) 2291–314.

Hartley,M Haste,J and Sethi,F (2019) Non-Conventional Pharmacological Formulations for Enhancing the Management of Acute Disturbance. *Journal of Psychiatric Intensive Care* **15** (2) 79–86.

Hirsch,SR, Link,CGG and Goldstein,JM (1996) ICI204,636: A New atypical Antipsychotic Medication. *British Journal of Psychiatry* **168** (Suppl 29]) 45–56.

Huhn,M, Nikolakopoulou,A, Schneider-Thoma,J, Krause, M, Samara,M, Peter,N, et al. (2019)Comparative Efficacy and Tolerability of 32 Oral Antipsychotics for the Acute Treatment of Adults with Multi-Episode Schizophrenia: A Systematic Review and Network Meta-Analysis. *Lancet* **394** (10202) 939–51.

Hunt,C, Issakidis,C and Andrews,G (2002) DSM-IV Generalized anxiety disorder in the Australian National Survey of Mental Health and Well-Being. *Psychological Medicine* **32** (4) 649–59.

Janssen-Cilag (2018a) *Summary of Product Characteristics – Xeplion 100 mg Prolonged Release Suspension for Injection (Paliperidone)*. High Wycombe: Janssen-Cilag Ltd. www.medicines.org.uk/emc/product/7653/smpc.

Janssen-Cilag (2018b)*Summary of Product Characteristics – Rispercal Consta 25 mg Powder and Solvent for Prolonged-Release Suspension for Injection (Risperidone)*. High Wycombe: Janssen-Cilag Ltd. www.medicines.org.uk/emc/product/1690/smpc.

Janssen-Cilag (2019) *Summary of Product Characteristics – Trevicta 175 mg Prolonged Release Suspension for Injection (Paliperidone)*. High Wycombe: Janssen-Cilag Ltd. www.medicines.org.uk/emc/product/7230/smpc.

Jones,PB, Barnes,TRE, Davies,L, Dunn,G, Lloyd,H, Hayhurst,KP, et al. (2006) A Randomized Controlled Trial of Effect on Quality of Life of Second Generation Versus First Generation Antipsychotic Drugs in Schizophrenia. *Archives of General Psychiatry* **63** (10) 1079–87.

Kahn,RS, Fleischhacker,WW, Boter,H, Davidson,M, Vergouwe,Y, Keet,IP, et al. (2008) Effectiveness of Antipsychotic Drugs in First Episode Schizophrenia and Schizophreniform Disorder: An Open Randomized Clinical Trial. *Lancet* **371** (9618) 1085–97.

Kane,J, Canas,F, Kramer,M, Ford,L, Gassamann-Mayer,C, Lim,P, et al. (2006) Treatment of Schizophrenia with Paliperidone Extended-Release Tablets: A 6-Week Placebo-Controlled Trial. *Schizophrenia Research* **90** (1–3) 147–61.

Kane,J, Honigfield,G, Singer,J and Meltzer,HY (1988) The Lozaril Collaboration Study Group. Clozapine for the Treatment-Resistant Schizophrenic: A Double-Blind

Comparison with Chlorpromazine. *Archives of General Psychiatry* **45** (9) 789–96.

Kapur,S and Remington,G (2000) Atypical Antipsychotics: Patients Value the Lower Incidence of Extrapyramidal Adverse Effects. *British Medical Journal* **321** (7273) 1360–1.

Kishimoto,T, Hagi,K, Nitta,M, Leucht,S, Olfson,M, Kane, JM, et al. (2018) Effectiveness of Long-Acting Injectable vs. Oral Antipsychotics in Patients with Schizophrenia: A Meta-Analysis of Prospective and Retrospective Cohort Studies. *Schizophrenia Bulletin* **44** (3) 603–19.

Leucht,S, Komossa,K, Rummel-Kluge,C, Corves,C, Hunger, H, Schmid,F, et al. (2009a) A Meta-Analysis of Head-to-Head Comparisons of Second-Generation Antipsychotics in the Treatment of Schizophrenia. *American Journal of Psychiatry* **166** (2) 152–63.

Leucht,S, Corves,C, Arbter,D, Engel,RR, Li,C and Davis,JM (2009b) Second-Generation Versus First-Generation Antipsychotic Drugs for Schizophrenia: A Meta-Analysis. *Lancet* **373** (9697) 31–41.

Leucht,S, Tardy,M, Komossa,K, Heres,S, Kissling,W, Salanti,G, et al. (2012) Antipsychotic Drugs Versus Placebo for Relapse Prevention in Schizophrenia: A Systematic Review and Meta-Analysis. *Lancet* **379** (9831) 2063–71.

Leucht,S, Cipriani,A, Spineli,L, Mavridis,D, Orey,D, Richter,F, et al. (2013) Comparative Efficacy and Tolerability of 15 Antipsychotic Drugs in Schizophrenia: A Multiple Treatments Meta-Analysis. *Lancet* **382** (9896) 951–62.

Lieberman,JA, Stroup,TS, McEvoy,JP, Swartz,MS, Rosenheck,RA, Perkins,DO, et al. (2005) Clinical Antipsychotic Trials of Intervention Effectiveness (CATIE) Investigators: Effectiveness of Antipsychotic Drugs in Patients with Chronic Schizophrenia. *New England Journal of Medicine* **353** (12) 1209–23.

Llorca,P-M, Abbar,M, Courtet,P, Guillaume,S, Lancrenon,S and Samalin,L (2013) Guidelines for the Use and Management of Long-Acting Injectable Antipsychotics in Serious Mental Illness. *BMC Psychiatry* **13** (1) 340.

Loebel,A, Cucchiaro,J, Xu,J, Sarma,K, Pikalov,A and Kane,J (2013a) Effectiveness of Lurasidone vs. Quetiapine XR for Relapse Prevention in Schizophrenia: A 12-Month, Double-Blind, Noninferiority Study. *Schizophrenia Research* **147** (1) 95–102.

Loebel,A, Cucchiaro,J, Sarma,K, Xu,J, Hsu,C, Kalali,AH, et al. (2013b) Efficacy and Safety of Lurasidone 80 mg/day and 160 mg/day in the Treatment of Schizophrenia: A Randomized, Double-Blind, Placebo- and Active-Controlled Trial. *Schizophrenia Research* **145** (1–3) 101–9.

Loebel,A, Cucchiaro,J, Silva,R, Kroger,H, Hsu,J, Sarma,K, et al. (2014a) Lurasidone Monotherapy in the Treatment of Bipolar I Depression: A Randomized, Double-Blind,

Placebo-Controlled Study. *American Journal of Psychiatry* **171** (2) 160–8.

Loebel,A, Cucchiaro,J, Silva,R, Kroger,H, Sarma,K, Xu,J, et al. (2014b) Lurasidone as Adjunctive Therapy with Lithium or Valproate for the Treatment of Bipolar I Depression: A Randomized, Double-Blind, Placebo-Controlled Study. *American Journal of Psychiatry* **171** (2) 169–77.

Loo,H, Poirier-Littre,MF, Theron,M and Fleurot,O (1997) Amisulpride versus Placebo in the Medium-Term Treatment of Negative Symptoms of Schizophrenia. *British Journal of Psychiatry* **170** (1) 18–22.

Marder,SR and Meibach,RC (1994) Risperidone in the Treatment of Schizophrenia. *American Journal of Psychiatry* **151** (6) 825–35.

Markowitz,JS, Candace,SB and Moore,TR (1999) Atypical Antipsychotics: Pharmacology, Pharmacokinetics, and Efficacy. *Annals of Pharmacotherapy* **33** (1) 73–85.

Medicines and Healthcare Products Regulatory Agency (MHRA)(2017) Clozapine: Reminder of Potentially Fatal Risk of Intestinal Obstruction, Faecal Impaction, and Paralytic Ileus. www.gov.uk/drug-safety-update/clozapine-reminder-of-potentially-fatal-risk-of-intestinal-obstruction-faecal-impaction-and-paralytic-ileus.

Medicines and Healthcare Products Regulatory Agency (MHRA) (2018) Valproate Use by Women and Girls: Information About the Risks of Taking Valproate Medicines During Pregnancy. www.gov.uk/guidance/valproate-use-by-women-and-girls.

Meltzer,HY, Cucchiaro,J, Silva,R, Ogasa,M, Phillips,D, Xu,J, et al. (2011) Lurasidone in the Treatment of Schizophrenia: A Randomized, Double-Blind, Placebo- and Olanzapine-Controlled Study. *American Journal of Psychiatry* **168** (9) 957–67.

Mortimer,A (1997) Treatment of the Patient with Long-Term Schizophreni. *Advances in Psychiatric Treatment* **3**: 339–46.

Muralidharan,K, Ali,M, Silveira,LE, Bond,DJ, Fountoulakis, KN, Lam,RW, et al. (2013) Efficacy of Second-Generation Antipsychotics in Treating Acute Mixed Episodes in Bipolar Disorder: A Meta-Analysis of Placebo-Controlled Trials. *Journal of Affective Disorders* **150** (2) 408–14.

National Association of Psychiatric Intensive Care and Low Secure Units (NAPICU) (2014) *National Minimum Standards for Psychiatric Intensive Care in General Adult Services.* Glasgow: NAPICU.

National Association of Psychiatric Intensive Care and Low Secure Units (NAPICU) (2020) *Managing Acute Disturbance in the Context of COVID-19.* Glasgow: NAPICU.

National Institute for Health and Care Excellence (NICE) (2009a) *Borderline Personality Disorder: Recognition and Management. Clinical Guideline [CG78].* London: NICE.

National Institute for Health and Care Excellence (NICE) (2009b) *Depression in Adults: The Treatment and Management of Depression in Adults. Clinical Guideline [CG90]*. London: NICE.

National Institute for Health and Care Excellence (NICE) (2011) *Generalised Anxiety Disorder and Panic Disorder in Adults: Management. Clinical Guideline [CG113]*. London: NICE.

National Institute for Health and Care Excellence (NICE) (2014a) *Antenatal and Postnatal Mental Health: Clinical Management and Service Guidance. NICE Clinical Guideline [CG192]*. London: NICE.

National Institute for Health and Care Excellence (NICE) (2014b) *Bipolar Disorder: Assessment and Management. NICE Clinical Guideline [CG185]*. London: NICE.

National Institute for Health and Care Excellence (NICE) (2014c) *Psychosis and Schizophrenia in Adults: Prevention and Management. Clinical Guideline [CG178]*. London: NICE.

National Institute for Health and Care Excellence (NICE) (2015) *Violence and Aggression: Short-Term Management in Mental Health, Health and Community Settings. NICE Guideline [NG10]*. London: NICE. www.nice.org.uk/guidance/NG10.

Nose,M, Barbui,C and Tansella,M (2003) How Often Do Patients with Psychosis Fail to Adhere to Treatment Programmes? A Systematic Review. *Psychological Medicine* 33: 1149–60.

Nutt,DJ and Blier,P (2016) Neuroscience-based Nomenclature (NbN) for Journal of Psychopharmacology. *Journal of Psychopharmacology* 30 (5) 413–15.

Organon Pharma (2021) *Summary of Product Characteristics – Sycrest 10 mg Sublingual Tablets (Asenapine)*. London: Organon Pharma (UK) Limited. www.medicines.org.uk/emc/product/7737/smpc.

Ostrom,M, Eriksson,A, Thorson,J and Spigset,O (1996) Fatal Overdose with Citalopram. *Lancet* 348 (9023) 339–40.

Otsuka (2020) *Summary of Product Characteristics for Abilify Maintena 400 mg Powder and Solvent for Prolonged-Release Suspension (Aripiprazole) Clozapine*. Wexham: Otsuka Pharmaceutics (UK) Ltd.

Paris,J (2000) Chronic Suicidality Among Patients with Borderline Personality Disorder. *Psychiatric Services* 53 (6) 738–42.

Patel,MX, Sethi,FN, Barnes,TR, Dix,R, Dratcu,L, Fox,B, et al. (2018) Joint BAP NAPICU Evidence-Based Consensus Guidelines for the Clinical Management of Acute Disturbance: De-Escalation and Rapid Tranquillisation. *Journal of Psychopharmacology* 32 (6) 601–40.

Paton,C (2002) Benzodiazepines and Disinhibition: A Review. *Psychiatric Bulletin* 26 (12) 460–2.

Paton,C and Okocha,CI (2004) Risperidone Long-Acting Injection: The First 50 Patients. *Psychiatric Bulletin* 28 (1) 12–14.

Paton,C and Okocha,CI (2005) Pharmacological Treatment of Borderline Personality Disorder. *Journal of Psychiatric Intensive Care Psychiatry* 1 (2) 105–16.

Perry,PJ, Miller,DD, Arndt,SV and Cadoret,RJ (1991) Clozapine and Norclozapine Plasma Concentrations and Clinical Response of Treatment-Refractory Schizophrenic Patients. *American Journal of Psychiatry* 148 (10) 231–5.

Pope,HG, McElroy,SL, Keck,P and Hudson,JI (1991) Valproate in the Treatment of Acute Mania: A Placebo-Controlled Study. *Archives of General Psychiatry* 48 (1) 62–8.

Robinson,D, Woerner,MG, Alvir,JM, Bilder,R, Goldman,R, Geisler,S, et al. (1999) Predictors of Relapse Following Response from a First Episode of Schizophrenia or Schizoaffective Disorder. *Archives of General Psychiatry* 56 (3) 241–7.

Royal College of Physicians (2017) *National Early Warning Score (NEWS) 2*. London: Royal College of Physicians. https://www.rcplondon.ac.uk/projects/outputs/national-early-warning-score-news-2.

Royal College of Psychiatrists (2014) *Consensus Statement on High-dose Antipsychotic Medication, CR190*. London: Royal College of Psychiatrists. www.rcpsych.ac.uk/files/pdfversion/CR190.pdf.

Royal College of Psychiatrists Psychopharmacology Committee (2017) *Use of Licensed Medicines for Unlicensed Applications in Psychiatric Practice*, 2nd ed. London: Royal College of Psychiatrists.

Srisurapanont,M, Sirijit,S, Maneeton,N and Maneeton,B (2015) Efficacy and Safety of Aripiprazole Augmentation of Clozapine in Schizophrenia: A Systematic Review and Meta-Analysis of Randomized Controlled Trials. *Journal of Psychiatric Research* 62: 38–47.

Taylor,D, Barnes,TRE and Young,AH (2018) (eds.) *The Maudsley Prescribing Guidelines in Psychiatry*, 13th ed. Chichester: Wiley Blackwell.

Taylor,D and Duncan,D (1995) The Use of Clozapine Plasma Levels in Optimizing Therapy. *Psychiatric Bulletin* 19: 753–5.

Tiihonen,J, Mittendorfer-Rutz,E, Majak,M, Mehtala,J, Hoti,F, Jedenius,E, et al. (2017) Real-World Effectiveness of Antipsychotic Treatments in a Nationwide Cohort of 29,823 Patients with Schizophrenia. *JAMA Psychiatry* 74 (7) 686–93.

Tollefson,GD, Beasley Jr,CM, Tran,PV, Street,JS, Krueger, JA, Tamura,RN, et al. (1997) Olanzapine Versus Haloperidol in the Treatment of Schizophrenia, Schizoaffective, and Schizophreniform Disorders: Results of an International Collaborative Trial. *American Journal of Psychiatry* **154** (4) 457–65.

Vieta,E, Reinares,M, Corbella,B, Benabarre,A, Gilaberte,I, Colom,F. et al. (2001) Olanzapine as Long-Term Adjunctive Therapy in Treatment-Resistant Bipolar Disorder. *Journal of Clinical Psychopharmacology* **21** (5) 469–73.

Waddell,L and Taylor,M (2008) A New Self-Rating Scale for Detecting Atypical or Second-Generation Antipsychotic Side Effects. *Journal of Psychopharmacology* **22** (3) 238–43.

Wilson,WH and Claussen,AM (1994) Seizures Associated with Clozapine Treatment in a State Hospital. *Journal of Clinical Psychiatry* **55** (5) 184–8.

Winston,AP (2000) Recent Developments in Borderline Personality Disorder. *Advances in Psychiatric Treatment* **6** (3) 211–8.

Yildiz,A, Vieta,E, Leucht,S and Baldessarini,RJ (2011) Efficacy of Antimanic Treatments: Meta-Analysis of Randomized, Controlled Trials. *Neuropsychopharmacology* **36**(2): 375–89.

Chapter 18

Rapid Tranquillisation

Ross Runciman, Steve Ireland and Brenda Wasunna-Smith

Introduction

This chapter looks at the evolving nature of rapid tranquillisation (RT) through the years and current evidence-based best practice. The authors define RT, including the complexities around its definition, and present views based on the review of international guidelines, literature and personal experience. The chapter provides details of the medications used for RT, considerations around administration, side effects and the implications of these. It also discusses considerations required following the administration of RT and emphasises the importance of rebuilding trust in the ongoing relationship between clinicians and the patients who have received RT.

RT is an invasive procedure, and before its use is considered, it is vital that clinicians have explored other non-invasive approaches to reduce the patient's arousal levels. This chapter highlights the importance of reflective practice, communication and a multi-disciplinary approach in decision-making regarding the administration and delivery of RT. Every hospital should have a robust RT policy that contains guidelines for the use of RT in that setting. All clinicians who administer RT should undergo training, preferably in a multi-disciplinary learning environment where they are able to share experiences and have discussions; every patient is an individual and one can never predict every single scenario requiring the consideration of RT use that would present itself. It is also important for clinicians to keep updated with any new guidance around the delivery of RT.

A Brief History of RT

The beginning point in any aspect of the history of psychiatry is to acknowledge at least three crucial dynamics.

Firstly is the challenge to psychiatrists writing the history of their own specialism, led by 'outsiders' such as Michel Foucault in the 1960s, whereby the linear narrative of progressive treatments was put in sharp contrast with his vision of the Enlightenment, leading to what he characterised as the 'great confinement' of those with mental illness into asylums. This began a revisionist history of mental health and decades of probing the speciality (Beveridge, 2014)

Secondly is the emergence of the history of psychiatry from the patient's perspective. This brought luminaries such as Roy Porter who, for example, worked with psychiatrist German Berrios to fundamentally change the narrative of the subject (Beveridge, 2014).

Thirdly, through the prism of anachronism, we try to understand the motive and ethics of previous centuries with our own contemporary framework. Therefore, in the Middle Ages, madness was seen as divine punishment, in the Renaissance as having natural causes and in the Enlightenment as having social and psychological origins (Burton, 2010).

With these factors recognised, we can now consider the difficulty of defining RT through history, as this is often viewed as a near equivalent to sedation or, indeed, often to restraint (Negroni, 2017). It was Thomas Szasz who, in 1957, characterised the newly emerging antipsychotics as 'chemical straightjackets' (Negroni, 2017). Although chemical restraint clearly is not directly equivalent to RT, it is closely related, and exploration of this relation gives access to a longer history of chemicals being used to sedate patients.

In the beginning of the nineteenth century, opiates, hyoscine and digitalis (hence digitalisation, an early shorthand term for RT) were used to sedate patients. Then, in 1869, chloral hydrate was created, replacing earlier chemicals deployed in mental health hospitals. However, soon doctors were reflecting that these approaches were not helpful and, in 1883,

Cameron stated, firstly, that such practices could be seen as 'chemical restraint' and secondly, that 'there are no facts to bear out the assumption that it is by excessive drugging we are enabled to avoid the use of restraining apparatus in our asylums (Cameron, 1883). Indeed, another contemporary, Dr George Savage, writing in 1887 at Bethlem Royal Hospital, described how he found most sedatives of little use when the patient is distressed, but stated there might be a role for chloral in order to 'tide over periods of excitement when some bodily complication is also threatening' (Savage, 1887).

Therefore, wrestling over both the ethics of using medicines or chemicals in restraint and risks of side effects is not new, and just as in the history of psychiatry in general, there is little evidence. Indeed, Cameron and Savage in the 1880s were pontificating the same ethical dilemmas, and the associated terminology was being examined again by Currier (2003) many years later.

After chloral, came paraldehyde in the 1880s. Then, the early twentieth century brought barbiturates amongst other sedatives for use in mental health hospitals. It is interesting to note that Allison and Moncrieff (2014) as well as Braslow (1997) assert that until the 1950s, there were only chemical restraints; then came antipsychotics with disease-modifying properties, which therefore justified the term RT. However, is the principle aim of RT to *treat* mental illness or to reduce risk or manage immediate distress in the patient?

Allison and Moncrieff (2014) analysed contemporaneous medical journal advertisements and psychiatry textbooks from the 1950s to 1980s as more medication was sold and indicated for managing acute disturbance, though only in the 1970s did the term 'rapid tranquillisation' emerge; 'digitalisation' was also still used. Their work is summarised in Table 18.1.

Therefore, the 1950s and 1960s witnessed the emergence of antipsychotics used for sedation, whereas from the 1970s onwards, specific medications were cited for their speed of efficacy in aiding with acute disturbance and sometimes for specific conditions.

Defining RT

Within the United Kingdom, the National Institute for Health and Care Excellence (NICE, 2015)

guidance, supported by the British Association of Psychopharmacology (BAP), define RT as being represented by parenteral administration only. This may stand in contrast to the experience of many inpatient nurses and other clinicians. *For instance, RT administered by injection if it is not accepted orally by the patient is considered RT as well.* There are similar characteristics to those present when an injection is administered (e.g. the formation of a restraint team and/or other coercive indications).

The authors consider that RT is a procedure that occurs when medication is administered for the purpose of calming acute disturbance in circumstances where the clinical decision has been taken that receiving the prescribed medication is essential. This is distinct from the concept of Pro Re Nata (PRN) medication, which is medication that is available for use on an as needed basis. PRN can be requested by the patient or offered by staff and is often utilised to calm escalating disturbance as part of a range of wider considerations. The major difference is that the patient could decline PRN without the clinical team using the authority afforded by law to insist the medication is received.

RT should only be utilised as part of a measured and proportionate approach to de-escalation. This commences with approaches aimed at de-escalation. RT may represent an unavoidable intervention where other less restrictive approaches have not succeeded. Further, this is a requirement within the Mental Health Act Code of Practice (Department of Health, 2015). All individuals should be treated using the 'least restrictive' principle underpinning any intervention. The administration route of RT medications is important. Parenteral RT can be a very distressing experience for the patient and presents several significant risks. The clinical team will often be faced with making difficult judgements within stressful situations leading to the patient requiring RT.

NICE (2015) defines RT as the use of medication by the parenteral route (usually intramuscular (IM) or, exceptionally, intravenous (IV)) if oral medication is not possible or appropriate and urgent sedation with medication is needed.

Within acute inpatient mental health practice, the clinical team is required to respond to acute behavioural disturbance in a range of ways, utilising a hierarchy of response. In view of the progressive nature of the response to acute disturbance from clinicians, it is helpful to consider this definition: RT

Table 18.1 Medications and their stated purposes (1950s to 1980s)

Decade	Medication	Stated use in advertisement (A) or textbook (T) or journal (J)
1950s	Reserpine	'remarkable calming and relaxing action' (A)
	Promazine	'controlling acute agitation' (A)
	Mepazine	'for control aggression, impulsiveness' (A)
	Trifluoperazine	'for the hallucinated, delusional and aggressive psychotic' (A)
	Chlorpromazine	'control of cases of manic excitement' (T)
1960s	Thioproperazine	'acute manic and other states of psychotic excitement'
	Haloperidol	'quickly controls the psychotic manifestations of schizophrenia'
	Chlorpromazine and Trifluoperazine	'useful in allaying turmoil and tension' (T)
	Barbiturates (oral) and Chlorpromazine (IM)	For use in psychiatric emergencies if alternative, non-medication options have been exhausted (T)
1970s	Chlorpromazine	'50-200 mg orally every two hours' to enable tranquillisation within 6 hours (J)
	Chlorpromazine and Haloperidol	'safely and effectively tranquilize violent, agitated and psychotic patients' (J)
	Perphenazine	'acutely disturbed patients' (J)
1980s	Droperidol	'rapid control of acute agitation' (A)
		With Allison and Moncrieff noting that droperidol was marketed for across mental health diagnoses and was produced by Janssen, which also made haloperidol.
	Lorazepam and Haloperidol	Allison and Moncrieff also state that haloperidol continued to be widely used as chlorpromazine was side-lined due to concerns around inducing hypotension, with lorazepam also emerging in its use in the 1980s.

is the reactive administration of medication (IM or oral) to manage unanticipated agitation or disturbance with the intended purpose of tranquilising the patient.

RT is an extremely intrusive and restrictive intervention that should be utilised as a last resort when dealing with violence and aggression. The response to a highly agitated patient can involve a range of de-escalation approaches and, as such, impending negotiation with the patient can lead to the acceptance of oral medication when the alternative of IM medication is presented to them. This definition is helpful for the clinical practicalities when balancing the least restrictive principle and engaging with acute agitation. Whilst it is acknowledged that coercive practice would still be taking place, the ability to deliver RT in oral form is a preferable outcome in the context of the least restrictive principle (Department of Health, 2015). There would also be increased scope for avoiding the physical restraint process as the negotiation progresses on a continuum.

It is important to consider and further explore the differentiation between PRN medication and RT medication. In terms of prescribing and administering medications, clinicians need to be able to develop a clear rationale for their use based upon the presenting situation. This approach will likely provide increased opportunity for more timely reviews of RT medication prescriptions, which is considered to be good practice. Further to this, given the clear prescription of both PRN and RT medications, there will be increased opportunities to monitor the specific use of medications over defined periods of time.

It is considered good practice to have a well-developed RT pathway in use where RT approaches are a possibility. The availability of a specific document or an area of the prescription chart dedicated to RT prescription and administration can assist with the monitoring of RT use. Healthcare organisations should also have a clear description of steps that clinicians can take to attempt to avoid the use of RT and a description of steps to take should RT have been administered to the patient.

Given that both PRN and RT medication can be administered via the same routes, the emphasis lies with the clinical team engaging in the situation with the patient and their decision regarding the necessity of the patient receiving the medication. As such, PRN can be described as a proactive approach to offer the patient a potential way to avoid increased agitation and will not be administered in conditions where the patient does not wish to accept it. PRN should be offered as one of a range of options to assist the patient in the progressive stages of their agitation levels increasing from their baseline presentation. Contrastingly, RT is a judged requirement for the patient to receive medication and will be administered regardless of route and to maintain safety of the patient and others. This judgement will be made by the clinicians involved in the presenting situation.

Considerations before Administration of RT

Clinical Assessment

The patient presentation on admission to hospital and any relevant history should be considered prior to the prescription of RT medications. During the process of assessing risk and the initial care plan for the patient, there may be historical information that can assist with the prescribing (i.e. previous violent behaviour, response to previous medications and any protective factors/helpful strategies for assisting the patient in times of disturbance).

Clear consideration should also be given to any pre-existing health conditions of concern and potential pregnancy. Obtaining allergy information is imperative, and any previous responses to medications will require exploration, for example, the patient may have received medications of similar type in the past. It is imperative that there are additional considerations given to the prescription of medications if the patient is neuroleptic naïve. Whether the patient has been able to consent to a physical examination and an ECG are also important factors to consider when prescribing.

Additionally, the clinical team will need to consider the potential impact of any illicit substance use on the patient and adjust the approach to managing disturbance accordingly. At the point of prescription, attention should be given to the possible interactions with other prescribed medications and an awareness of the total dose prescribed of each drug. The prescription chart itself may feature a medication such as a specific benzodiazepine in several locations on the same chart. This places greater emphasis on the clinician carrying out the administration of the medicine checking each location. RT and PRN medication prescriptions being separated adds to the increased number of locations for a valid prescription to be written.

Advanced Statements and Advanced Decisions

Prior to the administration of RT, the team will need to consider any advance statements or decisions recorded or made by the patient. Such statements/decisions need to be recorded in the clinical notes and should fit within the context of the patient's overall clinical care. The statement/decision should also clearly state what specific interventions the patient would refuse if their capacity is impaired at a future point (Department of Health, 2015). The advance statement/decision should be adhered to if deemed clinically appropriate to do so by the assessing clinical team. Should there be cogent reason to deviate from any advanced statement/decision, very clear documentation should be present and have followed multi-disciplinary team (MDT) review and analysis.

Covert Administration

Covert medication may also feature in the approach to RT, and the same principles with regards to decision-making for administration apply. Regarding covert medication, a clear protocol should be in place and defined within the organisation's Policy for Ordering, Prescribing and Administering of Medications (POPAM) document.

Reducing the Need for RT

By its nature, RT is a very intrusive approach and there should be strong emphasis on developing therapeutic relationships with the patient, individualised support plans and achieving a high level of understanding of the patient's circumstances. All steps possible should be taken to reduce conflict and disturbance, thus reducing the need for RT. The Restraint Reduction Network Training Standards (Ridley and Leitch, 2019) highlight the principles of this approach and the requirement for clinicians to be able to appraise the needs of patients and attempt to gain an understanding of their experiences. A specific care plan detailing the patient's preferences in terms of engagement and activity will be helpful, and the input from carers should also feature where this is possible (Duxbury et al., 2019).

The 'Safewards' model (Bowers, 2014) further supports the approaches to patient engagement and the creation of ward programmes focused on providing meaningful activity. The range of interventions within the 'Safewards' package also includes approaches to de-escalation, and each healthcare setting should have a fully developed training approach for staff which aims to deliver up-to-date practice designed to increase the skill base of clinicians who are likely to encounter patients in distress.

Ward activity programmes have been shown to decrease the need for restrictive practice, and therapeutic activity is directly associated with improved outcomes. This includes more structured activity such as the use of the gym and smaller activities such as ward coffee mornings and music groups. The focus on the patient's collaboration in the development and evaluation of their care plans has also displayed a positive effect in this area (RCP, 2021).

Cox et al. (2010) also note that intermittent psychiatric observations on wards are far more effective when combined with interventions such as therapeutic activity. This further supports the promotion of development of the therapeutic milieu as the first port of call in terms of reducing the need for RT interventions.

Reducing Distress When Administering RT

As previously discussed, the clinicians engaging with an agitated patient will be tasked with making the judgement of whether to administer RT. Given the intrusive nature of an IM injection, all efforts should be made to administer the medication via the least restrictive route and explore the potential for the patient to accept medication orally.

When engaging with the patient, the clinician with the best rapport with that individual could be considered to make the first approach and carefully explain the situation whilst offering the medication. There should be due consideration to the location at which this would be best carried out. For example, approaching a patient in a confined area may increase the patient's feelings of fear. In addition, immediate hazards in the surrounding area need to be considered. Potential hazards could include items that could be picked up quickly, no clear area enabling a rapid exit, other patients present in the vicinity and surroundings that make a physical intervention situation problematic (tight spaces, items on bed area,

etc.). For planned interventions, there will likely be increased potential to ensure that the area can be assessed in this way. If there is no time to plan the response, a member of the team can be deployed to focus on the safety of the area.

Following the reduction of prone restraint procedures in the United Kingdom, many providers have been able to demonstrate positive outcomes with decreased numbers of recorded prone restraint situations. Much of this improvement has been due to staff training and shifts away from the more traditional usage of the ventrogluteal injection site.

With regards to training as a whole, healthcare providers should have a clear approach and a focus on utilising any physical restraint procedure for the shortest amount of time possible and in the least restrictive way (Ridley and Leitch, 2019).

Restraint and Changing Culture

Terminology is complex and variable around restraint and restrictive practice. This area of acute care in mental health requires a careful balance of maintaining the patient's safety, the safety of those around them (including other patients and clinicians) and the patient's liberty and rights. This judicious balance obviously fluctuates depending on the severity and associated risks as a result of the patient's mental ill health in symbiosis with the environment (including clinicians, their experience and skills) in which they are cared for. It is in this context that RT can be considered a significant part of restraint (sometimes specified as chemical restraint) and therefore a form of restrictive practice.

Human Rights Legislation in Relation to RT

It is useful to begin thinking of how restraint in all forms impacts a patient's human rights. In the United Kingdom, the Equality and Human Rights Commission states that 'Restraint includes chemical, mechanical and physical forms of control, coercion and enforced isolation, which may also be called 'restrictive interventions' (Connolly et al., 2019).

Specifically, in terms of the European Convention on Human Rights, restraint relates to:

- Article 3: prohibition on torture, inhuman and degrading treatment
- Article 8: respect for autonomy, physical and psychological integrity

- Article 14: non-discrimination

The Commission (Equality and Human Rights Commission, 2019) further states that the principles for use of restraint are:

- 'Means of restraint and its duration must be necessary, and no more than necessary, to accomplish the aim'
- 'Requires consideration of whether there is a less intrusive measure that could reasonably achieve the aim'
- 'A fair balance has to be struck between the severity and consequences of the interference for the individual being restrained and the aim of the restraint'
- Restraint should be used 'as a last resort, where there is no viable alternative'

Further guidance is derived from the Mental Health Act Code of Practice which states how the primary mental health legislation (Department of Health, 2015) is put into action in European countries. The Code of Practice requires patients to have individualised care plans that operate at primary (which enhance patient quality of life and thus reduce the chance of behavioural disturbance), secondary (recognise early signs of impending behavioural disturbance to enable de-escalation) and tertiary levels (responses for staff when there is behavioural disturbance) (Department of Health, 2015).

These human rights, principles and strategies frame the approach to choosing *when* to use medication and *which* medication to use, with factors such as time to maximum plasma concentration (Tmax) carefully considered. For example, if a patient has stated before that haloperidol works very well for them when they are distressed by symptoms of their psychotic illness and are at immediate risk to others, but that injections are especially unhelpful for them, an oral version of haloperidol may be the least intrusive or restrictive action. Using an oral medication is a more patient-centred approach and in accordance with the Code of Practice as well as the human rights frameworks discussed previously.

Beyond the individual patient in the Code of Practice is the guidance to create a systematic approach to reducing restrictive practice in the healthcare organisation. This involves:

- Demonstrating 'organisational commitment to restrictive intervention reduction at a senior level'
- Using 'data relating to restrictive interventions (to) inform service developments'
- 'Continuing professional development for staff'
- Ensuring 'models of service which are known to be effective in reducing restrictive interventions are embedded into care pathways'
- Enabling 'service users are engaged in service planning and evaluation and how lessons are learned following the use of restrictive interventions (Department of Health, 2015)

Thus, the Code of Practice provides a set of standards to guide healthcare organisations to ensure they are systematically reducing restrictive practice. Organisations such as the Restraint Reduction Network unite a wide range of healthcare organisations and government bodies in the England and the United Kingdom to provide resources and materials to ensure restrictive practice is minimised in all healthcare settings.

Furthermore, in the United Kingdom, the National Collaborating Centre for Mental Health (NCCMH), a collaboration between the Royal College of Psychiatrists and University College of London, brought a quality improvement approach to systematically reduce restrictive practice in a project that took place simultaneously in 38 mental health wards across England (RCP, 2021). One of the three key measurables was the use of RT (alongside seclusion and physical restraint).

This same programme then became a stream in the National Health Service's National Patient Safety Improvement Programme, specifically the Mental Health Safety Improvement Programme, as a way of delivering the NHS Patient Safety Strategy (NHS England, 2021). Here, the same systematic approach to reducing restrictive practice is being used nationwide with the stated aim of 'reducing the incidence of restrictive practice in inpatient mental health and learning disability services by 50%' over a period of three years (NHS England, 2021).

Medication Used in RT

Consensus on the most effective medications for RT is very difficult to reach given the paucity of large trials, the varying definitions of RT and the variety of settings. Categorising the types of medications used is similarly complex as this leads back to the latter two factors of definition and settings. Therefore, taking a route-based approach allows for easier discussion of combinations of medications, which is an important consideration. However, efficacy alone is not the full picture; the reliability of the availability of medication, the ease of preparation as well as the clarity for colleagues under considerable stress as what to use are also amongst many other important factors.

Oral RT

As discussed earlier in this chapter, it is credible and helpful to consider that RT can be administered orally, as it is the intention with which the medication is given to the patient that is defining, rather than the route of administration. The reasons for choosing oral or IM administration are complex and should be considered for each patient. Furthermore, trial data for oral RT is sparse compared to the evidence available for the same medications administered via the IM route.

Inhaled RT

Given the aforementioned definitions of RT, all routes must be considered. Loxapine, a dibenzoxazepine tricyclic antipsychotic that can be delivered in oral and IM forms, has recently become available via an inhalation device. Inhaled loxapine provides another route that has assurances that the dose has been given (due to the delivery device). Limited trial data demonstrates some efficacy compared to placebo, but performance compared other medications is not known (Lesem et al., 2011).

Intramuscular RT vs Oral Routes

The majority of RT is usually delivered via IM route. Whilst there appears a clear advantage for many of the medications used in RT with regards to Tmax of IM vs oral (see Table 18.2), this is not always reflected in trial data of antipsychotics. Currier and Medori (2006) highlight that small studies have shown oral risperidone to be as effective and with less side effects at two hours than IM haloperidol. Similarly, oral medication was shown to be preferred by patients (Currier and Medori, 2006), which is a paramount concern, especially when this impacts the clinician–patient relationship and thus ultimately the patient's ongoing quality of care.

Intramuscular RT

Benzodiazepines

Lorazepam IM is widely used given its relatively short half-life and modest Tmax of around 1–1.5 hours. However, this is similar to the oral equivalent Tmax

at two hours; multiple studies have shown that there is little difference after 30 minutes of administration of IM vs oral medication as a monotherapy (Patel et al., 2018). Lorazepam has the most trial data of the benzodiazepines as RT but has been found to be slower to act than combined medications such as haloperidol and promethazine and, in some studies, has been shown to be less effective than olanzapine IM (Patel et al., 2018).

Midazolam IM by contrast has a Tmax of only 30 minutes, therefore using Tmax as the only measurement, it would seem that midazolam is more suitable for RT. However, absorption via IM can be erratic raising the risk of oversedation (Parker, 2015). Thus, use should be limited to where there is very close physical health monitoring available as well as access to a reversing agent such as flumazenil, such as an in an emergency department.

Antipsychotics

Haloperidol IM has weak evidence for use as monotherapy as RT despite its extensive use. Although Ostinelli et al. (2017) identify 41 trials, the number of participants is few, and the majority do not relate to real-world practice. In two trials, haloperidol IM was shown to offer no more tranquillisation than lorazepam IM. Furthermore, acute dystonia was a common side effect, leading to more complications for patients who are often already very distressed.

Olanzapine IM offers a potential alternative to haloperidol with a lower risk of acute dystonia and prolonged QT with similar efficacy (Baldaçara et al., 2011). However, in addition to the variable availability of injectable olanzapine in some countries, a study has shown that 1% of those given it may require intubation due to its unpredictable level of sedation (Cole et al., 2017). Again, this potentially limits its use in stand-alone psychiatric units without advanced physical monitoring and easy access to resuscitation facilities.

Aripiprazole IM could be viewed as offering a safer route for RT, however, there are much less studies than there are for haloperidol and they are of poor quality. Furthermore, olanzapine has been found to be superior in reducing agitation with aripiprazole compared to haloperidol, both producing similar numbers of side effects, whilst aripiprazole more likely needs a further dose (Ostinelli et al., 2018). Although the evidence is poor, the potential need to return for further doses of medication with a possible additional physical restraint for the patient is obviously distressing and detrimental to their overall care.

Droperidol IM is no longer available in some countries such as the United Kingdom due to risk of QT prolongation. However, Isbister et al. (2010) found it to be as effective as midazolam IM but needing less subsequent doses. In addition, their study found there was no increase in QT prolongation with droperidol compared to midazolam.

Levomepromazine IM has a Tmax of 30–90 minutes but with side effects of QT prolongation and hypotension. It is more well known for its use in terminal care (Patel et al., 2018). Evidence for use in RT is sparse, with small studies indicating that levomepromazine offered similar speed and efficacy but resulted in more side effects compared to olanzapine IM and haloperidol IM (Suzuki et al., 2013).

Combined IM Medications

Haloperidol and promethazine IM is a useful combination with evidence to suggest it is quick acting compared to lorazepam or haloperidol alone with a longer-lasting effect than olanzapine. One review highlights that this combination avoids the respiratory depression effects of midazolam and lorazepam, whilst the promethazine offers some protection against dystonia from the haloperidol (Huf et al., 2016). It should be noted there is little evidence for use of promethazine on its own as RT and that it has a similar Tmax (2-3 hours) whether given orally or via IM (Patel et al., 2018).

Haloperidol and lorazepam IM used together have little evidence to support them compared to monotherapy with either in contrast to haloperidol and promethazine; two studies with small numbers showed a little evidence that haloperidol and lorazepam IM were slightly more effective than haloperidol IM alone (Ostinelli et al., 2017).

Intravenous RT

In a psychiatric setting, the use of IV sedation without full resuscitation facilities including an anaesthetist and intensive care department is very risky. However, in emergency departments and more widely in physical health hospitals where the aforementioned clinicians and equipment are present, Table 18.2 illustrates the time taken for maximum absorption of the drugs utilised for RT.

Administration Considerations

Monitoring during Administration

Following the assessment of the surrounding area, there then needs to be due consideration given to the administration site should the patient be in a position where they are not able to accept oral medication. With the increased guidance pertaining to the avoidance of prone restraint, this position should only be used as a last resort. It is accepted, however, that responding to an unpredictable patient can lead to the potential for the patient to be contained in the prone position. With this in mind, it is important to note that practice should include a staff member assigned for the sole purpose of physical health monitoring throughout the scenario (Metherall et al., 2006). Regardless of the position of the patient during physical intervention, the allocated staff member should have access to a pulse oximeter and other equipment to monitor the physical health of the patient. The intervention should be ceased if the physical health of the patient is compromised, and the team involved will be guided by the staff member responding to physical observation of the patient.

Administration Site

Traditionally, physical intervention training in the United Kingdom had focused on securing the patient in the prone position and administering IM medications in the gluteus maximus muscle, but this approach has been changed based on the risk of positional asphyxia.

The access to the IM site is clearly an important consideration in the context of a physical intervention and, when an intervention is planned, every effort to ensure that the patient is restrained in the supine position should be made. The access to the quadricep muscle would then be presented and the patient can receive the medication in this area. The advantages of this include a significantly reduced risk of positional asphyxia, increased ability to communicate with the patient and the patient being able to communicate with staff whilst also being able to see those around them.

Administration and Clothing

Administering IM medication also presents challenges, such as the clothing a patient may be wearing,

Table 18.2 Tmax of medications commonly used in RT

Medication	Route	Formulation	Tmax
Aripiprazole	Oral	Tablet	3–5 hours
	Oral	Oro-dispersible	3–5 hours
	Oral	Liquid	3–5 hours
	IM	Injection	1 hour
Droperidol	Oral	Tablet	1–2 hours
	IM	Injection	< 30 minutes
	IV	Injection	Seconds/minutes
Haloperidol	Oral	Tablet	2–6 hours
	Oral	Liquid	2–6 hours
	IM	Injection	20–40 minutes
	IV	Injection	Seconds/minutes
Levomepromazine	Oral	Tablets	1–3 hours
	IM	Injection	30–90 minutes
Lorazepam	Oral	Tablets	2 hours
	IM	Injection	1–1.5 hours
	IV	Injection	Seconds/minutes
Midazolam	Buccal	Oro-mucosal solution	30 minutes
	IM	Injection	30 minutes
	IV	Injection	Seconds/minutes
Olanzapine	Oral	Tablet	5–8 hours
	Oral	Oro-dispersible	5–8 hours
	IM	Liquid	15–45 minutes
	IV	Injection	Seconds/minutes
Promethazine	Oral	Tablet	2–3 hours
	IM	Injection	2–3 hours
Risperidone	Oral	Tablet	1–2 hours
	Oral	Oro-dispersible	1–2 hours
	Oral	Liquid	1–2 hours

Adapted from Patel et al. 2018.

and many organisations now include training specific for administering IM medication into the quadricep muscle through clothing. Clearly, there should be thought about the potential for soiled clothing or other interference with the ability to safely deliver the medication into this area. Where there is potential for RT to be required, the clothing a patient may be wearing can be a very important factor in other ways, such as the potential for overheating and the potential to contribute to further distress levels for the patient when attempting to access an IM site.

A further factor when applying physical restraint with a patient for the purposes of safely administering RT is the likelihood of increasing the level of fear for the patient. This, in turn, can contribute to feelings of punishment or the possibility that historical abuse a patient may have been subjected to will resurface in terms of their expression of trauma during the scenario itself. Some medications can be administered into the deltoid muscle as well as both the ventrogluteal and quadriceps sites. The deltoid muscle can be a difficult one to secure in for the safe administration of the medication in a physical containment scenario, but the site can be a preferable one for the patient.

Side Effects of Medication

Considering the side effects of the medication used is of particular importance in RT. Some of the side effects are difficult to distinguish from the therapeutic benefit; however, there are three main areas that are of critical importance.

Respiratory Depression

Respiratory depression is characterised as slow (usually less than 10 breaths a minute) and ineffective breathing; however, a universal definition of this is very difficult to arrive at (Ko et al., 2003). Respiratory depression when taking benzodiazepines alone is rare: critically, when taken with alcohol, the risk of respiratory depression increases considerably (Kang and Ghassemzadeh, 2019). Similarly, when benzodiazepines are combined with other medications, such as haloperidol, the risk of respiratory depression again increases.

It is important to note that slow and ineffective breathing may represent other diagnoses including alcohol toxicity, hypoglycaemia, hypo- or hypernatremia, opiate toxicity or a stroke (Ko et al., 2003). Exclusion of these differential diagnoses is essential, but of course should not delay lifesaving treatment. The reversal of benzodiazepine can be achieved with flumazenil.

However, flumazenil is contraindicated in patients taking long-term benzodiazepines for epilepsy. Furthermore, the British National Formulary advises that flumazenil is administered in intensive care or during anaesthesia 'by, or under the direct supervision of, personnel experienced in its use' (Joint Formulary Committee, 2021). This obviously creates difficulties for most mental health hospitals where access to such specialists is likely limited. Therefore, it may be safest to assume that if the patient is presenting with respiratory depression, they will likely require transfer to an acute physical health hospital for closer monitoring and specialist intervention.

Neuroleptic Malignant Syndrome

Neuroleptic malignant syndrome (NMS) is characterised by 'rigidity, tremor, fever, dysregulated sympathetic nervous system hyperactivity, alterations of mental status, leukocytosis, and creatine kinase (CK) elevation' (Murri et al., 2015).

Although NMS can be difficult to predict and surprises even experienced clinicians, there are risk factors (see Table 18.3).

It is important to note the risk factors pertinent to RT that may increase the probability of NMS in these circumstances. These risks are to be balanced against the risk the patient poses to themselves or others.

All antipsychotics can cause NMS, although second-generation antipsychotics are less likely to lead to NMS with them also being more likely to present with atypical features (Murri et al., 2015) Therefore, another focus of RT is the use of well-known, first-generation antipsychotics that may confer additional risk of NMS.

Serotonin Syndrome

Serotonin syndrome (SS) is a 'triad of altered mental status, autonomic hyperactivity and neuromuscular abnormalities' (Francescangeli et al., 2019) which may include symptoms such as agitation, hallucinations, hyperthermia, tachycardia and muscle twitching (Racz et al., 2018). Not all the triad will be detectable for all patients.

Differentiating SS from NMS is not easy clinically, but as shown in Table 18.4, the speed of onset as well as the contrast of neuromuscular hyperactivity in SS vs neuromuscular hypoactivity in NMS is significant.

Causative agents include selective serotonin reuptake inhibitors (SSRIs), monoamine oxidase inhibitors (MAOIs), opioid analgesics, antiemetics and illicit drugs (such as ecstasy) (Francescangeli et al., 2019). However, more recent research indicates that second-generation antipsychotics may also be implicated in SS, especially when combined with the more well-known agents highlighted earlier (Racz et al., 2018).

This information needs to be held in mind when assessing patients following administration of

Table 18.3 Risk factors for NMS

Category	Variable
Pharmacological	Starting, stopping and changing dose of antipsychotics *High doses of antipsychotics* *Administration via the IM or IV route* *Polypharmacy, especially multiple antipsychotics* Co-prescribing with antidepressants, anticholinergics mood stabilisers and antiparkinsonian medications
Environmental	*Physical restraint* *Dehydration* *High temperature*
Demographics (Oruch et al., 2017)	Age 40+ years Males more than females (2:1) Comorbidities such as Lewy Body Dementia
Genetic and patient history	Previous NMS Family history of catatonia Muscle channelopathy (e.g. myotonic dystrophy)

Table adapted from Tse et al. 2015 with additions from Oruch et al. 2017 antipsychotics in RT, as it may be difficult to know for certain the other potential causes of SS the patient has ingested as well as to differentiate SS from NMS in the context of a likely complex presenting situation.

Intended Side Effects

The aim of RT is to reduce the immediate risk the patient poses to themselves or others. The sedative nature of medications used may therefore be useful under careful monitoring. Proportionate sedation may do this in the short term; however, it is crucial to recognise that this is separate from effective treatment for the underlying causative mental health presentation.

Extrapyramidal Side Effects

The most likely extrapyramidal side effect given the timescale is dystonia (Taylor et al., 2021). Dystonia can occur within hours of starting an antipsychotic or, indeed, minutes if delivered via IM or IV routes, especially pertinent in RT. Treatment consists mainly of anticholinergic drugs with a different route applicable depending on severity.

There is also the risk of acute akathisia developing following RT, although this would likely be from higher doses, which can occur within hours following administration (Taylor et al., 2021). The sensation akathisia produces of inner tension, restlessness and discomfort is very distressing for patients. First-line treatment includes changing the antipsychotic to one that is likely to cause less akathisia (e.g. quetiapine/olanzapine), reducing the dose or switching to monotherapy. Pharmacological treatment with propranolol amongst other medications are second-line options, but evidence is modest.

Considerations Following Administration of RT

A national survey reviewing 58 mental health trusts across England revealed less than a third of them could provide any evidence of an audit of post-RT administration physical health monitoring (Loynes et al., 2013). A further survey of an adult inpatient setting over a year showed that only 8.8% of patients had any physical observations recorded, with only one case completed fully as per protocol (Talukdar et al., 2016). The revelation that physical health observations and investigations are not

Table 18.4 Serotonin syndrome and neuroleptic malignant syndrome

Syndrome	Causative agent	Onset and resolution	Physical observations	Pupils	Mental state	Other clinical features
Serotonin syndrome	Serotonergic drugs	Sudden < 24 h Most resolve with 24 h of treatment (though 25% develop symptoms after > 24 h)	Hyperthermia (> 41.1°C), tachycardia, hypertension and tachypnoea	Mydriasis (dilation of the pupil)	Delirium, agitation and coma	Neuromuscular hyperactivity (tremor, myoclonus, hyperreflexia and clonus), diaphoresis and hyperactive bowel sounds
Neuroleptic malignant syndrome	Dopamine antagonists and dopamine withdrawal	Slower onset (days to weeks) Up to 10 days to resolve with treatment	Hyperthermia (> 41.1°C), tachycardia, hypertension and tachypnoea	Normal or mydriasis	Delirium, agitation	Neuromuscular hypoactivity ('lead-pipe' rigidity and bradykinesia) Hypoactive bowel sounds

Table adapted from Scotton et al. 2019

performed consistently coupled with poor compliance to guidance highlights an area of concern, given this is an essential aspect following this high-risk clinical procedure. This section of the chapter provides guidance on various aspects to consider post-RT administration.

General Considerations

RT is an invasive procedure that compromises the patient's autonomy and therefore it is paramount to provide high-quality clinical care not only before and during RT but also after giving it. We must be particularly mindful of the ongoing patient–clinician relationship which will need to be rebuilt following this procedure.

Physical Monitoring

After administration of RT, it is necessary to carefully monitor the patients' physical health due to potential complications arising from RT and/or physical interventions such as restraint. IM medications used in RT have the potential to cause serious physical side effects.

Physical observations include the patient's level of consciousness, respiratory rate, heart rate, oxygen saturation without additional oxygen, blood pressure, temperature and hydration status. The minimum level recommended by NICE is at least one recording each of blood pressure, pulse, respiratory rate and temperature within an hour following RT administration (NICE, 2015).

A recent study in the United Kingdom across 66 mental health services showed that in four out of five RT episodes, physical health monitoring following RT did not reach the minimum recommended level recommended by NICE (Paton et al., 2019). These finding suggest that there was a lack of targeting patients at risk of developing abnormal physical health parameters post RT.

If there has been a restraint as part of RT, the patient will need to be reviewed by both nursing and medical colleagues.

Physical monitoring protocols should include how often physical observations should be recorded, the parameters being measured and the different outcome pathways. It is reasonable to stop monitoring if normal parameters are recorded consistently for four hours. If abnormal parameters are recorded within the stipulated timeframe, then a medical

review should be requested. The frequency of physical monitoring should be adjusted according to the patient's physical state, for example, if a patient is sedated or unarousable it would follow that monitoring would be more frequent with a medical review being called and emergency procedures activated as appropriate.

The study by Paton et al. (2019) highlighted the varying distinct processes and training for guidelines relating to post-RT physical health monitoring, protocols for detecting the deteriorating patient and clinical systems to record nursing observations. This highlighted a case for streamlining these protocols and systems to improve care planning for individual patients.

Non-Contact Observations

It may be the case that it is difficult to get a full set of physical observations, including respiratory rate, heart rate, oxygen saturation levels, blood pressure, temperature and level of consciousness following administration of RT. Reasons for this include:

1. The patient remains in a state of high arousal posing an increased risk of assault to staff
2. Approaching the patient may antagonise the situation
3. The patient is resting/sleeping after a prolonged period without rest

In these cases, it is acceptable to complete non-contact observations, as these still provide useful information about the patient's physical response to RT.

Of note, a respiratory rate can still be calculated without touching or being too close to the patient and this, in many ways, is one of the most useful indicators of potential physical health deterioration given the first-line medications used for RT can cause respiratory depression.

Technology has evolved and Oxehealth has created Oxevision health monitors to enable clinicians to detect patient activity, heart rate and breathing rate through video on demand. This information is useful to guide the decision-making process regarding the need for further immediate assessment (Oxehealth, 2021).

The rationale and reason for not completing a full set of physical observations should be clearly documented. It is important to have a policy safeguarding the use of non-contact observations to ensure clinicians are informed and educated about the alternative practices they can adopt when a full set of observations is not possible.

Debriefing

Given the significance of RT, it is imperative to have a debrief to consider the event and the patient's experience of it. Debriefing can be done on an informal or formal basis. This process should ideally include the patient involved in RT, other patients who witnessed the incident/RT as well as all the staff members involved. The success of this process can underpin the rebuilding of the clinician–patient relationship following RT.

RT Audit and Practice Development

Given RT is a traumatic and potentially dangerous procedure undertaken for patients when they are very unwell and vulnerable, it is essential that healthcare organisations deliver RT in a safe and dignified way. This should be manifested in a comprehensive and regularly reviewed policy for RT. Similarly, repeated auditing and systemic quality improvement is required to maintain and improve the highest standards in the field of RT. Furthermore, effective mandatory training should be designed, delivered and received by an MDT, including discussions or simulations of anonymised clinical scenarios to foster learning from experience. Throughout each of these preceding elements, it is important to involve patients, as co-production will render the highest quality of care.

Conclusion

RT is a procedure that is carried out as a last resort following the consideration of all other alternatives. It is the responsibility of the MDT to ensure that they are equipped with the necessary skills to carry out effective de-escalation of patients in distress which minimises the need to use RT. In addition, interventions carried out in response to a patient's distress should always be proportionate to the situation a clinician is presented with.

Invariably, it is difficult to predict the nature of each and every potential scenario and thus the decision to administer RT should be the outcome of a multi-disciplinary discussion done in a safe, collaborative way to ensure the safety of both the patients and clinicians involved. The key to this is to ensure open channels of communication and discussion between the MDT present before, during and after RT. It is vital to consider the individual needs, risks, and presentation of each patient as well as the changeability of these factors over time, including a reflection of their preferences in the process when possible.

Clear, accurate and comprehensive documentation of all the discussions from before RT is administered to what happened during and following RT is required. This provides information and an explanation to everyone caring for the patient as to why the actions taken were necessary, thereby protecting both patients and clinicians.

Receiving RT is only a short period in a patient's overall care, but nonetheless it is a procedure that has lasting effects, including potentially traumatic memories for all involved. Therefore, debriefing of patients and colleagues as well as continuous improvement in the training, systems, policy and delivery of RT in all healthcare organisations is paramount.

References

Allison,L and Moncrieff,J (2014) 'Rapid Tranquillisation': An Historical Perspective on Its Emergence in the Context of the Development of Antipsychotic Medications. *History of Psychiatry* 25 (1) 57–69.

Baldaçara,L, Sanches,M, Cordeiro,DC and Jackoswski,AP (2011) Rapid Tranquilization for Agitated Patients in Emergency Psychiatric Rooms: A Randomized Trial of Olanzapine, Ziprasidone, Haloperidol Plus Promethazine, Haloperidol Plus Midazolam, and Haloperidol Alone. *Brazil Journal of Psychiatry* 33 (1) 30–9.

Beveridge,A (2014) The History of Psychiatry: Personal Reflections. *Journal of Royal College of Physicians Edinburgh* 44 (1) 78–84.

Bowers,L (2014) Safewards: A New Model of Conflict and Containment on Psychiatric Ward. *Journal of Psychiatric and Mental Health Nursing* 21 (6) 99–508.

Braslow,J (1997) Mental Ills and Bodily Cures: Psychiatric Treatment in the First Half of the Twentieth Century. Berkeley and Los Angeles: University of California Press.

Burton,N (2010) A Brief History of Psychiatry. In Burton,N (ed.), *Psychiatry*, 2nd ed. Chichester: Blackwell Publishing. pp. 3–10.

Cameron,RWD (1883) The Philosophy of Restraint in the Management and Treatment of the Insane. *Journal of Mental Science* 28 (124) 519–31.

Cole,J, Moore,JC, Dolan,BJ, O'Brien-Lambert,A, Fryza,BJ, Miner,JR, et al. (2017) A Prospective Observational Study of

Patients Receiving Intravenous and Intramuscular Olanzapine in the Emergency Department. *Annals of Emergency Medicine* **69** (3) 327–36.

Connolly,G, Evans,T, Leitch,S, MacDonald,A and Ridley,J (2019) Reducing Restrictive Interventions in People with 'Challenging' Behaviors. *Nursing Times* **115** (12) 42–6.

Cox,A, Hayter,M and Ruane,J (2010) Alternative Approaches to 'Enhanced Observations' in Acute Inpatient Mental Health Care. *Journal of Psychiatric and Mental Health Nursing* **17** (2) 162–71.

Currier,GW (2003) The Controversy over 'Chemical Restraint' in Acute Care Psychiatry. *Journal of Psychiatric Practice* **9** (1) 59–70.

Currier,G and Medori,R (2006) Orally Versus Intramuscularly Administered Antipsychotic Drugs in Psychiatric Emergencies. *Journal of Psychiatric Practice* **12** (1) 30–40.

Department of Health (2015) *Code of Practice: Mental Health Act 1983*. London: TSO. https://assets.publishing.service.gov.uk/government/uploads/system/uploads/attachment_data/file/435512/MHA_Code_of_Practice.PDF.

Duxbury,J, Baker,J, Downe,S, Jones,F, Greenwood,P, Thygesen,H, et al. (2019) Minimising the Use of Physical Restraint in Acute Mental Health Services: The Outcome of a Restraint Reduction Programme ('REsTRAIN YOURSELF'). *International Journal of Nursing Studies* **95**: 40–8.

Equality and Human Rights Commission (2019) *Human Rights Framework for Restraint: Principles for the Lawful Use of Physical, Chemical, Mechanical and Coercive Restrictive Interventions*.

Francescangeli,J, Karamchandani,K, Powell,M and Bonavia,A (2019) The Serotonin Syndrome: From Molecular Mechanisms to Clinical Practice. *International Journal of Molecular Sciences* **20** (9) 2288.

Huf,G, Alexander,J, Gandhi,P and Allen,MH (2016) Haloperidol Plus Promethazine for Psychosis-Induced Aggression. *Cochrane Database of Systematic Reviews* **11** (11) CD005146.

Isbister,GK, Calver,LA, Page,CB, Stokes,B, Bruant,JL and Downes,MA (2010) Randomized Controlled Trial of Intramuscular Droperidol Versus Midazolam for Violence and Acute Behavioral Disturbance: The DORM Study. *Annals of Emergency Medicine* **56** (4) 392–401.

Joint Formulary Committee (2021) 'Flumazenil', in *British National Formulary*. www.bnf.nice.org.uk/drugs/flumazenil/.

Kang,M and Ghassemzadeh,S (2019) *Benzodiazepine Toxicity*. Treasure Island (FL): StatPearls Publishing.

Ko,S, Goldstein,DH and VanDenKerkhof,EG (2003) Definitions of 'Respiratory Depression' with Intrathecal Morphine Postoperative Analgesia: A Review of the Literature. *Canadian Journal of Anaesthesia* **50** (7) 679–88.

Lesem,MD, Tran-Johnson,TK, Riesenberg,RA, Feifel,D, Allen,MH, Fishman,R, et al. (2011) Rapid Acute Treatment of Agitation in Individuals with Schizophrenia: Multicentre, Randomised, Placebo-Controlled Study of Inhaled Loxapine. *British Journal of Psychiatry* **198** (1) 51–8.

Loynes,B, Innes,J and Dye,S (2013) Assessment of Physical Monitoring Following Rapid Tranquillisation: A National Survey. *Journal of Psychiatric Intensive Care* **9** (2) 85–90.

Metherall,A, Worthington,R and Keyte,A (2006) Twenty-Four-Hour Medical Emergency Response Teams in a Mental Health In-Patient Facility: New Approaches for Safer Restraint. *Journal of Psychiatric Intensive Care* **2** (1) 21–9.

Murri,M, Guaglianone,A, Bugliani,M, Calcagno,P, Respino, M, Serafini,G, et al. (2015) Second-Generation Antipsychotics and Neuroleptic Malignant Syndrome: Systematic Review and Case Report Analysis. *Drugs in R&D* **15** (1) 45–62.

National Institute of Health and Care Excellence (NICE) (2015) *Violence & Aggression: Short-Term Management in Mental Health, Health, and Community Settings*. London: NICE.

Negroni,AA (2017) On the Concept of Restraint in Psychiatry. *European Journal of Psychiatry* **31** (3) 99–104.

NHS England (2021) The National Patient Safety Improvement Programmes. www.england.nhs.uk/patient-safety/patient-safety-improvement-programmes/#MHSIP.

Oruch,R, Pryme,IF, Engelson,BA and Lund,A (2017) Neuroleptic Malignant Syndrome: An Easily Overlooked Neurologic Emergency. *Neuropsychiatric Disease and Treatment* **13**: 161–75.

Ostinelli,EG, Brooke-Powney,MJ, Xue,L and Adams,CE (2017) Haloperidol for Psychosis-Induced Aggression or Agitation (Rapid Tranquillisation). *Cochrane Database of Systematic Reviews* **7** (7) CD009377.

Ostinelli,E, Jajawi,S, Spyridi,S, Sayal,K and Jayaram,MB (2018) Aripiprazole (Intramuscular) for Psychosis-Induced Aggression or Agitation (Rapid Tranquillisation). *Cochrane Database of Systematic Reviews* **1** (1) CD008074.

Oxehealth (2021) How Does Oxevision Work? (online) www.oxehealth.com/oxevision.

Patel,M, Sethi,FN, Barnes,TRE, Dix,R, Dractu,L, Fox,B, et al. (2018) Joint BAP NAPICU Evidence-Based Consensus Guidelines for the Clinical Management of Acute Disturbance: De-Escalation and Rapid Tranquillisation. *Journal of Psychopharmacology* **32** (6) 601–40.

Paton,C, Adams,CE, Dye,S, Delgado,O, Okocha,C and Barnes,TRE (2019) Physical Health Monitoring After Rapid Tranquillisation: Clinical Practice in UK Mental Health Services. *Therapeutic Advances in Psychopharmacology* **9**: 1–12.

Parker,C (2015) Midazolam for Rapid Tranquillisation: Its Place in Practice. *Journal of Psychiatric Intensive Care* **11** (1) 66–72.

Racz,R, Soldatos,TG, Jackson,D and Burkart,K (2018) Association Between Serotonin Syndrome and Second-Generation Antipsychotics via Pharmacological Target-Adverse Event Analysis. *Clinical and Translational Science* **11** (3) 322–9.

Ridley,J and Leitch,S (2019) *Restraint Reduction Network (RRN) Training Standards*. Birmingham: BILD Publications.

Royal College of Psychiatrists (RCP) (2021) Reducing Restrictive Practice Collaborative. www.rcpsych.ac.uk/improving-care/nccmh/reducing-restrictive-practice.

Savage,GH (1887) The Use of Sedatives in Insanity. *The Practitioner: A Journal of Therapeutics and Public Health* **XXXVIII.**, 32-36.

Scotton,WJ, Hill,LJ, Williams,AC and Barnes,NM (2019) Serotonin Syndrome: Pathophysiology, Clinical Features, Management, and Potential Future Directions. *International Journal of Tryptophan Research* **12**: 1–14.

Suzuki,H, Gen,K and Takahashi,Y (2013) A Naturalistic Comparison of the Efficacy and Safety of Intramuscular Olanzapine and Intramuscular Haloperidol in Agitated Elderly Patients with Schizophrenia. *Therapeutic Advances in Psychopharmacology* **3** (6) 314–21.

Talukdar,R, Ludlam,M, Pout,L and Lekka,NP (2016) Ensuring Patient Safety: Physical Health Monitoring in Rapid Tranquillisation for Aggression and Violence of Adult Acute Inpatients. *European Psychiatry* **33**: S170–1.

Taylor,DM, Barnes,TRE and Young,AH (2021) *The Maudsley Prescribing Guidelines in Psychiatry* Chichester: John Wiley & Sons. pp. 109–16.

Tse,L, Barr,AM, Scarapicchia,V and Vila-Rodriguez,F (2015) Neuroleptic Malignant Syndrome: A Review from a Clinically Oriented Perspective. *Current Neuropharmacology* **13** (3) 395–406.

Chapter 19

The Use of Seclusion in Mental Health Care

Roland Dix and Mathew Page

Introduction

Whether or not seclusion has a place within the treatment of the mentally disordered is one of the longest running debates in the history of mental health care, and it is likely to continue. Controversial deaths in mental health facilities and their subsequent inquiries will further fuel speculation as to how best to manage challenging behaviour. The Independent Inquiry into the Death of David Bennett (Norfolk, Suffolk and Cambridgeshire Strategic Health Authority, 2003) questioned whether the use of seclusion may have been preferable to prolonged restraint.

The use of seclusion is at least 2,000 years old and many of the related questions have remained consistent, persisting to the modern day. It is not the intention of this chapter to re-describe the moral, ethical and legal paradigms that have punctuated much of seclusion's history. The focus here is to provide an overview of the history of seclusion, its value or otherwise, its alternatives and the necessary supporting policies for its use. Finally, we offer a practical framework within which seclusion may be considered in the context of psychiatric intensive care units (PICUs).

For the purpose of this chapter, seclusion is defined as 'supervised confinement and isolation of a patient, away from other patients, in an area from which the patient is prevented from leaving, where it is of immediate necessity for the purposes of containment of severe behavioural disturbance which is likely to cause harm to others.' (Mental Health Act Code of Practice (Department of Health, 2015, para 26.103)). For a person to be considered 'secluded' does not depend upon them being locked alone in a room. This introduces additional layers of complexity to an already difficult subject.

Seclusion is widely used throughout the world (Mason, 1994). Not surprisingly, different cultures have different attitudes and, as a result, different variations on the use of seclusion (Al-Maraira and Hayajneh, 2019). While it would be unwise to completely ignore experiences of other countries, the emphasis of this chapter is the use of seclusion in the United Kingdom.

No attempt to deal with the use of seclusion can be completely divorced from the simple question of whether seclusion should be used or not (Dix, 2019). To do so would deny the emotive nature of issues innate to the subject. Having recognised this, the authors do not offer a definitive view of whether PICUs and low secure units (LSUs) should have seclusion, but rather provide a balanced guide to thinking, informing the decision-making process for anyone planning or operating such a service. The arguments for and against the use of seclusion are apparent throughout the chapter.

History of Seclusion

It is difficult to define an era that marks the birth of seclusion in management of mental disorder. The ancient Greeks had rooms designed to entice the mentally ill patient to sleep so that they would 'dream their way back to sanity' (Wells, 1972).

One early account of attempts at isolation of someone in evident distress can be found in Christian scripture dating to the early part of the first century CE: three of the Gospels have accounts of a man isolated from his community. In the words of St Mark, 'he lived among the tombs; and no one could restrain him anymore, even with a chain; for he had often been restrained with shackles and chains, but the chains he wrenched apart, and the shackles he broke in pieces; and no one had the strength to subdue him'.

Even in ancient times, physicians of the Roman Empire, such as Soranus, advocated a compassionate attitude towards the insane. He suggested that sufferers should be, as far as possible, protected from fear, anger and, most interestingly, blame (Nolan, 1993). This epoch in history may not only mark the first recorded use of seclusion but also the beginning of one of the longest debates in mental health care.

During the Middle Ages and Renaissance, different religions attached their own meanings to the disordered mind. The extent to which severe methods of management featured, including the use of seclusion, varied considerably (Mora, 1967). The eighteenth and nineteenth centuries saw a shift towards the institutional model for housing of the insane and, with it, brought the use of seclusion that more closely resembles modern-day methods (i.e. for management of the most disturbed behaviour). During the 1790s, Philippe Pinel demonstrated that his asylum, the Bicêtre in Paris, could operate without profound reliance on use of seclusion and restraint (Renvoize, 1991). Pinel was confident that with the correct method of communication, paying attention to the inmates' individuality and self-respect, *few* restraints were necessary (Hunter and Macalpine, 1963). While it is apparent that Pinel had demonstrated the value of de-escalation, it is difficult to overlook the use of the term 'few' which clearly signals that physical confinement was still deemed unavoidable in some circumstances. In Britain, William Tuke, a layman superintendent of the Retreat asylum in York, also advocated a more humane approach based upon his Quaker 'moral therapy' philosophy. In 1892, an interesting debate about the use of seclusion between Tuke and another British pioneer, John Conolly, quoted Tuke as arguing:

> If Conolly attached too much importance to this mode of treatment (*seclusion*), the other extreme, of regarding the padded room as never useful, is a very questionable position to take.
> (Cited by Angold, 1989)

In Howe and Sethi's (2018) analysis of the Victorian approach, it is noted that locked door seclusion was originally introduced as a means of reducing dependence on mechanical restraint and therefore represented an improvement in least restrictive options for managing disturbance. It is difficult to avoid the feeling that in the twenty-first century this debate is no nearer to a conclusion.

The latter half of the nineteenth century marked increased attempts to more clearly legislate for the legal and conceptual underpinnings of mental health care. There emerged several consistent themes, often in conflict with each other, attempting to improve the experience of the patient while at the same time addressing the fears of society. A number of attempts were made to balance the determined efforts by the medical profession to claim the scientific high ground, with lawmakers who argued that mental health care was a legal rather than medical concern (Rogers and Pilgrim, 1996). While this situation produced various degrees of focus on humane treatment of the patient, by and large, the experience of the patient remained unchanged with continued and unregulated use of mechanical restraint and seclusion.

During the 1920s, there was growing concern about conditions in many psychiatric hospitals, for staff and patients alike. Staff were expected to work 14 hours a day with only half a day off per month. In September 1922, tensions reached such a pitch that staff and patients of the Nottinghamshire County mental hospital joined forces in fighting against police who were sent there to restore order (Nolan, 1993).

In 1923, an inquiry at Hull Asylum reported on the lack of privacy, dirty conditions, patients having to bath in the same water and, most worryingly, 'patients being confined in dungeons for long periods of time'. Conditions for all within many of the institutions during the early 1920s left little time or interest in singling out the use of seclusion for debate, amongst what appeared to be far more important concerns. In 1923, Dr Montagu Lomax published his book *Confessions of an Asylum Doctor*. This book was highly critical of the conditions in many institutions, the appalling arrogance and behaviour of many medical superintendents and the barbaric methods of treatment, including the use of seclusion. A storm of debate resulted from the book's publication. Even amidst determined attempts by medical superintendents to discredit Dr Lomax, the Royal Commission recommended wide-reaching improvements which included limiting patient seclusion to certain clearly defined circumstances. Patients also had to be carefully monitored whilst in seclusion (Nolan, 1993). This was possibly the first appearance of standard regulation on the use of seclusion.

The outbreak of war in 1939 preoccupied much of the 1940s. Mental hospitals, as far as it was possible, were emptied to accommodate the wounded. This also resulted in a renewed interest in the science of mental illness, in particular the use of electroconvulsive therapy for the treatment of shell shock and depression (Merskey, 1991). Another addition included introduction of psychotherapeutic techniques. Even with these innovations, the widespread and unregulated use of seclusion continued. This is chillingly illustrated by the personal accounts of nurses working in hospitals during the 1940s, collected by Nolan (1993). One nurse recalls:

> Patients were subjected to hours and hours of endless boredom in the airing courts . . . We counted patients in and out . . . In side rooms, there were patients locked up for weeks on end; the staff had become so used to the screaming of these patients that they totally ignored it.

The 1950s saw the introduction of chlorpromazine, hailed by many as a miracle cure for psychosis. Even though the true efficacy of chlorpromazine remained in debate, a new era had dawned with many hospitals opening their doors during the 1950s and 1960s. Many wards now had open-door policies with new freedoms given to many patients, although for a significant minority of patients locked wards and seclusion continued.

In the 1960s and 1970s, new ideologies emerged, sometimes based on a deep scepticism of the discipline of psychiatry but always associated with social justice and the rights of those accommodated in institutions for long periods. Inspired by individuals such as R.D. Laing, the movement began to prevail across Europe leading to significant policy changes by governments. The career of Franco Basaglia, an Italian psychiatrist credited with the paradigm shift that sees that country in general, and Trieste specifically, operating one of the most liberalised and de-institutionalised models is described in detail by Foot (2015)

In 1983, a new UK Mental Health Act (MHA) resulted in the publication of the first associated Code of Practice in 1993 which made a determined attempt to finally regulate the use of seclusion. Further revisions of the Code of Practice were published, including in 2015. Within the United Kingdom, the Care Quality Commission (CQC) was designed to improve quality in mental health facilities, including regulating seclusion usage. This did not prevent re-emergence of mental hospital brutality scandals that riddled the 1970s. Appalling abuse of residents with learning disability was documented by an undercover reporter at the Winterbourne View hospital in 2011 (BBC, 2011).

As was the case in previous mental health abuse scandals, it seems that regulators had failed where investigative journalism had succeeded (Rogers and Pilgrim, 1996). It took another nine years before the CQC published a report on restraint and seclusion entitled 'Out of sight who cares', which catalogued a range of concerns, including prolonged use of seclusion with dubious justification (Rees and Milnthorpe, 2010).

During the 1990s, several often-polarised arguments were advanced resulting, in some cases, abolition of seclusion altogether in many hospitals. As far as PICUs are concerned, Beer et al. (1997) in their survey found that of 110 PICUs in the United Kingdom, 40% had no seclusion room. Of those that did have seclusion, 15 units admitted to having no written policy on its use. Department of Health figures for 2004 confirmed that of PICUs and LSUs, 50% continue not to have seclusion. The most recent national survey of UK PICUs (Pereira et al., 2021) recorded that 86% of surveyed PICUs reported having access to seclusion.

The press has also recorded deaths of secluded patients. In the United States and much of Europe, the use of mechanical restraint and seclusion remains a routine procedure in many modern psychiatric hospitals (Hamolia, 1995; Al-Maraira and Hayajneh, 2019). Appelbaum (1999) reported on 142 deaths in American seclusion rooms between 1988 and 1998. The US House of Representatives introduced the Patient Freedom from Restraint Act (Appelbaum, 1999). In Britain, the famous and disturbing case of the death of Orville Blackwood in seclusion left the panel of inquiry concluding that a 'macho culture' existed around the use of seclusion in Broadmoor Special Hospital (Prins, 1994). The Independent Inquiry into the Death of David Bennett (Norfolk, Suffolk and Cambridgeshire Strategic Health Authority, 2003) also comments on seclusion, this time not as a situation to be avoided but as a possible safer alternative to prolonged restraint. This point has also been raised by other authors such as Paterson et al. (2003), and these views will be more closely examined later in the chapter.

Within the United Kingdom, the Royal College of Nursing reported more than 33,000 assaults against mental health staff in 2017 (RCN, 2018). This report, just one amongst many, confirms that violence and its management in mental health care remain at the top of the agenda. A snapshot survey of the professional press between 2016 and 2021 showed more than 200 papers containing the word 'seclusion' in three popular mental health databases.

Amidst often passionate and polarised arguments presented by supporters and opponents of seclusion, one thing is clear: seclusion continues to be used in many hospitals, and when staff are in the position of having to manage serious aggression, one is often reduced to few options. This point was succinctly made by Mason (1994) who concluded his international review of seclusion with the following comments:

> When the patient is no longer susceptible to the paradigms of treatment, when they are in the throes of assault, when they are combatant – there remain only four things one can do: seclude them, restrain them, medicate them, or pass the problem on to someone else (transfer them).

The remainder of this chapter illuminates a path through the maze of argument surrounding the modern-day use of seclusion, which will guide the thinking of PICU/LSU staff.

Factors Affecting Seclusion Rates

Opponents of seclusion present arguments for its abolition which are profound and diverse. Seclusion continues to hold a precarious position in modern psychiatric hospitals and its continued use is under close scrutiny (Department of Health, 2021).

Seclusion is intended for use when there are no safe, less restrictive alternatives and solely for management of severe behavioural disturbance which is likely to cause harm to others (Department of Health, 2015). There is good evidence that factors other than the severity of behavioural disturbance affect rates of seclusion.

Disturbed Behaviour

The decision to implement seclusion is a complicated process that takes place in a short time. An examination of literature over 30 years reveals alarming variations in the rationale offered for the use of seclusion. Tooke and Brown (1992) found that both staff and patients viewed destructive, aggressive behaviour but also inappropriate sexual behaviour as the main reasons for seclusion. A review of 10 studies undertaken by Soloff et al. (1985) concluded that seclusion was most frequently used to contain disruptive, agitated or excited behaviour. Also, it was the clear belief of the staff that much of the behaviour represented

a serious risk of escalation into actual violence. The conclusion of this extensive review was that early use of seclusion dramatically reduced the incidence of actual violence.

Morrison and Lehane (1996) concluded that physical assaults on staff were the single most common cause for seclusion, closely followed by threats to staff, self-inflicted injury, damage to property, disturbed behaviour, physical assault on patients, threats to patients and 'self-seclusion'. Threat of assault was also confirmed as a significant factor by Kuivalainen et al. (2017). Moreover, physical assaults on staff and patients only accounted for one-third of the total episodes of seclusion. Surprisingly, most episodes were precipitated by non-violent behaviours (Morrison and Lehane, 1996).

During a yearlong study of the use of seclusion and restraint use in 82 medical centres in the United States, the primary reason given for its use was disruptive behaviour disturbing the ward environment, not necessarily violent behaviour itself. Closely following in descending order were patient agitation, physical and verbal aggression (Betemps et al., 1993).

Bowers et al (2017) completed a comprehensive evaluation study of PICU and seclusion usage. They found the most common reason for seclusion was aggression (typically aggression to objects but also verbal aggression, self-directed aggression and physical aggression), followed by psychiatric symptoms (e.g. delusion, disorientated, confused or disturbed behaviour), disruptive behaviour, attempting to abscond and medication refusal.

Ward Characteristics

General ward characteristics and staffing levels have also proven to significantly impact the use of seclusion. Staffing levels in particular have been the focus of many studies which have consistently found a strong correlation between increased staffing levels and reduced incidence of seclusion (Outlaw and Lowery, 1992; Morrison, 1995; Yurtbasi et al., 2021). Craig et al. (1989) found that staffing levels, education and experience in dealing with disturbed behaviour made a significant impact on the use of seclusion.

Unit Culture and Staff Attitudes

The link between attitudes and general unit culture with uptake of seclusion has long been established. De Cangas (1993) found that staff viewed seclusion use to be more affected by unit factors than variations in their own attitude and performance. In contrast, De Cangas and Shopflocher (1989) recorded that nursing staff held a positive attitude towards seclusion, were open minded about its implementation and believed that it was an effective intervention. Steele (1993) surveyed staff attitudes in four hospitals and revealed that 80% of staff claimed to refuse to consider seclusion until verbal intervention had been attempted and had failed. Most staff viewed seclusion as a last resort which had some therapeutic benefit. Plaskey and Coakley (2001) did report a dramatic reduction in reliance on seclusion after a package of education and procedural changes were made. Doedens et al. (2020) showed that an education programme could change staff perception of disturbed behaviour, although it did not achieve statistical significance in reducing seclusion rates.

Gerlock and Solomons (1983) established a correlation between staff attitude, ward culture and frequency of seclusion. Tolerance levels towards disturbed behaviours, anxiety levels, the need to control behaviour because of low staffing and perceptions of the therapeutic benefits of seclusion were all found to be highly significant. It is of no surprise that some staff teams are more motivated towards proactive interventions that can de-escalate behaviours which would otherwise warrant seclusion. Positive attitudes towards seclusion as a therapeutic treatment and low motivation towards creative interventions will undoubtedly result in higher rates of seclusion.

Forster et al. (1999) found that introducing an interdisciplinary quality improvement workgroup and associated training around issues of prevention of aggression and promotion of least restrictive methods of management significantly reduced the incidence of seclusion. Elzubeir et al. (2017) showed that a multidisciplinary, collaborative formulation of seclusion-ending indicators had potential to reduce total episodes and time spent in seclusion.

Patient Characteristics

Correlations between seclusion and patient characteristics such as gender, age and race have been established. Soloff and Turner (1981) found an alarmingly disproportionate number of black patients were being secluded.

Cullen et al. (2016) found that secluded patients in PICU were also more likely to be younger and legally detained relative to non-secluded patients; however, female sex increased the odds of seclusion.

Within the United Kingdom, the institute for race relations (Byrne et al., 2020) assert that people from Black, Asian and minority ethnic (BAME) groups are more likely than White British people to be detained compulsorily under mental health legislation or put in seclusion (Gajwani et al., 2016). Further, it is reported that Black people detained under mental health legislation are 29% more likely to be forcibly restrained than White patients. They are also 50% more likely to be placed in seclusion and more likely to be diagnosed as psychotic.

Summary of Important Factors that Affect Use of Seclusion

Key points

- Justifying the use of seclusion purely on the grounds of managing high levels of violence is simply not supported by the evidence.
- There is indication that seclusion can be used to supplement staffing levels.
- Staff attitudes to seclusion are important.
- Adequate staff training in seclusion is needed.
- There is an apparent over-representation of non-White patients in seclusion statistics.

Does Seclusion Have a Place in Contemporary Psychiatric Practice?

The arguments for and against seclusion are complex. Many authors have advanced both evidence and argument to support their particular viewpoint. In order to promote clarity and provide a context within which to consider the evidence, it is helpful to categorise the debate under three main headings.

Morality: There are those who believe that the use of seclusion is morally wrong. Put simply, it is held that within modern practice the procedure of locking a patient alone in a room cannot in principle be justified.

Consequentialism: There are those that maintain a consequent approach to ethical reasoning: that the decision whether or not seclusion is used results from a direct appraisal of the potential consequences that arise for the patient and others (Morrison and Lehane, 1995).

In other words, when faced with extreme aggression the end justifies the means and that, in some cases, seclusion may be the least damaging option for the patient as well as others.

Treatment: Some commentators have maintained that seclusion is a useful treatment modality (Orr and Morgan, 1995). They do not, in the first instance, overly concern themselves with moral or ethical debate but rather maintain that the practice can produce positive effects in the mental and behavioural state of the patient.

The Moral Argument

Within the literature it is not difficult to find examples of powerful condemnation of seclusion. Some commentators have described the practice as an 'archaic, controversial form of tyranny' and 'an embarrassing reality' in the management of mental disorder (Pileete, 1978; Rosen and DiGiacomo, 1978; Soloff, 1979). The Royal College of Nursing has been quoted to regard seclusion as an anti-therapeutic intervention that will ultimately become redundant (Topping-Morris 1994).

Although these comments are generally representative of the views held by opponents of seclusion, they do not in themselves provide a solid foundation from which to debate. The consistent themes are that seclusion is a very distressing patient experience (Noris et al., 1992; Tooke et al., 1992; Meehan et al., 2000; Griffiths 2001), and that it is outdated and outmoded. These views are fuelled by evidence that patients can perceive seclusion as a form of torture (Chamberlin, 1985; Jensen, 1985).

In a systematic literature review (Chieze et al., 2019), there was good evidence that seclusion and restraint have 'deleterious physical or psychological consequences'. This was especially apparent for patients with past traumatic experiences. Interestingly, compared to other coercive measures (notably forced medication), seclusion seemed to be better accepted, thus having relevance to the consequentialist argument.

The moral arguments opposing seclusion seem largely based on significant evidence that, when available, seclusion will be implemented with dubious rationale, inconsistently used and that its frequency is related to many other variables not necessarily dependent upon degrees of violence. The basic core of the moral argument is that if seclusion as an available option, patients will be secluded inappropriately,

suffer extreme distress and staff will not be motivated to develop superior methods of dealing with violence (Dix, 2017). It is reasonable therefore not to have seclusion at all.

Alternatives to Seclusion

Beauchamp and Childress (2019) defined the application of consequentialism to an ethical debate as 'the right act in any circumstance is the one that produces the best overall result, as determined from an impersonal perspective that gives equal weight to the interests of each affected party'. It is not difficult to see the attraction of this theory for supporters of seclusion as a method for managing violence. Verbal de-escalation, restraint, medication and the use of increased observation in an extra care area (ECA) have all been proposed as alternatives to seclusion (Kingdon and Bakewell, 1988; Myers, 1990; Kinsella and Brosnan, 1993; Donat, 1998; Department of Health, 2002; NAPICU, 2014; NICE, 2015; Dix, 2017). All these alternatives are covered in detail elsewhere in this volume. So far as they directly compare to seclusion, we examine evidence for their effectiveness as a preferable alternative to seclusion.

Verbal De-escalation

The value of verbal de-escalation in preventing actual physical assault has long been accepted (Infantino and Mustingo, 1985; Turnbull et al., 1990; Stevenson, 1991). Newman et al. (2018) showed a 92% reduction in use of seclusion in the 6 months following introduction of a de-escalation training programme. Lavender and Shepherd (1999) showed that of 127 violent incidents, 50% could be managed with verbal interventions alone. They reported seclusion being used in only two of the total incidents. A clinical trial demonstrated a drop in use of seclusion by 50% after introduction of a model of de-escalation (Morales, 1995). Following a change in seclusion policy in a secure unit, Torpy and Hall found a highly significant reduction in seclusion rates. They suggested that staff had become considerably more skilled at alternative interventions, in particular verbal de-escalation.

In line with the experience of many mental health nurses, most if not all advocates of de-escalation accept that at best the technique can only dramatically reduce, rather than eradicate, physical violence.

Although seclusion has been advocated as a quick and effective method of preventing progression towards physical assault, it must be accepted that a determined attempt at verbal de-escalation is an obvious first as well as often a very effective intervention.

Physical Restraint

The introduction of control and restraint (C&R) training to a medium secure unit showed several benefits (Parks, 1996). Seclusion was only used in 12% of the total number of violent incidents. It was suggested that staff were subsequently in the position to hold a patient safely until either verbal de-escalation or medication could work. This was balanced however with an increase in injuries to staff in comparison to figures before the introduction of C&R.

Physical restraint as an alternative to seclusion can in itself be a very problematic intervention. Chieze et al. (2019) indicated that restraint seemed to be less tolerated than seclusion which may have been perceived as 'non-invasive' in comparison to restraint.

Betemps and Buncher (1992) showed that some patients spent up to 72.2 hours in a single episode of mechanical restraint in American hospitals. In the United Kingdom, prolonged restraint has been known to result in sudden death from asphyxia (Parkes, 2002; Paterson et al., 2003). Indeed, many of the deaths that occur while a patient is in the seclusion room have been correlated with a violent struggle immediately before the patient was secluded (Kumar, 1997).

It may be reasonable to suggest that 40 minutes spent in a seclusion room may be preferable and safer for both the patient and staff compared to the same length of time spent in physical restraint. The evidence or otherwise supporting seclusion as a safer alternative to prolonged restraint is an extremely important issue. Restraint is covered elsewhere in this volume and readers are encouraged to read Chapter 20 to complement their understanding of seclusion.

Rapid Tranquillisation

Rapid tranquillisation (RT) is covered in Chapter 18, so we shall only briefly touch on its relevance to seclusion. Patel et al. (2018) produced detailed and comprehensive guidance on the use of RT, including seclusion as a related intervention. It is noted that seclusion should be considered when other interventions have failed to manage the risks. The

appropriate use of medication has been proposed as a method of reducing, or even eradicating, use of seclusion (Klinge, 1994). Not surprisingly Pilowsky et al. (1992) showed that when given intravenously, RT had eradicated the need for seclusion. Intramuscular RT has also proved highly effective, with only a small minority of cases requiring restraint or seclusion following its use. It is beyond question that RT is largely effective in calming an agitated, angry and potentially assaultive patient. However, there remain circumstances where seclusion is also considered required, either at the same time or instead of RT.

The Extra Care Area (ECA)

The use of an ECA in which a single patient may receive intensive nursing intervention is advocated in the National Minimum Standards for Psychiatric Intensive Care in General Adult Services (NAPICU, 2014) as a possible alternative to seclusion, and has become a popular method of managing acute disturbance (Dix, 1996, 2017, 2019; Kinsella and Brosnan, 1993). The principles of the ECA appear to fulfil much of the function of seclusion by removing a patient who is liable to assault others from the general ward population. It also has the advantage of keeping staff in contact with the patient through the aggressive episode so that they can develop and utilise the enhanced skills necessary for dealing with disturbed behaviour. The use of graded observation in concert with the ECA was reported by Kingdon and Bakewell (1988) to have successfully completely replaced seclusion. They reported no increase in violent incidents or any cases of refused admission as a result of a new non-seclusion policy.

Again, this method is also not without its problems. Kinsella and Brosnan (1993) reported occurrence of patients receiving positive reinforcement towards disturbed behaviour as a result of the special attention they receive from prolonged use of the ECA. The ECA can also be difficult for staff. In terms of the numbers of staff needed, there is a danger of creating a ward within a ward.

Summary of Seclusion Alternatives and Their Consequences

To summarise the seclusion debate within the context of consequentialism, alternatives to seclusion should be carefully appraised in relation to problems they themselves may cause. It is very easy to maintain a no seclusion policy while at the same time failing to recognise the possibility of equally undesirable and sometimes dangerous consequences of alternative interventions. The basic position of this philosophy is that while all possible action should be taken to avoid the need for seclusion, there are rare circumstances in which it remains the least damaging intervention. Of particular importance is the need for a detailed analysis of the cases of sudden death that occur during prolonged restraint (Paterson and Leadbetter, 2004).

Key points

- Verbal de-escalation is valuable in reducing and managing the incidence of assaults, although it cannot eradicate them.
- Physical restraint is effective for the immediate management of assault. When used for extended periods, it can be potentially dangerous for the patient and arguably is not preferable to seclusion.
- RT is effective in the immediate management of disturbed behaviour. There can be difficult delays (unless administered intravenously) in achieving sedation. There is also the possibility of severe side effects.
- The ECA is effective in containing a patient liable to assault others. It can be very expensive in terms of time and resources. There is also a possibility of producing a secondary behavioural disturbance in order to maintain intensive contact with the staff.

The Treatment Argument

Several authors have produced evidence that seclusion can promote positive mental and behaviour change in the patient (Mason, 1993; Orr and Morgan, 1995). In short, they advance the argument that, more than just a method of emergency management, seclusion can be an effective treatment. Before we examine some of this evidence, we must clearly state that the concept of seclusion as a treatment is simply not acceptable within the UK MHA Code of Practice (Department of Health, 2015), where paragraph 26.106 states that:

It (seclusion) not be used as part of a treatment plan.

It is difficult to identify recent published evidence that seclusion is an effective treatment. Much of the literature that does promote seclusion as treatment in more than 20 years old.

In the United States, Khan et al. (1987) concluded that patients who were exposed to low stimulation, mechanical restraint and seclusion experienced a significant reduction in psychotic symptoms. Hamolia (1995) again argues that seclusion can be therapeutic as a result of the patient being contained, removed from the circumstance in which they responded aggressively and receiving reduced sensory input. It has been suggested that seclusion is a place where the patient can learn to exercise control over their impulses. Sixty percent of the staff surveyed by Steele (1993) felt that seclusion had therapeutic as well as emergency management value. In a minority of the sample group, some studies of patients' perception of seclusion have recorded positive comments in relation to the experience of being secluded (Norris and Kennedy, 1992). Feelings such as safety, reassurance from the regular observations and time to reflect in the quiet of the seclusion room were reported.

The major problem with demonstrating that seclusion has any treatment value is the overwhelming evidence that staff and patients perceive seclusion very differently. Staff tend to underestimate the negative experience of the patient while simultaneously overestimating the positive effects. In addition, it is difficult to organise a robust research program for the empirical comparison of non-secluded patients with secluded patients against which therapeutic value may be measured.

To conclude the treatment argument, it is beyond question that most patients perceive seclusion as a negative experience. Much of the evidence for positive effects can easily be questioned in terms of its scientific rigour (Whittington and Mason, 1995). In any event, in the United Kingdom at least, this modality of 'treatment' is as good as outlawed by the MHA Code of Practice (Department of Health, 2015).

Policy for the Use of Seclusion

Throughout this chapter it has become clear that there can be wide variation on the use of seclusion. While it may have to be accepted that the very nature of aggression and the use of seclusion in its management will always produce variation in practice, it is inexcusable to maintain the seclusion option without a clear, agreed and well-thought-through policy.

Principles of a Working Seclusion Policy

Within the United Kingdom the definition of seclusion was changed in 2015 to include those who have been separated from their peers; seclusion is no longer dependent upon being locked alone in a room (Department of Health, 2015).

In certain circumstances, this has resulted in use of an ECA meeting the requirements for monitoring of seclusion. There has, however, been significant confusion around the monitoring of seclusion, particularly for those patients who are engaged in the ECA in the company of staff. An ECA is defined as 'a quiet, low-stimulus space for patients experiencing high levels of arousal during periods of disturbed behaviour' (NAPICU, 2014).

Professionals, faced with the prospect of having to seclude a patient, need to be knowledgeable regarding the legal framework applicable. Furthermore, the policy should be informed by evidence offered in the literature. This necessity may produce a degree of discomfort because the policy will need to cater to some potentially sensitive issues. These include, for example, staff attitudes, staffing levels and perceptions of age and ethnicity.

Legal Position: Common Law

Mental health staff are often dependent upon the application of the MHA and Code of Practice to define the extent to which they can restrain or detain patients.

However, there are statutory and common law powers of restraint and detention which can be relied upon by mental health professionals in their everyday care of patients (Parsons, 2023).

In Black v Forsey 1987 SLT 681 (Parsons, 2023), Lord Griffiths viewed one authority as 'imposing temporary confinement on a lunatic who has run amok and is a manifest danger either to himself or others – a state of affairs as obvious to a layman as to a doctor'. Lord Keith outlined the authority to detain where someone was mentally ill and likely to harm self or others. This judgement may also extend to the use of seclusion.

The Criminal Law Act 1967 allows use of reasonable force to prevent a crime or to effect/assist a lawful arrest. The power could be relevant to informal and detained patients permitting the use of reasonable force either to restrain the patient or place them in seclusion in self-defence or the defence of others or property (Parsons, 2023). However, it does not apply where the patient is not deemed capable of committing a crime because of their mental state.

Mental Health Act 1983

Seclusion is not covered by the 1983 MHA itself, although there is comprehensive guidance in the MHA Code of Practice (Department of Health, 2015). The extent to which the Code's requirements must be followed were specifically tested in case law Munjaz v Mersey Care 2003. The ruling required staff to adhere to the Code and only depart from it when a cogent' reason to depart from it can be demonstrated (Seligman et al., 2006). However, as a statutory document, if the Code's principles are not adhered to, then this evidence could be used in legal proceedings. The Code of Practice clearly states that seclusion should be used for the shortest period of time possible, and that it must not be used as a punishment, a treatment, because of staff shortages or because of self-harm or suicide risk.

The sole aim of seclusion is 'to contain severely disturbed behaviour which is likely to cause harm to others'.

Within the Code of Practice (Department of Health, 2015) the definition of seclusion was revised to no longer require a patient to be locked alone in a room in order for them to be considered to have been secluded. The definition of seclusion required only that the patient be isolated away from other patients in an area from which they are prevented from leaving. This presented some difficulties in clearly understanding when seclusion has occurred and differentiating it from other restrictive interventions, for example, restraint. It may be helpful within the United Kingdom to consider a patient being locked alone in a room as 'traditional seclusion'. Other approaches that do not involve being locked alone in room, while requiring the same regulation as traditional seclusion, are significantly different in that the patient always remains in the company of staff.

NAPICU (2016) published a position statement clarifying the issue of seclusion for those who were not locked alone in a room. It is proposed that once any physical restraint and de-escalation had concluded and the staff had taken the decision that the risks were such that the patient must still be separated from others, then seclusion had occurred.

The Evidence and Policy-Making

The published evidence sends clear messages in a number of areas that must be heard by policy-makers. They include accounting for varying attitudes of staff, the need to monitor the effects of staffing levels and perceptions of age and ethnicity. In addition, accurate records of all patient behaviours and ward environmental factors that preceded seclusion must be kept and regularly reviewed. In terms of audit, the authors suggest the input of professionals divorced from the unit, for both an independent perspective and credibility of the monitoring process.

A robust seclusion policy will require the decision-maker to give a clear description of what actually happened. This could be assisted by using agreed upon measures, such as assault rating scales such as those proposed by Lanza and Campbell (1991). These requirements aim to prevent vague rationale being used to implement seclusion. Moreover, they help the staff to focus on what level of real threat they are dealing with, hopefully diminishing impulsive reactions while under stress.

It is also helpful for policy to require staff to describe what alternative interventions were attempted, again promoting the emphasis of avoiding seclusion. The numbers of staff on duty and the patient's age and ethnicity are also helpful for audit purposes.

Conclusion

PICUs have now become established as essential facilities for engaging patients who present higher degrees of risk and disturbance. By definition, the PICU will often be the facility that has responsibility for the most disturbed patients (Beer et al., 1997). Already, many of these units house the only seclusion room in the hospital. There may be a danger of complacency resulting from the notion that seclusion has been hidden away in corners of PICUs rather than in view of all patients and staff in every general adult ward.

There are PICUs that operate successfully without using traditional seclusion (Dix, 2019). There is debate as to the efficacy of alternatives such as the ECA. We have seen throughout this chapter that seclusion continues to be an enormously complex issue. To date, the polarised positions held by many commentators have not been helpful in progressing into this millennium with any more clarity than the last.

Several important questions remain regarding the use of seclusion in the future of mental health services:

- How does seclusion compare with the alternatives of restraint and medication in terms of safety, in particular for the patient?
- Once a person has been secluded, are serious risks being managed, or are we just delaying the risks until seclusion is discontinued?
- How does the experience of being secluded affect the patient staff relationship?

In recent years, it has become increasingly difficult to discredit the use of seclusion purely on the basis of moral discomfort. There remains the need for detailed and objective analysis of the risk factors contained within prolonged restraint. The argument that a period in 'traditional seclusion' could be safer for the patient than prolonged restraint appears consistent with logical reasoning.

Much of the published analysis is undertaken from an academic foundation which often leaves unanswered questions for staff who actually face violence on a daily basis. To break from this tradition, the authors will conclude with thoughts based on first-hand experience of dealing with aggression both with and without traditional seclusion.

The need for, or the desirability of, traditional seclusion must be informed by systematic analysis of the evidence supporting least risk to the patient and staff, comparing traditional seclusion with all its alternatives. It is interesting that recent years may have seen seclusion again being favoured. Note must be taken of the Beer et al. (1997) PICU survey showing 40% of PICUs without seclusion and 2017 figures showing only 13% of PICUs without seclusion (Pereira et al., 2021)

Within many PICUs the use of the ECA as a direct alternative to locking a person alone in a room has been successful to the extent that some PICUs no longer have seclusion rooms at all. The debate does not rest here, however. The evidence is overwhelming. If you have traditional seclusion, eventually you will use it, and not always for the most extreme situations.

References

Al-Maraira,O and Hayajneh,F (2019) Use of Restraint and Seclusion in Psychiatric Settings: A Literature Review. *Journal of Psychosocial Nursing and Mental Health Services* **57** (4) 32–9.

Angold,A (1989) Seclusion. *British Journal of Psychiatry* **154** (4) 437–44.

Appelbaum,P (1999) Seclusion and Restraint: Congress Reacts to Reports of Abuse. *Psychiatric Services* **50** (7) 881–5.

BBC (2011) BBC One – Panorama, Undercover Care: The Abuse Exposed. www.bbc.co.uk/programmes/b011pwt6.

Beauchamp,T and Childress,J (2019) Principles of Biomedical Ethics, 8th ed. Oxford: Oxford University Press.

Beer,D, Paton,P and Pereira,S (1997) Hot Beds of General Psychiatry: A National Survey of Psychiatric Intensive Care Units. *Psychiatric Bulletin* **21** (3) 42–4.

Betemps,E and Buncher,M (1992) Length of Time Spent in Seclusion and Restraint by Patients at 82 VA Medical Centres. *Hospital and Community Psychiatry* **43** (9) 912–16.

Betemps,E. Somoza,E and Buncher,C (1993) Hospital Characteristics and Staff Reasons Associated with Use of Seclusion and Restraint. *Hospital and Community Psychiatry* **44** (4) 367–71.

Bowers,LA, Cullen,A, Achilla,E, Baker,J, Khondoker,M, Koeser,L, et al. (2017) *Seclusion and Psychiatric Intensive Care Evaluation Study (SPICES): Combined Qualitative and Quantitative Approaches to the Uses and Outcomes of Coercive Practices in Mental Health Services.* Southampton (UK): Health Services and Delivery Research.

Byrne,B, Alexander,C, Khan,O, Nazro,J and Shankley,W (2020) *Ethnicity, Race and Inequality in the UK: State of the Nation.* Bristol: Policy Press.

Care Quality Commission (CQC) (2020) A Review of Restraint, Seclusion and Segregation for Autistic People, and People with a Learning Disability and/or Mental Health Condition. CQC–464–102020.

Chamberlin,J (1985) An Ex-Patient's Response to Soliday. *Journal of Nervous and Mental Disease* **173** (5) 288–9.

Chieze,M, Hurst,S, Kaiser,S and Sentissi,O (2019) Effects of Seclusion and Restraint in Adult Psychiatry: A Systematic Review. *Frontiers in Psychiatry* **16** (10) 491.

Craig,C and Hix,C (1989) Seclusion and Restraint: Decreasing the Discomfort. *Journal of Psychosocial Nursing and Mental Health Services* **27** (7) 16–19.

Cullen,E, Bowers,L, Khondoker,M, Pettit,S, Achilla,E, Koeser,L, et al. (2016) Factors Associated with Use of Psychiatric Intensive Care and Seclusion in Adult Inpatient Mental Health Services. *Epidemiology and Psychiatric Sciences* **27** (1) 51–61.

De Cangas,J (1995) Nursing Staff and Unit Characteristics: Do They Affect the Use of Seclusion? *Perspectives in Psychiatric Care* **29** (3) 15–22.

De Cangas,J and Shopflocher,D (1989) The Practice of Seclusion and Factors Affecting Its Use. In Lo,C-H (ed.), Proceedings of the Sigma Theta Tau International Research Congress. Advances in International Nursing Scholarship Taipei: Sigma Theta Tau, p. 83.

Department of Health (2002) *Mental Health Policy Implementation Guide: National Minimum Standards in Psychiatric Intensive Care Units (PICU) and Low Secure Environments.* London: DOH.

Department of Health (2005) Survey of Physical Environments in PICU and LSUs in England and Wales.

Department of Health (2015) *Mental Health Act 1983: Code of Practice.* London: Department of Health.

Department of Health (2021) *Mental Health Units (Use of Force) Act 2018: Statutory Guidance for NHS Organisations in England, and Police Forces in England and Wales.* London: Department of Health.

Dix,R (2017) Seclusion: What's in a Name? *Journal of Psychiatric Intensive Care* **13** (2) 57–9.

Dix,R (2019) Restrictive Interventions and Seclusion: Time for Another Look. *Journal of Psychiatric Intensive Care* **15** (1) 1–3.

Dix,R and Williams,K (1996) Psychiatric Intensive Care Units, a Design for Living. *Psychiatric Bulletin* **20** (9) 527–9.

Doedens,P, Vermeulen,J, Boyette,L, Latour,C and de Haan,L (2020) Influence of Nursing Staff Attitudes and Characteristics on the Use of Coercive Measures in Acute Mental Health Services: A Systematic Review. *Journal of Psychiatric and Mental health Nursing* **27** (4) 446–59.

Donat,D (1998) Impact of a Mandatory Behavioural Consultation on Seclusion/Restraint Utilisation in a Psychiatric Hospital. *Journal of Behaviour Therapy and Experimental Psychiatry* **29**: 13–19.

Elzubeir,K and Dye,S (2017) Can Amount and Duration of Seclusion Be Reduced in Psychiatric Intensive Care Units by Agreeing SMART Goals with Patients? *Journal of Psychiatric Intensive Care* **13** (2) 109–16(8).

Foot,J (2015) *The Man Who Closed the Asylums: Franco Basaglia and the Revolution in Mental Health Care.* London: Verso.

Forster,PL, Cavness,C and Phelps,MA (1999) Staff Training Decreases Use of Seclusion and Restraint in an Acute Psychiatric Hospital. *Archives of Psychiatric Nursing* **13** (5) 269–71.

Gajwani,R, Parsons,H, Birchwood,M and Singh,P (2016) Ethnicity and Detention: Are Black and Minority Ethnic (BME) Groups Disproportionately Detained Under the Mental Health Act 2007? *Social Psychiatry and Epidemiology* **51**: 703–11.

Gerlock,A and Solomons,H (1983) Factors Associated with the Seclusion of Psychiatric Patients. *Perspectives in Psychiatric Care* **1** (2) 46–53.

Griffiths,L (2001) Does Seclusion Have a Role to Play in Modern Mental Health Nursing? *British Journal of Nursing* **10** (10) 656661.

Hammill,K (1987) Seclusion: Inside Looking Out. *Nursing Times* **83** (5) 38–9.

Hamolia,C (1995) Managing Aggressive Behaviour. In Stuart,G and Sundeen,S (eds.), *Principles and Practice of Psychiatric Nursing*, 5th ed. St Louis: Mosby. pp. 719–41.

Howe,A and Sethi,F (2018) Seclusion: The Untold Legacy of the Non-Restraint Movement in the UK. *Journal of Psychiatric Intensive Care* 14 (1) 5–13.

Hunter,R and Macalpine,I (1963) *Three Hundred Years of Psychiatry 1535–1860: A History Presented in Selected English Texts*. London. Oxford University Press.

Infantino,J and Mustingo,S (1985) Assaults and Injuries Among Staff With and Without Training in Aggression Control Techniques. *Hospital and Community Psychiatry* 36: 1312–4.

Jensen,K (1985) Comments on Dr. Stanley M. Soliday's Comparison of Patient and Staff Attitudes Towards Seclusion. *Journal of Nervous and Mental Disease* 173 (5) 290–1.

Jones,R (2021) The Mental Health Act Manual, 24th ed. London: Sweet & Maxwell.

Khan,A, Cohen,S, Chiles,J, Stowell,M, Hyde,T and Robbins, M (1987) Therapeutic Role of a Psychiatric Intensive Care Unit in Acute Psychosis. *Comprehensive Psychiatry* 28 (3) 264–9.

Kingdon,D and Bakewell,E (1988) Aggressive Behaviour: Evaluation of a Non-seclusion policy of a District Service. *British Journal of Psychiatry* 15: 631–4.

Kinsella,C and Brosman,C (1993) An Alternative to Seclusion? *Nursing Times* 89 (18) 62–4.

Klinge,A (1994) Staff Opinions About Seclusion and Restraint at a State Forensic Hospital. *Hospital and Community Psychiatry* 45 (2) 138–41.

Kuivalainen,S, Vehviläinen-Julkunen,K, Louheranta,O, Putkonen,A, Repo-Tiihonen,E and Tiihonen,J (2017) De-Escalation Techniques Used and Reasons for Seclusion and Restraint in a Forensic Psychiatric Hospital. *International Journal of Mental Health Nursing* 26 (5) 513–24.

Kumar,A (1997) Sudden Unexplained Death in a Psychiatric Patient – A Case Report: The Role of the Phenothiazines and Physical Restraint. *Medicine, Science, and the Law* 37 (2) 170–5.

Lanza,M and Campbell,R (1991) Patient Assault: A Comparison of Reporting Measures. *Quality Assurance* 5: 60–8.

Lavender,T and Shepherd,M (1999) Putting Aggression into Context: An Investigation into Contextual Factors Influencing the Rate of Aggressive Incidents in a Psychiatric Hospital. *Journal of Mental Health* 8 (2) 159–70.

Lomax,M (1922) *The Experiences of an Asylum Doctor*. London: George Allen & Unwin.

Mason,T (1993) Seclusion Theory Reviewed: A Benevolent or Malevolent Intervention? *Journal of Medicine, Science and the Law* 33: 1–8.

Mason,T (1994) Seclusion: An International Comparison. *Medicine, Science and the Law* 34 (1) 54–60.

Meehan,T, Vermeer,C and Windsor,C (2000) Patients' Perceptions of Seclusion: A Qualitative Investigation. *Journal of Advanced Nursing* 31 (2) 370–7.

Merskey,H (1991) Shell-shock. In Berrios,G and Freeman,H (eds.), *150 Years of British Psychiatry, 1841–1991*. London: Gaskell. pp. 245–67.

Mora,G (1967) History of Psychiatry. In Freeman,AM and Kaplan,HI (eds.), *Comprehensive Text Book of Psychiatry*. Baltimore: Williams and Wilkins.

Morales,T (1995) Least Restrictive Measures. *Journal of Psychosocial Nursing and Mental Health Services* 33 (10) 42–3.

Morrison,P (1990) A Multi-Dimensional Scalogram Analysis of the Use of Seclusion in Acute Psychiatric Settings. *Journal of Advanced Nursing* 15: 59–66.

Morrison,P (1995) Research on the Effects of Staffing Levels on the Use of Seclusion. *Journal of Psychiatric Mental Health Nursing* 2 (6) 365–6.

Morrison,P and Lehane,M (1995) Staffing Levels and Seclusion Use. *Journal of Advanced Nursing* 55: 1193–202.

Morrison,P and Lehane,M (1996) A Study of the Official Records of Seclusion. *International Journal of Nursing Studies* 33 (2) 223–35.

Musto,DF (1999) A Historical Perspective. In Bloch,S, Chodoff,P and Green,S (eds.), *Psychiatric Ethics*, 3rd ed. New York: Oxford University Press. pp. 1–23.

Myers,S (1990) Seclusion: A Last Resort Measure. *Perspectives in Psychiatric Care* 26 (3) 24–8.

National Association of Psychiatric Intensive Care Units and Low Secure Units (NAPICU) (2016) *Position on the Monitoring, Regulation, and Recording of the Extra Care Area, Seclusion, and Long-Term Segregation Use in the Context of the Mental Health Act 1983: Code of Practice*. Glasgow: NAPICU.

National Association of Psychiatric Intensive Care Units and Low Secure Units (NAPICU) (2014) *National Minimum Standards for Psychiatric Intensive Care in General Adult Services*. Glasgow: NAPICU.

National Institute for Care and Health Excellence (NICE) (2015) *Violence and Aggression: Short-Term Management in Mental Health, Health, and Community Settings*. London: NICE.

National Institute for Mental Health in England (NIMHE) (2004) *Mental Health Policy Implementation Guide: Developing Positive Practice to Support the Safe and Therapeutic Management of Aggression and Violence in Mental Health Inpatient Settings*. London: NIMHE.

Newman,J, Paun,O and Fogg,L (2018) Effects of a Staff Training Intervention on Seclusion Rates on an Adult Inpatient Psychiatric Unit. *Journal of Psychosocial Nursing and Mental Health Services* 56 (6) 23–30.

Nolan,P (1989) Face Value. *Nursing Times* **85** (35) 62–5.

Nolan,P (1993) *A History of Mental Health Nursing.* London: Chapman Hall.

Norfolk, Suffolk and Cambridgeshire Strategic Health Authority (2003) *Independent Inquiry into the Death of David Bennett.* Cambridge: Norfolk, Suffolk and Cambridgeshire Strategic Authority.

Norris,M and Kennedy,W (1992) The View from Within: How Patients Perceive the Seclusion Process. *Journal of Psychosocial Nursing and Mental Health Services* **30** (3) 7–13.

Orr,M and Morgan,J (1995) The Medical Management of Violence. In Kidd,B and Stark,C (eds.), *Management of Violence and Aggression in Health Care.* London: Gaskell.

Outlaw,FH and Lowery,BJ (1992) Seclusion: The Nursing Dhallenge. *Journal of Psychiatric Nursing and Mental Health Services* **30** (4) 13–17.

Parkes,J (1996) Control and Restraint Training: A Study of Its Effectiveness in a Medium Secure Psychiatric Unit. *Journal of Forensic Psychiatry* **7** (3) 525–34.

Parkes,J (2002) A Review of the Literature on Positional Asphyxia as a Possible Cause of Sudden Death During Restraint. *British Journal of Forensic Practice* **4** (1) 24–30.

Patel,MX, Sethi,F, Barnes,N, Thomas,R, Dix,R, Luiz,D, et al. (2018) Joint BAP NAPICU Evidence-Based Consensus Guidelines for the Clinical Management of Acute Disturbance: De-Escalation and Rapid Tranquillisation. *Journal of Psychiatric Intensive Care* **14** (2) 89–132(44).

Paterson,B, Bradley,P, Stark,C, Saddler,D, Leadbetter,D and Allen,D (2003) Deaths Associated with Restraint Use in Health and Social Care in the UK: The Results of a Preliminary Study. *Journal of Psychiatric and Mental Health Nursing* **10**: 3–15.

Paterson,B and Leadbetter,D (2004) Learning the Right Lessons. *Journal of Mental Health Practice* **7** (7) 12–15.

Paterson,B, Leadbetter,D and McComish,A (1998) Restraint and Sudden Death from Asphyxia. *Nursing Times* **94** (44) 62–4.

Pereira,SM, Walker,L and Dye,S (2021) A National Survey of Psychiatric Intensive Care, Low Secure and Locked Rehabilitation Units. *Mental Health Practice.*

Pilette,PC (1978) The Tyranny of Seclusion: A Brief Essay. *Journal of Psychosocial Nursing and Mental Health Services* **16** (10) 19–21.

Pilowsky,LS, Ring,H, Shine,PJ, Battersby,M and Lader,M (1992) Rapid Tranquillisation. A Survey of Emergency Prescribing in a General Psychiatric Hospital. *British Journal of Psychiatry* **160**: 831–5.

Plasky,P and Coakley,C (2001) Reducing the Incidence of Restraint and Seclusion. In Dickey,B and Sederer,LI (eds.), *Improving Mental Health Care: Commitment to Quality.* Washington: American Psychiatric Association.

Plutchik,R, Karasu,T, Conte,H, Siegel,B and Jerrett,I. Toward a Rationale for the Seclusion Process. *Journal of Nervous and Mental Disease* 166 (8) 571–9.

Prins,H (1994) *Report of the Committee of Inquiry into the Death of Orville Blackwood and a Review of the Deaths of Two Other Afro-Caribbean Patients.* London: Special Hospital Service Authority.

Parsons,A (2023) Powers of Restraint. Weightmans. www.weightmans.com/insights/powers-of-restraint/.

CQC (2020) A review of restraint, seclusion and segregation for autistic people, and people with a learning disability and/or mental health condition. October: CQC-464-102020

Renvoize,E (1991) The Association of Medical Officers of Asylums and Hospitals for the Insane, the Medico-Psychological Association, and Their Presidents. In Berrios, G and Freeman,H (eds.), *150 years of British Psychiatry, 1841–1991.* London: Gaskell.

Rogers,A and Pilgrim,D (1996) *Mental Health Policy in Britain: A Critical Introduction.* London: Macmillan Press Ltd.

Rosen,H and DiGiacomo,JN (1978) The Role of Physical Restraint in the Treatment of Mental Illness. *Journal of Clinical Psychiatry* **39**: 228–32.

Royal College of Nursing (RCN) (2018) *Report on Violence and Aggression in the NHS: Estimating the Size and Impact of the Problem.* London: Royal College of Nursing.

Seligman,M and Feery,D (2006) Lord Steyn's Lament. *Journal of Psychiatric Intensive Care* **2** (2) 111–17.

Soliday,SM (1985) A Comparison of Patient and Staff Attitudes Towards Seclusion. *Journal of Mental and Nervous Disease* **173**: 282–6.

Soloff,PH (1979) Physical Restraining and the Non-Psychotic Patient: Clinical and Legal Perspectives. *Journal of Clinical Psychiatry* **40**: 302–5.

Soloff,P, Gutheil,T and Wexler,J (1985) Seclusion and Restraint in 1985: A Review and Update. *Hospital and Community Psychiatry* **36** (6) 652–7.

Soloff,P and Turner,M (1981) Patterns of Seclusion. *Journal of Nervous and Mental Disease* **169** (1) 37–44.

Steele,R (1993) Staff Attitudes Toward Seclusion and Restraint, Anything New? *Perspectives in Psychiatric Care* **29** (3) 23–8.

Stevenson,S (1991) Heading Off Violence with Verbal De-escalation. *Journal of Psychosocial Nursing and Mental Health Services* **29** (9) 6–10.

Swett,C (1994) Inpatient Seclusion: Description and Causes. *Bulletin of the American Academy of Psychiatry and the Law* **22** (3) 421–30.

Tooke,S and Brown,J (1992) Perceptions of Seclusion: Comparing patient and staff Reactions. *Journal of Psychosocial Nursing and Mental Health Services* **30** (8) 23–6.

Topping-Morris,B (1994) Seclusion: Examining the Nurse's Role. *Nursing Standard* **8** (49) 35–7.

Turnbull,J, Aitken,J and Black,L (1990) Turn it Around: Short-Term Management of Aggression and Anger. *Journal of Psychosocial Nursing and Mental Health Services* **28** (6) 6–10.

Wells,D (1972) The Use of Seclusion on a University Hospital Floor. *Archives of General Psychiatry* **26** (5) 410–13.

Whittington,R and Mason,T (1995) A New Look at Seclusion: Stress, Coping, and the Perception of Threat. *Journal of Forensic Psychiatry* **6** (2) 285–304.

Yurtbasi,M, Melvin,G, Pavlou,C and Gordon,G (2021) Nurse and Patient Factors: Predicting Seclusion in Adolescent Psychiatric Units. *Journal of Child and Adolescent Psychiatric Nursing* **34** (2) 112–19.

Chapter 20

The Practice of Restraint and Physical Intervention

Roland Dix

Introduction

Virtually all societies have found the need for containment and control of behaviour by physical means. It is difficult to imagine a world without prisons, police and the periodic need for society to impose its collective standard of behaviour on individuals.

While most people share a degree of comfort with the notion of physical intervention to maintain law and order, its use under the justification of mental health 'care' is deeply troubling to many, with some arguing it has no place at all (Davis, 2004). Within the United Kingdom, recent years have seen renewed, determined efforts to reduce the use of restraint in mental health (Ridley and Leitch, 2019).

The first words in any discussion about restraint must include the methods of avoiding the need for its use wherever possible.

De-escalation, negotiation, meaningful activity programmes and the development of trusting relationships have been covered in detail elsewhere in this volume. The reader is advised to consider these issues as an essential first step. The focus here is confined to the activity of restraint, assuming that due attention has already been paid to the methods of avoiding the need for its use.

Restraint and Physical Intervention: The Questions

In mental health care, the use of restraint, both mechanical and interpersonal, has a long and chequered history. In recent years, the use of restraint has come under increasing scrutiny. In the United Kingdom and the United States, death during restraint has been increasingly reported (Appelbaum, 1999; Paterson et al., 2003). The death of David Bennett during restraint in a medium secure unit (MSU) (Paterson and Leadbetter, 2004) intensified the debate.

The inquest into the death of Seni Lewis following restraint by 11 police officers in a mental health ward considered the restraint used to be excessive, unreasonable and disproportionate. The death of Seni, aged just 23 years, resulted in the Use of Force Act 2018 (Department of Health and Social Care, 2021).

Society has become increasingly sensitive to the behaviour of professionals, particularly in relation to how they may exercise restrictive intervention towards others. Add to this the increasing trend towards videorecording events (by professionals and others), it is becoming increasingly common for statuary authorities to be subject to scrutiny. For these reasons, the coming years are likely to see major developments in the regulation of the practice of restraint in the United Kingdom. Restraint or 'physical intervention' is now considered part of the wider concept of 'restrictive interventions' described in the Mental Health Act (MHA) Code of Practice (Department of Health, 2015). Within the United Kingdom, the proposed replacement of the MHA is likely to focus clearly on liberty and least restriction.

While there is determined effort to regulate and reduce the use of restraint, at the same time, violence toward healthcare staff has become a major health and safety concern. From a figure of 65,000 assaults per year, Beech and Bowyer (2004) reported three times as many assaults against staff in UK mental health and learning disability units as compared to general health care.

Within the United Kingdom, the Royal College of Nursing (RCN) reported more than 33,000 assaults against mental health staff in 2017 (RCN, 2018). The Nuffield trust reported that 90.6% of staff working in mental health trusts had experienced a violent act during 2020 (Nuffield Trust, 2021).

There is no better time than now for a detailed examination of the issues surrounding restraint in mental health care. Providers of inpatient mental health care in general, and leaders of psychiatric intensive care units (PICUs) in particular, should be concerned with the following questions:

- What is the history and theoretical underpinning for systemised restraint?
- What are the law and ethics related to restraint?
- What is the evidence for the efficacy of some of the methods commonly in use?
- What principles underpin best practice?
- How do patients and frontline practitioners ensure that their experience inform future developments?

In terms of the theory and practice of physical intervention, the remainder of this chapter offers practical advice for service leaders and practitioners within inpatient environments.

History of Mechanical Restraint

The use of physical restraint has been a consistent feature within the history of mental health care. Before the advent of antipsychotic medication in the early 1950s, forcible confinement of patients often represented the first-line approach to the management of disturbed behaviour (Dix, 2004). The institutions of the nineteenth century record the use of a vast array of mechanical restraint equipment. Disturbing examples of their use include the story of James Norris, a former American Marine, who during the early nineteenth century spent 20 years shackled to a bed (Porter, 1991).

Industrialisation also brought ever-more elaborate pieces of equipment designed to restrict movement that were justified as treatment. Examples of these include machines capable of dropping a bound patient into hot and cold baths and spinning a patient around at high speed (Porter, 1991). Some of these 'therapy' sessions were many hours in duration and sanitised with the label of necessary treatment.

In the United Kingdom, increasing disquiet about practice in mental institutions fuelled momentum to abolish mechanical restraint. Reforms Initiated by Gardiner Hill and Charlesworth at the Lincoln Asylum in 1837 managed to reduce the number of patients kept under permanent mechanical restraint

from 39 to only 2 (Henderson, 1954). Subsequent decades saw increasing determination by reformist pioneers to eradicate the use of use of hobbles, chains and handcuffs.

The non-mechanical restraint philosophy of the British nineteenth-century reformists penetrated well into the 1960s and 1970s and led to the almost total abolition of mechanical restraint for the management of disturbed behaviour in the United Kingdom.

Mechanical restraints (including 4-point bed restraints) remain in regular use in many developed countries, including Europe and the United States (Cabral Iversen, 2009).

Within the United Kingdom, mechanical restraint is much less used than in some other developed countries, although the practice may have become more frequent in recent years. The UK health care regulator the Care Quality Commission (CQC) published a guide to physical and mechanical restraint (CQC, 2016).

The CQC commented: 'We recognise that the use of mechanical restraint may be considered to be the least restrictive intervention in some specific cases, and may present less risk to the individual than the alternative of prolonged manual restraint or transfer to a more restrictive setting.'

As we advance into the twenty-first century, within industrialised societies, there is considerable variation in attitude and philosophy regarding the use of mechanical restraint in mental health care. In the United Kingdom, the use of mechanical restraint is generally considered rare and applied only with special independent scrutiny from the CQC.

History and Development of Interpersonal Systemised Restraint in UK Mental Health Services

History also records staff having to physically take hold of patients during episodes of disturbed behaviour and aggression. Prior to 1981 in the United Kingdom, this often involved individual members of staff applying restraint in any way they could, often relying on superiority of numbers applying restraint in an uncoordinated fashion.

Many modern systems of interpersonal restraint have historical roots arising from the practice of martial arts. In 1882, the Japanese philosopher Jigoro Kano developed judo, a contact sport that modified the combat-orientated techniques of ju-jitsu to include methods of non-injury-inflicting systematised holds. These techniques allowed for one person to hold another person securely without inflicting injury to either. The principle and practice of other non-injury-inflicting methods of self-defence such as Aikido, developed by Morihei Ueshiba in 1942, also can be said to represent some of the technical under-pinning for many of the interpersonal restraint tech-niques taught in modern training programmes. This can be observed in many of the arm holds, wrist manipulation and techniques employed to restrict movement.

Recent decades have seen the introduction of sys-temised methods of physical restraint to mental health inpatient units (Lee et al., 2001). The UK prison service developed a systemised method of restraint in 1981 based on techniques developed from the martial arts and built on the experience of other organisations such as the police. Termed 'Control and Restraint' (C&R), this method aimed for the organised and safe restraint of prisoners relying on standard train-ing, regulation and teamwork.

During the 1970s, there was growing concern in UK mental health services regarding the ability and training of staff to safely deal with violence in psychi-atric hospitals (Brailsford et al., 1973; Bridges et al., 1981). The death in 1984 of Mr Michael Martin, a patient in Broadmoor high secure hospital, resulted in the publication of the Ritchie Report (1985). One of the report's main recommendations was that nursing staff should be properly trained in the use of C&R. Coincidently, only two days before the death of Mr Martin, a management team from Broadmoor Hospital had seen a demonstration of the prison ser-vice's new C&R method and immediately decided that it should be introduced to the hospital (Wright, 1999).

By the mid-1980s, training in C&R had also been introduced to UK MSUs. Several surveys confirm that the term C&R, with variations on its methodology, had become firmly ingrained in the spectrum of inpatient mental health settings (Gournay et al., 1998; Lee et al., 2001; UKCC, 2001) Training in the use of organised systems of restraint has become an accepted necessity within modern mental health prac-tice (Department Of Health, 2002; Department of Health, 2015; NICE, 2015).

Recent years have seen many different methods of systemised restraint introduced to mental health ser-vices within the United Kingdom (UKCC, 2001). Hitherto, it is not clear how many varieties of restraint training are actually in use. Lee et al. (2001) uncovered training in a 'wide variety of techniques' in their survey of staff working in PICUs and MSUs in England and Wales. Some unpublished surveys have suggested as many as 29 different methods of restraint are currently being taught to staff.

Nowadays, it is difficult to establish how many different restraint systems are being taught in the United Kingdom, let alone the rest of the world. The 2020 CQC report (CQC, 2020) of restraint use in mental health states: 'We found a variety of different types of physical restraint were used.' To improve consistency in practice within the United Kingdom, the restraint reduction network published training standards for restraint use (Ridley and Leitch, 2019). With such variation in practice, the overarching prin-ciples of lawful and safe practice must provide the starting point for the development of any restraint policy.

Law and Ethics Related to Restraint

Mental Health Act

Within the United Kingdom, one would expect the Mental Health Act 1983 (MHA) to be the starting point for the legality of restraint. However, the MHA does not specifically deal with the legal author-ity to restrain, and detailed guidance is only offered in the MHA Code of Practice (Department of Health, 2015).

While the Code is not a statutory document, the case of Munjaz (MHAC, 2005) concerned with the use of seclusion initially concluded that the code must be followed. Although this ruling was later challenged and modified by the court of appeal, the status of the code was strengthened to more than mere guidance (Seligman and Feery, 2006). In effect, practitioners need to demonstrate 'cogent reason' to deviate from the Code and thus it must be considered in all epi-sodes of restraint. The Code defines the circumstances in which restraint may be justified. These are sum-marised in Table 20.1.

The use of restraint to administer medical treat-ment in the absence of consent is also common within mental health inpatient units. For example, Shepherd et al. (2014) reported 2,267 episodes of rapid tranquillisation in two London NHS trusts (averaging 4 per day), 5 % of which involved the use of restraint.

Table 20.1 Code of practice (2015) guidance on justification and reasons for restrictive intervention including restraint

- To take immediate control of a dangerous situation where there is a real possibility of harm
- End or significantly reduce the danger to the patient or others

  The five most common reasons in the Code for restrictive intervention, including restraint:
- Physical assault by the patient
- Dangerous, threatening or destructive behaviour
- Attempts to escape or abscond
- Self-harm or risk of physical injury by accident
- Extreme and prolonged overactivity likely to lead to physical exhaustion

The code accepts that, in the appropriate circumstances, the MHA provides authority to administer treatment in the absence of consent. While there is no specific consideration of the use of restraint for this purpose in the code, restraint will at times be required.

Mental Capacity Act

The UK Mental Capacity Act 2005 allows for restraint, provided it is necessary and proportionate to the likelihood and seriousness of harm occurring and is in the person's best interests (Sethi et al., 2018).

Where a person lacks capacity and deprivation of liberty occurs, including the use of restraint, this should always be supported by a best interest meeting.

Criminal Law

The Criminal Law Act 1967 also allows for such force 'as is reasonable' in the prevention of a person committing a crime. This act provides a legal framework for the restraint of those who may or may not be subject to the MHA. When considering the concept of 'reasonableness', the Central Police Training and Development Authority (2003) advises that the question will need to be decided in each individual case. Further guidance offered to police officers include that force should only be used when considered an absolute necessity. In addition, the force should be as minimal as necessary and proportionate in intensity and duration to the perceived threat.

Human Rights Act

The Human Rights Act 1998 sets out 16 rights (Articles), all of which need to be considered in the care and treatment of people in hospitals. Some of these articles are particularly relevant to the practice of restraint. These include:

Article 3: Not using restrictive interventions that cause serious harm and safety risks or amount to inhumane or unusual treatment.

Article 8: Using proportionate restrictive measures

Article 2: Preservation of life

Article 5: Ensuring a legal basis for any action taken

Summary of the Legality for the Common Uses of Restraint in Mental Health

To summarise the law in relation to restraint in mental health, it may be helpful to consider the issues in terms of two general themes. Firstly, specific mental health practice guidance and law. Secondly, more general relevant issues contained within criminal and common law.

The MHA Code of Practice (Department of Health, 2015) offers detailed guidance, which, following the case of Munjaz, must be considered extremely important to the legality of restraint. In addition, the use of restraint for the enforcement of treatment for those subject to the MHA must first ensure that the Code's advice about informed consent is carefully considered.

If challenged in the civil courts, failure to provide informed consent may result in practitioners having difficulty accounting for their actions when justifying the use of restraint for the enforcement of treatment. The application of the relevant sections of the MHA does not in itself afford the right to use restraint in the delivery of treatment. The MHA contains the legal authority in specific circumstances to enforce treatment having first properly considered the consent guidance contained in the Code of Practice.

The second consideration can be said to arise from the application of criminal and common law. Within the United Kingdom, the common authorities are now largely enshrined the in the Mental Capacity

Act 2005. The common law doctrine of necessity provides authority to take steps that are reasonable and proportionate to protect a patient or others from harm. The Criminal Law Act 1967 provides a legal basis for physical intervention in the prevention of the committing of a crime. This is also relevant in issues of self-defence (Jones, 2004). The key here is the concept of 'reasonableness', meaning that actions should be proportional in intensity and duration to the level of threat for which physical intervention is being applied.

Evidence and Efficacy for Methods of Interpersonal Restraint

The lack of consistency in the methods of restraint presents major obstacles to an empirical evaluation of current practice. However, there may be other more significant challenges for researchers aiming to produce quality evidence in the use of restraint.

The randomised controlled trial (RCT) is the widely accepted gold standard of evidence for interventions used in health care. It is not difficult to advance the argument that the use of restraint simply cannot be tested using the RCT design. One cannot imagine nor expect ethical approval for a study using techniques that may inflict serious injury in order to compare them with techniques that may not. The UKCC (2001) comprehensive review on managing inpatient violence states:

We could find no high-quality studies that evaluate either the use of restraint or seclusion in those with mental illness

Much of the theoretical underpinning for the use of systemised restraint can be said to arise from common sense. Put simply, it is preferable for staff to act in a consistent, coordinated fashion in relation to restraint rather than using an improvised, spontaneous approach. Parkes' (1996) evaluation of the introduction of C&R to an MSU showed a reduction in the need for seclusion. This may suggest that staff felt more confident in their ability to effectively deal with aggression because of their C&R training. Interestingly, Parkes' (1996) evaluation also noted an increase in injuries to staff as compared to the period before the introduction of C&R. To date, it appears that there simply is not sufficient systematic evaluation of restraint practice to draw any reliable conclusions about efficacy.

Stewart et al. (2009) concluded that up to five episodes of manual restraint per month might be expected on an average 20-bed ward, with manual restraint lasting about 10 minutes. They also showed that patients tend to be restrained face down on the floor, with restrained patients more likely to be young, male and detained under mental health legislation.

Lepping et al. (2016), in their detailed caparison of restraint data from four countries, concluded that patient related-data were remarkably similar between countries, although type and length of restraint varied significantly. Sethi et al. (2018) attempted to establish safer restraint positions based on available literature. No firm conclusions or recommendations were made.

Safety

The very nature of aggression and restraint must be considered as somewhat unpredictable in terms of how each episode will ultimately unfold. It may be impossible to account for all potential variables when attempting to bring an often highly charged and frightening episode of physical aggression or disturbance under safe control. In order to maximise the safety of the person being restrained, several considerations have been proposed (Parkes, 2002; Paterson et al., 2004; MacPherson et al., 2005; Metherall et al., 2006). It is helpful to consider these factors under two broad headings: factors that are innate to the person being restrained and factors that may emerge as a product of the restraint process.

Safety Factors Innate to the Person Being Restrained

Wherever possible, it is important that staff have a detailed knowledge of the person who may be subject to restraint. This is helpful not only for maximising the potential for avoiding the need for physical intervention in the first place, but also to diminish the likelihood of injury or collapse. Table 20.2 is a list of issues reported as significant to maintaining the safety of a person being restrained.

In most circumstances, it should be possible for staff to complete an assessment of the factors in Table 20.2 before restraint is applied. PICU patients will often be known to staff, and where acute disturbance is possible, an early multidisciplinary review of the risk factors can be undertaken. This can also provide opportunity to include the patient in a discussion of how best to help them through an episode of acute disturbance,

Table 20.2 Factors increasing the risk of injury and cardiac/respiratory failure during restraint

Pre-existing medical conditions, especially cardiac or respiratory conditions (e.g. heart disease, asthma)
Pre-existing skeletal or muscular injury or disease
Pregnancy
Extreme fear as a function of delusional beliefs
Obesity
Substance misuse
High doses of medication

Table 20.3 Safety considerations that may emerge from the process of restraint

Prolonged restraint: the longer restraint is applied, the more risk of collapse or injury
The prone position: restraint in the face-down position
Seated restraint with patient head forward
Increased body temperature: resulting from prolonged struggling and close proximity with shared body heat.
Weight, pressure or holds to any part of the body restricting air way, breathing or circulation.

including the notion of advanced directives in the methods of management.

Beyond the factors that the patient brings to the episode of restraint, the restraint process itself also requires scrutiny to identify safety concerns that may emerge. It requires no great extension of common sense to recognise that even for an otherwise fit and healthy person, a violent struggle also poses serious risks. To manage these risks, constant awareness is required from staff involved in the restraint, which is often no easy task when their attention will inevitably be focused on bringing the situation under control.

Factors That Affect Safety During the Restraint Process

Authors such as Parkes (2002), Paterson et al. (2004), MacPherson et al (2005), Metherall et al. (2006), the report on the death of David Bennett, and the National Institute for Health and Care Excellence (NICE, 2017) offer guidance on how to recognise higher-risk situations that may arise during the restraint process. Metherall et al. (2006) described the creation of medical emergency response teams (MERTs) available to respond quickly to episodes of restraint over a 24-hour period. The MERT includes an assessor trained on intermediate life support standards, whose sole role is to monitor the physical condition of the patient being restrained. Table 20.3 outlines the considerations important to maintaining safety during the restraint process.

It is extremely important that a person independent of the restraint process is present with the sole purpose of monitoring the physical condition of the patient. In the event of prolonged restraint, a careful balance needs to be drawn between the risk to the patient of continuing restraint and the

Table 20.4 Main functions of the MERT assessor during a restraint episode

- The MERT assessor function is independent to the restraint process and is carried out in conjunction with the staff member responsible for holding the head of the patient during the restraint episode.
- The MERT assessor will monitor the airway, respirations and circulation of the patient and whenever possible utilise pulse oximetry.
- The MERT assessor will ensure that the patient's well-being is monitored and physical observations are recorded.
- The MERT assessor will assess physical observations against a pre-arrest call criteria.

risk of further assault if restraint is discontinued. In some circumstances, this may need to be weighed against early discontinuation of restraint while accepting some risk of further assault. The role of the MERT assessor is to be aware of all the physical risk factors associated with restraint and to implement the functions listed in Table 20.4 (Metherall et al., 2006; NICE, 2017). While accepting the lack of quality evidence about the efficacy of restraint methods, there can be little excuse for not paying close attention to the known factors that impact the safety of the patient during the restraint process. Metherall et al.'s (2006) concept of provision for close physical monitoring of the patient under restraint must be considered as a core principle underpinning best practice. Moreover, such provision is also recommended in NICE (2017) practice guidance. It also provides a solid foundation on which to build an audit for improving standards. This philosophy can be easily extended to the safety of staff, which also needs a robust system of monitoring and audit, probably best described within existing health and safety and human resource procedures.

Dignity

No matter how robust the justification, the experience of being physically restrained will often be perceived by the patient as a significant assault on their dignity. In many cases where restraint is necessary, there will be opportunity to take meaningful and practical steps towards promoting the dignity of the person. In some cases, the need for restraint may arise spontaneously leaving little time for planning. Often, however, there will be time to consider how best minimise the distress that will likely result Chieze et al., 2019). A simple step is to carefully consider the location for restraint, minimising the likelihood that the process will be observed by onlookers. The gender of the staff applying restraint should also be the same as the person being restrained. In the case of giving rapid tranquilisation (RT) while under restraint, it will often be necessary to expose embarrassing parts of the body, in particular the upper outer quadrant of the buttock. The combination of being restrained while clothing is removed has the obvious potential to be perceived as sexual assault. Every effort should be made, particularly in female patients, to ensure a gender match between staff and patient.

The practice of safer restraint must be considered in multifactorial terms, only one component of which is the holding techniques themselves. Of equal importance is the close physical monitoring of the patient's condition. Also of great importance is making every effort to preserve as much dignity for the person as possible. Possibly the most important and difficult variable arising from the process of restraint may be the ability to remain intimately and simultaneously in touch with the changing levels of risk both to and from the patient and discontinuing restraint at the earliest possible moment.

Leadership and Restraint

Episodes of acute disturbance and aggression are amongst the most challenging situations that mental health staff will encounter. Fear and anxiety are often close companions to highly charged situations that may culminate in restraint. If left unchecked, these emotions will often result either in lost opportunities for early de-escalation or increased potential for overreaction with the application of restraint.

Within a ward community, the fear that arises from aggression is often highly infectious, although so can be the confidence needed to engage it. Without skilled leadership in taking forward crisis resolution strategies, situations will often become much worse than they may have needed to be. Leadership is an essential part of both avoiding the need for restraint and, where absolutely necessary, for its minimum and safe application. Unlike management, it is extremely difficult to set out a list of definitive measures that can be applied to produce effective clinical leaders for dealing with crises. The following may be a reasonable starting point:

- Highly developed communication skills
- Ability to empathise with the patient and the wider staff team
- Creative thinking toward options for resolving crises
- A willingness to take the initiative and lead from the front
- Effective training
- Role modelling a calm and receptive attitude
- Flexibility in overcoming potential conflict
- Willingness to take risks in allowing frustration discharge without quick resort to physical intervention
- Facilitating the patient and other staff in crisis resolution skills
- Effective post-incident debrief with honest reflection on learning points
- Experience

The PICU maybe an ideal learning environment in which much of the preceding can be cultivated toward producing effective leaders. Most importantly, the atmosphere and ward culture that encourages insight and reflection amongst staff allows for the development of creative methods of dealing with acute crises.

Conclusion

Throughout this chapter, we have seen that the practical and conceptual issues associated with restraint of patients with mental health problems remain complex. Possibly the biggest challenge to advancing practice is trying to achieve an intimate understanding of the basic human issues that arise when a staff group has the authority to lay hands upon a person within the context of health care. Liberty is generally considered amongst humanity's most valued possessions. The physical removal of an individual's free body movement must be considered as one of the most severe infringements on civil liberty.

It is not difficult for each of us to imagine the fear, loss of dignity and helplessness which we would inevitably experience when our free movement is taken from us. When you are the subject of systemised restraint, you will feel and be at the mercy of others. It is no wonder anger is also a very familiar companion to the spectacle of restraint.

Many mental health nurses will have witnessed the distressing effects of systemised restraint on the recipient. In most cases, the efficiency of restraint applied by well-trained staff often leaves the patient feeling that they cannot resist its application, which is all the more distressing when applied to enforce treatment to a person already experiencing mental torment.

The tragic death of Mr David Bennett during restraint is a stark reminder of how badly wrong an episode of difficult restraint can go. It must also be remembered that a member of staff was knocked unconscious prior to Mr Bennett's restraint. No doubt extreme fear was present in all during that tragic incident. The distress resulting from the management of acute disturbance with the need for restraint has many victims, including the staff or others who may happen to bear witness to its occurrence.

The death of Mr Seni Lewis during restraint represents the most stark and unequivocal remainder of the responsibility that professionals have for maintaining safety.

Given the incredibly high human cost of episodes of restraint, what can be done to improve practice? First and foremost, front-line staff and patients who have first-hand experience of situations involving restraint must join together and define the future practice agenda.

In many organisations, senior service managers and other policy-makers can be so divorced from the reality of aggression and restraint that the enormously complicated issues are reduced to no more than statistics and graphs. Policy and practice must be informed by detailed understanding of the nature of situations and process of restraint. That said, it must also be recognised that, when used effectively, big picture data is a key component of practice development and service improvement. The advent of the MERT assessor in monitoring patient safety is a direct example of developing practice within a detailed understanding of the issues.

Finally, even with major advances in de-escalation and understanding of many of the ways in which institutions can diminish confrontation, circumstances where restraint is unavoidable are inevitable. Such are the potential human, risk and safety issues for all the people involved that restraint in all of its complexity must remain at the top of service leader's agenda.

References

Andoh,B (1995) Jurisprudential Aspects of the "Right" to Retake Absconders from mental Hospitals in England and Wales. *Science, Medicine and Law* **35** (3) 225–30.

Appelbaum,P (1999) Seclusion and Restraint: Congress Reacts to Reports of Abuse. *Psychiatric Services* **50** (7) 881–5.

Beech,B and Bowyer,D (2004) Management of Aggression and Violence in Mental Health Settings. *Mental Health Practice* **7** (7) 31–7.

Brailsford,D and Stevenson,J (1973) Factors Related to Violent and Unpredictable Behaviour in Psychiatric Hospitals. *Nursing Times* **69** (3) 9–11.

Bridges,W, Dunane,P and Speight,I (1981) The Provision of Post-Basic Education in Psychiatric Nursing. *Nursing Times* **77** (52) 141–4.

Cabral Iversen,V (2009) Mechanical Restraint – A Philosophy of Man, a Philosophy of Care, or No Philosophy at All? A Question from Norway. *Journal of Psychiatric Intensive Care* **5** (1) 1–4.

Care Quality Commission (CQC) (2020) Out of Sight – Who Cares? A Review of Restraint, Seclusion, and Segregation for Autistic People, and People with a Learning Disability and/or Mental Health Condition. www.cqc.org.uk/publications/themed-work/rssreview.

Care Quality Commission (CQC) (2016) *Brief Guide: Restraint (Physical and Mechanical)*. CQC.

Central Police Training and Development Authority (2003) *Personal Safety Manual*. Harrogate: Centrex.

Chieze,M, Hurst,S, Kaiser,S and Sentissi,O (2019) Effects of Seclusion and Restraint in Adult Psychiatry: A Systematic Review. *Front Psychiatry* **10**: 491.

Davis,P (2004) Critical Thoughts on Restraint in Hospital *Mental Health Nursing* **24** (3) 20–1.

Department of Health (2002) *Mental Health Policy Implementation Guide: National Minimum Standards in Psychiatric Intensive Care Units (PICU) and Low Secure Environments*. London: DOH.

Department of Health (2015) *Mental Health Act 1983: Code of Practice*. London: Department of Health.

Department of Health and Social Care (2021) *Mental Health Units (Use of Force) Act 2018*. London: Department of Health and Social Care.

Dix,R (2004) Advances in the Management of Acute Schizophrenia and Bipolar Disorder: Impact of the New Rapid-Acting Atypical Intramuscular Formulations of Treatment Choice. *Therapeutic Focus* 5–10.

Gournay,K, Ward,M, Thornicroft,G and Wright,S (1998) Crisis in the Capital: In patient Care in Inner London. *Mental Health Practice* 1: 10–18.

Henderson,D (1954) *A Text-Book of Psychiatry*. Oxford University Press: London.

Hoar,S (1997) *The A–Z of Judo*. Ippon Books Ltd: Bristol.

Jones,R (2004) *Mental Health Act Manual*, 9th ed. London: Sweet and Maxwell.

Lee,S, Wright,S, Sayer,J, Parr,AM, Gray,R and Gournay,K (2001) Physical Restraint for Nurses in English and Welsh Psychiatric Intensive Care and Regional Secure Units. *Journal of Mental Health* 10 (2) 151–62.

Lepping,P, Masood,B, Flammer,E and Noorthoorn,E (2016) Comparison of Restraint Data from Four Countries. *Social Psychiatry Psychiatric Epidemiology* 51 (9) 1301–9.

Macpherson,R, Dix,R and Morgan,S (2005) A Growing Evidence Base for Management Guidelines: Revisiting Guidelines for the Management of Acutely Disturbed Psychiatric Patients. *Advances in Psychiatric Treatment* 11 (6) 404–15.

Mental Health Act Code of Practice (1999) Department of Health and Welsh Office. London. The Stationary Office.

Mental Health Act Commission (MHAC) (2005) The House of Lords *Munjaz* Ruling. MHAC Policy Briefing for Commissioners. Issue 12. https://assets.publishing.service .gov.uk/government/uploads/system/uploads/attachment_ data/file/231709/1255.pdf.

Metherall,A, Worthington,R and Keyte,A (2006) The Introduction of Medical Emergency Response Teams to a Mental Health In-patient Hospital. *Journal of Psychiatric Intensive Care*. In press.

Middlewick,J (2000) Use of Restraint Techniques on Acute Psychiatric Wards: Legal, Ethical, and Professional Issues. *Mental Health Care* 3 (8) 271–3.

National Institute for Health and Care Excellence (NICE) (2015) *Violence and Aggression: Short-Term Management in Mental Health, Health and Community Settings. NICE Guideline [NG10]*. London: NICE. www.nice.org.uk/guid ance/NG10.

National Institute of Care and Health Excellence (NICE) (2017) *Violent and Aggressive Behaviours in People with Mental Health Problems*. London: NICE.

National Institute for Mental Health (NIMH) (2004) *Mental Health Policy Implementation Guide – Developing Positive Practice to Support the Safe and Therapeutic Management of Aggression and Violence in mental Health In-patient Settings*. London: DOH Publications.

Nuffield Trust (2021) Violence in the NHS: Quality Watch. www.nuffieldtrust.org.uk/resource/violence-in-the-nhs.

Parkes,J (1996) Control and Restraint Training: A Study of Its Effectiveness in a Medium Secure Unit. *Journal of Forensic Psychiatry* 7 (3) 525–34.

Parkes,J (2002) A Review of the Literature on Positional Asphyxia as a Possible Cause of Sudden Death During Restraint. *British Journal of Forensic Practice* 4 (1) 24–30.

Paterson,B and Leadbetter,D (2004) Learning the right lessons. *Mental Health Practice* 7 (7) 12–15.

Paterson. B, Stark. C, Sadler. D, Leadbetter. D, Allen. D (2003) Restraint-Related Deaths in Health and Social Care in the UK: Learning the Lessons. *Mental Health Practice* 6 (9) 10–17.

Porter,R (ed.) (1991) *The Faber Book of Madness*. London: Faber and Faber.

Royal College of Nursing (RCN) (2018) *Report on Violence and Aggression in the NHS: Estimating the Size and the Impact of the Problem*. London: Royal College of Nursing.

Ridley,J and Leitch,S (2019 *Restraint Reduction Network (RRN) Training Standards*. Birmingham: BILD Publications.

Ritchie,S (1985) *Report to the secretary of state for social services concerning the death of Michel Martin*. London: SHSA.

Seligman,M and Feery,D (2006) Lord Steyn's Lament. *Journal of Psychiatric Intensive Care* 2 (2) 111–17.

Sethi,F, Parkes,J, Baskind,E, Paterson,B and O'Brien,A (2018) Restraint in Mental Health Settings: Is It Time to Declare a Position? *British Journal of Psychiatry* 212 (3) 137–41.

Shepherd,N Parker,C and Arif,N (2014) Pattern of Rapid Tranquillisation and Restraint Use in a Central London Mental Health Service. *Journal of Psychiatric Intensive Care* 11 (2) 78–83.

Stewart,D, Bowers,L, Simpson,A, Ryan,C and Tziggili,M (2009) Manual Restraint of Adult Psychiatric Inpatients: A Literature Review. *Journal of Psychiatric and Mental Health Nursing* 16 (8) 749–57.

United Kingdom Central Council (UKCC) for Nursing, Midwifery and Health Visiting (1999) *Nursing in Secure Environments*. England: University of Central Lancashire.

United Kingdom Central Council (UKCC) for Nursing, Midwifery and Health Visiting (2001) *The Recognition Prevention and Therapeutic Management of Violence in Mental Health Care*. London: Health Services Research Department.

Wright,S (1999) Physical Restraint in the Management of Violence and Aggression in In-Patient Settings: A Review of the Issues. *Journal of Mental Health* 8 (5) 459–72.

Management of the Mental Health Emergency in the Community

Mathew Page and Matthew Truscott

Introduction

In this chapter we explore where the psychiatric intensive care unit (PICU) story often begins: in the community. Mental health problems by their nature are multifaceted; crises often emerge in a chaotic maelstrom of history, trauma, genetic vulnerability, illicit substances, economic deprivation, social exclusion and misfortune. What happens at each and every stage will impact on what happens next. Practitioners and experts with lived experience will often be able to identify moments when, if something had been different, the crisis could have been calmed and the adverse effects avoided.

Within this chapter, we provide an account of specialist PICU experience with the associated skills and knowledge from the inpatient setting for intervening as early as possible in mental health emergencies. By offering solutions which ensure the right help is available as soon as possible, it has been found that the need for more restrictive interventions can be avoided; mental health care being consistent with other branches of clinical services in upholding the maxim that 'prevention is better than cure'. The emerging evidence for the various models for providing a healthcare response to a mental health crisis point to a reduced stigma and use of force (de Jong et al., 2022).

This chapter considers the whole pathway from home/the wider community to PICU with a focus on ensuring that healthcare solutions are provided to healthcare emergencies. We describe what has developed over time in the United Kingdom, the legal powers that are involved and specifically the police powers under Section 136 of the Mental Health Act 1983 (MHA) (Legislation.gov.uk, 1983). We also discuss best practice within a service model that involves use of specialist mental health practitioners able to

respond to crises in the same way as the rest of the emergency services.

Recognising that there is still a role for physical spaces where safety and security are offered, we describe the various models for Health-Based Places of Safety (HBPoS) and examine the pathway into PICU where it is indicated.

History

As has been discussed elsewhere in this book, it is likely that the problem of what to do with people whose distress prevents them operating within normal societal conventions is as old as the formation of society itself.

The first methods of support would likely have been at the community level and were probably a mixture of the innate kindness many humans share with each other and the draconian restrictions of the day. While religious houses (monasteries) exercised a role in caring for the sick, which may have included people with mental health problems, there is unlikely to have been much coordinated planning.

Care started being organised in a more centralised manner in 1247 when the Priory of St Mary of Bethlehem (later known variously as Bedlam and Bethlem) was formed.

While we have relatively detailed accounts from the records of how the early institutions were organised (Nolan, 1993), what is less clear is what the route into hospital in the first place might have been.

The County Asylums Act of 1808 began the programme, refined in the County Asylums Act of 1845, to ensure each county had a functioning specialist institution for the care of people who were mentally unwell, avoiding their incarceration in prisons and workhouses.

Even in the mid-nineteenth century, 'home treatment' was being advocated as a viable alternative to the restrictions of hospital treatment in the first *Handbook for the Instruction of Attendants on the Insane* (Medico-Psychological Association, 1884)

It was in the same era that the first reference to what we might see as a 'crisis intervention' was enshrined in English law.

Section 68 of the Lunatic Asylum Act (1853) stated the following:

Every Constable, Relieving Officer, or Overseer, shall apprehend and take before a Justice, any lunatic not a pauper (poor person), wandering at large. Any Justice hearing information on oath that a lunatic was wandering, shall order a Constable, to apprehend and bring before him the lunatic. And any Constable, having knowledge that any lunatic, is not under proper care and control, or is cruelly treated or neglected by any person having charge of him, shall within three days give information on oath to Justice. The Justice may either visit and examine such person, and make enquiries himself, or a medical man to do so and report.

The lineage between this particular statute and the modern MHA provisions under Section 136 (power for a police office to detain a person in public appearing in need of mental health assessment) is plain to see. As in many aspects of life, the Victorian era saw the foundations of some of the standards we now take for granted.

The Mental Health Act 1959 further refined the law to reflect the powers of professional police constables throughout the country in wording that largely went unaltered into the 1983 Act.

Throughout most of this time, mental health care was largely considered the remit of the grand Victorian asylums, but in the latter part of the twentieth century, with changes in medical knowledge, societal sensibilities and the burden of public expenditure, things were changing as people with mental illness were expected to live in the community being supported by health and social care professionals to do so.

Contemporary Legislation

The general themes of this chapter will be of interest to practitioners involved in the support of people during mental health emergencies throughout the world. Out of necessity, the discussion around the legal aspects of this work will focus on the law in England and Wales

Section 136 of the MHA is the primary piece of legislation used in responding to a mental health

emergency outside of hospital. It gives the following authority:

If a person appears to a constable to be suffering from mental disorder and to be in immediate need of care or control, the constable may, if he thinks it necessary to do so in the interests of that person or for the protection of other persons –

(a) remove the person to a place of safety within the meaning of section 135, or
(b) if the person is already at a place of safety within the meaning of that section, keep the person at that place or remove the person to another place of safety

Many developed countries around the world will also have similar provisions. In the United Kingdom, the Mental Health Act 1983 (Legislation.gov.uk, 1983) defines a place of safety as:

- Residential accommodation provided by a local social services authority
- A hospital
- A police station
- An independent hospital or care home for mentally disordered persons
- Any other suitable place

A key aspect of Section 136 is the statutory time limit of 24 hours for detention at a place of safety. Of relevance to those responding, the mental health emergencies are the locations from which an individual can be detained. These can broadly be defined as anywhere other than a residential property and its associated garden and buildings.

Police forces in England and Wales, in the year ending March 2022, recorded 36,500 instances where Section 136 was used. Of these, 68% of detainees were removed to an HBPoS, 29% to an Accident and Emergency department and 0.8% to a police station (Home Office, 2022).

A less used but equally relevant power is enshrined in Section 135 of the Mental Health Act 1983 (Legislation.gov.uk, 1983) which allows an approved mental health professional to apply to a justice of the peace for a warrant which enables a constable to remove a person from a residential address to a place of safety.

O'Brien et al. (2018) recognise that the nature of Section 136 creates a complex interaction between the criminal justice system and health and social care. The responsibilities of the police, the provision of an

HBPoS and subsequent formal assessments make this one of the most resource-intensive and costly interventions in the mental health system. The involvement of the police and ambulance service in such serious situations as the use of Section 136 raises questions about the availability of training and support offered as well as highlights that a lack of integrated operating can cause frustration to professionals and adverse experiences for services users (Genziani et al., 2020)

The use of an agency primarily concerned with the prevention and detection of crime and maintenance of public order in responding to a mental health emergency continues to be challenged, and while a police station is legally available as a place of safety, the Mental Health Act 1983 (Places of Safety) Regulations (2017) (Legislation.gov.uk, 2017) significantly limit this possibility. These regulations require that only those at most risk of serious injury or death to themselves or others might be considered as appropriately detained in a police station. Children may not be detained at a police station under any circumstances. The drive to offer HBPoS as an alternative to police custody, even before the regulatory change, has been suggested to have contributed to changes in perception of when Section 136 might be used. Pugh and Laidlaw (2016), who reviewed data in one locality, point to an increasing number of people being detained with a decreasing proportion requiring onward detention in hospital.

One area which raises challenges for mental health practitioners and policy-makers is the number of people who are subject to multiple detentions under Section 136. Adewusi et al. (2022) conducted an analysis of a five-year period in one London trust which found that 1,767 individuals had been detained, with 81 having been detained three or more times. The analysis of patient characteristics for the cohort of 'repeat attenders' points to diagnoses of personality disorder, self-harm and self-reported trauma and abuse. Burgess et al. (2017) similarly found a prevalence of personality disorder and substance misuse diagnoses amongst those who were most frequently detained and least likely to be in longer-term secondary mental health care. The fact that many of the people in this cohort are often discharged back to the community without an admission reinforces the need to look systemically at solutions/service offers beyond those currently being used.

Providers of HBPoS may sometimes encounter difficulties at the end of the 24-hour-period of detention. Up to the 2017 revisions of the Mental Health Act 1983 (Legislation.gov.uk, 1983), a period of detention lasted up to 72 hours; this was changed to 24 hours to ensure that people received the help they needed as soon as possible. The realities of the current mental health system are such that an inpatient bed is not always available. This can lead to delays which potentially breach the 24-hour-detention. The difficulty of detaining someone who is waiting for a bed beyond 24 hours is significant. Ramesh and Kripalani (2021) note that there is inconsistent practice between providers relying on common law, the Mental Capacity Act 2005 (Legislation.gov.uk, 2005) and unlawful detention to manage this situation. Case law and national guidance may help to resolve this in due course. In the meantime, Ramesh and Kripalani (2021) suggest the need for duty of candour with the patient and their family and a clearly documented clinical review and decision at the point where the detention lapses.

Central to service and policy design should be the lived experience of people who use services. When those services are focussed on the most acute point of a mental health crisis, collecting information can be problematic; however, through retrospective interviews, Goodall et al. (2019) gathered instructive feedback on what can improve the experience for those detained. The findings include more obvious practices such as good communication and kindness, but perhaps most saliently, people knowing what to expect during what is quite likely to be a complicated set of personal, clinical and legal issues to understand. The sense of powerlessness and instances where force was used were associated with the most negative parts of the whole experience. Sondhi et al. (2018) also found that there were recurrent themes amongst those who attended a place of safety, including process or procedural issues, the professional–patient relationship and the importance of a supportive therapeutic environment. Further research and development in this area should serve to improve the experience of those being detained where the use of Section 136 cannot be avoided altogether.

Planning and Designing a Health-Based Place of Safety

Operational Models

While it is essential that all systems should have an HBPoS, it is fair to say that there is a significant degree of variation in service models.

There are several factors in play that will determine the type of model and this, in turn, is likely to determine how and how frequently it is used.

Prior to beginning any process of commissioning an HBPoS, a clear strategy should be developed which includes the voices of those with lived experience. This chapter focuses on the need to provide prompt and proportionate support to someone experiencing the beginning of a mental health crisis and in so doing it is anticipated that the use of Section 136 and therefore HBPoS will be minimised. Given that all mental health systems should be seeking to minimise restriction and promote independence, it is likely this would form the basis of any strategy. Nonetheless, local variation arising from organisational culture, geography and cost will all impact on the shape of the service.

It is probably true to say that HBPoS service models vary on a continuum between 'come alive' models, which are only opened up when required, and specialist units, which are permanently staffed and run similarly to inpatient wards.

The alternative is for the place of safety function to be provided by another service with a dual function such as an inpatient ward or assessment unit.

Interestingly there are some parallels in how HBPoS models have developed with the development of PICU as a specialism since the 1990s. Dix (2022) reflects on the journey from non-specialist, under-resourced responses to acute disturbance to purpose-built facilities with the specialist staff groups we see today.

There are merits and risks associated with all the models currently in use, and we discuss these later in the chapter.

The 'come alive' model works most effectively when the use of Section 136 is kept to an absolute minimum. It is likely that its nature of only physically opening up in extremis contributes to a psychology amongst all parts of the system to minimise its use. However, where processes and relationships between organisations are the best developed, the 'come alive' model can be effective. The risk of switching to it without supporting practice and culture is that staff brought from other areas (such as a crisis team) may become overwhelmed and distracted from other important aspects of their work.

The specialist unit can look immediately attractive as having the greatest level of clinical skill and most operational resilience. Such units require high levels of capital investment and significant recurrent funding for staffing; although it isn't the financial costs that create the biggest risk here, it is the 'build it and they will come' phenomena or so-called supply-led demand. Having a dedicated service with a skilled workforce will lead to high levels of confidence in all other parts of the system, which is more likely to mean that people will be taken to the unit and left there for longer than they could have been. It is also true to say that once a system has such a unit it will always be very difficult to scale it back.

The dual function service can mitigate some of the risks identified; however, the nature of a mental health crisis that includes Section 136 can mean that it becomes the predominant concern of the service at the expense of patients who are there in different circumstances.

Decision-makers contemplating what type of model to develop in their area should be afforded a degree of latitude based on a range of factors which might be unique. Issues including travel time and proximity to other services such as the police and emergency departments will all influence what the most effective solution will be.

As health care in England moves towards much greater cooperation and integration with partners, it is hoped that further opportunities for improved models will emerge. The early anecdotal reports from mental health urgent assessment centres which mix the skills of the ambulance service, mental health triage, place of safety and psychiatry and approved mental health professionals suggest that an integrated approach allows for a more nuanced response which upholds the principle of least restriction.

Physical Environment

The operational model will drive what type of environment will be provided. The anticipated duration of someone's stay will be a key determining factor. For example, when assessments are completed and a plan is enacted within a couple of hours, there is no need to provide someone with a bedroom and a bed.

Some aspects of PICU design (described by Dix and Page, 2023) may be relevant considerations in providing an appropriate building; however, the risk of building it like a PICU is that everyone will treat it like a PICU. Environmental principles of stress reduction described by Ulrich et al. (2018) are likely to be of relevance to people in the most distressed state when detained on a Section 136.

In addition to offering the most therapeutic milieu possible, other considerations must also be made. These include:

- Infection prevention and control (cohorting of people with viral symptoms)
- Single-sex space
- Assessment space
- Office space for multiple agencies to work in
- Ambulance access and parking
- Clinical space for physical health care
- Space for supporting riskier/disturbed behaviour

Workforce Model

Like the building, the workforce model will follow the operational model. Nurses and support workers are likely to be essential in any such model, as they have the requisite skill set for providing a therapeutic safe setting 24 hours a day, but other disciplines will also add significant value when immediately on hand.

Under the Mental Health Act 1983 (Legislation. gov.uk, 1983), those detained under Section 136 will require a medical assessment and one completed by an approved mental health professional. When these experts are co-located in the service, assessments are timelier and more robust holistic therapeutic plans are developed.

Availability of clinicians with skills in physical health care will increase the capability and capacity of the service and avoid the need for problematic transfers to general medical services. Given that mental health crisis can often be associated with injury of one kind or another, being able to provide a level of care in such situations is highly advantageous.

Procedures and Practice

Whichever delivery model is developed, the need for carefully negotiated and tested procedures is essential. More so than most other areas of mental health care, the HBPoS will require the interaction of several agencies whose practice will all need to be enshrined in procedures. It is not possible to provide an exhaustive list, but those developing a service will need to consider such issues as:

- Acceptance and conveyance of detainees
- Search procedures
- Police involvement in the management of disturbance
- Transfer to general medical services

- Management of complex care such as children or people with a learning disability
- Onward transfer and conveyance

Time spent contingency/scenario testing before a unit is operational is very likely to reap dividends in the months and years that follow.

Interface with the PICU

Being detained under Section 136 does not necessarily indicate a likelihood of an onward transfer to an assessment or treatment section (Sections 2 and 3, respectively) of the Mental Health Act 1983 (Legislation.gov.uk, 1983). In the year ending March 2022, of 21,000 people detained in an HBPoS in England, only 3,500 went on to be detained formally in hospital (NHS Digital, 2022).

There are a range of potential outcomes for people who are detained and the majority are often discharged back into the community. Some will be offered an informal admission to hospital, with the minority detained.

Further data analysis is required to identify precise numbers transferring from a HBPoS to a PICU, but clinical experience highlights that not only is this a frequent admission route, but it is also potentially the most problematic.

As in most aspects of health care, good relationships are at least as important as good procedures. The development of a clear process for establishing the need for PICU via screening and clinical assessment must be supported by the ready sharing of information, advice and support between the two services.

All PICUs will have their own process for deciding who should be admitted. The HBPoS team will need to ensure that they have a process for referral which dovetails precisely with that of the PICU. Where the HBPoS and PICU are co-located in a hospital, many of the potential inter-service challenges can be mitigated. For larger trusts across bigger geography, these challenges should not be underestimated. Opportunities such as rotational posts, shared team building/training and regular partnership meetings are all strategies which might be helpful in building a positive connection between the two services.

Once the decision has been made and a bed identified on a PICU, the transfer should be immediately arranged. There will need to be clear local policies and procedures that maintain the privacy and dignity of the patient at all times. It may be possible for the transfer to occur by walking between adjacent units; however, where distance is likely to be problematic or there is a risk of absconding, vehicular transport should be used.

Bed finding and transport availability can both be limiting factors in ensuring that the 24-hour statutory time limit is met. Procedures should be in place which ensure ready access and prioritisation for those detained in an HBPoS.

Where possible the practitioner who has developed the best rapport with the patient in the HBPoS should travel to the PICU to allay their understandable anxieties and ensure the highest standard of handover is presented to the PICU team.

Development of a Cross-Organisational Mental Health Emergency Service: One Service Model

Model Delivery

Over the last decade or so several innovative solutions have been tested based on providing a greater level of mental health expertise into emergency services' response to incidents. These have had varying levels of resources and collaboration between different service types and, as was evident in the early days of psychiatric intensive care, a lack of standardised approach and definitive evidence base. In the southwest of England a number of trials were undertaken which have led to the development of a sophisticated mental health Emergency Services Triage (EST) team, a strategic and operational partnership between the ambulance service, police and mental health trust.

The principle of 'parity of esteem' between mental and physical health was first enshrined in the Health and Social Care Act (Legislation.gov.uk, 2012). The Health and Care Act (Legislation.gov.uk, 2022) further requires that the concept is upheld in how services are delivered. This principle should inform any service model when considering how to respond to an emergency situation, which will often have a complex mix of dynamic factors that may include both physical and mental health issues. Systems must design intelligent responses to people in need that can adapt and offer a multi-layered clinical response as early in the patient journey as possible.

In the development of a new service which can respond to complex demand, the best outcomes are usually achieved when there is a unified system response that can adjust and provide different approaches, skills and experience depending on the need of the person in crisis.

The EST service emerged from the knowledge gained by having mental health clinicians (mental health nurses, social workers or occupational therapists) from the NHS mental health trust work with police in the control room as well as participate in police community response by riding along with officers. The potential for such services to be beneficial is recognised in the literature, but the significant variances in all aspects of delivery still make comparisons difficult (Puntis et al., 2018). Nonetheless, such services are generally supported by the police and found by service users to be less traumatising and stigmatising than previous approaches (Kirubarajan et al., 2018)

There were several challenges in providing a police-based mental health service, including:

- Lengthy police vetting preventing the use of temporary staff
- Mental health staff feeling isolated from peer supervision in the police environment
- Using specialist mental health staff to review a high volume of low-priority calls

A working group involving key representatives from the mental health trust, police and fire and ambulance services undertook detailed analysis of emergency calls and incidents to help determine a preferable service model. One of the most salient pieces of learning was that in many cases multiple services would become involved for the same person in crisis, often without knowing that the other was attending or having any mechanism for agreeing a shared response. For incidents where Section 136 of the MHA was being considered, this could be particularly complicated.

A cross-organisational review proved highly useful in realising particular issues, for example, when police officers are deployed to the scene of an incident and then have to wait for an extended time for an ambulance to become available, this could set in motion a series of decisions which might lead to greater restriction, poorer outcome and adverse experience for the individual service user.

The dispatch of a 'generic' ambulance to mental health-related calls was often a poor outcome for the person in distress. Ambulances arriving to these calls were not well equipped to respond to a mental health crisis and were found to convey the person to emergency department more often than not. This would result in a further delay for the distressed person waiting to see a mental health specialist in the emergency department.

The review identified some core tenets for a successful service redesign in the 999 call pathway:

1) Establishing a joint vision and commitment to an agreed service design across the entire emergency pathway
2) Combining provider organisations' approaches through a strategic partnership
3) Allowing bespoke data collection
4) Designing a workforce model that supports recruitment and retention
5) Identifying a clear and lean governance pathway to support agility and growth
6) Developing a model that can intervene as early in the call pathway as possible, ideally from a 999 (UK emergency telephone number) control room

The group agreed that successful operational delivery would require the clinical staff to work to the following priorities:

1) Pre-dispatch (early intervention) mental health advice and support that can coordinate and operate across all of 999
2) Pro-active (not relying on referral) and fast response to the scene of a mental health 999 call to offer specialist decision-making as early as possible

The service uses a hub-and-spoke model to work across the entire 999 emergency pathway (Figure 21.1). Mental health staff based at the ambulance service Emergency Operations Centre (EOC) manage the 'spokes' which consist of mental health response teams that could arrive at speed at different locations. The clinical team rotates around the varying functions which ensures team consistency and eliminates the deskilling sometimes found when specialist services are established.

In addition to mental health and ambulance staff, the EST relies on the presence of a police link officer, enabling access to the police call management system. The integration between police and ambulance control systems enables duplicate calls to quickly be identified and decisions to be made as to which service needs to respond. This has the dual benefit of better-coordinated care for the person in crisis and more efficient use of resources.

Enabling a deployment of specialist mental health practitioners to the scene of an incident alongside other emergency services is a core element of the EST service. In addition to a standard car-based street triage, an ambulance service rapid response vehicle is used to minimise journey times. The ambulance service provides the emergency care assistant who both drives and assists with physical healthcare issues and the mental health trust provides the specialist practitioner. Both practitioners are supported by the specialist clinical advice (available via the EOC).

Information Sharing between Organisations

Any integrated way of working will require the free flow of appropriate information between individuals and organisations. This fundamentally requires highly functional operational solutions, most likely reliant on digital platforms, and clearly articulated and agreed governance arrangements.

Real-time information from the emergency services (999) call, clinical information and other intelligence systems will all be helpful in enabling decisions as to which service should be dispatched. Access to clinical records can be more problematic when emergency services operate over multiple networks using differing record systems. Individuals and sometimes organisations can sometimes become quite paralysed by concerns about sharing information. Interestingly, Pope et al. (2022) found that the majority of service users were positive about the practice on the basis it is likely to reduce the use of arrest and promote more positive interactions. The issue is fundamentally about the balance of safety with the right of privacy (Sougias et al., 2022)

Ultimately, information sharing must be planned in advance through the development of formal information-sharing agreements which have been signed off by all relevant organisations. These documents will ensure information sharing occurs when it is necessary and appropriate.

The main clinical and operational value in effective information sharing includes:

1) Triangulating the response to calls open to multiple emergency services at the same time
2) Manually reviewing the 999 calls and identifying incidents that may benefit from a mental health response

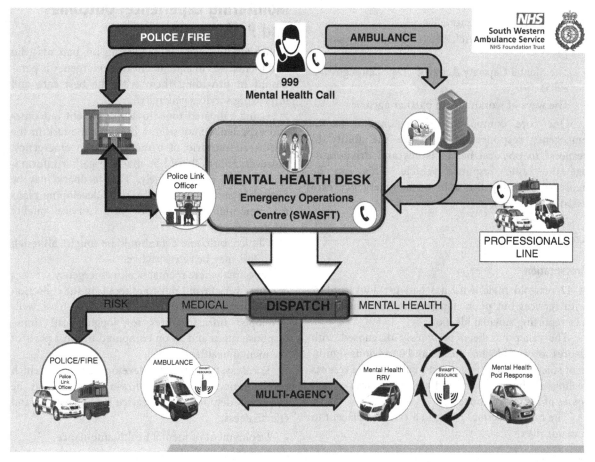

Figure 21.1 999 mental health call flow

3) Identifying and providing consistent care to 'high-impact users' or frequent callers who often interact with a range of emergency and healthcare services

Workforce Skills Requirements for the Mental Health Emergency in the Community

Telephone-based clinical work, especially in emergency situations which can often involve working with third parties who themselves are in shock or distressed, is highly taxing for any practitioner. In creating a team with a deployable function in the form of a mental health rapid response vehicle, duties can be rotated in a way that aims to minimise stress and compassion fatigue, so called burn out, that can adversely affect emergency services personnel (Renkiewicz and Hubble, 2022).

Similar to the recognition of PICU as a specialism distinct from other forms of acute mental health care, emergency mental health care requires a specific set of skills. These include:

- Conducting an assessment of the person in need
- De-escalation
- Supporting families, carers and third-party witnesses
- Being able to operate in the dynamic environment of the open street
- The ability to respond to traumatic incidents involving suicide and serious injury
- Supporting other staff with medical emergencies that may relate to the incident

In addition to these skills, a broad range of knowledge is needed including:

- Mental health conditions
- Pharmacological treatments
- The Mental Health Act 1983 (Legislation.gov.uk, 1983)
- The Mental Capacity Act 2005 (Legislation.gov.uk, 2005)
- The ways of working with partner agencies

One core component of the mental health emergency response is to ensure the ability to respond to physical health issues and drive/manage the rapid response vehicle. This can be achieved by using the skills of an emergency care assistants (ECAs).

Case vignette

Presentation

A 42-year-old male, who has had previous contact with services but poor engagement, calls into NHS 111 reporting suicidal ideation.

The caller has been previously diagnosed with depression and alcohol misuse and a previous significant suicide attempt in context of alcohol. He reports feelings of hopelessness and rejection amid recent losses of his job relationship.

The caller describes being in a vehicle adjacent to a major river.

Intervention

A mental health clinician in service of the NHS 111 system completed a remote assessment with the caller to assess presentation and risk. The assessment included reviewing the caller's mental health record and general practitioner notes, as well as risks considered high and requiring an emergency response. The clinician discussed the case and transferred the caller to the 999 system, and an emergency mental health rapid response vehicle was dispatched.

Result

The mental health clinician arrived at the scene within 30 minutes, as the case was considered high risk. The man was assessed and referred to the crisis team using a trusted assessment pathway. Police were not required to wait at scene and thus Section 136 was not needed. The caller was provided treatment at home and admission to hospital was avoided.

Monitoring Experience, Outcomes and Performance

Understanding what is happening for patients who find themselves in a mental health emergency is paramount in providing them with the best care and improving services generally.

Using validated tools to assess patient outcomes and experience may seem a burdensome task in the fast-paced scenario of a mental health emergency, however, efforts should be made to gather information, even if retrospectively. This feedback may be critical in such important tasks as developing plans for potential future crises and service quality improvement.

Clinical outcome data should be sought, although again this may be retrospective.

One area where mental health emergency services compare very favourably to others is in the collection of performance data. The 999 services have well-developed infrastructures for logging call times, response times and so on compared to most parts of the mental health system.

Local systems should develop data sets which reflect their needs. The following metrics may be helpful in demonstrating service responsiveness and effectiveness:

- Deployment of mental health ambulance
- Use of Section 136
- Specialist mental health advice sought by police prior to decision to detain
- Means of conveyance
- Time taken to complete assessment
- Time taken to find a bed
- Total time detained at an HBPoS

Conclusion

In this chapter, the authors considered, perhaps paradoxically, how best to avoid the need for PICU in the first place. Central to any progressive mental health system is the principle of 'least restriction', perhaps more positively framed as promoting independence. By providing clinical interventions when they are needed as someone's journey intersects with the emergency services, the use of the restrictions of MHA Section 136 can be avoided.

Most aspects of the health and care system are operating under significant pressure, often in excess

of what they were designed to deliver. Judicious investment of clinical resource and effort into the right
services can avoid unwanted consequences, reduce
trauma and result in better outcomes for individuals.

The development of specialist services to respond
to mental health emergencies, reducing the need to
rely on the police and mainstream ambulance is novel
and highly innovative. Just like the development of
PICUs over the last three decades, this emergent specialism will benefit from the leadership of passionate
experts prepared to invest effort in further advances
and establishing a high-quality evidence base.

References

Adewusi,L, Mark,I, Wells,P and O'Brien,A. (2022)
A Retrospective Cohort Study Describing Characteristics of
Those Repeatedly Detained Under Section 136 of the
Mental Health Act Over a 5-Year Period and the
Association With Past Abuse. *Medicine, Science and the Law*
62 (2) 124–33.

Burgess,JL, White,SJ and O'Brien,A (2017) Retrospective
Cohort Follow-Up Study of Individuals Detained Under
Section 136. *British Journal of Psychiatry: Open* **3** (6) 281–4.

de Jong,IC, van der Ham,LAJ and Waltz,MM (2022)
Responding to Persons in Mental Health Crisis: A Cross-
Country Comparative Study of Professionals' Perspectives
on Psychiatric Ambulance and Street Triage Models.
Journal of Community Safety and Well-Being (7) 36–S44.

Dix,R (2022) The National Association of Psychiatric
Intensive Care Units: 25 years not out. *Journal of Psychiatric
Intensive Care* **18** (1) 5–6.

Dix,R and Page,M (2023) Physical Environment. In Dix,R,
Dye,S and Pereira,SM (eds.), *Psychiatric Intensive Care*, 3rd
ed. (in print).

Genziani,M, Gillard,S, Samuels,L and Chambers,M (2020)
Emergency Workers' Experiences of the Use of Section 136
of the Mental Health Act 1983: Interpretative
Phenomenological Investigation. *British Journal of
Psychiatry Bulletin* **44** (6) 250–4.

Goodall,T, Newton,E, Larkin,M (2019) What are the critical
incidents that affect how people cope with being detained
under Section 136 of the Mental Health Act (1983, 2007)?
International Journal of Psychiatry in Clinical Practice **23** (3)
194–206.

Home Office (2022) Police Powers and Procedures: Other
PACE Powers, England and Wales, Year Ending
31 March 2022. (online) www.gov.uk/government/statis
tics/police-powers-and-procedures-other-pace-powers-eng
land-and-wales-year-ending-31-march-2022/police-power
s-and-procedures-other-pace-powers-england-and-wales-y
ear-ending-31-march-2022#detentions-under-section-136-
of-the-mental-health-act-1983.

Kirubarajan,A, Puntis,S, Perfect,D, Tarbit,M, Buckman,M
and Molodynski,A (2018) Street Triage Services in England:
Service Models, National Provision, and the Opinions of
Police. *British Journal of Psychiatry Bulletin* **42** (6) 253–7.

Legislation.gov.uk (2022) Health and Care Act 2022.
(online) www.legislation.gov.uk/ukpga/2022/31/contents/
enacted.

Legislation.gov.uk (2012) Health and Social Care Act 2012.
(online) www.legislation.gov.uk/ukpga/2012/7/contents/
enacted.

Legislation.gov.uk (2005) Mental Capacity Act 2005.
(online) www.legislation.gov.uk/ukpga/2005/9/contents.

Legislation.gov.uk (1983) Mental Health Act 1983. (online)
www.legislation.gov.uk/ukpga/1983/20/contents.

Legislation.gov.uk (2017) Mental Health Act 1983 (Places of
Safety) Regulations (2017). (online) www.legislation.gov.uk/
uksi/2017/1036/contents/made.

Medico-Psychological Association (1884) *Handbook for the
Instruction of Attendants on the Insane.* London: Balliere
Tindall.

NHS Digital (2022) Mental Health Act Statistics, Annual
Figures, 2021–22. (online) https://digital.nhs.uk/data-and
-information/publications/statistical/mental-health-act-stat
istics-annual-figures/2021-22-annual-figures

Nolan,P (1993) *A History of Mental Health Nursing.*
Cheltenham: Stanley Thornes.

O'Brien,A, Sethi,F, Smith,M and Bartlett,A (2018) Public
Mental Health Crisis Management and Section 136 of the
Mental Health Act. *Journal of Medical Ethics* **44** (5):349–53.

Pope,LG, Warnock,A, Perry,TH, Langlois,S, Anderson,S,
Boswell,T, et al. (2022) Information Sharing Across Mental
Health Service Providers and Criminal Legal System
Stakeholders: Perspectives of People with Serious Mental
Illnesses and Their Family Members. *Social Science &
Medicine* **307**(C).

Pugh,D and Laidlaw,J (2016) Sections 135 and 136: Running
a health-based place of safety in Gloucestershire. *Medicine,
Science and the Law* **56**(2):99–106.

Puntis,S, Perfect,D, Kirubarajan,A, Bolton,S, Davies,F,
Hayes,A, et al. (2018) A Systematic Review of Co-Responder
Models of Police Mental Health 'Street' Triage. *BMC
Psychiatry* **18** (1) 256.

Ramesh,Y and Kripalani,M (2021) Section 136: The 'Grey
Zone' After the 24-Hour Validity Period Lapses. *British
Journal of Psychiatry: Advances* **27**(1) 62–4.

Renkiewicz,GK and Hubble,MW (2022) Secondary
Traumatic Stress in Emergency Services Systems (STRESS)
Project: Quantifying and Predicting Compassion Fatigue in
Emergency Medical Services Personnel. *Prehospital
Emergency Care* **26** (5) 652–63.

Sondhi,A, luger,L, Toleikyte,L and Williams,E (2018)
Patient Perspectives of Being Detained Under Section 136 of

the Mental Health Act: Findings from a Qualitative Study in London. *Medicine, Science and the Law* **58** (3)159–67.

Sougias,K, Fernbacher,S and Lim,I (2022) Safety Over Privacy: Family Violence, Information Sharing, and Mental Health Care. *Australasian Psychiatry* **30** (5) 604–7.

Ulrich,RS, Bogren,L, Gardiner,SK, and Lundin,S (2018) Psychiatric Ward Design Can Reduce Aggressive Behavior. *Journal of Environmental Psychology* **57**: 53–66.

United Kingdom Parliament (1808) *County Asylums Act*. London: UK Parliament.

United Kingdom Parliament (1845) *County Asylums Act*. London: UK Parliament.

United Kingdom Parliament (1853) *Lunatic Asylums Act*. London: UK Parliament.

United Kingdom Parliament (1959) *Mental Health Act*. London: UK Parliament.

Chapter 22

PICU for the Care of Young People

Mathew Page

Introduction

This chapter provides an overview of how the concept of psychiatric intensive care can be applied when caring for young people. The term 'young people' is used collectively throughout this chapter to describe anyone younger than the age of 18.

At its heart, psychiatric intensive care practice has a desire to look after people when they are at their most vulnerable. When those needing support are still in their formative years, vulnerabilities can be even greater, requiring the highest standards of clinical person-centred care.

In highlighting some additional considerations and distinct clinical and legal issues, this chapter provides practitioners with guidance and acts as a stimulus for further research and practice development.

Due to the present paucity of research or published literature in this field, the chapter leans heavily on the work of the multidisciplinary group that developed the National Minimum Standards (NMS) for Psychiatric Intensive Care Units for Young People (NAPICU, 2015).

History and Development of PICU for Young People

The development of PICU as a concept for the care of young people tracks a similar journey to the development of the specialism within general adult services, albeit some 20 years later. For many years, the problem of how to care for young people whose presentation could not be safely supported within a 'general adolescent unit' was met with a variety of answers. These often mirrored practice in adult services prior to the development of agreed definitions and the first National Minimum Standards (Department of Health, 2002).

'Come-alive' facilities, 'high-dependency' areas and a proliferation of other solutions were characterised by a lack of clinical specialism and an over-reliance on temporary staffing. Young people were not always being well served at a time in their lives and in their treatment journey when they should have been expecting excellence.

Aside from these issues of definition and the lack of recognition of the need for specialist care, in the United Kingdom at least, there has been a gulf between services for children (usually referred to as child and adolescent mental health services [CAMHS]) and adult services. The variation, characterised by differences in thinking and clinical formulation, service models and treatment thresholds, casts a long shadow. This has prompted the transition from CAMHS to adult services to be a priority area for transformation in the Community Mental Health Framework in England (NHSE et al., 2019). Sadly, the stark separation between CAMHS and adult services may have meant that some opportunities for shared learning and improvement have been missed. This perhaps explains why the first set of UK National Standards for PICU for Young People were published 13 years after their adult equivalent.

In England, the responsibility for commissioning PICU services for young people generally sits within different structures to comparable adult services. Where adult services are usually commissioned at the Integrated Care Board (local) level, services for young people fall under the remit of NHS England. The logic of this structure being that numbers of such beds required is comparably lower, hence they are provided in a way to cover a larger geographical area. While NHS units are generally provided in a structure that relates to population needs, independent healthcare providers, who offer a significant amount of the UK bed stock, need to consider other commercial factors such as the availability of affordable estate. This mixed provider landscape means that at the present time, young people needing such care may be placed a very long way from their home, family and friends, with all of the associated challenges that this brings. Having received extensive feedback from young people, their families and carers, the elimination of inappropriate out-of-area placements and improvements in local bed availability are now key goals for NHS England. This has been reflected within the National Implementation Plan (NHS England, 2019). A move to bring commissioning closer home under so-called 'Provider Collaborative' arrangements aims to positively address many of these issues through more local cooperation and partnerships involving both NHS and independent sector units.

These commissioning changes, the provision of a national service specification (NHSE, 2018) and the publication of National Minimum Standards (NAPICU, 2015) all seek to ensure that, rather than allow a growth of ill-defined untested solutions, care is optimised by ensuring it is evidence based and operating to the highest standards.

Admission Criteria

In any unit the description of admission criteria must be very carefully considered, as such specifics define how the unit will operate and what it seeks to achieve. In the case of PICU for young people, perhaps the most important criteria is that the unit must be solely for the care of children as defined in law and in the United Nations Convention on the Rights of the Child (United Nations Children's Fund UK, 1989) which defines a child as 'any person under the age of 18'.

Practitioners familiar with adult psychiatric intensive care may be struck by some particular differences within that specialism. When working with young people, there is generally much greater diagnostic uncertainty. Issues which are more readily identified as psychosis, neurodevelopmental or personality based in later life may not be so easily defined as such in younger people. The condition will often not be fully formed in young people and will be further complicated by the context of other biological and social stressors associated with childhood and adolescence.

Nonetheless, overarching principles which should apply to all mental health care are relevant. These include ensuring that care is always provided in the least restrictive environment possible, that admission decisions are based on thorough clinical and risk assessment and that treatment goals are agreed and clearly defined.

The age range for which most units cater is usually between 12 and 18 years. Developmentally, these six years can represent significant differences in all aspects of the young person's life, in particular physical, psychological and social developmental changes (Christie and Viner, 2005). In light of this, units should give due consideration to the mix of patients on the ward in order to ensure that no individual or group of young people are put at risk or disadvantaged.

Care and Support

Participation, Involvement and Co-production

Placing young people at the centre of decisions about their own care requires a positive culture, not just within the unit, but also through the governance of the whole provider organisation.

This type of approach is generally referred to as 'Co-production' which is defined as 'an ongoing partnership between people who design, deliver and commission services, people who use the services and people who need them' (National Collaborating Centre for Mental Health, 2019). Mayer and McKenzie (2017) found that not only, as widely accepted, did a well-managed co-production approach positively affect social capital, self-esteem, self-efficacy and life skills, but it also fundamentally positively impacted on young people's personal identity structure.

As well as ensuring that individual young people can define their own goals and work with clinicians to develop a plan to achieve them, the PICU should ensure that the collective voice of young people is heard. This is likely to require such mechanisms effective as community meetings, as described by Smith and Hartman (2003), and clear responses to suggestions and feedback.

In a well-functioning young people's PICU, young people should be involved in the leadership by helping select and recruit staff and contributing to staff appraisal and development.

In its staff skill mix, published information and so on, the PICU should ensure cultural competence and demonstrate the range of language and literacy of the young people who use the service.

Pharmacological Interventions

The National Minimum Standards suggest two useful maxims for consideration when prescribing psychotropic medication (NAPICU, 2015). The first is that 'young people are not small adults', that is to say that the nuances of dose size and pharmacokinetics cannot simply being calculated as proportionate to that of a larger adult. Separate formularies such as the British National Formulary for Children (NICE, 2021) exist specifically to address these complexities.

The second piece of advice is to 'start low and go slow' (NAPICU, 2015). Caution is key, as the adverse side effects of many medications should be avoided if a treatment plan is going to be agreeable to the young person and their family.

The highest standards of information provision, physical health monitoring, observation of side effects and symptoms must all be upheld in order to ensure young people are kept safe and effectively treated.

Psychiatric intensive care practice often relies on judicious use of rapid tranquilisation (RT) which is defined as the 'use of medication by the parenteral route (usually intramuscular or, exceptionally, intravenous) if oral medication is not possible or appropriate and urgent sedation with medication is needed' (NICE, 2015). When caring for young people, perceived need for such an intervention can be just as great as in adult services; however, as the Guidelines for the Clinical Management of Acute Disturbance: De-escalation and Rapid Tranquillisation (Patel et al., 2018) note, there is a paucity of evidence to support how this should be undertaken. The principles described in the National Minimum Standards (NAPICU, 2015) should be considered by any clinician who is considering such an intervention.

Psychological Support

Consistent with any restrictive environment, the purpose of treatment within a PICU for young people should be to rapidly get to a state where they can continue their treatment journey in a service with greater freedoms.

The multidisciplinary team (MDT) should work with the young person and their family to agree on a plan which upholds the key principles characterised in the "SMART" mnemonic; goals should be Systematic,

Measurable, Attainable, Realistic and Timely (Doran, 1981). It is likely that the young person will benefit from a plan which emerges from an agreed formulation, and this may require different disciplines to contribute using their professional knowledge and expertise.

A predominance of emotional dysregulation and associated lack of behavioural self-control amongst young people requiring inpatient admission has prompted the development of dialectical behaviour therapy (DBT) practice within the specialism. Flynn et al. (2019) describe how this model has a demonstrable efficacy amongst this population and, given the likely continued prevalence of such presentations, the model seems set to be core to the offer within any PICU caring for young people. Some units may go so far as to base their entire therapeutic approach around this model and its theories.

The current paucity of research into therapeutic interventions within the PICU for young people begs questions of how the evidence base for the specialism can be urgently developed.

Recognising that psychological support is not the sole responsibility of one discipline but within the remit of the whole MDT, research by Foster and Smedley (2019) analysed the range of interventions offered to young people in a PICU by mental health nurses. They found that they generally fell into one of seven broad categories:

- Emotional containment
- Communication
- Attachment
- Personal qualities and self-management
- Furnishing with skill
- Environmental
- Managing and modulating risk

The research reinforces the critical role that mental health nurses play within PICU therapeutic provision and provides an indication of what skill set should be present or developed within such units.

Educational Provision

One of the chief distinctions between an adult PICU and a unit for young people is the need for education to be part of the routine of the service. In the United Kingdom, young people must receive an education until they are 16 years old and, even when unwell, adjustments should be made in order that learning can continue.

In practice this means that all inpatient services for young people including PICU must have access to suitable personnel and resources. This may be particularly important when lengths of stay become extended.

The logistics of providing holistic education within a PICU cannot be underestimated; provision can be according to different structures and can be quite variable (Department for Education, 2018). Consideration should be given to distinct dedicated space; information technology and the hours of operation must work in union with healthcare assessment and intervention. The need for education does also provide an opportunity for multidisciplinary, person-centred, planning to ensure that the young person's own aims of what they wish to achieve in terms of education and treatment can, as far as possible, align.

A final consideration is that of regulatory compliance and ensuring that in addition to meeting the standards laid down by healthcare regulators such as the Care Quality Commission (CQC), education regulators such as the Office for Standards in Education, Children's Services and Skills (OfSted) are satisfied. Including both agencies in the design and commissioning process is likely to reduce the possibility of problems later.

Restrictive Interventions

A common misconception in the specialism of PICU is that the expertise is borne out of enhanced training and environmental resources to restrict and contain people. The paradox is, of course, that when done well, the efforts of everyone involved in delivering the intensive care are invested in avoiding the use of those very restrictions. This simple flipping of logic turns the concept of a 'lock-up' ward, which patients would rightly dread, into a wholesome, therapeutic space in which distress can be eased. The Restraint Reduction Network's (2021) scope of what constitutes a restrictive intervention includes:

- Physical
- Environmental (seclusion/long term segregation)
- Mechanical (e.g. cuffs/splints)
- Chemical (e.g. PRN and routine chemical restraints)
- Psycho-social (e.g. coercion/bullying)
- Other restrictive practices – includes a broader range of practices that also negatively impact on quality of life (e.g. institutional models of care)

This relative breadth of what is considered restrictive is a sobering reminder to PICU practitioners that they exercise enormous responsibility in the lives of young people. They must always seek to maximise what is considered therapeutic and only use that which is restrictive for the minimum possible time and only when absolutely essential.

Recent decades have seen considerable changes in perceived acceptability of restrictive interventions. Practice which was commonplace not long ago, such as 'pain-compliance' (the application of pain during restraint in order to compel someone to behave differently), are now an anathema in the models of restraint in health and custodial settings responsible for children and young people (Taylor, 2020). It must be hoped that this progress continues not only on ethical grounds but because there is little to support its use in the evidence.

All PICUs for young people should have a designated restraint reduction leader within their organisational hierarchy and there must be multidisciplinary programme, co-produced with young people, aimed at improving practice in the area.

Anyone working in institutional mental health care is well advised to understand the concept of the 'total institution' (Goffman, 1961), and be reminded that much of that which has the pretence of being part of the therapeutic regime can actually be considered to be unnecessarily restrictive. The Mental Health Act Code of Practice (Department of Health, 2015) suggests that 'blanket restrictions' exist when rules or policies are applied in the absence consideration of individual risk assessment. The most effective PICUs for young people will be able to demonstrate a holistic approach to care which dispenses with such restrictions and focuses on a pathway of support towards the least restrictive environment and, ultimately, the young person flourishing within the community.

The nature of institutions means that there is a risk of institutional abuse of all types. The scale of this problem is difficult to assess and is mainly performed by studying serious case reviews and other inquiry reports; the use of unnecessary restrictions amounting to abuse is not quantified anywhere. In 2021, the organisation Article 39 undertook a freedom of information investigation in England. It found that, on average, there were 32 allegations against adults working in young people's care settings per local authority area per year (Article 39, 2021). While the outcomes of these cases are not known, the numbers indicate that further improvements are required for the sake of young people and those who care for them.

The potential for institutional mechanisms to become abusive is clear and is a risk as old as the concept of institutions themselves. For this reason, the management of restrictive interventions much receive the closest possible attention.

Legal and Associated Considerations

The legal means under which young people are treated in a PICU will vary from country to country. That said, the law as applied in England and Wales may be representative of many of the issues which arise internationally.

The primary legal distinction compared to adult PICU is the role of parents. As part of the admission process, those with parental responsibility must be accurately identified so that they can be appropriately involved in decisions about the young person's care.

There are separate considerations where a young person is the responsibility of a local authority/government. Parents of course do not have absolute rights over their children; it is easy to imagine how, in the complex psychology of a PICU admission, disagreements can emerge. In English and Welsh law, a child's right to make decisions about their own medical treatment is considered in the context of their capacity. This is perhaps best summarised in Lord Scarman's ruling as follows (often referred to as 'Gillick competence') (United Kingdom House of Lords, 1985):

> As a matter of Law the parental right to determine whether or not their minor child below the age of sixteen will have medical treatment terminates if and when the child achieves sufficient understanding and intelligence to understand fully what is proposed.

PICU practitioners are likely to find themselves regularly involved in complex decision-making where the young person's wishes and capacity, parental preferences, clinical opinion and mental health legislation all intersect in informing treatment decisions.

The Mental Health Act 1983, while specific to England and Wales, publishes a Code of Practice (Department of Health, 2015) which contains guidelines, which could inform young people's mental health care anywhere. These include principles of:

- Best interests
- Welfare

- Personal preferences
- Least restriction
- Being close to home
- Access to education
- Dignity
- Privacy and confidentiality

National Standards and Future Developments

Having identified a lack of clarity around the definitions and provision for the emerging discipline of PICU for young people, in 2015 the National Association for Psychiatric Intensive Care and Low Secure Units (NAPICU) published its National Minimum Standards (NAPICU, 2015). These standards represent the first attempt to describe best practice within such services and aim to reduce unwarranted variation, which occurs when services are allowed to develop without reference to each other.

There continues to be a paucity of research into the specialism, and practitioners should be encouraged to seek to investigate and report innovative practice in the expectation of advancing the evidence base. While the evidence base is slim, related areas such as acute mental health units for young people and adult PICU can offer valuable perspectives on the opportunities to further improve care.

Innovation, although welcome, is best undertaken with reference to the best available published expertise such as the National Minimum Standards or similar work such as the Quality Network for Inpatient CAMHS Standards (Royal College of Psychiatrists, 2021). Young people requiring PICU are the most vulnerable amongst us, therefore great care must be taken to ensure that developments in practice reflect their best interests and not other less worthy motivations such as free market principles or a complex commissioning environment.

Case vignette

Frankie is a 16-year-old in the care of foster parents who has been in receipt of CAMH services for 10 years. The working formulation within her community team is complex and involves emotional dysregulation, mood (affective) components and possible autistic spectrum condition. There have been several incidents of self-harm that have required hospital attendance, including overnight stays.

One Friday evening after an episode of significant distress, her foster parents find her unrousable with a ligature around her neck. She is taken to hospital by ambulance, and during the journey, she attempts to exit the vehicle on several occasions. At the emergency department, it is clear that her physical injuries are minor, and while waiting for the liaison team to assess, she leaves the unit, knocking a health care assistant to the ground as she goes.

A police constable on duty at the hospital exercises his powers under Section 136 of the MHA and, after consultation with the liaison team, she is taken to a Health Based-Place of Safety (HBPoS). The physical and procedural restrictions of the HBPoS prove more compounding for the situation and her self-harm behaviour escalates further. After an assessment under the Mental Health Act (1983) she is detained under Section 2 and transferred to the local CAMHS unit.

Despite some initial settling of problematic behaviour, the busyness of the environment prompts a further escalation of self-harm, antagonising other young people and attempts to abscond. A gatekeeping assessment for the PICU concludes that the less populated environment, access to quiet spaces and higher nursing ratio may mean that a transfer could be beneficial.

The PICU clinical model is based on the principles of Dialectical Behaviour Therapy. Whilst reluctant initially, some successful rapport building by her named nurse enables Frankie to accept that the clinical team may have some support that may help her. After extensive 1:1 work over the first few days with her named nurse, occupational therapist and psychologist, she agrees to join the daily group programme and attends regularly.

While on the PICU, her emotional dysregulation continues; episodes are usually associated with difficult interactions with others, often relating to contacts from home or issues to do with education. Initially, the team try several tactics to contain this; using a debriefing approach after a difficult instance which culminated in physical restraint, a shared care plan is developed. As trust and confidence builds, the destructive nature of the behaviour associated with it reduces. Her greater self-awareness also means that, for the first time, she will consider working with someone to establish whether autism is a viable diagnosis.

After six weeks, Frankie's transfer is carefully managed back to the acute ward, from where, after a further two weeks, she returns to her foster home with daily visits from the CAMHS intensive team. She becomes a regular attender at the community DBT group and is soon able to use her own experiences to speak positively to other young people.

Conclusion

The specialism of PICU for young people is still a relatively new one. This chapter has identified some of the key considerations for those working in such a unit. The recognition that PICU for young people are not exactly comparable to adult PICUs and need to be distinct from other admission wards for young people is key in ensuring that services are developed optimally and that appropriate research and practice development are undertaken.

One principle which is consistent in all branches of inpatient mental healthcare is that of 'least restriction'. It must be hoped that in further developing and improving PICU for young people clinical practice, a context emerges in which young people are only placed in such environments when all other options have been excluded and that due to the quality of service available, the young people's clinical presentation improves as swiftly as possible so that they can move to a less restrictive care setting.

References

Article 39 (2021) *Abuse in Children's Institutional Settings: How Much is Known?* https://article39.org.uk/wp-content/uploads/2021/12/Abuse-in-institutional-settings-how-much-is-known-2021-Final-15-Dec-2021.pdf.

Christie,D and Viner,R (2005) Adolescent Development. *British Medical Journal* **330** (7486) 301–4.

Department for Education (2018) *Education in Inpatient Children and Young People's Mental Health Services: Research Report.* London: Department for Education.

Department of Health (2002) *National Minimum Standards for General Adult Services in Psychiatric Intensive Care Units (PICU) and Low Secure Environments* London: Department of Health.

Department of Health (2015) *The Mental Health Act 1983: Code of Practice 2015.* London: Department of Health.

Doran,GT (1981) There's a S.M.A.R.T. Way to Write Management's Goals and Objectives. *Management Review* **70** 35–6.

Flynn,D, Kells,M, Joyce,M, Corcoran,P, Gillespie,C, Suarez, C, et al. (2019) Innovations in Practice: Dialectical Behaviour Therapy for Adolescents: Multisite Implementation and Evaluation of a 16-Week Programme in a Public Community Mental Health Setting. *Child and Adolescent Mental Health* **24** (1) 76–83.

Foster,C and Smedley,K (2019) Understanding the Nature of Mental Health Nursing Within CAMHS PICU: 1. Identifying Nursing Interventions That Contribute to the Recovery Journey of Young People. *Journal of Psychiatric Intensive Care* **15** (2) 87–102.

Goffman,E (1961) *Asylums: Essays on the Social Situation of Mental Patients and Other Inmates.* New York: Anchor Books.

Mayer,C and McKenzie,K (2017) '. . . It Shows That There's No Limits': The Psychological Impact of Co-Production for Experts by Experience Working in Youth Mental Health. *Health and Social Care in the Community* **25**: 1181–9.

National Association of Psychiatric Intensive Care and Low Secure Units (NAPICU) (2015) *National Minimum Standards for Psychiatric Intensive Care Units for Young People.* Glasgow: NAPICU. https://napicu.org.uk/wp-content/uploads/2014/08 /CAMHS_PICU_NMS_final_Aug_2015_cx.pdf.

National Collaborating Centre for Mental Health (2019) *Working Well Together: Evidence and Tools to Enable Co-production in Mental Health Commissioning.* London: National Collaborating Centre for Mental Health.

NHS England (2018) *Service Specification: Tier 4 CAMHS Psychiatric Intensive Care Unit (PICU).* www.england.nhs .uk/wp-content/uploads/2018/02/camhs-psychiatric-inten sive-care-unit-service-specification-v2.pdf.

NHS England (2019) *NHS Mental Health Implementation Plan 2019/20 – 2023/24.* www.longtermplan.nhs.uk/wp-co ntent/uploads/2019/07/nhs-mental-health-implementa tion-plan-2019-20-2023-24.pdf.

NHS England and NHS Improvement and the National Collaborating Centre for Mental Health (2019) *The Community Mental Health Framework for Adults and Older Adults.* www.england.nhs.uk/wp-content/uploads/2019/09/ community-mental-health-framework-for-adults-and-older-adults.pdf.

National Institute for Health and Care Excellence (NICE) (2015) *Violence and Aggression: Short-Term Management in Mental Health, Health and Community Settings.* London: NICE.

National Institute for Health and Care Excellence (NICE) (2021) BNF for Children. www.pharmaceuticalpress.com/ products/bnf-for-children/.

Patel,MX, Sethi,FN, Re Barnes,T, Dix,R, Dratcu,L, Fox,B, et al. (2018) Joint BAP NAPICU Evidence-Based Consensus Guidelines for the Clinical Management of Acute Disturbance: De-Escalation and Rapid Tranquillisation. *Journal of Psychopharmacology* **32**(6) 601–40.

Restraint Reduction Network (2021) Our Scope. https://res traintreductionnetwork.org/about

Royal College of Psychiatrists (2021) Quality Network for Inpatient CAMHS Standards for Services Eleventh Edition. www.rcpsych.ac.uk/docs/default-source/improving-care/cc qi/quality-networks/child-and-adolescent-inpatient-ser vices-(cahms)/qnic-standards-11th-ed.pdf? sfvrsn=ab861d11_4.

Smith,L and Hartman,D (2003) Implementing a Community Group on an Adolescent Psychiatric Intensive Care Unit. *Mental Health Practice* **6** (5) 14–17.

Taylor,C (2020) *A Review of the Use of Pain-Inducing Techniques in the Youth Secure Estate.* https://assets.pub lishing.service.gov.uk/government/uploads/system/upload s/attachment_data/file/893193/charlie-taylors-review-pain-inducing-techniques.pdf.

United Kingdom House of Lords (1985) Gillick Respondent and West Norfolk and Wisbech Area Health Authority First Appellants and Department of Health and Social Security Second Appellants. www.bailii.org/uk/cas es/UKHL/1985/7.html.

United Nations Children's Fund UK (1989) *The United Nations Convention on the Rights of the Child.* New York: United Nations.

Female-Only PICUs

Joana Ferreira Marques de Paiva and Shanika Balachandra

Introduction

A psychiatric intensive care unit (PICU) is defined as a ward with higher levels of staff per patient, responsible for managing and caring for patients experiencing an acute deterioration of their mental health and displaying symptoms and behaviours that cannot be safely managed in an acute psychiatric setting, namely, aggression to themselves or others (Brown et al., 2008). They tend to be locked wards with seclusion facilities for the most aggressive and agitated patients (Bowers et al., 2008).

When PICUs were first designed, they were mixed wards, meaning they had both male and female patients, like other psychiatric inpatient settings. However, over the years, single-sex PICUs began to emerge as research started showing that men and women had different characteristics and needs that could not be equally accommodated on a mixed ward.

This chapter focuses specifically on female PICUs and why they were created, reports on some female-specific characteristics of such wards and describes some of the special provisions that are in place for women accessing mental health services in the United Kingdom.

History and Development of Female PICUs

In the United Kingdom, PICUs were created in the 1990s and they were mixed-sex wards. Studies of those PICU populations over the years showed that the majority of service users were men (as much as 85% of admissions, according to some studies) Brown et al., 2008; O'Brien et al., 2013; Archer et al., 2016), in their 20s and 30s (Cullen et al., 2018) and most frequently diagnosed with acute psychosis, particularly schizophrenia (Brown et al., 2008; O'Brien et al., 2013). Also, Black, Asian and minority ethnic (BAME) backgrounds, particularly Black ethnicities,

were overrepresented (Bowers et al., 2008; Brown et al., 2008), and these men were more likely to be unemployed, to have past and/or current history of drug/alcohol misuse, of significant abuse/violent behaviour and damage to property, and to not be in an intimate relationship (Brown et al., 2008; Cullen et al., 2018). Table 23.1 shows characteristics from three of the mentioned studies.

These findings demonstrated the overall greater need for male PICU beds than female ones. It also meant that research conducted on PICUs, along with treatment and management approaches, were created based on a majority male population and findings were generalised to women service users. This was based on the held belief at the time that women were not a 'special group' but part of the mainstream and, therefore, should be treated accordingly (Satel, 1998). Regarding PICUs more specifically, with the clear majority of its service users being men, the question of whether the number of women requiring intensive care admission was enough to justify their own female-only PICU wards was a contentious topic.

With the turn of the millennium, concerns started being raised that women accessing mental health services did not have the same characteristics and needs as those of men and, therefore, they were not receiving appropriate care (Archer et al., 2016). Kohen (2001), for example, argued that psychiatric services had failed to consider that women suffer from certain gender-specific mental illnesses such as postpartum depression and psychosis and that by using mainstream approaches to psychiatric care, mental health services were dismissing important factors that could affect the management and outcomes of treatment for women. The authors pointed out that women had higher incidence and prevalence of depression, generalised anxiety disorder (GAD), panic attacks, deliberate self-harm (DSH), dysthymia and seasonal affective disorders. The Department of Health (Department of

Table 23.1 Summary of some of the demographic characteristics of the cohort of patients studied in three research articles.

Variable	Brown et al. (2008) – Prospective survey of patient demographics at seven English PICUs	O'Brien et al. (2013) – Admissions to the two PICUs at South West London and St George's MH NHS Trust for 1 year (April 2009 – March 2010)	Cullen et al. (2018) – Demographic data of patients admitted to PICUs at SLaM NHS Foundation Trust over five years (April 2008 – April 2013)
Gender (%)			
Male	78.5	84.6	74
Female	21.5	15.4	26
Mean Age (years)	35	38	25 – 34
Ethnicity (%)			
Caucasian	74	58	28
Black	18	31	63
Asian/Other	8	11	9
Diagnosis (%)			
Schizophrenia	55	53	36
Affective disorder	24	26	27
Drug-induced psychosis	5	8	-
Personality disorder	5	5	3
Other	8	8	9

Health, as cited in Archer et al., 2016) also mentioned that aspects of safety, privacy and dignity for women were not being considered by mental health services and therefore psychiatric treatments were providing a disservice to this population.

Such arguments lead to a growing interest in studying the female population accessing mental health services, including in PICU settings.

Brown et al. (2008) studied the population of seven different PICUs in England over a period of approximately a year and a half and reported on obvious gender differences that were identified. He found that women tended to be slightly older than their male counterparts (34–36 years old at time of admission), were more likely to be in a relationship and less likely to have history of substance/alcohol misuse, but were more likely to engage in DSH (although these incidences were not more severe than those of male patients) and to have a primary diagnosis of personality disorder (PD), whereas they were less likely to have diagnosis of schizophrenia.

O'Brien et al. (2013), who studied the population of two PICU wards at the South West London and St

George's Mental Health NHS Trust over a period of one year, also concluded that women were more likely to have a diagnosis of PD and prolonged admissions when compared to men (mean length of stay in a PICU of 83.9 days for women compared to 35.3 days for men).

Archer et al. (2016) conducted a literature review of the female population of PICUs and low secure units (LSUs) and reported that women tended to have fewer convictions but more mental health admissions when compared to men, were more likely to have been admitted from another hospital rather than prison, were more likely to have diagnosis of PD (particularly emotionally unstable PD [EUPD]) and depression, and were less likely to misuse substances. They were also more likely to have other mental health comorbidities, such as eating and anxiety disorders (Coid et al., 2000, as cited in Archer et al., 2016) and of having history of physical and sexual abuse in the past (Long et al., 2001). Contrary to their male counterparts, they were more likely to be in a relationship at time of admission.

Regarding their treatment needs, women appeared to respond better to being in a stimulating and structured environment where there was a routine to their day with activities to keep them occupied throughout. Patients' relationship with the staff was emphasised as an important factor for recovery, and patients stressed the importance of feeling heard, understood and respected by all team members. In terms of management of risks in PICU environment, women appeared to present with significantly higher levels of aggression towards themselves and others and to be more likely to require seclusion and be prescribed mood stabilisers.

Balachandra and Benson (2014) studied the PICU population at St Charles Hospital, part of the Central and North West London NHS Trust in London that has both male and female-only wards. They reported that the female PICU population tended to exhibit more incidents of DSH and violence towards others, which translated to a significantly greater use of both oral and intra-muscular (IM) rapid tranquilisation (RT) on the female ward, along with stricter requirements for the use of physical restraint when administering RT to women.

This research showed that, despite the fact women make up a minority of PICU admissions, they do have their own specific mental health issues, needs and expectations that cannot be met in a mixed PICU ward, validating the need for gender-specific PICUs.

In the United Kingdom, there are currently between 20 and 30 female-only PICUs (NAPICU, 2016). They have only been around for about one decade, meaning they are still a relatively new mental health service and therefore ongoing research needs to be conducted so that women continue to receive the best quality of care in a PICU setting.

Gender-Specific Considerations for Female PICUs

A pervasive problem mentioned by most women accessing mental health services is that they suffer from a lack of self-esteem and confidence. This does not simply translate to women feeling uncomfortable about their bodies and physical appearance; it is more pervasive than that. The lack of self-esteem leads to many women believing that they are not capable of caring for themselves and/or of getting better, which, in extreme cases, leads to feelings of worthlessness and hopelessness about their futures.

There are also certain life pressures that disproportionately affect women, such as the pressure to get married while one is still relatively young (a fact that is more prevalent within certain cultures), the expectation to have children and be a good mother and pressure to conform to the ideal of normality that exists within the cultural sphere that one is brought up in. Therefore, having a mental illness might cause strained family relationships, strain in a marriage and even impact on a woman's assessment of their role as a mother.

From a female PICU perspective, all these factors play a role in the management of patients and need to be addressed as part of a wider treatment plan for each individual woman. PICUs offer a myriad of ward groups and activities, including music groups, art groups, reading groups, dancing groups, beauty groups, cooking sessions and psychology sessions. The purpose of all these is severalfold; having different daily activities allows women to pick and choose the ones they like and offers a routine to their day and an escape from the medicalised ward environment they are in. These activities/groups are also a safe space and, at times, the only way that many women find to be able to express themselves, when they struggle to do so verbally. The groups are also designed to help support women's self-esteem, where they are encouraged to attend and engage in the activities in meaningful ways and receive positive feedback for their achievements, however small. In beauty groups, for example, women get to have their hair cared for, makeup applied and/or receive a manicure or pedicure. However small and 'superficial' this group might sound, being able to feel that their outer appearance is beautiful and matches their inner self a bit more can go a long way in raising women's self-esteem and encourage their compliance with their pharmacological treatment. This is particularly important given that most psychotropic medication is associated with side effects that are considered by a lot of women as unacceptable, such as weight gain and hair loss.

PICUs also have occupational therapists (OTs) that not only help organise and manage a number of these activities but are also responsible for assessing patients' capacity to complete activities of daily living (ADLs). OTs also provide support to those women that have difficulties in some of these areas while in an inpatient setting so that they can be better prepared for life after discharge.

PICUs also offer psychological support. This is a space where women can start talking about past and current trauma, develop coping mechanisms for managing stress and anger management skills and work further on their self-esteem.

Postpartum Acute Presentations

The perinatal period, identified by the World Health Organization (WHO, 2010) as time from pregnancy up to one year after delivery of the baby, is associated with a significant risk for women to develop a mental health illness, either as a first psychiatric presentation or severe recurrence of previous mental illness (Griffiths et al., 2019). It includes the postpartum period, which is the time from delivery of the baby to six weeks after birth. As many as 20% of woman will develop mental health difficulties during this period and four in 1000 will require inpatient admission to a psychiatric facility (Gillham and Wittkowski, 2015).

There are three main postpartum presentations: maternal 'blues', postpartum depression and postpartum psychosis. Only the last two are considered acute presentations.

Maternal 'Blues'

Maternal 'blues' commonly begin within the first couple of days after delivery and are characterised by feelings of fatigue, tearfulness and depressed affect. It affects 50%–85% of women after delivery (Le et al., 2015), but the symptoms tend to be mild and usually self-resolve within 10 days. Management is supportive, including routine follow-up by midwives and family support.

Postpartum Depression (PPD)

Postpartum depression (PPD) refers to a non-psychotic depressive episode characterised by depressed mood, anhedonia, social withdrawal, lack of motivation and somatic symptoms (loss of libido, weight loss and anorexia or weight gain and hyperphagia, low energy and sleep disturbances such as insomnia or hypersomnia) that represent a significant change from normal behaviour and cause impairment of functioning, lasting for a minimum of two weeks (Robertson et al., 2003; Sadock and Sadock, 2010). PPD is therefore defined as major depression that occurs during the postpartum period and affects 10%–13% of new mothers (Sit et al., 2006).

Diagnosing PPD is paramount because women often experience feelings of worthlessness, inability to think or concentrate and guilt associated with intrusive thoughts of wanting to harm their baby, of being a bad mother and of thinking about death and/or suicide (Doucet et al., 2009).

There are a few documented risk factors associated with increased risk of development of PPD, such as previous diagnosis of PPD or depression, absence of close relationships, feelings of depression or anxiety during pregnancy, being from low-income social strata and rapid return to work (Murray et al., 2003).

Management of PPD is similar to treatment of major depression, including antidepressants and psychological interventions. Many women request non-pharmacological treatments, such as cognitive behavioural therapy (CBT), interpersonal psychotherapy and psychodynamic therapy, due to concerns of transferring medication to their baby through breastfeeding (Doucet et al., 2009). However, most patients require a combination of the two. Side effects of medication are the same as for non-breastfeeding women.

In terms of prognosis, women tend to have a prolonged course of PPD due to late diagnosis, but once treatment is commenced, recovery usually occurs within 12 weeks, with 25% of patients developing a future major depressive episode outside the postpartum period and around 41% developing PPD in a subsequent pregnancy (Doucet et al., 2009).

Postpartum Psychosis (PPP)

Postpartum psychosis (PPP) is characterised by early (within two to three days after delivery) and sudden onset of mood swings, delusional thinking (including paranoid, grandiose and bizarre delusions), thought disorder, severe confusion and grossly disorganised behaviour that represent a dramatic change from previous normal functioning; PPD affects one to two women in 1000 (Sit et al., 2006). Even though PPP has been classified as severe depression and delusions (Sadock et al., 2010), a significant body of research proposed that PPP actually represents an episode of bipolar affective disorder (BPAD) triggered by childbirth (Murray et al., 2003; Sit et al., 2006; Doucet et al., 2009).

Women usually start by developing mood disturbances, from mania to significant mood swings, closely followed by onset of psychotic symptoms such as thought broadcast/withdrawal/insertion, paranoid/persecutory or bizarre delusions, delusion of grandeur and reference and visual or command auditory hallucinations to hurt oneself or the baby (Doucet et al., 2009).

The main risk factor for development of PPP is a previous episode of PPP (incidence of one in seven women) and diagnosis of BPAD or schizoaffective disorder, particularly if these women stop their mood stabilisers during pregnancy (Sit et al., 2006).

As with PPD, PPP requires quick diagnosis and treatment, as it is associated with a 70-fold increase risk of maternal suicide, increased risk of harming others due to fear that baby will be taken away and risk of neonaticide (Sit et al., 2006).

PPP is a psychiatric emergency. Consequently, women suffering from it generally require inpatient management, whether in an acute ward, a mother-and-baby unit (MBU) or even in a PICU setting (Bergink et al., 2016). First-line treatment is pharmacological with mood stabilisers, particularly lithium (Bergink et al., 2012), antipsychotics and electroconvulsive therapy (ECT) (Bergink et al., 2016).

Generally speaking, there is an overall good prognosis for women with PPP, with more than 75% of them having only one episode of PPP and remaining symptom free afterwards (Protheroe, 1969, as cited in Sit et al., 2006).

Risks for Mother and Baby of Acute Postnatal Presentations

Mental illness during postpartum period can have significant impacts for the mother, the baby and their relationship. Maternal mental illness is associated with a twofold increased risk of foetal death or stillbirth, inability of the mother to detect cues from the baby, inadequate breastfeeding, marked behavioural problems and lower IQ of their children at four years and increase risk of maternal self-harm, maternal suicide, infanticide and even neonaticide (Murray et al., 2003; Sit et al., 2006; Elkin et al., 2009).

Positive Outcomes for Mother and Baby of Prompt Treatment of Postpartum Acute Presentations

Currently, recommendations for women with postpartum disorders that require inpatient admission aim to keep the baby with the mother whenever possible in MBUs, unless there are specific reasons for not doing so (Stephenson et al., 2018). These are specialised units that provide joint admissions of mothers and babies for inpatient treatment and monitoring of the mother–infant relationship. BMUs provide individualised treatment programmes from a multidisciplinary team (MDT), including antenatal and postnatal care for mother and baby, management of maternal mental illness and physical health, pharmacological interventions for pregnant and breastfeeding women, developmental assessment of babies, psychological therapies, occupational therapy and support for mothers to develop independent living skills and assessment of and assistance with social needs.

According to Stephenson et al. (2018), women that were admitted to MBUs with a postpartum illness had significant improvement in their mental health symptoms and their relationship with their babies. In addition, their ability to understand and appropriately respond to their babies' cues also improved significantly.

MBUs are not just available for women with PPP. Women with established severe and enduring mental illnesses (such as schizophrenia and BPAD) who experience or are at high risk of relapse during the perinatal period, women with other psychiatric conditions (such as anxiety disorder or obsessive-compulsive disorder) whose symptoms become disabling in the perinatal period and women with bonding or attachment difficulties secondary to maternal mental illness are also treated in BMUs (McKay, 2022; RCPsych, 2018).

However, not all perinatal maternal mental illness can be managed in an MBU. Women denied access to such a unit usually include women who have very aggressive behaviour that might pose a risk of harm or injury to their own or other babies, women with severe learning disability or substance misuse who do not have a comorbid severe enduring mental illness, women who are not capable of independently caring for their infant even with reasonable support (such as women who need to live in supported accommodation) and women who just need an assessment of their ability to parent, but who do not need treatment for a serious or complex mental illness.

For those women who cannot access MBUs but still require inpatient care given the severity of their mental illness, placement in acute psychiatric wards, such as PICUs, is the alternative. They cannot have their baby with them, but the aim of the admission is similar, which is to treat the mental illness and return the mother to her baby as quickly and as safely as possible.

Provision for Special Family Needs Including Access to Children and Infants

Many women admitted to mental health units, including PICUs, have children. Therefore, PICU staff must be well aware of safeguarding procedures and work closely with MBUs, perinatal services, child and family services (CFS) and child and family court (CFC) to ensure the welfare of children from mothers admitted to the intensive care ward.

As PICUs are not like MBUs, children are invariably separated from their mother. Therefore, a big role of PICU staff is to work closely and in partnership with CFS to ensure that mothers and children can keep in touch as much as possible.

Provisions for mothers and children to meet need to be in place, as PICUs are not an environment that any child should be exposed to. Mothers should therefore have access to a family room within the psychiatric hospital premises so they can safely see their children face to face when they are well enough and when it is safe to do so under appropriate staff supervision.

It is important for PICU staff to understand that many women admitted to mental health units have had or will have children taken away from them. This is particularly common in women admitted to PICUs. Certain dates or times of the year can, therefore, be triggers for woman and lead to deterioration/relapse in their mental health, and staff need to keep this in mind and be sympathetic and empathetic towards the patients. This is also one of the main reasons why it is important to support these patients in engaging with psychology to discuss such situations, as they can affect their mental health for years to come.

Clinical Considerations for Comorbidity with Personality Disorders

Personality disorders are inflexible and enduring patterns of behaviour in response to different personal and social situations, which are ' . . . extreme or significant deviations from the way in which the average individual in a given culture perceives, thinks, feels and, particularly, relates to others' and often cause subjective distress and problems in social functioning (WHO, 1992).

Dissocial personality disorder (DPD), also known as antisocial PD is characterised by 'disregard for social obligations, and callous unconcern for the feelings of others (. . .) low tolerance to frustration, a low threshold for discharge of aggression (. . .) and a tendency to blame others' (WHO, 1992).

EUPD, also known as borderline PD, is characterised by a 'definite tendency to act impulsively and without consideration of the consequences; the mood is unpredictable and capricious. There is a liability to outbursts of emotion and an incapacity to control the behavioural explosions. There is a tendency to quarrelsome behaviour and to conflicts with others, especially when impulsive acts are thwarted or censored' (WHO, 1992).

Both DPD and EUPD are prevalent diagnoses within the population accessing mental health services. EUPD is much more prevalent in women (71%–73% of diagnoses) and affects 10% of outpatient and 20% of inpatient psychiatric patients, versus only 1% of the general population (Widiger and Weissman, 1991; Linehan and Heard, 1999). It also one of the most common psychiatric diagnoses in female prisoners (Singleton et al., 1998).

DPD is very prevalent in the prison populations, being diagnosed in 63% of male remand prisoners, 49% of sentenced men and 31% of female prisoners (Singleton et al., 1998).

Both disorders are linked to higher rates of mental disorder, such as anxiety, depression and substance abuse disorders (Moran, 1999; Trull et al., 2000).

Management of EUPD

Current guidelines recommend that patients with a diagnosis of EUPD should be managed in the community by specialised PD services that can offer patients the adequate management and support they require (NICE, 2009; Stapleton and Wright, 2019; Gintalaite-Bieliauskiene et al., 2020). Evidence for treatment is based on psychological interventions, with dialectical behavioural therapy (DBT) and group therapy having the most statistically significant positive effects on these cohort of patients (Lied et al., 2014). Pharmacological therapies have a role in management of crisis but have not shown consistent therapeutic benefit in the long run.

However, patients with EUPD may occasionally require admission to a mental health facility, usually in context of a period of crisis, when risk of significant self-harm or suicide cannot be safely managed in the community (Gintalaite-Bieliauskiene et al., 2020). As per NICE Quality Standards guidelines (NICE, 2013), such admissions should be pre-agreed between the patient and all care teams involved and have as main aims to provide a safe environment for patients, manage the crisis, stabilise the patients and prepare them for quick return back to the community. The rationale against prolonged admissions stems from patients' poor coping skills to deal with past traumas and life stressors. When in hospital, engaging in self-harming behaviour or threatening/attempting suicide can lead to feelings of 'reward' by the increased nursing care and supervision patients receive, which reinforces their maladaptive coping mechanisms and can lead them to regress in their behaviour (Livesley, 2003; Steinert et al., 2010). According to Paris (2004), another problem with inpatient admissions for this cohort of patients is that they may start seeking hospital admission as yet another unhelpful coping strategy when they cannot cope with stress and 'even if suicidality is reduced by admission, (...) patients often continue to have chronic suicidal ideation after discharge'.

Patients diagnosed with EUPD tend to have long history of contact with mental health services and multiple and prolonged admissions, including to PICU wards (Gintalaite-Bieliauskiene et al., 2020). Even though a significant number engage in self-harming behaviours (Gintalaite-Bieliauskiene et al., 2020), and about 9%–10% of those that threaten suicide are successful (Stone; Paris & Zweig-Frank, as cited in Paris, 2004), overall their outcomes are positive, with 75% patients requiring inpatient admissions experiencing remission of their symptoms within six years of follow-up (Zanarini et al., 2003).

From a practical point of view, many women with a diagnosis of EUPD in crisis end up being admitted to a female PICU due to the high perceived risks to self and others. However, female PICUs are very acute wards, where the environment is often chaotic and distressing and therefore not conducive to the kind of management required by EUPD patients. The literature has also showed that a significant number of mental health professionals have negative stereotypical views of EUPD patients, often times described as difficult and manipulative individuals who are actually in control of their behaviours and use them for attention seeking (Woollaston and Hixenbaugh, 2008;

Bodner et al., 2011), which has contributed to a degree of suboptimal care of these patients, particularly in wards where work pressures and time restraints are a particular burden (Weight and Kendal, 2013).

Strategies used by PICU wards to provide EUPD patients with the support, containment and routine that they require to manage their crises include segregating patients to reduce their expose to a chaotic ward environment, creation of behavioural plans around maladaptive stress responses, access to psychological therapies and encouragement to engage in ward activities and groups in order to maintain a daily routine while ensuring clear and continual communication between patients and staff. Along with the daily interactions with patients, PICU teams also maintain regular contact with patients' community teams to achieve the goals for admission set by NICE.

Management of DPD

There is limited evidence-based treatment for DPD. Interventions used focus on different areas, from management of the personality disorder to treating comorbid disorders, such as depression, anxiety or substance abuse, and managing symptoms and behaviours associated with DPD such as impulsivity and aggression (NICE, 2009).

Pharmacological options can be used in patients with other psychiatric comorbidities such as anxiety and depression. Use of medication in these cases should be in line with guidelines for the treatment of such conditions. There is no evidence for use of medication solely for the purpose of managing DPD symptoms.

Psychological interventions, such as group-based cognitive and behavioural interventions, can help address emotional dysregulation, impulsive and aggressive behaviours and help reduce offending behaviour. Such interventions should be offered both in community and institutional settings.

As with EUPD, the aim is to treat DPD patients in the community setting. Inpatient admissions to mental health services should be brief and reserved for crisis management or the treatment of comorbid disorders. As per NICE guidelines, 'admission to inpatient services solely for the treatment of antisocial personality disorder or its associated risks is likely to be a lengthy process and should be under the care of forensic/specialist personality disorder services'.

References

Archer,M, Lau,Y and Sethi,F (2016) Women in Acute Psychiatric Units, Their Characteristics and Needs: A Review. *BJPsych Bulletin* 40: 266–72.

Balachandra,S and Benson,V (2014) Men are from Mars, Women are from Venus. National Association of Psychiatric Intensive Care and Low-Secure Units – NAPICU – Local Quarterly Meetings 2016 Presentations. https://napicu.org.uk/membership/presentations/local-quarterly-meetings–2014/.

Bergink,V, Bouvy,PF, Vervoort,JSP, Koorengevel,KM, Steegers,EAP and Kushner, S. (2012) Prevention of Postpartum Psychosis and Mania in Women at Risk. *American Journal of Psychiatry* 169: 609–15.

Bergink,V, Rasgon,N and Wisner,KL (2016) Postpartum Psychosis: Madness, Mania, and Melancholia in Motherhood. *American Journal of Psychiatry* 173: 1179–88.

Bodner,E, Cohen-Fridela,S and Iancuc,I (2011) Staff Attitudes toward Patients with Borderline Personality Disorder. *Comprehensive Psychiatry* 52: 548–55.

Bowers,L, Jeffery,D, Bilgin,H, Jarrett,M, Sympson,A and Jones,J (2008) Psychiatric Intensive Care Units: A Literature Review. *International Journal of Social Psychiatry* 54 (1) 56–68.

Brown,S, Chhina,N and Dye,S (2008) The Psychiatric Intensive Care Unit: A Prospective Survey of Patient Demographics and Outcomes at Seven English PICUs. *Journal of Psychiatric Intensive Care* 4 (1–2) 17–27.

Cullen,AE, Bowers,L, Khondoker,M, Pettit,S, Achilla,E, Koeser,L, et al. (2018) Factors Associated with Use of Psychiatric Intensive Care and Seclusion in Adult Inpatient Mental Health Services. *Epidemiology and Psychiatric Sciences* 27: 51–61.

Doucet,S, Dennis,C, Letourneau,N and Robertson Blackmore,E (2009) Differentiation and Clinical Implications of Postpartum Depression and Postpartum Psychosis. *Journal of Obstetric, Gynaecologic and Neonatal Nursing* 38: 269–79.

Dzikiti,C (2016) Introduction to NAPICU & the Commissioning of Female PICU Beds in England. National Association of Psychiatric Intensive Care and Low-Secure Units – NAPICU – Local Quarterly Meetings 2016 Presentations. https://napicu.org.uk/local-quarterly-meetings-2016-presentations/.

Elkin,A, Gilburt,H, Slade,M, Lloyd-Evans,B, Gregoire,A, Jhonson,S, et al. (2009) A National Survey of Psychiatric Mother and Baby Units in England. *Psychiatric Services* 60 (5) 629–33.

Gillham,R and Wittkowski,A (2015) Outcomes for Women Admitted to a Mother and Baby Unit: A Systematic Review. *International Journal of Women's Health* 7: 459–76.

Gintalaite-Bieliauskiene,K, Dixon,R and Bennett,L (2020) A Retrospective Survey of Care Provided to Patients with Borderline Personality Disorder Admitted to a Female Psychiatric Intensive Care Unit. *Journal of Psychiatric Intensive Care* 16 (1) 35–42.

Griffiths,J, Taylor,BL, Morant,N, Bick,D, Howard,LM, Seneviratne,G, et al. (2019) A Qualitative Comparison of Experiences of Specialist Mother and Baby Units versus General Psychiatric Wards. *BMC Psychiatry* 19: 1–15. DOI: https://doi.org/10.1186/s12888-019-2389-8.

Kohen,D (2001) Psychiatric Services for Women. *Advances in Psychiatric Treatment* 7: 328–34.

Le,T, Bhushan,V, Sochat,M, Sylvester,P, Mehlman,M and Kallianos,K (2015) *First Aid for the USMLE Step 1 2015: A Student-to-Student Guide*. USA: McGraw Hill Education.

Lied,K, Zanarini,MC, Schmahl,C, Linehan,MM and Bohus, M (2004) Borderline Personality Disorder. *Lancet* 364: 453–61.

Linehan,MN and Heard,H (1999) Borderline Personality Disorder: Costs, Course, and Treatment Outcomes. In Miller,N and Magruder,K (eds.), *The Cost-Effectiveness of Psychotherapy: A Guide for Practitioners, Researchers and Policy-Makers*. New York: Oxford Press. pp. 291–305.

Livesley,JW (2003) *Practical Management of Personality Disorder*. London: Guilford Press.

Long,C, Hall,L, Craig,L, Mochty,U and Hollin,CR (2011) Women Referred for Medium Secure Inpatient Care: A Population Study Over a Six-Year Period. *Journal of Psychiatric Intensive Care* 7 (1) 17–26.

McKay,A (2022) *Bed Management Policy January 2019*. Camden and Islington NHS Foundation Trust. www.candi.nhs.uk/sites/default/files/Bed%20Management%20Policy%20%20s140%20update%20November%202021.pdf.

Moran,P (1999) The Epidemiology of Antisocial Personality Disorder. *Social Psychiatry and Psychiatric Epidemiology* 34 (5) 231–42.

Murray,L, Cooper,C and Hipwell,A (2003) Mental Health of Parents Caring for Infants. *Archives of Women's Mental Health* 6 (2) 71–7.

National Institute for Health and Care Excellence (NICE) (2013) Self-Harm. Quality Standard [QS34]. www.nice.org.uk/guidance/qs34.

National Institute for Health and Care Excellence (NICE) (2009) Antisocial Personality Disorder: Prevention and Management – Clinical Guideline 77 [CG77]. www.nice.org.uk/guidance/cg77.

O'Brien,A, Cramer,B, Rutherford M and Attard,D (2013) A Retrospective Cohort Study Describing Admissions to a London Trust's PICU Beds Over One Year: Do Men and Women Use PICU Differently? *Journal of Psychiatric Intensive Care* 9 (1) 33–9.

Paris,J (2004) Is Hospitalisation Useful for Suicidal Patients with Borderline Personality Disorder? *Journal of Personality Disorders* 18 (3) 240–7.

Robertson,E, Celasun,N and Stewart,DE (2003) Risk Factors for Postpartum Depression. In Stewart,DE, Robertson,E, Dennis,C -L, Grace,SL and Wallington,T (eds.), *Postpartum Depression: Literature Review of Risk Factors and Interventions*. Toronto: University Health Network.

Royal College of Psychiatrists (RCPsych) (2018) Mother and Baby Units (MBUs). www.rcpsych.ac.uk/mental-health/treatments-and-wellbeing/mother-and-baby-units-(mbus).

Sadock,BJ and Sadock,VA (2010) *Kaplan & Sadock's Pocket Handbook of Clinical Psychiatry*. USA: Lippincott Williams & Wilkins and Wolters Kluwer.

Satel,SL (1998) Are Women's Health Needs Really Special? *Psychiatric Services* **49**: 565. DOI: https://doi.org/10.1176/ps.49.5.565.

Singleton,N, Coid,J, Bebbington,P, Jenkins,R, Brugha,T, Lewis,G, et al. (1998) *The National Survey of Psychiatric Morbidity among Prisoners and the Future of Prison*. London: The Stationery Office.

Sit,D, Rothschild,AJ and Wisner,KL (2006) A Review of Postpartum Psychosis. *Journal of Women's Health* **15** (4) 352–68.

Stapleton,A and Wright,N (2019) The Experiences of People With Borderline Personality Disorder Admitted to Acute Psychiatric Inpatient Wards: A Meta-Synthesis. *Journal of Mental Health* **28** (4) 443–57.

Steinert,T, Lepping,P, Bernhardsgrütter,BR, Conca,A, Hatling,T, Janssen,W, et al. (2010) Incidence of Seclusion and Restraint in Psychiatric Hospitals: A Literature Review and Survey of International Trends. *Social Psychiatry and Psychiatric Epidemiology* **45** (9) 889–97.

Stephenson,LA, Macdonald,AJD, Seneviratne,G, Waites,F and Pawlby,S (2018) Mother and Baby Units Matter: Improved Outcomes for Both. *British Journal of Psychiatry Open* **4**: 119–25.

Trull,TJ, Sher,KJ, Minks-Brown,C, Durbin,J and Burr,R (2000) Borderline Personality Disorder and Substance Use Disorders: A Review and Integration. *Clinical Psychology Review* **20** (2) 235–53.

Weight,EJ and Kendal,S (2013) Staff Attitudes Towards Inpatients with Borderline Personality Disorder. *Mental Health Practice* **17** (3) 34–8.

Widiger,TA and Weissman,MM (1991) Epidemiology of Borderline Personality Disorder. *Hospital and Community Psychiatry* **42** (10) 1015–21.

Woollaston,K and Hixenbaugh,P (2008) 'Destructive Whirlwind': Nurses' Perceptions of Patients Diagnosed with Borderline Personality Disorder. *Journal of Psychiatric and Mental Health Nursing* **15** (9) 703–9.

World Health Organization (WHO) (1992) *The ICD-10 Classification of Mental and Behavioural Disorders: Clinical Descriptions and Diagnostic Guidelines*. Geneva: WHO.

World Health Organization (WHO) (2010) *WHO Technical Consultation on Postpartum and Postnatal Care*. Geneva: WHO. p. 12. www.ncbi.nlm.nih.gov/books/NBK310595/.

Zanarini,MC, Frankenburg,FR, Hennen,J and Silk,KR (2003) The Longitudinal Course of Borderline Psychopathology: 6-Year Prospective Follow-Up of the Phenomenology of Borderline Personality Disorder. *American Journal of Psychiatry* **160**: 274–83.

The Complex Needs Patient

Sanjith Kamath and Vishelle Kamath

Introduction

For clinicians, one of the more enjoyable aspects of working in a psychiatric intensive care setting is the opportunity to work with patients who present with an incredibly wide variety of clinical problems and challenges. These issues span a broad spectrum of complexity, with each individual patient requiring a highly personalised approach to care being delivered quickly and efficiently to enable them to move to a less restrictive setting. However, increasingly, the case is that the resources and support required to manage complexity, which is often manifested through comorbidity and additional problems, are inadequate or simply lacking.

The phrase 'complex needs patient' is often used by clinicians to describe a patient who presents with challenges and needs that require management approaches that are resource intensive and multi-focused. Unfortunately, the phrase can also be used pejoratively, and in the authors' experience, particularly when an effective management strategy eludes the treating team either through lack of resource, capacity or expertise. These individuals are often passed from service to service, with high costs to services across the board. In this chapter, we seek to define 'complex needs patients', recognising that for many clinicians the phrase refers to those individuals who present with severe mental illnesses together with other comorbid challenges including, but not limited to, serious physical illness, substance misuse or addiction, social problems including a lack of support, homelessness as well as problematic, absent or abusive relationships and the presence of another comorbid mental illness.

These patients present a significant treatment challenge to mental health workers within psychiatric intensive care facilities. One reason for this is that the

treatment of the symptoms of their mental illness alone is often insufficient to deliver holistic improvement, a sustained reduction of risks and increased mental, physical and social wellbeing required to effectively support these individuals to truly begin their recovery journey. This can result in difficulties in achieving consistent treatment goals, with delayed discharges and long lengths of stay within the psychiatric intensive care service along with other treatment issues (see Box. 24.1). During this time, these individuals continue to present with high levels of distress and agitation, displaying verbal or physical aggression, and can be responsible for impacting the milieu and relation security across the unit.

In this chapter, we explore and try to understand possible aetiological factors of complexity as well as its background and characteristics and discuss useful treatment modalities. Lastly, we consider the impact that the Covid-19 pandemic has had both in terms of disease presentation and the impact it has had on services.

Definition and Characteristics

The complex needs patient is a theory which has arisen within multidisciplinary healthcare settings over the past decade. A concept clarification study concluded that the term 'complex needs' goes beyond its precursors, 'multimorbidity' or 'poly-pathology',

---

Box 24.1 Challenges of managing complex needs patients within a PICU

- Poor mental health outcomes
- Delayed discharges
- Long lengths of stay
- High levels of risk to themselves and others
- Influencing the dynamic across the PICU

Acknowledgement to Harriet Stedman

Table 24.1 Evolving concept of complex needs patient

Historical	Now
Multimorbidity – based on health diagnosis	Complex – interface between biopsychosocial elements
Linear	Dynamic and changeable
Predictable	Random
Health interventions	Biopsychosocial approach

Box 24.2 Other terms used to describe complex needs patients

- New long-stay patient
- Young chronics
- Difficult to treat
- Treatment resistant
- Dual or multiple diagnosis
- Challenging behaviour

encompassing factors outside of healthcare diagnoses (Loeb et al., 2015; Manning and Gagnon, 2017). Stemming from complexity science in the 1980s, the concept redefines multiple diagnoses from linear and predictable to dynamic and contextual (Martin and Félix-Bortolotti, 2010), as illustrated in Table 24.1.

Other terms used to describe complex needs patients are shown in Box 24.2.

Systems theory describes the interdisciplinary relationship between physiological, psychological, socio-economic and environmental components within the treatment and diagnoses of patients within a psychiatric intensive care unit (PICU) (Knudsen and Vogd, 2014). The needs-based approach (Beer et al., 2008) remains relevant both in terms of diagnosis and consideration of intervention strategies.

Patients with complex care needs (PCCNs) can be considered as individuals experiencing a severe mental health illness with one or more additional problems, as demonstrated in Box 24.3 (Beer et al., 2001; Bujold et al., 2017). Additional problems include another mental health disorder, medical problems such as diabetes, cardiovascular or respiratory conditions, substance misuse, mild learning difficulties, homelessness, issues related to ethnicity, sexuality or gender, forensic history or a history of abuse. Most of these individuals will have a diagnosis of a psychotic illness, associated with treatment resistance, the presence of negative symptoms and cognitive impairment.

Consequently, due to these multiple issues, these individuals present with severe impairment in their everyday functioning, with behaviours that challenge, compounded by poor engagement (Beer, et al., 2008; Killaspy, 2014).

Typically, these patients spend in excess of 6–8 weeks in a PICU and are described as 'hard to place' due to challenging behavioural problems, often manifesting as aggression, agitation or treatment resistance (Beer et al., 2001; Pereira et al., 2021).

Characteristics

Psychiatric patients with complex needs were first defined by Mann and Cree (1976) as 'long-stay' patients. These patients remained in hospital continuously for between 1 and 5 years, with two-thirds of these patients requiring further treatment within hospital and the remaining one-third being able to be discharged to an alternative placement but having more complex or challenging disorders than other residents in these placements (Mann and Cree, 1976). In other studies, long-stay patients are described as individuals who consistently occupy a bed on a PICU or an acute psychiatric ward for a minimum of 6 months. Typically, these patients, occupy around one-fifth of all acute beds and pose challenges when it comes to discharge, often requiring referral to more intense rehabilitation units or permanent residential homes (Commander and Rooprai, 2008). Patients are often noncompliant with medication and/or treatment plans or are 'treatment-resistant' due to the delusions or confabulations surrounding the reason they are in hospital and receiving treatment. 'Treatment resistance' infers that the individual has had no benefit from interventions like medication, psychological therapies or even electroconvulsive treatment (Howes et al., 2017). Individuals who are noncompliant are likely to have worse outcomes and require longer stays in hospital (Kleinsinger, 2010). The complex needs patient remains within this healthcare environment, either in an acute ward, PICU or residential home, presenting with one or more additional problem, as outlined in Box 24.3.

Severe Mental Illness and an Additional Mental Health Illness

The leading cause of disability in the United Kingdom is mental health illness. The disease burden for mental

Box 24.3 Characteristics of complex needs patients

Severe mental illness *plus* one or more of the following:

- Another mental health problem
- Substance abuse
- Mild learning difficulty
- History of abuse
- History of brain injury
- Medical problems
- Homelessness
- Lack of social support
- Problems related to ethnicity

Table 24.2 Comorbid mental illnesses

Primary Mental Illness	Common Comorbid Mental illnesses
Borderline personality disorder	• Depression • Anxiety • Substance misuse
Bipolar affective disorder	• Anxiety disorders • Impulse control disorders • Substance misuse disorders
Schizophrenia	• Depression • Anxiety • Substance misuse

health illness is about 23% higher than cancer and cardiovascular disease, which have a disease burden of about 16% (Knapp et al., 2011). The impact of this extends beyond those to the individual themselves and their families to economic and social costs. The economic and social costs in England were estimated by Knapp et al. (2011) to be around £105 billion each year.

The National Institute for Mental Health (2021) defines a severe mental illness as 'a mental, behavioural, or emotional disorder resulting in serious functional impairment, which substantially interferes with or limits one or more major life activities'.

Patients with multiple psychiatric comorbidities in a PICU setting present healthcare professionals with challenges related to their assessments, diagnosis, treatment options and treatment response. Community discharge pathways commonly align to single diagnosis streams, posing further difficulties in discharging planning.

Comorbidity with a personality disorder and other mental illness is common and has an adverse effect on the course of the illness and treatment outcomes (Tyrer et al., 2015). These personality disorders include borderline personality disorder and antisocial personality disorder. These may typically coexist with depression, anxiety and substance misuse. Of patients with a borderline personality disorder, 96% will have a mood disorder in their lifetime, with 71% to 83% experiencing depression (Zanarini et al., 1998; McGlashan et al., 2000).

Comorbidity rates of other mental illnesses in bipolar affective disorder are also high. Concurrent

illnesses are illustrated in Table 24.2. For example, in bipolar disorder, coexisting conditions include anxiety disorders, impulse-control disorders and substance misuse (Parker, 2010). Anxiety disorders that occur with bipolar affective disorder include panic attacks, agoraphobia, generalised anxiety disorder, obsessive compulsive disorder and social phobias. Impulse control disorders include attention deficit hyperactivity disorder (ADHD), oppositional defiant disorder and conduct disorder (Parker, 2010). The National Comorbidity Survey Replication (NCS-R) reported that patients had a sixfold increased lifetime comorbidity of any anxiety disorder (Merkangas et al, 2010). A similar pattern was observed for impulse control disorders and substance misuse disorders.

There is substantial psychiatric comorbidity with schizophrenia, which complicates the clinical picture (Pincus et al., 2004). Concurrent depression may complicate the clinical picture as well, appearing as negative symptoms (Green et al., 2003). Anxiety symptoms may compound paranoia. There is also an association between cannabis abuse and worsening psychotic symptoms (Buckley et al., 2009).

The multimorbidity of mental health problems increases not only the complexity of patient care but also overall outcome, length of stay and ability to rationalise pharmacological interventions.

Severe Mental Illness and Substance Abuse

In the United States, mental illness and substance use disorders have an estimated lifetime prevalence of 4%–17%, with all of the associations found between mood disorders and drug use to be statistically significant in both institutionalised and non-institutionalised patients (Conway et al., 2006; Pary et al., 2017). Research indicates that the diagnosis of a psychiatric disorder may increase the risk of further substance misuse, greater contributing to the presentation of the patients psychiatric and behavioural symptoms. Moreover, for psychiatric inpatients, the risk of suicide and self-harm is greater and the length of stay is longer for individuals with substance use disorders than those without a history of substance abuse (Miller et al., 2016).

Severe Mental Illness and Learning Disabilities

The rate of learning disability in the general population is about 1%, but these individuals develop severe mental illness at a rate that is much faster than that in the general population (Buckles et al., 2013). This is further compounded by increasing risk profiles due to a proportion of these individuals who present with challenging behaviours, including behaviours that threaten the physical safety of themselves or others (Emmerson et al., 2001).

The interplay between mental illness and intellectual impairment results in this group of patients being moved between generic mental health services and those specialist services for learning disability, with capacity challenges in the latter often being a driver. There are also difficulties in diagnosing and assessing, resulting in delays in identifying and implementing appropriate treatment interventions. While the accurate identification of the underlying aetiology of challenging behaviours is essential to achieve positive treatment outcomes, this can also be problematic. It is important to recognise that this may include an organic illness or a mental illness in its own right.

Additional challenges within a PICU setting for individuals with a learning disability and mental illness include the requirements to support communication or sensory needs, which can be difficult in an environment that is often noisy with staff teams that may not have the skills or expertise and resources to meet those specific to an individual with a learning disability. The situation can be further exacerbated because of difficulties with finding teams who can secure appropriate discharge pathways that can meet the bespoke needs of these individuals with comorbidity.

Severe Mental Illness and History of Abuse

A history of sexual abuse is associated with an increased lifetime risk of a variety of different psychiatric disorders (Chen et al, 2010). These include depression, anxiety, PTSD and eating disorders. Sexually abused individuals may present with various medical and psychiatric symptoms and thus a coordinated approach aligned to the principles of trauma-informed care in the assessment and management of these individuals is helpful in achieving holistic outcomes. In a landmark longitudinal study in mental health epidemiology, Feletti (2002) examined how Adverse Childhood Experiences (ACEs) such as child abuse, neglect and household dysfunction (e.g. caregiver substance abuse, serious mental illness) correlated with long-term mental and physical health conditions. There was a strong proportionate relationship between ACE scores and lifelong medical and mental health problems and early mortality rates. The frequency and exposure to violence has also been shown to have a strong correlation to developing a mental illness (Ribeiro et al., 2009). Staff understanding and experience of strategies to prevent re-traumatisation is essential in a PICU setting. Exposure of staff to trauma within the work environment also needs to be considered to enable them to better care for individuals with complex needs.

Severe Mental Illness and an Acquired Brain Injury

Developing a severe mental illness after an acquired brain injury, in someone with an existing mental illness, is common and adds a degree of complexity, particularly in a PICU setting. Moderate to severe traumatic brain injury is associated with an increased initial risk of mental illness, whereas mild traumatic brain injury is usually associated with persistent mental health problems (Fann et al., 2004).

People with mental disorders themselves have a higher risk of having a traumatic brain injury (Liao et al., 2012). This is even more so in the group of patients receiving advanced psychiatric health care, with medication and psychiatric visit frequency highly correlated with traumatic brain injury, as demonstrated in a study by Liao et al. (2012).

Patients with a traumatic brain injury can present with physical, sensory, cognitive and behavioural and

Box 24.4 Effects of traumatic brain injury

Physical

- Motor impairment – e.g. limb weakness
- Swallowing difficulties
- Speech impairments
- Balance problems
- Falls
- Seizures
- Urinary incontinence
- Faecal incontinence

Cognitive

- Attention deficits
- Concentration problems
- Difficulties with immediate recall
- Short- and long-term memory deficits

Behavioural

- Agitation
- Aggression
- Sexually inappropriate behaviours
- Disinhibition

Sensory

- Blurred vision
- Partial or total blindness
- Ringing in the ears
- Deafness
- Impaired taste
- Loss or altered smell
- Increased sensitivity to sound or light

Psychiatric

- Lability of mood
- Depression
- Anxiety
- Psychosis

psychiatric symptoms (see Box 24.4). Physical symptoms include headache, nausea, fatigue, speech difficulties, loss of balance, swallowing problems, motor impairment and urinary or faecal incontinence. Sensory problems include blurred vision, ringing in the ears, changes in taste and impaired smell and increased sensitivity to sound or light. Cognitive issues include short- and long-term memory problems and difficulties with concentration and attention. Behavioural and psychiatric symptoms may include mood changes, lability of mood, anxiety, depression, psychosis, agitation, aggressive and sexually inappropriate behaviours.

Severe Mental Health Illness and an Additional Medical Problem

Patients living with severe mental disorders such as bipolar disorder, schizophrenia or emotionally unstable personality disorder have poorer physical health status and a shorter life expectancy than the general population, in part due to physical comorbidities (Doherty and Gaughran, 2014). Research indicates that the development of a physical morbidity in addition to a mental

health problem contributes to an individual's social isolation, thus magnifying their mental distress.

Studies focussing on mortality in patients with psychosis-related disorders have indicated that individuals with a diagnosis of schizophrenia may die up to 18 years sooner than the general population (Tiihonen et al., 2009). Whilst a variety of factors including obesity, hypertension, poor oral health and diabetes all contribute to the significantly shortened life expectancy, cardiovascular disease is the leading cause for the excess mortality. In addition, individuals aged 18–49 years with complex mental health illnesses have an elevated mortality risk of 300% resulting from coronary heart disease (Osborn et al., 2007). These findings were replicated in other studies which controlled for confounding factors such as socio-economic status and medication (Merrick and Merrick, 2007). Similar findings have been observed in patients with bipolar disorder, major depressive disorder, PTSD and anxiety symptoms, indicating that there is a shared aetiology between mental health disorders and coronary heart disease (De Hert et al., 2018). This shared aetiology may contribute to the increased risk of individuals with a psychotic illness carrying a cardiac mortality risk of twice the general population (Osby et al., 2001).

In addition to cardiovascular diseases, individuals with severe mental health diagnoses are more likely to develop diabetes (prevalence of 10% vs 6% in the general population), which is associated with a poor prognosis (Gonzalez et al., 2008; Diabetes.co.uk, 2019). Medication non-adherence is common in individuals with mental health disorders and diabetes. In particular, individuals with depressive disorders are unlikely to self-manage treatment plan due to decreased levels of self-care (Lin et al., 2006; Koopmans et al., 2009). Thus, the presence of a psychiatric comorbidity alongside diabetes increases healthcare usage and the need for longer stays in psychiatric intensive care units and other hospital settings (Albrecht et al., 2012).

In an inpatient setting like the PICU, these issues are best addressed through the adoption of integrated care models which provide better holistic outcomes for patients. The benefits of this approach have been cited in several documents and papers and by the Kings Fund (Naylor et al., 2016). These include an increased life expectancy for individuals with serious mental illness and a reduction of acute hospital utilisation for mental health service users with possible saving or re-investment opportunities created from decreased acute hospital utilisation. Another benefit cited is a reduction in healthcare inequalities, thereby achieving parity of esteem of physical and mental health, as a result of improved proactive, preventative care. However, achieving this in a PICU can be challenging.

Severe Mental Illness and Homelessness/Low Socio-Economic Status

Severe mental illness is a large contributing factor to someone's socio-economic and residential status. Homeless population studies have found that the prevalence of psychiatric disorders, such as schizophrenia and bipolar disorder, have increased significantly in the past three decades. However, it remains unclear as to the causative relationship between the two factors, as each heightens the effect of the other (North et al., 2004; Tulloch et al., 2012). Moreover, homelessness has a significant impact (45% increase) on a patient's length of stay following admission, as finding suitable housing or residential schemes for these individuals may increase their discharge time.

This may place a strain on the individual's mental stability as well as the funding and resources of the PICU they have been admitted to.

Issues Relating to Ethnicity and Gender

Ethnicity

A study analysing the characteristics of patients admitted into PICUs found that a 'typical PICU patient' surfaced. This patient was typically male, detained, belonged to an ethnic minority and had a history of previous detentions and forensic incidents. This resulted in an overrepresentation of ethnic minorities (55%) within PICU settings, the reason for which remains unclear (Feinstein and Holloway, 2002; Kasmi, 2007). In addition, Black patients are significantly more likely to receive a diagnosis of schizophrenia during inpatient psychiatric care than White patients yet are less likely to receive the necessary help within mental health services (Hamilton et al., 2015).

Gender

Psychiatric epidemiological studies have found that there is a greater prevalence of anxiety and mood-related disorders in women, while there is a greater prevalence of substance use and antisocial personality disorders in men (Grant and Weissman, 2007). Moreover, when considering admissions to PICUs, women are significantly less likely to be admitted to a PICU than men (31% to 69% respectively), and women which are admitted tend to be referred from an open ward, whereas men are more likely to be admitted directly from the community. In addition, men are more likely to be admitted to PICUs for aggressive or challenging behaviours alongside substance misuse (Grube, 2007; Mustafa et al., 2013).

Typically, PICUs are separated into single-sex wards (male or female) which raises gender-sensitive issues for those identifying as transgender or gender fluid. Whilst single-sex wards are designed to be safer in protecting vulnerable individuals from exploitation, the provision of a gender-sensitive approach within psychiatric intensive care will allow fewer gender-fluid individuals to be overlooked, without jeopardising the other vulnerable individuals within the unit (Archer et al., 2016).

Forensic History

Forensic-psychiatric histories are common inpatients within the PICU environment, which poses a complexity to the patient's length of stay, discharge and treatment plans, as everything must be regulated by the Ministry of Justice. Patients detained on criminal sections do not tend to have a time limitation on their stay, with their discharge largely depending on the risk they pose to the community and themselves. A significant number of mentally disordered offenders will require lifelong psychiatric care, with minimal progress with their treatment, due to non-compliance in therapy and often complex poly-diagnoses (Vorstenbosch et al., 2014; Huband et al., 2018).

Treating and Managing Complex Needs Patients

Mental health needs for this patient group can be complex, enduring and deep-rooted. Thus, the priority of treatment in any setting should focus on early intervention to help prevent more serious problems from occurring.

To best support people presenting with complex needs is to collaborate with them to deliver individualised support that will meet their needs. This allows for shared responsibility in the recovery process and empowers individuals to make decisions and choices about their lives as well as increase confidence and promote their independence.

Treatment plans should be developed in collaboration with individuals to focus on holistic recovery with co–produced goals, as shown in Table 24.3.

The view of all stakeholders central to the individual are also important to consider. Box 24.5 lists key stakeholders who have expressed goals themselves.

The effective management and treatment of patients with complex needs requires time to allow teams to develop authentic relationships with the patient, broadening the skill set and membership of the care teams and being able to communicate across sectors. This includes in-depth integration across all disciplines, including pharmacology, psychology, occupational therapy, physical health services and physiotherapy, substance abuse services, social services and local community teams. The pathway should operate as a 'whole system, integrated care pathway' between inpatient and community settings (Killaspy, 2014). This will allow for evidenced-based treatments

Table 24.3 Goals for patients with complex mental health issues

Goals	Management focus
Short Term	• Assess risk and focus on safety • Crisis intervention • Stabilise living situation • Address treatment needs
Medium Term	• Coordinate services/agencies/sectors involved

Long Term	• Treatment of presenting issues, for example:
	  – individual therapy
	  – family therapy
	  – group therapy
	  – medication management
	  – transition planning

(Wolfson et al, 2009)

Box 24.5 Stakeholder goals

Staff

- To provide an intensive service that is durable and sustainable
- To continue to support people as their needs change
- To adapt the environment to sustain change
- To improve physical health and life expectancy.

Service users

- To learn life skills
- To get you standing on your feet again
- To be free

Carers

- To relieve distress
- To provide a place of safety for vulnerable people
- To help make the outside world safer for service users by educating the public.

within inpatient units, as well as sustaining community living for those discharged from PICUs. The multidisciplinary or transdisciplinary team must articulate a holistic care plan, which addresses all aspects of the individual's issues, and is aimed at recovery, focusing not only on getting the individual back to their community placement with their families but also ensuring the discharge is successful (Wolfson et al., 2009). All staff should deliver their specialist interventions within the collaborative framework of the recovery approach.

The provision of integrated community care for this group of patients is key in preventing long stays on a PICU or acute admission ward. To this end, the Royal College of Psychiatrists published a commissioning guide to support local rehabilitation care pathways to address this (Royal College of Psychiatrists, 2011). The pathway aligns to that described by Killaspy et al. (2005), as a '"whole system, integrated care pathway" across inpatient and community settings provided by statutory and non-statutory health and social care sectors'.

In relation to the use of medication, many people are admitted to a PICU because they have not responded adequately to medications, often including those prescribed for 'treatment resistance'. The ability to find the best medication regime to minimise symptoms without producing distressing side effects is key.

Recent Intervention

In response to finding solutions to deal with people with complex mental health issues, a group of general practitioners in London and Hackney decided to tackle this by setting up a new service. The groundbreaking Primary Care Psychotherapy Consultation Service (PCPCS), implemented and run by the Tavistock and Portman NHS Foundation Trust, is the result of that innovation. It offers help for a range of needs, close to home, often in people's own general practitioners' surgeries, rather than in remote clinics. The service offers a range of psychological therapies, joint consultations with general practitioners and training for primary care staff to enhance their capacity to help. As The report by Parsonage et al. (2014) asserted that it can change people's lives and dramatically improve their health and well-being.

A study by van der Meer et al. (2021) reviewed a process of a new intervention called 'This is me' (TiM) through user-centred design. TiM helped some individuals to reflect on their identity and appeared to benefit the relationship between the service users and the mental health professionals. The study concluded that TiM is a promising tool for supporting people with serious mental illness in

redeveloping a multidimensional identity and a renewed sense of purpose.

The Danish Health and Medicines Authority assembled a group of experts to develop a national clinical guideline for patients with schizophrenia and complex mental health needs (Banndrup et al., 2016). A guideline development group (GDG) recommended that the interventions in Box 24.6 should be offered routinely.

Impact of Managing People with Complex Mental Health Needs

Responding and managing individuals with complex mental health needs impacts on all stakeholders differently, as detailed in Box 24.6, with the impact shown in Box 24.7.

Impact of COVID-19

The coronavirus pandemic which spread across the globe in 2020 has resulted in profound mental health consequences. It was found that most patients admitted for psychiatric hospitalisation in Swiss emergency departments displayed more severe symptoms, including suicidal ideation or behaviour, psychomotor agitation and behavioural disturbances (Ambrosetti et al., 2021). Furthermore, in the United Kingdom, the NHS saw a significant 11.8% increase in formal detention under the Mental Health Act during the lockdown period (the period

---

Box 24.6 Recommended interventions

- Antipsychotic maintenance therapy
- long-acting injectable antipsychotics
- Family intervention
- Assertive community treatment
- Neurocognitive training
- Social cognitive training
- Cognitive behavioural therapy for persistent positive and/or negative symptoms
- Combination of cognitive behavioural therapy and motivational interviewing for cannabis and/or central stimulant abuse
- SSRI or SNRI add-on treatment for persistent negative symptoms

Box 24.7 Impact

For people providing services

- Pressure
- Feeling overwhelmed
- Exhaustion
- Motivated to find support

For people presenting with complex mental health needs

- Frustration
- Confusion
- Exhaustion
- Looking for ways to get attention and support

For families and supports

- Frustration
- Confusion
- Exhaustion
- Motivated to find support

during which government-imposed restrictions to contain the spread of the pandemic were at their most intense). The most significant increase in admissions were for patients (both men and women) with schizoaffective disorders (Davies and Hogarth, 2021). Additionally, when comparing the number of mental health admissions to acute medical units in 2020 with those in 2019, results show a significant increase in the number of admissions, with the pandemic being a significant stressor in individuals suffering from anxiety disorders (Grimshaw and Chaudhuri, 2021). Following studies that showed an increase in admissions following suicide attempts, researchers found that the pandemic increased the risk of mental health crises due to a variety of environmental stressors, both for individuals already suffering from complex mental health disorders and those who were not already known to mental health services. Contributing factors included self-isolation; fear, avoiding seeking services; financial stress and employment loss; increased access to means; and an increased risk of domestic violence (Gunnell et al., 2020).

COVID-19 is a highly transmissible virus, which has resulted in an increased complexity within PICUs, due to the close living quarters of patients and staff as well as the often-close contact during behavioural crises that is required to disengage patients in an agitated state (Brown et al., 2020, p. 19). Furthermore, individuals who lack the mental capacity to carry out basic personal care regimes may struggle to understand the severity of the disease and the requirement for frequent handwashing and social distancing to prevent transmission, thus increasing the likelihood of COVID-19 transmission within the wards. Moreover, often patients on some antipsychotic medications have an increased risk of pneumonia and respiratory infections, making them particularly vulnerable to the virus (Kuo et al., 2013). When considering the isolation of patients during COVID-19, it is important to refer to the Mental Health Act, as it states, 'MHA powers must not be used to enforce treatment or isolation for any reason unrelated to the management of a person's mental health', thus raising issues surrounding the legislation of isolating patients for physical health, potentially against their will (Brown et al., 2020).

The pandemic raised issues surrounding staff shortage, as staff have had to work from home, isolate or take time off to prevent COVID-19 transmission, with NHS staff absences in April 2020 being the highest ever recorded, as well as issues of staff burnout. Studies observed meaningful changes in work-related burnout associated with having different roles during the pandemic, with limited training or various equipment concerns. Moreover, reductions in non-COVID19 have resulted in an unequal spread of workload across the NHS, with some staff feeling underutilised and others feeling overworked (Gemine et al., 2021). The integration within psychiatric services of health and social care services has also been under strain during the pandemic. The Health Select Committee found that while the United Kingdom has a 10-year plan for funding within the NHS, there is no plan or long-term funding for social care, with fewer staff to handle the increasing workload (Open Access News, 2021).

References

Albrecht,JS, Hirshon,JM, Goldberg,R, Langenberg,P, Day, HR, Morgan,DJ, et al. (2012) Serious Mental Illness and Acute Hospital Readmission in Diabetic Patients. *American Journal of Medical Quality* 27 (6) 503–8.

Ambrosetti,J, Macheret,L, Folliet,A, Wullschleger,A, Amerio,A, Aguglia,A, et al. (2021) Impact of the COVID-19 Pandemic on Psychiatric Admissions to a Large Swiss Emergency Department: An Observational Study. *International Journal of Environmental Research and Public Health* 18 (3) 1174.

Archer,M, Lau,Y and Sethi,F (2016) Women in Acute Psychiatric Units: Their Characteristics and Needs: A Review. *BJPsych Bulletin* **40** (5) 266–72.

Baandrup,L, Rasmussen,JO, Klokker,L, Austin,S, Bjørnshave,T, Bliksted,V, et al. (2016) Treatment of Adult Patients with Schizophrenia and Complex Mental Health Needs: A National Clinical Guideline. *Nordic Journal of Psychiatry* **70** (3) 231–40.

Beer,MD, Pereira,SM and Paton,C (2001) *Psychiatric Intensive Care*, 1st ed. Cambridge: Cambridge University Press.

Beer,MD, Pereira,SM and Paton,C (2008) *Psychiatric Intensive Care*, 2nd ed. Cambridge: Cambridge University Press.

Brown,C, Keene,A, Hooper,C and O'Brien,A (2020) Isolation of Patients in Psychiatric Hospitals in the Context of the COVID-19 Pandemic: An Ethical, Legal, and Practical Challenge. *International Journal of Law and Psychiatry* **71**: 101572.

Buckles,J, Luckasson,R and Keefe,E (2013) A Systematic Review of the Prevalence of Psychiatric Disorders in Adults With Intellectual Disability, 2003–2010. *Journal of Ment Health Research and Intellectual Disabilities* **6**: 181–207.

Buckley,PF, Miller,BJ, Lehrer,DS and Castle,DJ (2009) Psychiatric Comorbidities and Schizophrenia. *Schizophrenia Bulletin* **35** (2) 383–402.

Bujold,M, Pluye,P, Légaré,F, Haggerty,J, Gore,GC and El Sharif,R (2017) Decisional Needs Assessment of Patients With Complex Care Needs in Primary Care: A Participatory Systematic Mixed Studies Review Protocol. *BMJ Open* **7** (11) e016400.

Chen,LP, Murad,MH, Paras,ML, Colbenson,KM, Sattler, AL, Goranson,EN, et al. (2010) Sexual Abuse and Lifetime Diagnosis of Psychiatric Disorders: Systematic Review and Meta-Analysis. *Mayo Clinic Proceedings* **85** (7) 618–29.

Commander,M and Rooprai,D (2008) Survey of Long-Stay Patients on Acute Psychiatric Wards. *Psychiatric Bulletin* **32**(10) 380–3.

Conway,KP, Compton,W, Stinson,FS and Grant,BF (2006) Lifetime Comorbidity of DSM-IV Mood and Anxiety Disorders and Specific Drug Use Disorders: Results from the National Epidemiologic Survey on Alcohol and Related Conditions. *Journal of Clinical Psychiatry* **67** (2) 247–57.

Davies,M and Hogarth,L (2021) The Effect of COVID-19 Lockdown on Psychiatric Admissions: Role of Gender. *BJPsych Open* **7** (4) e112.

De Hert,M, Detraux,J and Vancampfort,D (2018) The Intriguing Relationship Between Coronary Heart Disease and Mental Disorders. *Dialogues in Clinical Neuroscience* **20** (1) 31–40.

Diabetes.co.UK (2019) Diabetes Prevalence. Website. www.diabetes.co.uk/diabetes-prevalence.html.

Doherty,AM and Gaughran,F (2014) The Interface of Physical and Mental Health. *Social Psychiatry and Psychiatric Epidemiology* **49** (5) 673–82.

Emerson,E, Kiernan,C, Alborz,A, Reeves,D, Mason,H, Swarbrick,R, et al. (2001) The Prevalence of Challenging Behaviours: A Total Population Study. *Research in Developmental Disabilities* **22**: 77–93.

Fann,JR, Burington,B, Leonetti,A, Jaffe,K, Katon,WJ and Thompson,RS (2004) Psychiatric Illness Following Traumatic Brain Injury in an Adult Health Maintenance Organization Population. *Archives of General Psychiatry* **61** (1) 53–61.

Feinstein,A and Holloway,F (2002) Evaluating the Use of a Psychiatric Intensive Care Unit: Is Ethnicity a Risk Factor for Admission? *International Journal of Social Psychiatry* **48** (1) 38–46.

Felitti,VJ (2002) The Relation Between Adverse Childhood Experiences and Adult Health: Turning Gold into Lead. *The Permanente Journal* **6** (1) 44–7.

Gemine,R, Davies,GR, Tarrant,S, Davies,RM, James,M and Lewis,K (2021) Factors Associated with Work-Related Burnout in NHS Staff During COVID-19: A Cross-Sectional Mixed Methods Study. *BMJ Open* **11** (1) e042591.

Gonzalez,JS, Peyrot,M, McCarl,LA, Collins,EM, Serpa,L, Mimiaga,MJ, et al. (2008) Depression and Diabetes Treatment Nonadherence: A Meta-Analysis. *Diabetes Care* **31** (12) 2398–2403.

Grant,BF and Weissman,MM (2007) Gender and the Prevalence of Psychiatric Disorders. In Narrow,WE, First,MB, Sirovatka,PJ and Regier,DA (eds.), *Age and Gender Considerations in Psychiatric Diagnosis: A Research Agenda for DSM*-V. Arlington: American Psychiatric Association. pp. 31–45.

Green,A.I, Canuso,CM, Brenner,MJ and Wojcik,JD (2003) Detection and Management of Comorbidity in Patients with Schizophrenia. *Psychiatric Clinics of North America* **26** (1) 115–39.

Grimshaw,B and Chaudhuri,E (2021) Mental Health-Related Admissions to the Acute Medical Unit During COVID-19. *Clinical Medicine* **21** (1) e77–9.

Grube,M (2007) Gender Differences in Aggressive Behavior at Admission to a Psychiatric Hospital. *Aggressive Behavior* **33** (2)97–103.

Gunnell,D, Appleby,L, Arensman,E, Hawton,K, John,A, Kapur,N, et al. (2020) Suicide Risk and Prevention During the COVID-19 Pandemic. *Lancet Psychiatry* **7** (6) 468–71.

Hamilton,JE, Heads,AM, Cho,RY, Lane,SD and Soares,JC (2015) Racial Disparities During Admission to an Academic Psychiatric Hospital in a Large Urban Area. *Comprehensive Psychiatry* **63**: 113–22.

Howes,OD, McCutcheon,R, Agid,O, de Bartolomeis,A, van Beveren,NJM Birnbaum,ML, et al. (2017) Treatment-resistant schizophrenia: Treatment Response and

Resistance in Psychosis (TRRIP) working group consensus guidelines on diagnosis and terminology. *American Journal of Psychiatry* 174: 216–29.

Huband,N, Furtado,V, Schel,S, Eckert,M, Cheung,N, Bulten,E, et al. (2018) Characteristics and Needs of Long-Stay Forensic Psychiatric Inpatients: A Rapid Review of the Literature. *International Journal of Forensic Mental Health* 17 (1) 45–60.

Kasmi,Y (2007) Characteristics of Patients Admitted to Psychiatric Intensive Care Units. *Irish Journal of Psychological Medicine* 24 (2) 75–8.

Killaspy,H, Harden,C, Holloway,F and King,M (2005) What Do Mental Health Rehabilitation Services Do and What Are They For? A National Survey in England. *Journal of Mental Health* 14: 157–65.

Killaspy,H (2014) The Ongoing Need for Local Services for People With Complex Mental Health Problems. *Psychiatric Bulletin* 38 (6)257–9.

Kleinsinger,F (2010) Working with the Noncompliant Patient. *The Permanente Journal* 14 (1) 54–60.

Knapp,M, McDaid,D and Parsonag,M (2011) *Mental Health Promotion and Mental Illness Prevention: The Economic Case.* London: Department of Health and Social Care.

Knudsen,M and Vogd,W (2014) *Systems Theory and the Sociology of Health and Illness: Observing Healthcare.* Oxford: Routledge.

Koopmans,B, Pouwer,F, de Bie,RA, vanRooij,ES, Leusink, GL, and Pop,VJ (2009) Depressive Symptoms Are Associated With Physical Inactivity in Patients With Type 2 Diabetes: The DIAZOB Primary Care Diabetes Study. *Family Practice* 26 (3) 171–3.

Kuo,C-J, Yang,SY, Liao,YT, Chen,WJ, Lee,WC, Shau,WY, et al. (2013) Second-Generation Antipsychotic Medications and Risk of Pneumonia in Schizophrenia. *Schizophrenia Bulletin* 39 (3) 648–57.

Liao,C, Chiu,W, Yeh,C, Chang,HC and Chen,TL (2012) Risk and Outcomes for Traumatic Brain Injury in Patients with Mental Disorders. *Journal of Neurology, Neurosurgery, and Psychiatry* 83:1186–92.

Lin,EHB, Katon,W, Rutter,C, Simon,GE, Ludman,EJ, Von Korff,M, et al. (2006) Effects of Enhanced Depression Treatment on Diabetes Self-Care. *Annals of Family Medicine* 4 (1) 46–53.

Loeb,DF, Binswanger,IA, Candrian,C and Bayliss,EA (2015) Primary Care Physician Insights into a Typology of the Complex Patient in Primary Care. *Annals of Family Medicine* 13 (5) 451–5.

Mann, S. A. and Cree, W. (1976) 'New' Long-Stay Psychiatric Patients: A National Sample Survey of Fifteen Mental Hospitals in England and Wales 1972/3. *Psychological Medicine* 6 (4) 603–16.

Manning,E and Gagnon,M (2017) The Complex Patient: A Concept Clarification. *Nursing & Health Sciences* 19 (1) 13–21.

Martin,CM and Félix-Bortolotti,M (2010) W(h)ither Complexity? The Emperor's New Toolkit? Or Elucidating the Evolution of Health Systems Knowledge? *Journal of Evaluation in Clinical Practice* 16 (3) 415–20.

McGlashan,TH, Grilo,CM, Skodol,AE, Gunderson,JG, Shea,MT, Morey,LC, et al. (2000) The Collaborative Longitudinal Personality Disorders Study: baseline Axis I/II and II/II diagnostic co-occurrence. *Acta Psychiatrica Scandanavia*102: 256–64.

Merikangas,KR, Akiskal,HS, Angst,J, et al. (2007) Lifetime and 12-month prevalence of bipolar spectrum disorder in the National Comorbidity Survey Replication. *Archives of General Psychiatry* 64: 543–52.

Merikangas,K, He,J, Burstein,M, Swanson,S, Avenevoli,S, Cui,L, et al. (2010) Lifetime Prevalence of Mental Disorders in U.S. Adolescents: Results from the National Comorbidity Survey Replication–Adolescent Supplement (NCS-A). *Journal of the American Academy of Child & Adolescent Psychiatry* 49 (10) 980–9.

Merrick,J and Merrick,E (2007) Equal Treatment: Closing the Gap. A Formal Investigation into Physical Health Inequalities Experienced by People with Learning Disabilities and/or Mental Health Problems. *Journal of Policy and Practice in Intellectual Disabilities* 4 (1) 73–73.

Miller,KA, Miller,KA, Hitschfeld,MJ, Lineberry,TW and Palmer,BA (2016) How Does Active Substance Use at Psychiatric Admission Impact Suicide Risk and Hospital Length-of-Stay? *Journal of Addictive Diseases* 35 (4) 291–7.

Mustafa,FA, Bayatti,Z and Faruqui,RA (2013) Gender Differences in Referral Pathways and Admissions to a Psychiatric Intensive Care Unit in a County Psychiatric Hospital in the UK. *International Journal of Social Psychiatry* 59 (2) 188–9.

National Institute of Mental Health (2021) Mental Illness. www.nimh.nih.gov/health/statistics/mental-illness.

National Mental Health Development Unit (2011) *In Sight and in Mind: A Toolkit to Reduce the Use of Out of Area Mental Health Services.* Royal College of Psychiatrists.

Naylor,C, Das,P, Ross,S, Honeyman,M, Thompson,J and Gilbert,H (2016) *Bringing Together Physical and Mental Health: A New Frontier for Integrated Care.* London: The Kings Fund.

Open Access News (2021) Committee Report Finds NHS 'Burnout Is Widespread Reality'. www.openaccessgovernment.org/nhs-burnout/112353/.

North,CS, Eyrich,KM, Pollio,DE and Spitznagel,EL (2004) Are Rates of Psychiatric Disorders in the Homeless Population Changing? *American Journal of Public Health* 94 (1) 103–8.

Osborn,DPJ, Levy,G, Nazareth,I, Petersen,I, Islam,A and King,MB (2007) Relative Risk of Cardiovascular and Cancer Mortality in People with Severe Mental Illness from the United Kingdom's General Practice Research Database. *Archives of General Psychiatry* **64** (2) 242–9.

Osby,U, Brandt,L, Correia,N, Ekbom,A and Sparén,P (2001) Excess Mortality in Bipolar and Unipolar Disorder in Sweden. *Archives of General Psychiatry* **58** (9) 844–50.

Parker,GB (2010) Comorbidities in Bipolar Disorder: Models and Management. *Medical Journal of Australia* **193** (4) S18.

Parsonage,M, Hard,E and Rock,B (2014) Managing Patients with Complex Needs: Evaluation of the City and Hackney Primary Care Psychotherapy Consultation Service. Centre for Mental Health.

Pary,R, Patel,M and Lippmann,S (2017) Depression and Bipolar Disorders in Patients with Alcohol Use Disorders, *Federal Practitioner* **34** (Suppl 2) 37S–41S.

Pereira,S, Walker,L and Dye,S (2021) A National Survey of Psychiatric Intensive Care, Low Secure and Locked Rehabilitation Units. *Mental Health Practice* **24** (4).

Pincus,HA, Tew,JD and First,MB (2004) Psychiatric Comorbidity: Is More Less? *World Psychiatry* **3** (1) 18–23.

Ribeiro,WS, Andreoli,SB, Ferri,CP, Prince,M and Mari,JJ (2009) Exposure to Violence and Mental Health Problems in Low and Middle-Income Countries: A Literature Review. *Brazilian Journal of Psychiatry* **31** (Suppl 2) S49–57.

Tiihonen,J, Lonnqvist,J, Wahlbeck,K, Klaukka,T, Niskanen,L and Haukka,J (2009) 11-Year Follow-Up of Mortality in Patients With Schizophrenia: A Population-Based Cohort Study (FIN11 Study). *Lancet* **374** (9690) 620–7.

Tyrer,P, Reed,GM and Crawford,MJ (2015) Classification, Assessment, Prevalence, and Effect of Personality Disorder. *Lancet* **385** (9969) 717–26.

Tulloch,AD, Khondoker,MR, Fearon,P and David,AS (2012) Associations of Homelessness and Residential Mobility with Length of Stay after Acute Psychiatric Admission. *BMC Psychiatry* **12**: 121.

Van der Meer,L, Jonker,T, Wadman,H, Wunderink,C, van Weeghel,J, Hendrika,G, et al. (2021) Targeting Personal Recovery of People with Complex Mental Health Needs: The Development of a Psychosocial Intervention Through User-Centred Design. *Frontiers in Psychiatry* **12**: 635514.

Vorstenbosch,ECW, Bouman,YH, Braun,PC and Bulten,EB (2014) Psychometric Properties of the Forensic Inpatient Quality of Life Questionnaire: Quality of Life Assessment for Long-Term Forensic Psychiatric Care. *Health Psychology and Behavioral Medicine* **2**(1) 335–48.

Wolfson,P, Holloway,F and Killaspy,H (2009) Enabling recovery for people with complex mental health needs. A template for rehabilitation services. Faculty report FR/RS/1 Faculty of Rehabilitation and Social Psychiatry of the Royal College of Psychiatrists November 2009.

Zanarini,MC, Frankenburg,FR, Dubo,ED, Sickel,AE, Trikha,A, Levin,A et al. (1998) Axis I Comorbidity of Borderline Personality Disorder. *American Journal of Psychiatry* **155**:1733–9.

Zubair,UB and Brown,R (2021) Audit of Documentation of Forensic History on Admission Form in a Psychiatric Intensive Care Unit. *Journal of the College of Physicians and Surgeons–Pakistan* **30** (6) 707–9.

Psychiatric Intensive Care in General Hospital Settings

Jim Welch, Karen Williams and Emma Phillips

Introduction

Beer et al. (2008) state that 'Psychiatric intensive care is for patients compulsorily detained, usually in secure conditions, who are in an acutely disturbed phase of a serious mental disorder.' At first glance, it might seem that psychiatric intensive care would rarely be required in general hospitals. However, the 2017 National Confidential Enquiry into Patient Deaths (NCEPOD) *Treat as One* report into care of 552/11980 patients in English hospitals with co-existing mental health problems found 13/552 had been restrained, 11 had been given rapid tranquilisation (RT), 8 had made significant self-injury attempts and 23 had required the input of hospital security staff. The report made several recommendations to improve the care and treatment of patients with mental health diagnoses admitted to general hospitals.

It is perhaps not surprising that many patients with mental disorders are regularly admitted to general hospitals. Raj et al. (2014) found that 37.6% of people with severe mental health symptoms also have a long-term physical condition; this compares with 25.3% of people with no or few symptoms of a mental health problem. People with mental disorders in general hospitals include patients with pre-existing psychiatric diagnoses admitted with an unconnected acute illness and patients admitted for medical/surgical treatment of the consequences of mental disorder (e.g. self-injurious behaviour or refeeding in anorexia nervosa). However, the commonest causes of acute ill mental health requiring intensive psychiatric attention in general hospitals arise as a result of physical illness causing psychiatric and behavioural disturbance (e.g. delirium, drug and alcohol withdrawal, head injury and limbic encephalitis) in patients with or without known psychiatric disorder.

In this chapter we describe the types of clinical situations that can arise in the general hospital that need intensive psychiatric care along with principles and practice of treatment. We highlight the conditions that commonly occur, particularly in patients that require ongoing care in the general hospital and cannot easily be diverted to psychiatric services because of the nature of their physical illness and/or treatment. We also discuss some of the pharmacological issues in managing patients on complex treatment regimens or with challenges to usual pharmacokinetics and pharmacodynamics.

We explain the use of RT/emergency sedation in the general hospital and the specific circumstance of patients admitted to general hospital critical care. We also cover the legal aspects of care of patients lacking in capacity/refusing treatment.

We discuss the special challenges of delivering psychiatric care in the general hospital, including organisational barriers that limit access to psychiatric clinical records and medication/environmental factors that create additional obstacles for managing patients with challenging behaviours. General hospitals are often busy, noisy, uncomfortable and cramped. There are few areas of privacy or opportunities for diverting or therapeutic activities and nearly all general hospital care is delivered at the bedside where potentially dangerous medical equipment is within reach of the patients.

We highlight staff factors affecting good psychiatric treatment, including the lack of knowledge about psychiatric conditions and their management and low confidence in providing treatment to mental health patients. This can be further complicated by using agency mental health practitioners to provide intense and potentially intrusive supervision and monitoring and the use of police to manage behaviour. We also describe how mental health liaison teams work in the general hospitals.

Challenges of the General Hospital

Staff Factors

The *Five Year Forward View for Mental Health* (Independent Mental Health Taskforce, 2016) states: 'For far too long, people of all ages with mental health problems have been stigmatised and marginalised, all too often experiencing an NHS that treats their minds and bodies separately.' The report highlights that one in four adults will experience a mental health problem in any given year.

Liaison psychiatry is a subspecialty within psychiatry that provides psychiatric assessment and treatment for patients who might be experiencing distress on medical wards or in the emergency department (ED) (Scott et al., 2017). Psychiatric liaison teams have been developing in scope and breadth across the United Kingdom, but there remain significant differences in service models and staffing depending on location and support from commissioning authorities. Whilst investment in psychiatric liaison services has improved in recent years, they continue to suffer from underfunding when compared to equivalent physical health services.

The Psychiatric Liaison Accreditation Network (PLAN) standards are recognised as the benchmark by which psychiatric liaison services are assessed and the *Five Year Forward View for Mental Health* (Independent Mental Health Taskforce, 2016) set an expectation that 50% of general hospitals would achieve a 'Core24' standard by 2021. This standard requires that a psychiatric liaison service is staffed 24/7 and can respond to ED referrals within one hour and a non-urgent (inpatient) referral within 24 hours. PLAN also defines criteria for more comprehensive services; cost savings of £4 for every £1 invested have been independently evaluated for the Rapid Assessment Integrated Discharge service model, one type of comprehensive psychiatric liaison service (Parsonage and Fossey, 2011).

The provision of psychiatric care within a general hospital setting poses unique and complex challenges. While core medical training contains specific elements on assessing mental state, the education of adult registered nurses in the United Kingdom largely avoids mental health and illness, focussing on the physical presentation of the individual.

Registered nurses therefore qualify with little or no core psychiatric knowledge and skills. Healthcare assistants are trained 'on the job', often by nursing staff that have their own poverty of knowledge.

Liaison psychiatry services have an important role in supporting patients within the general hospital, but they do not take over the care of patients. Rather, they provide consultation, so there is a need to develop approaches to shared care with medical and surgical colleagues. Organisational, hospital and ward culture have significant impact on the provision of high-quality care, and compassion fatigue is significant in all staff groups (Peters, 2018).

Staff who experience greater levels of exposure to the suffering of others are significantly more likely to experience compassion fatigue, which is most clearly observed in EDs and medical admission units. The frequent exposure to patients in psychiatric or social crisis where self-injury or substance misuse results in a need for emergency care can result in these patients receiving prejudicial treatment.

The value of clinical supervision has been well evaluated and described (Davenport, 2013; Care Quality Commission, 2010, Outcome 14, p. 134) as a proactive method of enabling professionals at risk of burnout or compassion fatigue to reflect upon practice and plan for continuing development. It should be closely linked to appraisal and embedded within organisational governance structures. It should not be confused with performance management or line management function. Supervision is an opportunity for a professional who has another person's development as their priority to engage in a supportive, reflective and confidential relationship with that person.

While clinical supervision is well embedded in psychiatric and social work professions in the United Kingdom, it has attracted limited attention within the general hospital setting. Steps are being taken to re-evaluate this position in favour of greater support for general hospital professionals, in part driven by the numbers leaving the caring professions, which has been exacerbated by the COVID-19 pandemic.

A basic mental health awareness programme should be considered statutory/mandatory for all employees (NCEPOD, 2017) and should be linked to annual appraisal. Staff engagement in mental health education cannot be over-valued, but the training must meet the needs of the individual practitioner, and these needs will vary greatly depending on the role of that person (NCEPOD, 2017). Educational programmes need to capture those differences and offer a bespoke role-based experience. A brief non-exhaustive description of topics is shown in Table 25.1.

Liaison psychiatry teams can support general hospital management to develop and deliver bespoke training for staff, but this should be factored into the commissioning of services and form a key element of the general hospital's overarching mental health strategy.

Risk Assessment and Enhanced Care

The effective and reliable assessment of risk is central to the safety of the individual, hospital staff, patients and other visitors.

The National Institute for Health and Care Excellence (NICE) clinical guidance (NICE, 2004) advocated that EDs should incorporate the Australasian Mental Health Triage tool (Broadbent et al., 2007), a recommendation echoed by the Royal College of Emergency Medicine in 2021(Swires-Hennessy and Hayhurst, 2021). This tool applies equivalent priority status to patients with mental health and physical health needs, including standards for senior review and comprehensive risk assessment which can be governance assured. This initial assessment also dictates the immediate level of supervision required to maintain the safety of the patient and staff. This may range from routine (15 minutes) to enhanced.

Treat as One (NCEPOD, 2017) and the RCEM (Swires-Hennessy and Hayhurst, 2021) determined that the standard for referral to psychiatric liaison services should be that the patient is 'medically fit for assessment', not 'medically fit for discharge'. Enhanced and comprehensive psychiatric liaison services (but not Core24 services) are resourced to enable the co-streaming of mental and physical health needs, according priority to both. Patients are seen by both services and are in receipt of the support of both physical and mental health care from point of arrival to discharge.

Levels of patient observation outside of psychiatric settings are limited in their gradation, usually moving from routine ward-based observations straight to 1:1 care, with little in between. In practical terms, the delivery of 1:1 care, where needed, has either been delegated to security staff or agency registered mental health nurses (RMNs), often with limited therapeutic value. These staff are usually temporary, and their performance is not managed by the host organisation; thus, the experience of individual patients varies greatly. RMNs are often allocated to one person for a whole day without access to meaningful distraction or occupation to support them.

'Enhanced Care' is a term used to describe a model to improve the delivery and efficacy of 1:1 observation. Patients are re-assessed for risk by the treating team on a daily basis. Those designated as representing a high risk to self or others will be allocated 1:1 care, as is usual in a general hospital setting, but consideration is given to whether the person would benefit from RMN or enhanced trained general hospital staff, who may be based on and familiar with the ward. Families are engaged in the process where it is safe to do so and this is supported by an individualised history, such as the Alzheimer's Society 'This is me' document, wherever possible. The Enhanced Care model also makes suggestions of methods of distraction/occupation.

A key element of this model is the use of Antecedent–Behaviour–Consequence (ABC) methodology. In this methodology, patient behaviours are recorded against standardised criteria at 15-minute intervals, or when any change from their baseline presentation is observed. This record is subsequently examined, enabling the treating team to identify person-specific factors in both escalation

Table 25.1 Topics which may be covered in mental health training for general hospital staff

Mental Health Act	Mental Capacity Act
Basic mental health awareness	Delirium
De-escalation skills	Dementia
Personal resilience and well-being	Depression and anxiety
Detoxification (alcohol, substance misuse)	Adjustment disorder
Brief psychological interventions	Refeeding in eating disorders
Risk assessment and positive risk-taking	Post-traumatic stress disorder
Self-harm and suicide	Personality disorders
Grieving	Postnatal disorders
Trauma-informed care	Somatisation

and de-escalation. Individualised care plans are then developed to reflect the strengths, opportunities and challenges relevant to the individual.

Local efforts to improve quality have shown significant improvement in patient experience following the implementation of the Enhanced Care policy. Agency costs have been significantly reduced and staff who would historically have had limited roles now describe a greater satisfaction in their work. Of equal, if not greater importance, patients describe better quality care. There have also been reductions in contacts with the restraint team and emergency sedation in pilot sites (publication pending).

Readers interested in further exploration of the Enhanced Care concepts are invited to contact the authors.

Environmental Factors

The management of the environment poses significant challenges in the general hospital setting and these challenges can be specific to the wards/departments to which the patient presents.

EDs are by their very nature busy, noisy and frenetic and this can be counter-therapeutic and even escalatory for patients in mental or social crisis. There has been significant debate as to whether alternative spaces should be developed for patients in mental health crisis. During the COVID-19 pandemic, several sites explored Mental Health Crisis Hubs/ED Diversion Schemes, prompting a position statement from National Health Service (NHS) England and NHS Improvement in October 2020 which broadly criticises the practical application of the concept (NHS England and NHS Improvement, 2020).

EDs should have an assessment area that is safe for patients and staff and is conducive to a valid mental health assessment (Swires-Hennessy and Hayhurst, 2021). Standards for this accommodation are described by the Psychiatric Liaison Accreditation Network (PLAN) (Baugh et al., 2020). This room, which should not serve dual purpose, should be a safe, quieter space with risk assessment and mitigation in place to maintain the safety of patients and staff alike. Furniture should be fit for purpose and not able to be used as projectiles.

Accommodation elsewhere in the estate can be equally challenging. Most wards will have a small number of private (side) rooms where confidential conversations can be had with confidence. However, these rooms are likely to be allocated to patients in need of barrier nursing or infection control measures. Patients with delirium will benefit from the quiet of a side room, but, conversely, may be more confused by the lack of orientation to external reality. The Enhanced Care model offers an opportunity to observe patients during a change in accommodation to evaluate whether the change has been beneficial.

Careful consideration should be given to moving patients with cognitive decline/delirium across wards or hospital sites. Clinical deterioration can often follow changes in placement, and even minor inconsistency in treatment plans can give rise to significant symptomatic deterioration (Goldberg et al., 2015). Despite these recommendations, patients continue to experience moves in response to challenges with bed occupancy and ED flow.

Most patients are likely to be accommodated in open bays with little privacy and where the culture is one of having confidential conversations behind curtains that do nothing to block sound. Other confidential spaces are often multi-purpose and in equally high demand. Biopsychosocial assessment and the mental healthcare planning process should be patient-centric and should not be engaged in unless confidentiality can be assured. General hospitals have a duty to ensure that suitable accommodation is available.

Psychiatric liaison services can offer an additional perspective in supporting general hospitals in developing their estate, whether that be supporting ligature risk-assessment or designing dementia-friendly spaces within older adult medical settings. Mental health services are familiar with the potential impact of proxemics and the need to factor in low-stimulus areas with increased individual space. Psychiatric liaison services should also be embedded within the host governance structures, including safeguarding, restraint or 'violence and aggression' (as it is frequently described in general hospital settings), finance, performance and serious incident investigation.

Legal Frameworks in the General Hospital Setting

The legal frameworks used for managing physical ill health are generally based around the patient's informed and competent consent to any hospital stay or treatment that is recommended.

In England and Wales, this is underpinned by The Mental Capacity Act 2005 (MCA), an act of parliament that aims to provide a legal framework for acting and making decisions for adults (older than 16 years) who lack the capacity or competence to make such decisions for themselves. Scotland and Northern Ireland have their own capacity legislation (The Adults with Incapacity (Scotland) Act 2000 and The Mental Capacity Act (Northern Ireland) 2016), and many other jurisdictions around the world have similar legal frameworks to help guide clinicians as to decision-making in scenarios where patients are unable to act or decide for themselves.

The UK Acts all contain a similar overriding principle, namely a presumption of capacity in adults older than the age of 16, which can only be overturned on evidence of impaired capacity. The onus is on clinicians to perform and document an adequate assessment demonstrating why the patient may lack capacity. In the MCA this includes a two-stage test:

1. A rationale for suspecting the patient may lack capacity identified by the questions:

    a. Is there an impairment of or disturbance in the functioning of the person's mind or brain?

    b. Is the impairment or disturbance sufficient that the person lacks the capacity to make that particular decision?

2. The 'functional' test – the person is then considered to lack capacity (about that specific decision) if they are unable to:

    a. Understand information about the decision to be made

    b. Retain that information in their mind

    c. Use or weigh-up the information as part of the decision process

    d. Communicate their decision

There are also similar principles following an assessment which determines that the person is lacking capacity, including that actions taken thereafter must 'benefit' or be in the 'best interests' of the person, that the 'least restrictive' option to provide benefit must be taken and that views of the person and significant others should be considered.

The Deprivation of Liberty Safeguards (DoLS) are part of the Mental Capacity Act 2005 in England and Wales. 'They are due to be updated and will be entitled 'Liberty Protection Safeguards (LPS). These safeguards provide a procedure (proscribed by law) which must be followed by hospitals or care homes to safeguard instances in which patients may be deprived of their liberty in order to provide care.

A procedure such as this is required by Article 5 of the Universal Declaration on Human Rights (the 'right to liberty'), and other jurisdictions have similar processes. Patients who lack capacity to agree to treatment or care and who are under continuous supervision and control; are trying to leave or would be prevented from leaving if they did attempt to do so; are in receipt of invasive procedures such as covert medication, intravenous or nasogastric procedure; and so on should be referred for their care to be reviewed under the DoLS process.

Treat as One (NCEPOD, 2017) highlighted significant opportunities for improvement in the legal aspects of care in general hospitals. Mental illness may pose challenges to clinicians' assessing a patient's capacity for interventions, treatment or hospital stay when they are not familiar with considering the impact of, for example, low mood or psychotic symptoms on decision-making capacity. These factors typically affect the 'using and weighing' of information; while the patient may be able to understand, retain and repeat back information that clinicians are giving them, strong depressive or anorexic cognitions may 'tip the scales' irrevocably for that patient, such that genuine 'weighing in the balance' is no longer possible. Similar conundrums can be encountered with patients who have harmed themselves, who are sometimes described as 'having capacity' to leave hospital despite expressing strong thoughts to harm themselves further.

Liaison psychiatry input into these scenarios is frequently beneficial. Mental health clinicians also have expertise in knowing when to use mental health versus mental capacity legislation, which is relevant in many jurisdictions.

Department of Critical Care

The Department of Critical Care (DCC) admits and treats many patients with psychiatric disorder who are heavily sedated during their admission, either by their condition (e.g. drug overdose/head injury) or because they have been effectively anaesthetised when more conventional RT medications have failed to calm a highly disturbed delirious patient. The court of appeal judgement in the Ferreira case (2017) judged that life-saving treatment in the intensive care unit (ICU) should not usually raise issues of deprivation of liberty; however, in the process of recovery, DoLS and MHA might need to be considered for patients with underlying mental health conditions (Baharolo et al., 2018).

Psychiatric liaison teams may be called when the patient is to be woken up because the patient may have been sedated for some days or may have been administered multiple sedatives, including drugs such as clonidine and dexmedetomidine, as well as anaesthetic agents, benzodiazepines and one or more antipsychotics (often at or above British National Formulary (BNF) limits).

Principles of managing this situation include:

- Planning for the process of waking the patient up when there are plenty of senior staff on duty
- Ensuring mental health staff (and if possible, family or friends) available
- Continued treatment of delirium or psychiatric illness
- Tapered withdrawal of other medication
- A clear treatment plan for mental health alongside attention to physical condition

Post discharge, patients may require additional psychological input for post-delirium flashbacks and intensive care post-traumatic stress disorder (PTSD) symptoms.

Clinical Situations Needing Psychiatric Intensive Care

Many physical illnesses (notably neurological) have neuropsychiatric sequelae. Mental health professionals should play a key role in the multidisciplinary assessment of psychiatric or 'behavioural' symptoms, including delirium, in the general hospital setting; this may occur via one-off assessment or more consistent 1:1 mental health nursing. Medical teams are encouraged to seek input from liaison psychiatry teams, including detailed neuropsychiatric assessment, a greater understanding of premorbid personality, mental illness, developmental difficulties or altered cognition prior to the new symptoms, mental state examination and use of standardised assessment scales to help understand any changes.

In treatment, common themes predominate regarding use of non-pharmacological approaches first; 'behaviours that challenge' should be approached initially with good nursing care.

Delirium

The most common neuropsychiatric presentation in general hospitals is delirium. Prevalence on medical wards may be as high as 20%–30%, with between 10%

and 50% of surgical patients developing delirium (NICE, 2010b). Delirium ('acute confusional state', 'encephalopathy') typically presents with fluctuating consciousness and reduced cognition and altered perceptions, has an acute onset (1–2 days) and can take several weeks to resolve, even once the causative insult has been remedied. There are 'hyperactive', 'hypoactive' and 'mixed' types.

Risk factors include:

- Age > 65 years
- Premorbid dementia or cognitive impairment
- Severe physical illness
- Hip fracture

Delirium is a serious condition, predisposing to longer length of hospital stay, more hospital-acquired complications (falls, pressure sores, poor nutrition), increased incidence of dementia, increased likelihood of move to long-term care and death.

Treatment for delirium focuses on identifying and treating the underlying cause. Using the 'PINCHME' mnemonic (see Table 25.2) can be helpful (Pryor and Clarke, 2017).

There is very little evidence-base for psychotropic prescribing in delirium. NICE Clinical Guideline 103 recommends the short-term use of haloperidol (licensed in the BNF for management of acute delirium when non-pharmacological treatments are ineffective) at a low dose (BNF, 2021). Usually, a starting dose of haloperidol 0.5 mg twice daily is appropriate in the elderly. Avoid benzodiazepines due to risk of falls or worsening delirium.

Alcohol Dependence Syndrome

Patients at high risk of serious complications from alcohol withdrawal should be admitted to the general hospital (NICE, 2021a). There were 1.3 million alcohol-related admissions to general hospitals in

Table 25.2 'PINCHME' mnemonic to aid recall of causes of delirium

P	Pain
I	Infection, inflammation
N	Nutrition
C	Constipation
H	Hydration
M	Medication
E	Environment

England in 2018–2019 (i.e. 7.4% of all hospital admissions) (NHS Digital, 2020).

Alcohol detoxification can be complicated by delirium tremens, Wernicke-Korsakoff syndrome and alcohol withdrawal seizures. Of these conditions, delirium tremens is the most likely to give rise to acute behavioural disturbance.

Good alcohol withdrawal management using NICE-approved symptom-led detoxification treatment (Clinical Guideline 100) can prevent most complications, but sometimes patients may present to hospital some days after beginning a planned or unplanned alcohol reduction in the community. The patient may be highly agitated and delirious and unable to give an accurate history. Blood tests such as gamma-glutamyl transferase, mean corpuscular volume (MCV), carbohydrate-deficient (CD) transferrin and phosphatidylethanol (PEth) alcohol testing with corroborative history may help make the diagnosis.

Patients with established delirium tremens should be managed in the general hospital. Note that under-treated delirium tremens carries significant mortality risk. The onset of delirium tremens is usually 48–72 hours into the detoxification/alcohol reduction and can last up to 72 hours. In addition to signs of delirium (sudden onset, fluctuating levels of cognition and orientation), patients may experience paranoid ideation, intense fear and visual hallucinations. They may become highly disturbed, frightened and attempt to leave. 'Violence and aggression' (restraint) teams and even the police are often deployed to manage agitation.

Management of delirium tremens should include medical treatment with high-dose, long-acting benzodiazepines (e.g. 100 mg diazepam daily), with the dose being titrated down after delirium has passed. Short-acting parenteral benzodiazepines may be used if the patient is unable to take oral medication. High-dose parenteral vitamin B1 (e.g. Pabrinex two pairs of vials three times daily for a minimum of three days) should be given to treat potential thiamine deficiency (thus avoiding Wernicke-Korsakoff syndrome) and antipsychotics may also be required to manage psychotic symptoms (e.g. haloperidol 2.5 mg *bd*).

Many patients with delirium tremens also have co-existing causes of delirium, including infections, head injury, electrolyte imbalances and hypoglycaemia; it is important to identify and treat these, avoiding diagnostic overshadowing. Likewise, it is important to identify and treat underlying mental health difficulties and other co-existing substance use disorders.

As with other delirium cases, the patient's capacity should be carefully assessed and consideration should be given to using mental capacity legislation (generally preferable) or mental health legislation (if an underlying psychiatric disorder is suspected or condition does not settle quickly). Careful nursing, use of 1:1 support, good lighting, consistency of staff and regular observations should be used. After completion of detoxification, patients should be referred to community treatment services for relapse prevention therapy and medication.

Substance Misuse

Hospital admissions where drug-related mental and behavioural disorder was a primary or secondary diagnosis increased by 3% to 99,782 between 2018 and 2019 and 2019 and 2020 (NHS Digital, 2021). Drugs of misuse fall into the following general categories: opioids, anxiolytics, empathogens, dissociative drugs, stimulants and hallucinogens. Patients may present to EDs for intoxication states or overdose.

It can be practically very difficult to identify what drug(s) have been used due to patient reluctance to give an accurate history due to fear or actual ignorance of what has been used. Corroboration via urine drug screens might be difficult and can be inaccurate if the drug was taken very recently. Drug effect can also be unpredictable and in some cases paradoxical.

Opiates

The generation of patients dependent on illicit opioids is getting older and frailer. Many will present to general hospitals because of conditions associated with their chronic drug use, such as injection-related infections, blood borne viruses (BBV), leg ulcers, osteoporosis and chronic pain. Co-existing use of alcohol, cigarettes and other psychoactive drugs are common.

Opioid withdrawal syndrome is not itself associated with delirium, but patients can become dysphoric and uncomfortable if their opioid needs are not met. However, a need for drug stabilisation or detoxification in the absence of another condition is not a reason for hospital admission. Unfortunately, many hospital staff lack confidence in prescribing for this group of patients. Sub-optimal management of dependence and pain can lead to continued drug use in the hospital, putting patients at risk of overdose and leaving hospital prematurely. Patients may demonstrate aggressive behaviour that is difficult to manage, and co-existing personality disorder diagnosis can lead to splitting of ward teams. Continued use of stimulant drugs may also exacerbate aggression.

The principles of good management for this group of patients includes prescribing adequate substitute opioid medication to prevent withdrawal symptoms using the Clinical Opioid Withdrawal Scale (COWS), treating and managing other substance dependence (e.g. alcohol, benzodiazepine, nicotine) and prescribing appropriate analgesia. The use of behavioural contracts can cause differences amongst staff and may have limited use, however, good communication about treatment planning and the ward expectations of the patient and their visitors is recommended. Attention to housing and social issues and organised discharge planning are also essential. On discharge all patients should be warned about the risk of drug overdose and ideally given a supply of the opiate antagonist naloxone as well as referred to community drug services.

Benzodiazepines

Benzodiazepines are commonly misused with medication being purchased via the Internet, leading to difficulties in determining the doses that users are taking. Use of benzodiazepines is reported to have increased throughout the pandemic (Gili et al., 2021). People who are physically dependent on benzodiazepines may present in acute withdrawal in an agitated and anxious state and, in some cases, with risk of epileptiform fits and psychosis.

Treatment includes symptom-led management of withdrawal symptoms with long-acting benzodiazepines using a similar method to managing alcohol withdrawal, with antipsychotics used to manage psychotic symptoms.

Patients with benzodiazepine intoxication will typically present with depression of central nervous system, drowsiness and so on, but paradoxical reactions can occur, albeit infrequently, and the patient might be overactive and agitated. This is managed through intensive nursing. The drug flumazenil might also be helpful.

Stimulant Use and Dependence

Stimulant use is associated with elevated mortality, BBV infection, poor mental health, suicidality and violence (Farrell et al., 2019). Patients may present to the ED with schizophreniform psychosis and it might be difficult to ascertain the cause of psychosis. RT may be required with short-acting benzodiazepines as first-line therapy and judicious use of antipsychotics and may involve care by the hospital 'violence and aggression' or restraint team. Stimulant users may also present with serotonin syndrome (autonomic changes, hyperpyrexia, movement disorder, agitation and seizures). Treatment for this is largely supportive, with close monitoring. Periactin/cyproheptadine can reduce serotonin levels.

Other 'Special Cases'

As a general rule, other neuropsychiatric symptoms should be assessed and managed much like their psychiatric syndrome counterparts (i.e. antidepressants for depression, antipsychotics for psychosis, cognitive enhancers for cognitive deficits, etc.).

RT for patients with most medical illnesses can follow usual protocols, taking into consideration drug interactions or patient-specific factors. As with delirium and alcohol withdrawal, management should always include non-pharmacological measures and de-escalation prior to consideration of medication. There are occasions where, due to underlying physical or mental illness, clinicians should deviate from usual 'rules' or emergency sedation protocols. Several of these examples are outlined in the sections that follow, with corresponding evidence-base for management of agitation, behavioural disturbance or psychiatric symptoms in these 'special cases'.

Behavioural and Psychological Symptoms in Dementia

Patients should be assessed for causes including underlying ill physical health, pain, hunger, medication side effects, delirium and underlying ill mental health (anxiety, depression, etc.) with appropriate interventions thereafter.

As with delirium, antipsychotics for behavioural and psychological symptoms in dementia (BPSD) should be considered only for those who are at risk of harming themselves or others or those experiencing agitation, hallucinations or delusions causing marked distress. As well as physical agitation or aggression, 'harm' may include inability to be concordant with care, nutrition or other factors, such as putting themselves at risk of hospital acquired infections (including COVID-19).

Repetitive shouting, wandering or pacing, touching objects and social withdrawal are not symptoms which tend to respond to antipsychotics.

The Banerjee report (2009) illustrated risks and benefits of using atypical antipsychotics in those with BPSD. For 1,000 people treated for 12 weeks, 91–200 showed clinically significant improvement in symptoms. This was weighed against the evidence of an additional 10 deaths, 18 cerebrovascular adverse events and 58–94 people with gait disturbance.

General principles suggest avoiding typical antipsychotics. Use the lowest dose for the shortest possible time and review the need regularly. Monitor electrocardiogram (ECG) if possible for risk of prolonged QTc. Risperidone is licensed in Alzheimer's disease for 'the short-term treatment (up to 6 weeks) of persistent aggression in patients with moderate to severe Alzheimer's dementia unresponsive to non-pharmacological approaches and when there is a risk of harm to self or others' (BNF, 2021). If risperidone is contra-indicated or ineffective, alternative antipsychotics can be considered. For prescribing in Lewy body dementia and the 'Parkinson's plus' syndromes, see appropriate NICE guidance (quetiapine may be useful as may clozapine or cholinesterase inhibitors) and the 'Movement Disorder' section below.

Limbic Encephalitis

'Limbic encephalitis' was a term first used in 1968 to describe a neuropsychiatric syndrome comprising acute-onset hallucinations, seizures and memory disturbance with evidence of medial temporal lobe inflammation. Similar cases were noted in earlier literature, primarily associated with malignancies, especially oat cell lung carcinoma and thymus, testicular, colon, uterine and ovarian cancers (i.e. a paraneoplastic syndrome with autoantibodies) (Rickards et al., 2014). By the 2000s, similar syndromes in the absence of malignancy were described (e.g. Vincent et al., 2004). The term is now used to describe a range of encephalitides with prominent psychiatric symptoms, mainly of autoimmune origin.

The evidence base for treatment has advanced in the last decade and research continues. Those with underlying malignancy can show full remission or cure following tumour removal (Mann et al., 2012). Those with high antibody titres respond well to immunosuppression and intravenous (IV) immuno globulins. Plasma exchange may be helpful.

Collaboration with neurology is essential. Some patients relapse following withdrawal of steroids; for these patients, steroid-sparing immunosuppression (e.g. azathioprine or methotrexate) may be considered. There is modest evidence for rituximab, cyclophosphamide and mycophenalate. Investigation with positron emission tomography (PET) or magnetic resonance imaging (MRI) scan, possibly in a serial fashion to identify slow-growing microtumours, may be needed.

Symptomatic treatment of psychiatric symptoms remains anecdotal (Rickards et al., 2014). Research increasingly suggests avoidance of antipsychotics, as they can exacerbate movement disorders. This may confuse the clinical picture, which, even without neuroleptic treatment, can include autonomic instability, elevated creatinine kinase (CK) and rigidity similar to malignant catatonia/neuroleptic malignant syndrome (NMS). As with the catatonia spectrum, benzodiazepines are the treatment of choice and electroconvulsive therapy can be considered if response to benzodiazepines is inadequate.

Patients presenting with acute-onset psychiatric symptoms, associated with seizures, dyskinesias and blood abnormalities (especially hyponatraemia) should lead to a high index of suspicion for these disorders and prompt collaboration with neurology colleagues.

Head Injury

Brain injury can occur through a variety of mechanisms, the most common being traumatic or anoxic/hypoxic injury. There is more literature about the neuropsychiatric manifestations of traumatic brain injury (TBI), and it is unclear whether common principles can be extrapolated between the two disorders. Prognosis can be variable and difficult to predict, with cognitive improvements occurring even up to two years following the event.

TBI can lead to a plethora of neuropsychiatric symptoms, ranging from irritability and anxiety to mania and psychosis. Impaired cognition is very common. Some symptoms (e.g. apathy, irritability, emotional lability, fatigue, insomnia and cognitive impairment) may be manifestations of the actual injury, whilst others, particularly anxiety or depression, can result from insight into the losses or life changes resulting from event. As with other neurological illnesses, complications such as seizures should be considered as a cause of symptoms, as well as side effects or interactions from other medication (e.g. levetiracetam for post-TBI seizures may worsen irritability or even lead to psychotic symptoms) (Vaishnavi et al., 2009).

There is limited evidence base for neuroleptic medications, but the principle of using the drug most suited to similar psychiatric syndromes predominates. It is better to 'start low, go slow', as the injured brain may respond differently to neuroleptic medications, particularly adverse effects. Sometimes doses like those for non-injured brains may be required. Reassessment of symptoms using standardised testing may be helpful. Avoid medications which worsen delirium, including heavy sedation (benzodiazepines) and anticholinergics. Antipsychotics should only be used cautiously; typical antipsychotics such as haloperidol may reduce neuronal recovery. There is some evidence base for non-psychotropic medications, for instance propranolol for isolated aggression without other mood changes. Psychological or psychotherapeutic input may be useful for patients well enough to engage in these, and patient support groups can also help.

It is important to note that there is a growing body of literature associating TBI with pre-existing attention-deficit hyperactivity disorder (ADHD) and suggesting that these patients have worse outcomes following TBI (Bonfield et al., 2013).

Movement Disorders

Parkinson's Disease Psychosis and BPSD in Dementia with Lewy Bodies/Parkinson's Disease Dementia

Patients presenting with parkinsonian-spectrum symptoms including idiopathic Parkinson's disease (IPD), multisystem atrophy (MSA), progressive supranuclear palsy (PSP) and dementia with Lewy bodies (DLB) tend to be extremely sensitive to antipsychotic medications. Extreme caution is required when considering medication for agitation in these patients.

People with parkinsonian syndromes are at risk of a wide range of neuropsychiatric symptoms, including depression, cognitive decline and psychosis. Psychotic symptoms are generally considered a consequence of L-dopa treatment; as illnesses progress, a balance should be sought between acceptable control of motor symptoms versus tolerability of agitation/delusions/hallucinations. However, psychosis was a recognised complication even before the introduction of L-dopa (Thanvi et al., 2005). Psychosis can significantly reduce quality of life, is often extremely difficult to manage for caregivers and is the most important risk factor for transfer to a care home in IPD. It is also associated with reduced survival.

After non-pharmacological measures, initially attempt reduction in one or more antiparkinsonian agents before adding further medications. Agents added most recently should generally be removed first, then those with least antiparkinsonian efficacy (e.g. anticholinergics, selegiline, amantadine). Next in order are dopamine agonists, catecholamine-O-methyltransferase inhibitors and L-dopa. Note that dopamine agonists are much more likely to cause psychosis than L-dopa (Kyle and Bronstein, 2020).

If this does not work, consider adding the following drug treatments:

- Atypical antipsychotics
  - Typical antipsychotics tend to cause severe worsening of parkinsonian motor symptoms and should be avoided.
  - Newer atypicals work via non-selective antagonism at dopaminergic and serotonergic receptors and hence cause less extrapyramidal side effects. Clozapine, quetiapine, risperidone, aripiprazole and olanzapine are all efficacious in trials. Risperidone, olanzapine and aripiprazole can lead to worsening of parkinsonian symptoms. Risperidone and olanzapine are associated with sedation. There may be a class-effect of increased stroke risk in elderly patients with cognitive changes; this has been demonstrated with olanzapine and risperidone. Clozapine is probably the most effective and does not cause worsening of parkinsonian symptoms. Its use is fairly limited in the United Kingdom due to need for monitoring because of agranulocytosis. Quetiapine is favoured by many specialists due to its side effect profile. Studies are conflicted as to its efficacy. Doses should be very low and incrementally increased only slowly (e.g. 12.5 mg *bd* for quetiapine, 6.25 mg *bd* for clozapine). QTc prolongation is possible, and ECG should ideally be taken at baseline and for intermittent monitoring.
- Acetylcholinesterase inhibitors
  - Open-label studies of donepezil and rivastigmine have shown benefit in patients

with IPD by improving cognitive and functional abilities, as well as resolution in behavioural problems and visual hallucinations.

- 5-HT3 receptor antagonists
  - One small short-term study showed improvement in hallucinations, confusion, delusions and associated functional impairment with ondansetron. It was well tolerated without any worsening of parkinsonian symptoms. More rigorous studies have not been completed.

Huntington's Disease

This autosomal dominant trinucleotide repeat neuro-degenerative genetic illness has a wide variety of neuropsychiatric symptoms, which alongside cognitive and motor changes are a core feature of the disorder. In one study, 98% of patients exhibited neuropsychiatric symptoms, the most prevalent being dysphoria, agitation, irritability, apathy and anxiety (Goh et al., 2018). Symptoms ranged from mild to severe and were unrelated to dementia and chorea. Depression and psychosis are also common presentations.

Haloperidol, olanzapine, risperidone and quetiapine can all be used to suppress the chorea in Huntington's disease (unlicensed indications). In the case of agitation, it is often useful to increase the dose of antipsychotic medication the patient is already taking (Paulsen et al., 2001).

Epilepsy

Aggression or agitation can occur with epilepsy, but it is likely that agitation in people with epilepsy is no more prevalent than in the general population. Factors such as organic brain disease, low socioeconomic status, increased likelihood of intellectual disability, lower educational attainment, comorbid psychiatric disease and medication may all confer increased risk. There can be a clear chronological relationship between seizures and violent behaviour, the main risk occurring if the patient suffers post-ictal psychosis. Violence as a purposeful manifestation of seizures is extremely unusual.

Comorbid psychiatric disorders are common, with depression the commonest with rates of 20%–55% and as high as 80% in some studies (Elnazer and Agrawal, 2017) There is some evidence that irritability and aggression are more common in depression with epilepsy than in idiopathic depression. Some psychotropics (in particular tricyclics and chlorpromazine) can lower seizure threshold and may therefore increase likelihood of seizures and post-ictal symptoms. Selective serotonin reuptake inhibitors (SSRIs), haloperidol and sulpiride are generally considered safe in epilepsy.

There is case report evidence for new-onset psychotic symptoms following initiation of some antiepileptic drugs, including carbamazepine, lamotrigine, levetiracetam and gabapentin. Levetiracetam, topiramate, tiagabine and vigabatrin also have case report evidence for new-onset depressive symptoms. There is reasonable evidence associating a wide range of antiepileptic drugs with agitation and aggression, most notably levetiracetam. Clinicians should look for temporal correlation with initiation of medication or dose increases.

Given the wide differential of causes of agitation/aggression, clinicians should focus on history, detailed neuropsychiatric examination and investigation to identify pathophysiology to best direct treatment. Start with confirmation of diagnosis and type of epilepsy, followed by consideration of potential risk factors such as comorbid psychiatric diagnosis, history of head trauma, brain surgery (including for epilepsy itself), cerebrovascular events, type of seizures and changes to or instigation of new antiepileptic medication. Electroencephalogram and neuroimaging may be helpful in establishing causation.

Treatment should focus on optimising seizure control and treating comorbid psychiatric disorders. Psychological interventions such as anger management and relaxation training can be helpful. If this fails, consider psychotropic medication, bearing in mind interactions and effects on seizure control. There is no randomised controlled trial evidence for specific psychopharmacological management of agitation/aggression in epilepsy. An approach such as in TBI is followed, using atypical antipsychotics (risperidone, quetiapine, olanzapine or aripiprazole) in low doses as a first-line therapy. Beta blockers may be helpful in reducing hyperarousal, restlessness and anxiety appear to have little impact on seizure threshold in trials; however, depression may be a rare side effect of propranolol. Avoid benzodiazepines if possible due to risk of dependence and possibility of withdrawal seizures.

Neuroleptic Malignant Syndrome (NMS) and Malignant Catatonia

Neuroleptic malignant syndrome (NMS) is a life-threatening complication associated with treatment with or abrupt withdrawal of psychotropic medications, usually dopamine antagonists. It is idiosyncratic and not dose related. The cause is uncertain but may relate to sympathetic hyperactivity occurring as a result of dopamine blockade, likely in the context of genetic predisposition and environmental factors. 'Full-blown' NMS probably represents the extreme of a range of related symptoms. Some patients can present with milder symptoms; asymptomatic increases in CK are fairly common. Incidence and mortality are difficult to establish. Incidence with typical antipsychotics is likely < 1% and may be even less with atypicals, though there are case reports of occurrence with all available drugs, even newer agents like zisprasidone, aripiprazole and paliperidone. NMS can sometimes be seen with antidepressants and lithium. Combinations of antipsychotics and SSRIs or cholinesterase inhibitors may increase risk. NMS-type syndromes induced by atypical antipsychotic/SSRI combinations may share symptoms and pathogenesis with serotonin syndrome.

NMS is characterised by hyperthermia, muscle rigidity, altered mental state, autonomic lability (fluctuating blood pressure, tachycardia and diaphoresis) and hypermetabolism, as well as elevated CK. Risk factors include rapid dose increase/decrease, organic brain disease, alcoholism, psychomotor agitation and dehydration.

NMS and malignant catatonia share common features and treatment pathways, although it is likely the pathobiology is separate, with NMS being a subcortical motor phenomenon and catatonia being a cortical psychomotor problem (Vancaester and Santens, 2007).

Catatonia is a reasonably common (up to 10%) feature of psychiatric illness (particularly in schizophrenia and the psychotic affective syndromes). The more common subtype is 'retarded', with immobility, mutism, staring, rigidity and many soft neurological signs (e.g. waxy flexibility). Excited catatonia is less common, where patients develop prolonged periods of psychomotor agitation (Rasmussen et al., 2016).

In both disorders, milder cases can be managed in psychiatric units if CK remains low and patients can be monitored carefully for autonomic instability and renal impairment. Treatment comprises withdrawal of antipsychotics (in catatonia, ongoing treatment with antipsychotics during an episode can increase risk of NMS) and high-dose benzodiazepines. In NMS, more severe symptoms require general hospital admission, including critical care, rehydration, cooling (if needed), treatment with dopamine agonists (bromocriptine/dantrolene) and sedation with benzodiazepines. Intubation and ventilation can sometimes be required. Ongoing psychotic symptoms may require treatment with ECT to avoid antipsychotic use. In catatonia, the main risks are those associated with immobility and poor nutrition/hydration (dehydration, malnutrition, deep vein thrombosis, pulmonary embolism, pneumonia and other infections, pressure ulcers and muscle contractures).

Restarting antipsychotics is required in most instances. Between five days and two weeks is suggested prior to re-challenge, allowing time for symptoms of NMS or catatonia to resolve completely. Consider using an antipsychotic unrelated to that previously associated with triggering NMS or a drug with low dopamine affinity (quetiapine or clozapine). Aripiprazole (a partial agonist) is another option. Avoid depot (of any kind) and high-potency typical antipsychotics. 'Start low and go slow', monitoring physical observations.

HIV-Associated Neuropsychiatric Symptoms

Highly active antiretroviral therapy (HAART) has reduced HIV-related morbidity and dramatically improved life expectancy. Patients with co-existing mental illness and HIV are at increased risk of contracting and transmitting HIV (and being tested for HIV).

Studies of patients with HIV have found a high prevalence of comorbid depression and substance misuse, and the prevalence of bipolar disorder is thought to be four times that of the general population. Psychosis is found in 6%–17%, and persecutory, grandiose and somatic delusions are the most common neuropsychiatric presentation (Harris et al., 1991). HIV-associated neurocognitive disorder (HAND) covers a spectrum of impairment caused by HIV from asymptomatic to severe interference with everyday life (Knights et al., 2018).

The consensus of Freudenrich et al. (2010) recommended and noted:

- Citalopram/escitalopram for depression, quetiapine for psychosis and mania and clonazepam for anxiety
- Patients with HIV are more susceptible to movement disorders
- Several HAART medications and antipsychotics are metabolised via cytochrome p450
- Lithium is not recommended due to HIV-induced nephropathy
- Carbamazepine should be avoided due to pancytopenia
- Psychosocial interventions and exercise are useful for most

Anorexia Nervosa

Eating disorder patients admitted for medical refeeding pose their own special set of considerations due to physical comorbidities and extremes of body mass index (BMI). Anorexia nervosa is a serious illness with the highest mortality of any psychiatric condition. Physical risks of low BMI include hypothermia, weakness, bradycardia, postural hypotension, delayed gastric emptying, electrolyte abnormalities (commonly hypokalaemia due to purging behaviours or hyponatraemia due to water loading, but also acute kidney injury and magnesium and phosphate abnormalities), liver function abnormalities and pancytopaenia. Cardiac function can be compromised, with valvular dysfunction, conduction abnormalities and dysregulation of peripheral blood vessels all possible complications. Refeeding syndrome poses its own risks, and guidelines for refeeding are variable with underfeeding, which is also a significant possibility due to risk-aversive policies leading to low calorie intake initially.

Patients may fear weight gain so intensely that illness drives them to extreme attempts to avoid feeding, or to counteract it, including exercise (or micro-exercise), hiding food, manipulating nasogastric tube feeding, weight manipulation (e.g. via fluid loading or holding weights) or other purging behaviours. These behaviours can be extremely difficult to manage in the general hospital environment, and 1:1 nursing is usually needed. Other measures such as restricting access to bathrooms, other patient's fluids and so on may be required.

Comorbidity with other psychiatric conditions is common, including autism spectrum disorders, anxiety and obsessive-compulsive disorders. Suicidal ideation and self-injurious behaviour are also not uncommon. All attempts should be made to enable refeeding of low-weight patients by oral and consensual means, however, feeding under restraint may occasionally be necessary. Often this necessitates utilising limited restraint trained staff in the general hospital. If restraint must be used, it should be with careful planning and the instances of feeding reduced to the minimum safe number.

Medications such as benzodiazepines or atypical antipsychotics (often olanzapine is used due to its propensity to encourage weight gain) can be used to manage anxiety. Emergency sedation can occur as per usual protocols, but should be used cautiously, particularly if there are already ECG abnormalities (Robinson and Rhys Jones, 2018). The newly revised MEED guidelines are helpful for all professionals (RCPsych CR233, 2022)

Renal Impairment and the Dialysed Patient

Altered renal function, whether via acute kidney injury or chronic kidney disease, can affect the pharmacodynamics of prescribed medications. Most psychotropic medications are metabolised via the liver, so the impact is less than for renally excreted drugs. Reduced dosing should be considered for patients needing medication to manage agitation or other neuropsychiatric symptoms. Lithium is the main renally excreted psychotropic, and careful monitoring of levels and symptoms of toxicity is required in renal impairment. As lithium itself is nephrotoxic, discussion about withdrawal of lithium treatment, usually in conjunction with community psychiatric teams, may be needed if renal function is too poor to continue medication.

Patients who are being treated with renal replacement therapy pose a different risk in that dialysis may actively be removing the drug from their system, with a possible impact on mental state. There is case report evidence of patients with epilepsy well controlled by valproate experiencing breakthrough seizures when commenced on dialysis. It is reasonable to extrapolate that patients requiring mood stabilisation with valproate may experience dosing difficulties.

Some patients, particularly in the critical care environment where delirium is common, may be receiving continuous renal replacement therapy (CRRT). There is very little evidence base for psychotropic dosing in CRRT, and although consideration of renal impairment is required in research trials, research on CRRT is not mandated (Bouajram and Awdishu, 2021).

Jim Welch et al.

End-Stage Liver Disease and Hepatic Encephalopathy

The liver is the organ in the human body with the most functions. Most psychotropic drugs are metabolised by the liver. Liver failure impacts on all stages of pharmacokinetics, including absorption (portal vein flow), metabolism (liver enzymes), distribution (protein binding) and elimination (bile). Understanding of these processes reduces risk of psychotropic toxicity. To complicate matters, psychotropic drugs are the second most important group implicated in hepatotoxicity (after antibiotics/antifungals).

End-stage liver disease can also result in psychiatric symptoms via hepatic encephalopathy or psychological adjustment to life-limiting disease. Use psychotropics cautiously in this patient group, who may be particularly prone to further toxicity or adverse effects. In particular, benzodiazepines and opiates can build up and worsen encephalopathy.

Various studies have classified antidepressants into those with higher risk of hepatotoxicity (tricyclic antidepressants, nefazodone, venlafaxine, duloxetine, sertraline, bupropion, trazodone and agomelatine) and lower-risk agents (citalopram, escitalopram, paroxetine and fluvoxamine).

First-generation/typical antipsychotics, particularly chlorpromazine, are well documented as causing hepatotoxicity. Haloperidol, whilst structurally similar to phenothiazines, seems to be lower risk. Severe hepatotoxicity is rarely seen with atypical antipsychotics, although asymptomatic increases in liver enzymes and bilirubin can be seen. If antipsychotic prescribing is necessary in patients with severe liver disease, it is advisable to use lower-risk medications and monitor liver function tests (Telles-Correia et al., 2017).

Pregnancy and the Puerperium

Perinatal mental health care is a vast topic, much of which is outside the scope of this book. Pregnant women have been called the last true 'therapeutic orphan' (Wisner, 2012) due to the lack of clinical trials undertaken during pregnancy and breastfeeding.

Around half of pregnancies are unplanned, and the sensitive period for cardiac malformations is in the third to fourth week of pregnancy, before a person may even realise that they are pregnant. Psychotropic prescription therefore needs careful discussion with persons of childbearing potential, except where the patient may lack capacity to be involved. If there is any suspicion of pregnancy, RT using benzodiazepines in the first trimester may be safer. Avoid valproate and carbamazepine except as a last resort due to risks of teratogenicity and prescribe pregnancy prevention for patients where these treatments cannot be avoided.

Mental ill-health is an independent risk factor for pregnancies resulting in congenital malformations, stillbirth and neonatal death; thus, avoiding medication is not necessarily the goal. Avoid abrupt discontinuation of medication and discuss with specialist teams where possible.

Pregnancy results in physiological changes affecting pharmacokinetics, as shown in Table 25.3.

Side effects such as constipation and orthostatic hypotension may be exacerbated (Cox, et al., 2017).

Consider the trimester of pregnancy and the effect of medication on the neonate. Avoiding medication during the first trimester reduces the risk of teratogenicity. Individual drugs have specific issues around delivery and afterwards, including neonatal toxicity, withdrawal monitoring and treatment. Of these, the most common are:

- neonatal sedation following third trimester administration of benzodiazepines or 'Z' drugs – 'floppy infant syndrome' and neonatal withdrawal
- poor neonatal adaptation syndrome in neonates exposed to antidepressants including SSRIS in the late third trimester (though this is usually transient and self-limiting)
- persistent pulmonary hypertension of the newborn following maternal SSRI treatment, which is rare (2–6 per 1000) but can be fatal

Table 25.3 Pharmacokinetic changes during pregnancy

Absorption	Delayed gastric emptying, longer intestinal transit time – decreased absorption Late pregnancy – reduced peripheral blood flow – reduced absorption IM drugs
Metabolism	Increased cardiac output but changes in tissue delivery – more blood to uterus, less to liver Altered liver enzymes – increased activity CP450, CYP2D6 and CYP3A4, decreased activity CYP1A2
Distribution	Increased plasma volume, body fat and extracellular fluids – increased volume of distribution
Elimination	Increased renal blood flow and glomerular filtration rate – increased renal excretion

320

- lithium toxicity and hypoglycaemia in babies whose mother's received lithium therapy
- opiate withdrawal in infants with maternal opiate substance misuse.

Huybrechts' (2016) cohort study of 1.3 million pregnant women showed no clear evidence that any antipsychotic is a teratogen, but there is some evidence of increased risk of cardiac malformations with risperidone doses greater than 2 mg.

Consider medications which may be safe in breastfeeding when initiating medication during pregnancy. Every drug has a relative infant dose (RID), which is determined by dividing the baby's dose via milk (mg/kg/day) by the mother's dose in mg/kg/day (Hale, 2020). RID of < 10% is generally considered safe; most drugs are < 1%. Also consider medication half-lives, lipid solubility (breast milk is fatty and therefore concentrates lipophilic drugs including psychotropics) and prematurity or other developmental issues in the newborn. Sertraline is generally considered the safest of the SSRIs, with RID of 0.4%–2.2%. Fluoxetine has a RID score of 1.6%–14% and should be used with caution. Clozapine has a low RID score but may cause severe haematological sequelae and thus should be avoided. Lithium has a RID score of 0.87%–30% and should be avoided.

Pre-emptively plan for RT where possible and do not seclude individuals afterwards. Collaborate closely with paediatrics, anaesthetics and obstetrics in the perinatal period. Adapt restraint procedures to avoid possible harm to the foetus and discomfort to the mother (e.g. using left lateral positioning). Choose an antipsychotic or a benzodiazepine with a short half-life; in the third trimester, consider neonatal effects (extrapyramidal symptoms if an antipsychotic is used, floppy baby syndrome with benzodiazepines) (NICE, 2014).

Consider promethazine for sleep/sedation as there is evidence-base for use in hyperemesis which showed no increased risk of congenital malformations.

Conclusion

All the medical disorders mentioned in this chapter have the potential to give rise to the need for intensive psychiatric care within a wide variety of medical and surgical specialist settings. Many of the emergency situations can be ameliorated (and the need for intervention with emergency sedation reduced) by early identification of mental health conditions, enhanced nursing care and environment modification, following guidelines on managing delirium and other common conditions and close collaboration between general hospital staff and psychiatric liaison teams.

References

Alzheimer's Society (2022) *This is Me*. London: Alzheimer's Society. www.alzheimers.org.uk/sites/default/files/2020-03/this_is_me_1553.pdf.

Baharlo,B, Bryden,D and Brett,SJ (2018) Deprivation of Liberty and Intensive Care: An Update Post Ferreira. *Journal of the Intensive Care Society* **19** (1) 35–42.

Banerjee,S (2009) *The Use of Antipsychotic Medication for People with Dementia: Time for Action. A Report for the Minister of State for Care Services*. London: Department of Health.

Baugh,C, Blanchard,E and Hopkins,I (2020) *Psychiatric Liaison Accreditation Network (PLAN) Quality Standards for Liaison Psychiatry Service*, 6th ed. London: RCPsych CCQI Publications.

Beer,MD, Pereira,SM and Paton,C (2008) *Psychiatric Intensive Care*, 2nd ed. Cambridge: Cambridge University Press.

Bonfield,CM, Lam,S, Lin,Y and Greene,S (2013) The Impact of Attention Deficit Hyperactivity Disorder on Recovery from Mild Traumatic Brain Injury. *Journal of neurosurgery Pediatrics* **12** (2) 97–102.

Bouajram,RH and Awdishu,L (2021) A Clinician's Guide to Dosing Analgesics, Anticonvulsants, and Psychotropic Medications in Continuous Renal Replacement Therapy. *Kidney International Reports* **6** (8) 2033–48.

British National Formulary Joint Formulary Committee (2021) *BNF 82 (British National Formulary): September 2021–March 2022*. London: Pharmaceutical Press.

Broadbent,M, Moxham,L and Dwyer,T (2007) The Development and Use of Mental Health Triage Scales in Australia. *International Journal of Mental Health Nursing* **16** 6 413–21.

Care Quality Commission (2010) *Essential Standards of Safety and Quality*. London.

Cox,Henshaw and Barton,J (2017) *Modern Management of Perinatal Psychiatric Disorders*, 2nd ed. London: RCPsych Publications.

Davenport,D (2013) The Basics of Clinical Supervision. *Nursing in Practice* www.nursinginpractice.com/professional/the-basics-of-clinical-supervision/.

Elnazer,HY and Agrawal,N (2017) Managing Aggression in Epilepsy. *BJPsych Advances* **23**: 253–64.

Farrell,M, Martin,NK, Stockings,E, Borquez,A, Cepeda,JA, Degenhardt,L, et al. (2019) Responding to Global Stimulant Use: Challenges and Opportunities. *Lancet* **10209**: 1652–67.

Freudenreich,O, Goforth,HW, Cozza,KL, Mimiaga,MJ, Safren,SA, Bachmann,G, et al. (2010) Psychiatric Treatment of Persons with HIV/AIDS: An HIV-Psychiatry Consensus Survey of Current Practices. *Psychosomatics* **51**: 480–8.

Gili,A, Bacci,M, Aroni,K, Nicoletti,A, Gambelunghe,A, Mercurio,I, et al. (2021) Changes in Drug Use Patterns During Covid-19 Pandemic in Italy: Monitoring a Vulnerable Group by Hair Analysis. *International Journal of Environmental Research and Public Health* **18**: 1967.

Goh,AM, Wibawa,P, Loi,SM, Walterfang,M, Velakoulis,D, Looi,JC (2018) Huntington's Disease: Neuropsychiatric Manifestations of Huntington's Disease. *Australasian Psychiatry* **26** (4) 366–75.

Goldberg,A, Straus,SE, Hamid,JS and Wong,CL (2015) Room Transfers and the Risk of Delirium Incidence Amongst Hospitalized Elderly Medical Patients: A Case–Control Study. *BMC Geriatrics* **15**: 69.

Hale,TW (2020) *Hale's Medications & Mothers' Milk 2021: A Manual of Lactational Pharmacology*, 19th ed. New York: Springer Publishing.

Harris,MJ, Jeste,DV, Gleghorn,A and Sewell,DD (1991) New-Onset Psychosis in HIV-Infected Patients. *Journal of Clinical Psychiatry* **52** (9) 369–76.

HM Government (2005) The Mental Capacity Act 2005. www.legislation.gov.uk/ukpga/2005/9/contents.

Huybrechts,KF, Hernandez-Diaz,S, Patorno,E, Desai,RJ, Mogun,H, Dejene,SZ, et al. (2016). Antipsychotic Use in Pregnancy and the Risk for Congenital Malformations. *JAMA Psychiatry* **73** (9) 938–46.

Independent Mental Health Taskforce (2016) *The Five Year Forward View for Mental Health*. London: NHS England.

Knights,J, Chatziagorakis,A and Buggineni,SK (2018) HIV Infection and Its Psychiatric Manifestations: A Clinical Overview. *BJPsych Advances* **23** (4) 265–77.

Kyle,K and Bronstein,JM (2020) Treatment of Psychosis in Parkinson's Disease and Dementia with Lewy Bodies: A Review. *Parkinsonism & Related Disorders* **75**: 55–62.

Mann,A, Machado,N, Liu,N, Mazin,A, Silver,K and Afzal,K (2012) A Multidisciplinary Approach to the Treatment of Anti-NMDA-Receptor Antibody Encephalitis: A Case and Review of the Literature. *Journal of Neuropsychiatry and Clinical Neurosciences* **24** (2) 247–54.

National Confidential Enquiry into Patient Outcome and Death (NCEPOD) (2017) *Treat as One: Bridging the Gap between Mental and Physical Healthcare in General Hospitals*.

NHS Digital (2020) *Statistics on Alcohol, England 2020*. https://digital.nhs.uk/data-and-information/publications/statistical/statistics-on-alcohol/2020.

NHS Digital (2021) *Statistics on Drug Misuse, England 2020*. https://digital.nhs.uk/data-and-information/publications/statistical/statistics-on-drug-misuse/2020.

NHS England and NHS Improvement (2020) *Mental Health Crisis / A&E Diversion Hubs: NHS England National Finding and Position as at October 2020*. London: NHS England & Improvement.

National Institute for Health and Care Excellence (NICE) (2004) *Self Harm in Over 8's: Short Term Management and Prevention of Recurrence [CG16]*. London: NICE www.nice.org.uk/guidance/cg16.

National Institute for Health and Care Excellence (NICE) (2010a) *Alcohol-Use Disorders: Diagnosis and Management of Physical Complications [CG 100]*. London: NICE www.nice.org.uk/Guidance/CG100.

National Institute for Health and Care Excellence (NICE) (2010b) *Delirium: Prevention, Diagnosis and Management [CG103]*. London: NICE. www.nice.org.uk/Guidance/CG103.

National Institute for Health and Care Excellence (NICE) (2014) *Antenatal and Postnatal Mental Health: Clinical Management and Service Guidance [CG192]*. London: NICE www.nice.org.uk/guidance/cg192.

Parsonage,M and Fossey,M (2011) *Economic Evaluation of a Liaison Psychiatry Service*. London: Centre for Mental Health.

Paulsen,JS, Ready,RE, Hamilton,JM, Mega,MS, and Cummings,JL (2001) Neuropsychiatric Aspects of Huntington's Disease. *Journal of Neurology, Neurosurgery, and Psychiatry* **71** (3) 310–4.

Peters,E (2018) Compassion Fatigue in Nursing: A Concept Analysis. *Nursing Forum* **53** (4) 466–80.

Pryor,C and Clarke,A (2017) Nursing Care for People with Delirium Superimposed on Dementia. *Nursing Older People* **29** (3) 18–2.

Raj,D, Stansfeld,S, Weich,S, Stewart,R, McBride,O, Brugha,T, et al. (2014) Comorbidity in Mental and Physical Illness. In McManus,S, Bebbington,P, Jenkins,R and Brugha,T (eds.), *Mental health and wellbeing in England: Adult Psychiatric Morbidity Survey 2014*. Leeds: NHS Digital.

Rasmussen,SA, Mazurek,MF and Rosebush,PI (2016) Catatonia: Our Current Understanding of Its Diagnosis, Treatment, and Pathophysiology. *World Journal of Psychiatry* **6** (4) 391–8.

Rickards,H, Jacob,S, Lennox,B and Nicholson,T (2014) Autoimmune Encephalitis: A Potentially Treatable Cause of Mental Disorder. *Advances in Psychiatric Treatment* **20** (2) 92–100.

Robinson,P and Rhys Jones,W (2018) MARSIPAN: Management of Really Sick Patients with Anorexia Nervosa. *BJPsych Advances* **24** (1) 20–32.

Royal College of Psychiatrists (2022). Medical emergencies in eating disorders (MEED). [CR233]. London RCPsych https://www.rcpsych.ac.uk/improving-care/campaigning-for-better-mental-health-policy/college-reports/2022-college-reports/cr233.

Scott,J, Aitken,P, Peters,T and Kumar,K (2017) Liaison Psychiatry Explained. *BMJ* **357**: j1757.

Swires-Hennessy,K and Hayhurst,C (2021) *Mental Health in Emergency Departments: A Toolkit for Improving Care.* London: The Royal College of Emergency Medicine.

Taylor,DM, Barnes,TRE and Young,AH (2018) *The Maudsley Prescribing Guidelines in Psychiatry*, 13th ed. Nashville: John Wiley & Sons.

Telles-Correia,D, Barbosa,A, Cortez-Pinto,H, Campos,C, Rocha,NBF, and Machado,S (2017) Psychotropic Drugs and Liver Disease: A Critical Review of Pharmacokinetics and Liver Toxicity. *World Journal of Gastrointestinal Pharmacology and Therapeutics* **8** (1) 26–38.

Thanvi,BR, Lo,TCN and Harsh,DP (2005) Psychosis in Parkinson's disease. *BMJ Journals Postgraduate Medical Journal* **81**: 644–6.

Vaishnavi,S, Rao,V and Fann,JR (2009) Neuropsychiatric Problems After Traumatic Brain Injury: Unraveling the Silent Epidemic. *Psychosomatics* **50** (3) 198–205.

Vancaester,E and Santens,P (2007) Catatonia and Neuroleptic Malignant Syndrome: Two Sides of a Coin? *Acta Neurolologica Belgica* **107** (20) 47–50.

Vincent,A, Buckley,C, Schott,JM, Baker,I, Dewar,BK, Detert, N, et al. (2004) Potassium Channel Antibody Associated Encephalopathy: A Potentially Immunotherapy Responsive Form of Limbic Encephalitis. *Brain* **127**: 701–12.

Wisner,KL (2012) The Last Therapeutic Orphan: The Pregnant Woman. *American Journal of Psychiatry* **169** (6) 554–6.

Chapter 26

An Overview of International Perspectives on PICUs

Angus McLellan and Andrew Molodynski

A Brief History of Psychiatric Intensive Care

Mental illness has always affected people, but care and treatments have only become available much more recently. For millennia, mental illness was considered to have a supernatural or religious cause. Many people were subjected to degrading and inhumane behaviour such as trepanning, drowning and burning. Many of these acutely unwell individuals would now be cared for in psychiatric intensive care units (PICUs) (where they exist). Records show hospitals existing for those with mental illness from as early as the ninth century, but it wasn't until the eighteenth century that any coordinated provision was considered. This provision was initially in the form of so- called insane asylums where there was little care and treatment but where people were kept apart and 'hidden' from the rest of society.

The United Kingdom was the first country to coordinate a wider approach. The 'Lunacy Act' in 1845 (Unsworth, 1993) made it mandatory for every county in the United Kingdom to construct an asylum that then had to have a physician. France and the United States also started to develop a systematic approach and by the end of the nineteenth century several countries had done the same. As treatments such as insulin coma therapy and lobotomy were trialled and then disproved (though not always taken out of use), de-institutionalisation and a focus on treatment and rehabilitation in the community came to the fore in the latter half of the twentieth century.

PICUs were first described in the 1970s in the United Kingdom, Australia, the United States, and Canada. These were smaller open-plan wards with more staff to allow for more detailed and personalised care. Since their introduction, PICUs have looked after the most unwell and distressed patients. Little literature exists about the use of PICUs globally and their use varies significantly. In the United Kingdom, such units are available in almost all NHS trusts and the UK Royal College of Psychiatrists has published a set of standards for PICUs (Rodriguez et al 2023). This is a notable contrast to countries where systematic mental health care doesn't exist, let alone specialist PICUs. Some countries use high-dependency psychiatric units rather than PICU. Others rely on the criminal justice system to 'manage' such patients. This global disparity highlights the importance of continuing to develop systems for mental health care that avoid unnecessary and damaging persecution, and incarceration-specialised services such as PICUs play a crucial role in this.

The National Association of Psychiatric Intensive Care and Low Secure Units (NAPICU) was formed in the United Kingdom in 1996. This is a multidisciplinary organisation whose goal is to 'advance the care and treatment of people . . . through promoting and sharing good practice, providing education and training, encouraging clinicians to establish networks, and by undertaking research and audit'. It was the first organisation to take a truly global approach to providing high-quality care for patients in PICU or low secure services and establish a set of standards (NAPICU, 2014) to guide the creation and maintenance of such resources (NAPICU, 2014). NAPICU continues to share experience, research and education, all of which are key in improving global standards for PICU.

Demographics of Patients in PICUs

Whilst the demographics of patients in PICUs can vary significantly due to policy, mental health legislation, resource provision and local practice, PICUs are widely considered to have patients who experience severe mental illness and who present the greatest risk to themselves and/or others.

A 2008 study of English PICUs (Brown et al., 2008) reported that most patients were male (78.5%) and Caucasian (74%). Whilst the majority were Caucasian, 26% of those admitted were non-Caucasian compared to a national population rate of just 5.5% at the time. Patients from Black ethnic groups were significantly over-represented (18% vs 2% population rate) compared to Caucasian and Asian ethnicities despite illness rates being broadly the same. This may speak to a wider issue around experience of and attitudes towards those with mental illness in different ethnic groups. A study of PICU patients in Egypt (Okasha et al., 2021) reported roughly equal numbers of male and female patients and suggests differences in practice according to gender internationally. While there may be some issues specific to the United Kingdom or Egypt, it is reasonable to suggest that ethnicity and gender have an impact in general on whether somebody is admitted to PICU.

The English study showed that 92% of admissions were unemployed and 89% were not in an intimate relationship, highlighting levels of social isolation and likely poor support systems. According to both studies, the majority of patients admitted to PICU had a diagnosis of either schizophrenia (55% and 44%) or mania (20% and 26%), though other illnesses such as depression, personality disorder and substance dependence were also represented, as shown in Table 26.1. Of total admissions, 84% a history of violence towards other people or towards property, 40% had experienced self-harm, and 97% of patients were detained under the UK Mental Health Act (MHA) (the UK's mental health law).

These figures are in keeping with other research published in this area. Those admitted to PICU are very likely to be socially isolated, have drug or alcohol problems and/or have a history of violence. This suggests that access to better social support, substance misuse treatment and de-escalation techniques could reduce the necessity of PICU for many.

PICU in High-Income Group Countries

The Quality Network for Psychiatric Intensive Care Units (QNPICU) organised by the Centre for Quality Improvement within the UK Royal College of Psychiatrists (Townsed and Georgiou, 2020) and the Australasian Health Infrastructure Alliance (AHIA,

Table 26.1 Factors associated with PICU admission

Current or historic factors	Admissions to PICU with this characteristic
Schizophrenia	55%/44%
Bipolar affective disorder	20%/26%
Depression	4%
Personality disorder	5%
Drug misuse	71%
Alcohol misuse	58%
Polysubstance misuse	49%
Violence to person	79%
Violence to property	66%
Previous hospital admission	80%
Previous PICU admission	55%

2015) has produced guidelines for standards of care in PICU (NAPICU, 2017). These set a minimum standard to be adhered to for high-quality and consistent care across assessment, admission, treatment and discharge. Assessment should involve close liaison with the referring team, ensuring that the patient meets criteria for admission and will not be unnecessarily deprived of their liberty. Admission should involve clear goal setting with the aim of time-limited management of an acute change in behaviour attributable to mental illness that can only be managed in PICU. If admission is not appropriate, the PICU team should offer advice on further management. Management should include both physical and mental health assessment and treatment. Risk assessment and management, diagnosis, communication, levels of supervision, pharmacological, psychological and all other management options should be explored within the correct legal framework. Discharge should be considered from the point of admission with clear goals and objectives agreed between all. Patient and carer involvement in all stages is crucial to ensure a patient-centred and holistic approach.

The standards also cover staffing and advocate a multidisciplinary approach and minimum staffing levels. Environment is important with single ensuite rooms recommended when risk assessed as appropriate and no more than 14 beds per ward. The physical environment should be designed in a way that works for all and include a garden and extra care space. Day-to-day running should be based on a sound policy and leadership philosophy with the aim of maximising safety, therapy and security alongside clinical audit and quality improvement. This is crucial to demonstrate and maintain high-quality, effective care. A focus on patient and carer experience including clear and timely communication, the opportunity for involvement in all aspects of care and the consideration of patient and carer feedback are crucial.

Urgent health issues including current medication should be considered within the first 24 hours and all other concerns should be addressed within 7 days. Weekly reviews of treatment in a multidisciplinary fashion, always considering the opinions and wishes of the patient and their carer(s), is recommended. Increased staffing levels are also advocated for to allow for increased one-to-one time with patients.

Given that PICUs are used for the most distressed patients and those with an inherently higher risk of harm to themselves or others, they are often considered a place of increasing restraint. Whilst practice varies, there is some evidence that the opposite is true due to the higher levels of resources available (Georgieva et al., 2010). Increased staff-to-patient ratios can allow more time for patients to verbally de-escalate, reducing the need for more restrictive interventions. The availability of seclusion (an area separate from the main ward) has also been shown to reduce violence and the need for restraint, though it is also coercive. One study of an acute psychiatric ward in India showed that family members were most likely to be the victims of violence from mentally unwell people, but that restrictions were more likely to be placed on someone after they assaulted a staff member (Danivas et al., 2016). The first finding suggests that the specially trained staff in a PICU can more effectively de-escalate a situation and highlights the importance of staff training, but training in such techniques is mostly limited to high-income group (HIG) countries (Raveesh and Lepping, 2019). Development of new strategies and techniques is also important, as shown by the High and Intensive Care (HIC) model from Holland that integrates community care and open communication into the PICU care structure (Voskes et al., 2021).

Everyone agrees that mental health is one of the most stigmatised areas within health care. Patients, families, professionals, communities, government and the media all play significant roles in reducing

or perpetuating stigma. One study in the United States (Carpenter-Song et al., 2010) showed that 'European Americans' were more likely to express and understand mental illness within the biopsychosocial model, whereas African American and Latino participants were more likely to describe 'non-biomedical' interpretations of mental illness. All groups reported experiencing stigma relating to their mental illness. Latino participants reported that a diagnosis of mental illness could be 'very socially damaging'.

Medication is an important aspect of treatment within the PICU setting. Several guidelines for rapid tranquilisation (RT) exist, and one paper (Nadkarni et al., 2015) identified guidelines from the United Kingdom, United States, Canada, Australia and New Zealand. Interestingly, these guidelines all contained different recommendations, with some encouraging use of benzodiazepine medications as first line and others supporting the use of antipsychotic medication primarily. Whilst it is good that such guidelines exist, disparities remain, and further research and global collaboration is required to help establish a consistent evidence-based approach.

The Lived Experience of Being in a PICU

The biopsychosocial model is widely used throughout psychiatry and is no less important here. The increased time and the specialist input available in this setting should provide a platform for excellent patient-centred and holistic care.

A study examining the experiences of those admitted to PICU (Salzman-Erikson et al., 2017) gives an alternative perspective on what it is like to be cared for in a PICU. Some patients felt shocked when first admitted. They described the environment as often highly restricted with everything locked. They reported that staff spent less time talking with them and sharing information compared to non-PICU wards, leading to poor understanding of the goals of treatment. Patients also felt that their freedom and autonomy were reduced, suggesting a paternalistic approach. Unfortunately, some patients described their PICU experience as more like prison which tells us there is still much work to be done in reducing institutional effects.

Whilst this experience is certainly not universal, important themes are there. Whilst those in PICU are undoubtedly some of the most unwell, this does not necessarily follow that their freedom and autonomy should be significantly less than others. Open and honest communication, supportive and collaborative care and clear goals should be standard practice in establishing a therapeutic relationship, even (or perhaps especially) in the most challenging circumstances.

Management of Mental Illness in Non-Healthcare Settings Globally

Having considered some standards for best practice with regards to PICU, one would hope they would be applied globally. Unfortunately, this is far from the case. Many countries rely upon their criminal justice systems to manage mentally unwell people. There is no doubt some excellent practice in some prisons, but grotesque human rights breaches have been widely reported, such as patients being chained to their beds, kept in cages, secured in concrete rooms with a hole in the floor as a toilet and subjected to abuse that seems unthinkable (Kleinman, 2009). Shackling is another troubling method used to 'treat' those with mental illness. One first-hand report states:

> I've been chained for five years. The chain is so heavy. It doesn't feel right; it makes me sad. I stay in a small room with seven men. I'm not allowed to wear clothes, only underwear. I have to go to the toilet in a bucket. I eat porridge in the morning and if I'm lucky, I find bread at night, but not every night .... It's not how a human being is supposed to be. A human being should be free. (Human Rights watch 2020)

Such practice is often due to a lack of appropriate mental health care and poor understanding of the nature of mental illness.

In many countries the role of psychiatric institutions is not to focus on the treatment and rehabilitation of those with mental illness. Rather it is to 'protect' the public from these 'dangerous' individuals. Less overtly, even in countries with developed mental health care systems, many with mental illness still end up in prison or have very little choice in their treatment, for example, in Saudi Arabia where capacity to consent is considered but legislation does not meet World Health Organization (WHO) standards (Carlisle, 2018). Such things remind us that we still have a long way to go. PICUs can play an important

role in this journey, as they provide diagnosis, treatment and support rather than simply punitive, coercive measures.

A study of Chinese families in Australia (Hsiao et al., 2006) outlined their expectations of what are considered 'appropriate' behaviours and how symptoms of mental illness can be seen as 'inappropriate'. This in turn alienates people with these experiences from the family and their wider social support. This is likely to be exacerbated for patients admitted to PICU given that they are generally the most unwell and distressed. Additional sensitivity to cultural issues in this population are undoubtedly important.

Rates of mental illness are higher in prisoners than in the general population, especially rates of psychosis (3.5% of prisoners in high-income nations and 5.5% in low- and middle income countries (LAMICs) have a psychotic illness) (Fazel et al., 2018). Up to 90% of prisoners have experienced mental illness and many have more than one diagnosable condition. Patients with mental illness die earlier than those without, and keeping the mentally ill in prison with reduced access to healthcare services exacerbates this problem. We also know that prisons do not stop or prevent drug use and, indeed, can make it more likely. Investing in the treatment and care of those with severe mental illness results in not only health benefits but also economic benefits (Mclellan and Molodynski, 2023). The increased prevalence of mental illness in prison in LAMICs may be related to several factors such as lack of funding for mental health services, misunderstanding of severe mental illness and stigma. PICUs could be a way to change this. Rather than the severely ill being thrown into prison, a consistent and caring approach would allow for better identification, diagnosis and treatment of mental illness. Mental health services within prisons can also help with this by ensuring that mentally unwell prisoners have timely access to the correct support.

Global Differences in Mental Healthcare Resources

With limited data available concerning the use of PICUs globally, we are left to draw conclusions about the care provided to the most unwell by considering the funding allocated and resources available to those with mental illness. It is universally accepted that mental illness hits the poor hardest, a group who also have poor access to care.

The WHO's *Mental Health Atlas* (WHO, 2017) revealed that only 37% of member states regularly compiled mental health-specific data. This means poor awareness of the rates, management and burden of mental illness. Without this information, effective mental health policy and care cannot happen. Only 20% of countries had the resources or infrastructure in place to monitor whether their plans and policies were working. A key step in improving this will be to establish regular data collection in every country; 72% of countries had a policy or plan around mental health but only 48% were up to date with international and regional human rights standards. This decreased further to just 39% of countries having mental health law that protected individuals' human rights.

Mental health workers are a precious resource. Some LAMICs have less than one mental health worker per 100,000 population while there are up to 72 per 100,000 elsewhere. There are similar inequalities regarding the availability of mental health beds, with less than 7 per 100,000 in LAMICs to more than 50 per 100,000 elsewhere (Eurostat, 2018). In child and adolescent psychiatry, the figures fall as low as 0.2 beds per 100,000. The makeup of the mental health workforce shows significant variation in the availability of psychiatrists, mental health nurses, social workers and psychologists. Reducing this variation and uplifting numbers overall, possibly with an agreed minimum level, would help those with mental illness access the right support. Spend per capita varies greatly depending upon the wealth of a country and factors such as political priorities. Problems with mental healthcare systems are by no means confined to LAMICs, with France reporting an increase in mental illness in prisons after a move to de-institutionalise those in mental health hospitals (Velpry et al., 2014). Figure 26.1 (reproduced from WHO, 2017) shows that spending decreases significantly outside of the HIG countries and spending in LAMICs is more focussed on inpatient treatment and hospitals.

Treatment of existing mental illness is crucial, but in the longer term prevention and early detection is what will move things forward the most. Fast access to personalised and evidence-based care is vitally important. Whilst we need to remain cautious of the untoward use of mental health policy, such as diagnoses of sluggish schizophrenia (Wilkinson, 1986), a diagnosis assigned to those with unfavourable political views,

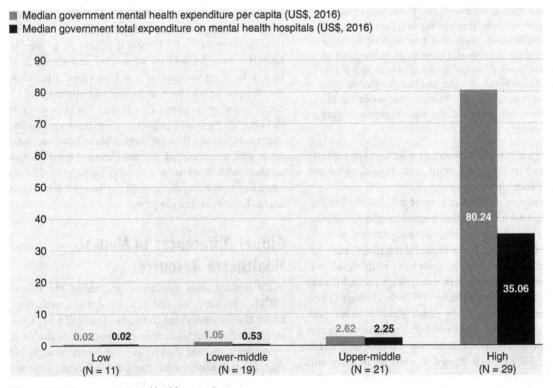

Figure 26.1 Government mental health expenditure

such things must not discourage the expansion of mental health services globally to meet the pressing need.

Another profound difference between healthcare systems is cost to the patient. This includes the wide range of treatment that is fully funded by taxation (such as the NHS in the United Kingdom) to fully privatised health care where the patient picks up the entire cost, even when treatment is against their will. Suicide was the second leading cause of death in 15–29-year-olds in 2016, and we already know that those with mental illness are more likely to experience significant physical illness and earlier death than those without. Mental illness is the leading cause of disability in the United Kingdom, accounting for 22.8% of the total burden (Department of Health, 2011). A compassionate healthcare system should look for ways to reduce this burden that falls unequally and generally on the most vulnerable in society.

Legal Frameworks for the Management of Mental Illness

A legal framework is crucially important in a coordinated national approach to mental illness. This must ensure that those whose decision-making is impaired receive the treatment they need while there are safeguards in place to prevent the exploitation and abuse which has been and remains so prevalent.

Mental health law is in place in 75% of countries (covering 69% of the global population). Half of these frameworks have been implemented or updated in the last 30 years. Given the changes in societal attitudes and norms over this time, a significant proportion of the world's population is exposed to mental health law that is not fit for purpose and many countries have no safeguards at all. One study looking at Commonwealth countries (Fistein et al., 2009) showed significant variations in mental health law and in its application. Mental health law is often paternalistic with little opportunity for the patient and those around them to state their opinion and be heard. Given the move towards collaborative care in many countries, legislation needs to evolve to keep pace with this. The upcoming changes to the MHA in the United Kingdom, for example, seem like progress.

In the United Kingdom, the MHA allows for people to be detained in hospital or in the community for assessment and treatment of their mental illness if it is thought to be proportionate and if treatment is available. All detained patients have a right to an appeal by a panel of independent experts with the support of a lawyer. Whilst not perfect, this demonstrates that it is possible to offer some protection for people from the effects of their mental illness whilst maintaining safeguards to prevent abuse. In countries where mental health law is non-existent or out of date, people may be held indefinitely against their will with no right to appeal, no representation and no access to treatment.

Mental health law is not just about the detention of patients. It can also mandate the safeguards and standards required for treatment. One study focussing on mental health governance in LAMICs showed a willingness to enact appropriate mental health law, but several barriers such as finance, resources and stigma meant that either no action or inadequate action was taken (Petersen et al., 2017). Other research has reported that only judicial intervention brings effective change, emphasising the importance of government and policymakers in developing and maintaining good mental health care (Raja et al., 2021). Spreading knowledge and experience is one way of tackling these difficulties, and the *WHO Resource Book on Mental Health, Human Rights and Legislation* (WHO, 2005) provides a framework for countries creating or updating legislation to ensure not only adherence to human rights law but also the application of best practice and care. Their Quality Rights work package also supports humane care within a legal framework (WHO, 2019).

Conclusion

Mental illness has always been highly stigmatised, and this leads to individuals, societies, families and government not giving people the care and respect they deserve. Things are steadily changing, and this should be reflected in systems of care. Asylums and the detention of the mentally ill in prison should be consigned to the past, and resources such as PICU are a requirement for a humane mental healthcare system.

The extra resources available in PICUs can lead to reduced restraint, better therapeutic relationships and (most importantly) reduced morbidity and mortality for the most unwell. PICUs should be present in every country in a way that makes them accessible to those in need. Budget holders may argue that there is not enough money, but the money saved by interventions such as PICU will accrue over time and may well outweigh the start-up costs. Standards that have been developed so far are a good starting point but need refining and pushing internationally. Whilst a balanced approach is important, a global agreement on levels of funding for mental health care as a proportion of GDP should be pursued vigorously.

Mental health law must protect and care for those with mental illness rather than locking them away simply for the protection of others. There is too much international variation in mental health law. Establishing more consistent, supportive and human rights-compliant law that focuses on prevention and treatment rather than punishment is an urgent need. PICU, not prison, should be the resource of choice for those in mental health crisis with behaviour that poses a risk.

Tackling stigma, prejudice and persecution experienced by those affected by mental illness will reduce the burden placed upon them. Rather than hiding mental illness and having poorer outcomes, people with mental illness must receive effective, evidence-based treatment early. Too many disparities exist between people of different ethnicity and cultural background. More must be done to change this. Education is important, and all staff should play a role in this as advocates for our patients and their families. Given that PICU care decisions are not immune to bias, we must always self-reflect and look to challenge our own thinking and decision-making to ensure that fair and appropriate decisions are made. As PICU is not present in many countries, existing PICU clinicians can help by sharing their experience and knowledge with countries and regions where such resources do not exist.

A truly global approach is the only way forward. This may mean starting with information and knowledge sharing, but we must all aspire to better care in the longer term. The PICU can be one place where such global change is driven. Looking after the most unwell patients can give a unique insight into the roles and responsibilities of everyone involved, and there is no one better place to ensure that our most unwell and vulnerable people are looked after in the most caring, compassionate way possible.

References

Australasian Health Infrastructure Alliance (AHIA) (2015) *Australasian Health Facility Guidelines. Part B - Health Facility Briefing and Planning. 0137 – Mental Health Intensive Care Unit.* North Sydney: AusHFG.

Brown,S, Chhina,N and Dye,S (2008) The Psychiatric Intensive Care Unit: A Prospective Survey of Patient Demographics and Outcomes at Seven English PICUs. *Journal of Psychiatric Intensive Care* 4 (1–2) 17–27.

Carlisle,J (2018) Mental Health Law in Saudi Arabia. *BJPsych International* 15 (1) 17–19.

Carpenter-Song,E, Chu,E, Drake,RE, Ritsema,M, Smith,B and Alverson,H (2010) Ethno-Cultural Variations in the Experience and Meaning of Mental Illness and Treatment: Implications for Access and Utilization. *Transcultural Psychiatry* 47 (2) 224–51.

Danivas,V, Lepping,P, Punitharani,S, Gowrishree,H, Ashwini,K, Raveesh,BN, et al. (2016) Observational Study of Aggressive Behaviour and Coercion on an Indian Acute Ward. *Asian Journal of Psychiatry* 22: 150–6.

Department of Health (DOH) (2011) *No Health without Mental Health: A Cross Government Mental Health Outcomes Strategy for People of all Ages.* London: Department of Health.

Eurostat (2018) Number of Psychiatrists: How Do Countries Compare? Website. https://ec.europa.eu/eurostat/web/products-eurostat-news/-/DDN-20181205-1.

Fazel,S and Seewald,K (2018) Severe Mental Illness in 33,588 Prisoners Worldwide: Systematic Review and Meta-Regression Analysis. *British Journal of Psychiatry* 200 (5) 364–73.

Fistein,EC, Holland,AJ, Clare,ICH and Gunn MJ (2009) A Comparison of Mental Health Legislation from Diverse Commonwealth Jurisdictions. *International Journal of Law and Psychiatry* 32 (3) 147–55.

Georgieva,I, de Haan,G, Smith,W and Mulder,CL (2010) Successful Reduction of Seclusion in a Newly Developed Psychiatric Intensive Care Unit. *Journal of Psychiatric Intensive Care* 6 (1) 31–8.

Hsiao,FH, Klimidis,S, Minas H and Tan,ES (2006) Cultural Attribution of Mental Health Suffering in Chinese Societies: The Views of Chinese Patients With Mental Illness and Their Caregivers. *Journal of Clinical Nursing* 15 (8)

King,DB, Viney,W and Woody,WD (2007) *A History of Psychology: Ideas and Context*, 4th ed. Boston: Pearson.

Kleinman,A (2009) Global Mental Health: A Failure of Humanity. *Lancet* 374 (9690) 603–4.

Human Rights Watch (2020) Living in Chains. Website. www.hrw.org/report/2020/10/06/living-chains/shackling-people-psychosocial-disabilities-worldwide.

McLellan,A and Molodynski,A (2023) The Mental Health of Prisoners: An International Overview. In Gogineni,RR, Pumariega,AJ, Kallivayalil,R, Kastrup,M and Rothe,EM (eds.), *The WASP Textbook on Social Psychiatry*. Oxford: Oxford University Press.

Nadkarni P, Jayaram M, Nadkarni S, Rattehalli R, Adams C, Rapid Tranquilisation: a global perspective, BJPsych Int. 2015 Nov; **12**(4): 100–102, Nov. 2015.

National Association of Psychiatric Intensive Care and Low Secure Units (NAPICU) (2017) *Design Guidance for Psychiatric Intensive Care Units*. Glasgow: NAPICU International Press. https://napicu.org.uk/wp-content/uplo ads/2017/05/Design-Guidance-for-Psychiatric-Intensive-Care-Units-2017.pdf.

National Association of Psychiatric Intensive Care and Low Secure Units (NAPICU) (2014) *National Minimum Standards for Psychiatric Intensive Care in General Adult Services*.

Okasha,TA, Sabry,WM, Zaki,NH, Rabie,MA and Elhawary, YA (2021) Characteristics and Outcomes of Patients Admitted to the First Psychiatric Intensive Care Unit in Egypt. *South African Journal of Psychiatry* **27**: 1527.

Petersen,I, Marais,D, Abdulmalik,J, Ahuja,S, Alem,A Chisholm,C, et al. (2017) Strengthening Mental Health System Governance in Six Low- and Middle-Income Countries in Africa and South Asia: Challenges, Needs, and Potential Strategies. *Health Policy and Planning* **32** (5) 699–709.

Raja,T, Tuomainen,H, Madan,J, Mistry,D, Jain,S, Easwaran, K, et al. (2021) Psychiatric Hospital Reform in Low- and Middle-Income Countries: A Systematic Review of Literature. *Social Psychiatry and Psychiatric Epidemiology* **56** (8) 1341–57.

Raveesh,BN and Lepping,P (2019) Restraint Guidelines for Mental Health Services in India. *Indian Journal of Psychiatry* **61**(Suppl 4) S698–705.

Rodriguez,K, Webster,M, Herbert,R and Ivanov,M (2023) *Standards for Psychiatric Intensive Care Units*, 3rd ed. London: Royal College of Psychiatrists.

Salzmann-Erikson,M and Soderqvist,C (2017) Being Subject to Restrictions, Limitations and Disciplining: A Thematic Analysis of Individuals' Experiences in Psychiatric Intensive Care. *Issues in Mental Health Nursing* **38** (7) 540–8.

Unsworth,C (1993) Law and Lunacy in Psychiatry's 'Golden Age'. *Oxford Journal of Legal Studies* **13** (4) 479–507.

Velpry,N and Eyraud,B (2014) Confinement and Psychiatric Care: A Comparison Between High-Security Units for Prisoners and for Difficult Patients in France. *Culture, Medicine and Psychiatry* **38** (4) 550–77.

Voskes,Y, van Melle,AL, Widdershoven,G, van Mierlo, AFMM, Bovenberg,F and Mulder,C (2021) High and Intensive Care in Psychiatry: A New Model for Acute Inpatient Care. *Psychiatric Services* **72** (4) 475–77.

World Health Organization (WHO) (2005) *Resource Book on Mental Health, Human Rights and Legislation*. Geneva: WHO.

World Health Organization (WHO) (2017) *Mental Health Atlas*. Geneva: WHO.

World Health Organization (WHO) (2019) *WHO QualityRights Initiative – Improving Quality, Promoting Human Rights*. Geneva: WHO.

Wilkinson,G (1986) Political Dissent and 'Sluggish' Schizophrenia in the Soviet Union. *British Medical Journal* **293** (6548) 641–2.

Index

Printed in the United States
by Baker & Taylor Publisher Services